MEDICAL RADIOLOGY

Diagnostic Imaging and Radiation Oncology – Softcover Edition

Editorial Board

Founding Editors   L. W. Brady, M. W. Donner (†),
                             H.-P. Heilmann, F. H. W. Heuck

Current Editors

Diagnostik Imaging   A. L. Baert, Leuven
                             F. H. W. Heuck, Stuttgart
                             J. E. Youker, Milwaukee

Radiation Oncology   L. W. Brady, Philadelphia
                             H.-P. Heilmann, Hamburg

Springer
Berlin
Heidelberg
New York
Barcelona
Hong Kong
London
Milan
Paris
Singapore
Tokyo

Radiological Diagnosis of Breast Diseases

With Contributions by

D.D. Adler · L.W. Bassett · M. Bauer · R.J. Brenner · M.J.M. Broeders · N.D. De Bruhl
S. Delorme · G.W. Eklund · S.A. Feig · M. Friedrich · H.-J. Frischbier · D.P. Gorczyca
A.G. Haus · R.E. Hendrick · H. Junkermann · M. Lanyi · E.B. Mendelson · J.-W. Oestmann
E.D. Pisano · I. Schreer · R. Schulz-Wendtland · E.A. Sickles · J. Teubner · C.E. Tobin
P. Tontsch · A.H. Tulusan · A.L.M. Verbeek · D. von Fournier · L.J. Warren Burhenne

Edited by

Michael Friedrich and Edward A. Sickles

Foreword by

Friedrich H.W. Heuck

With 297 Figures in 597 Separate Illustrations, Some in Color

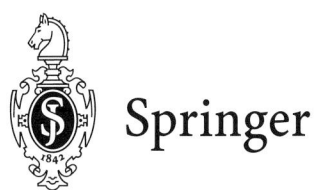

MICHAEL FRIEDRICH, MD
Professor
Abteilung für Radiologie und Nuklearmedizin
Krankenhaus Am Urban
Dieffenbachstraße 1
10967 Berlin
Germany

EDWARD A. SICKLES, MD
Professor
Department of Radiology, Box 1667
University of California Medical Center
San Francisco, CA 94143-1667
USA

MEDICAL RADIOLOGY · Diagnostic Imaging and Radiation Oncology

Continuation of
Handbuch der medizinischen Radiologie
Encyclopedia of Medical Radiology

ISSN 0942-5373
ISBN 3-540-66339-8 Springer-Verlag Berlin Heidelberg New York

Library of Congress Cataloging-in-Publication Data applied for

Die Deutsche Bibliothek – CIP-Einheitsaufnahme
Radiological diagnosis of breast diseases / with contributions by D.D. Adler ... Ed. by Michael Friedrich and Edward A. Sickles. Foreword by Friedrich H.W. Heuck. – Berlin; Heidelberg; New York; Barcelona; Hong Kong; London; Milan; Paris; Singapore; Tokyo: Springer, 2000. (Medical radiology). ISBN 3-540-66339-8. Radiological diagnosis of breast diseases. – 2000

This work is subject to copyright. All rights are reserved, whether the whole or part of the material is concerned, specifically the rights of translation, reprinting, reuse of illustrations, recitation, broadcasting, reproduction on microfilm or in any other way, and storage in data banks. Duplication of this publication or parts thereof is permitted only under the provisions of the German Copyright Law of September 9, 1965, in its current version, and permission for use must always be obtained from Springer-Verlag. Violations are liable for prosecution under the German Copyright Law.

© Springer-Verlag Berlin · Heidelberg 2000
Printed in Germany

The use of general descriptive names, registered names, trademarks, etc. in this publication does not imply, even in the absence of a specific statement, that such names are exempt from the relevant protective laws and regulations and therefore free for general use.

Product liability: The publishers cannot guarantee the accuracy of any information about dosage and application contained in this book. In every individual case the user must check such information by consulting the relevant literature.

Cover-Design: Joan Greenfield, New York

Typesetting: Best-set Typesetter Ltd., Hong Kong

SPIN: 10741593   21/3135-5 4 3 2 1 – Printed on acid-free paper

Foreword

This book has been edited by two of the best known experts in the field of breast diseases. It was in 1975 that MICHAEL FRIEDRICH, Professor of Radiology at the Free University of Berlin, commenced his efforts to develop and improve mammography so as to allow the early diagnosis of breast cancer. The outstanding results that he has achieved have led to awards from the German Radiological Society (the Hermann-Holthusen-Ring) and the Medical High School, Hannover (the Johann-Georg-Zimmermann Prize).

EDWARD ALLEN SICKLES, Professor of Radiology and Chief of the Breast Imaging Section at the University of California San Francisco, has since 1976 devoted much effort to comparison of the different methods of diagnostic radiology of the breast, including ultrasonography and magnetic resonance imaging. He has received many distinctions and important awards in recognition of his studies. Professor Sickles is one of the leading radiologists in this field of research in the United States, and is well known all over the world.

The aim of both editors has been to produce a modern textbook that covers all of the special methods of diagnostic imaging of the breast and analyzes the typical patterns presented by the various disease entities that are encountered. In addition, the criteria of differential diagnosis are highlighted. All of the authors emphasize the importance of clinical efforts, including screening projects, to achieve the early diagnosis and treatment of breast cancer. Some of the contributors also discuss the role of fine-needle aspiration and biopsy in rendering diagnosis more reliable. It is to be stressed that the decision to employ surgery or radiation therapy in the treatment of breast cancer is of critical importance, given the potential effects on the personal lives and well-being of patients. This book, written by recognized experts, provides an up-to-date overview of all questions relating to diseases of the breast.

Stuttgart   F.H.W. HEUCK

Preface

While the incidence of breast cancer continues to rise in Europe and the United States, there are subtle hints that, since 1989, the mortality from this disease may have been decreasing in the United States, possibly due to earlier diagnosis through the increased use of screening mammography.

This volume on the *Radiological Diagnosis of Breast Diseases* in the series *Medical Radiology*, edited by A.E. Baert (Leuven, Belgium), F.H.W. Heuck, (Stuttgart, Germany), and J.E. Youker (Milwaukee, USA) and published by Springer-Verlag, Heidelberg, is a joint project involving American and European authors renowned in the field of breast diagnosis, whose willing cooperation we have been fortunate to enlist. The volume is intended to provide the most recent information on the radiological diagnosis of breast diseases, thereby complementing existing textbooks and updating knowledge on this topic.

A thorough knowledge of breast cancer epidemiology and the pathological basis of breast disease is a prerequisite for the interpretation of results obtained with the various breast imaging procedures. The first two chapters give a comprehensive overview of these topics.

The introduction of breast cancer screening programs on a national scale in the United States and Europe requires highly developed quality assurance programs with mammography of the highest technical and diagnostic quality. Several excellent contributions address these problems. Furthermore, expert reading and interpretation are crucially important for mammography to be successful in the early diagnosis of breast cancer. Several chapters on the differential diagnosis of the various mammographic signs of breast cancer and the diagnostic strategy to limit the rate of false-positive results provide an excellent update on this subject.

The complementary imaging modalities of ultrasonography and contrast-enhanced magnetic resonance imaging are described in two comprehensive chapters. All image-guided biopsy methods used for the assessment of possibly malignant mammographic findings are described in two further chapters.

Because of the widespread introduction of breast conservation therapy and breast implant surgery, the role of the radiologist is constantly being redefined, with new diagnostic issues in the preoperative phase during local staging of breast cancer, as well as in the postoperative follow-up. Two contributions deal extensively with these topics.

The still controversial interpretation of recent results from various mammography screening projects in the United States and Europe, as well as their design and implementation, is extensively discussed in two excellent contributions. Finally, in view of the increasing political and economic pressures on medicine in the United States and Europe, we have also included a contribution on the medicolegal aspects of breast diagnosis.

As editors of this volume we wish to express our thanks to the series editors for their invitation to work on this project. We would like to thank all our colleagues for their excellent contributions and collaboration. We also wish to thank the staff of Springer-Verlag (Ms. U. Davis and Mr. R. Mills) for their patience, understanding, and invaluable assistance during the preparation of the manuscripts.

Berlin/San Francisco

M.A. FRIEDRICH
E.A. SICKLES

Contents

1 Breast Cancer Epidemiology and Risk Factors
   M.J.M. Broeders and A.L.M. Verbeek 1

2 Mammographic-Pathological Correlations
   A.H. Tulusan 13

3 Technical Aspects of Screen-Film Mammography
   A.G. Haus 33

4 Current Legislation on Mammography Quality Assurance
   R.E. Hendrick 57

5 Digital Mammography
   J.-W. Oestmann 65

6 The Art of Mammographic Postioning
   G.W. Eklund 75

7 Differential Diagnosis of Microcalcifications
   M. Lanyi 89

8 Imaging Evaluation of Spiculated Masses
   D.D. Adler 137

9 The Management of Nonpalpable Circumscribed Breast Masses
   E.D. Pisano 149

10 Management of Lesions Appearing Probably Benign at Mammography
   E.A. Sickles 167

11 Radiation Risk of Mammography
   S.A. Feig and R.E. Hendrick 173

12 Echomammography: Technique and Results
   J. Teubner 181

13 Doppler Sonography of Breast Tumors
   S. Delorme 221

14 Magnetic Resonance Imaging of the Breast
   M. Friedrich 229

15 Prebiopsy Localization of Nonpalpable Breast Lesions
   H. Junkermann and D. von Fournier 283

16 Fine-Needle Aspiration and Core Biopsy
   M. Bauer, P. Tontsch, and R. Schulz-Wendtland 291

17	Imaging the Breast After Radiation and Surgery E.B. Mendelson and C.E. Tobin	299
18	Imaging After Breast Implants N.D. DeBruhl, D.P. Gorczyca, and L.W. Bassett	319
19	Breast Cancer Screening Projects: Results I. Schreer and H.-J. Frischbier	333
20	Breast Cancer Screening: Gereral Guidelines, Program Design, and Organization L.J. Warren Burhenne	347
21	Medicolegal Aspects of Breast Imaging R.J. Brenner	367

Subject Index 379

List of Contributors 385

1 Breast Cancer Epidemiology and Risk Factors

M.J.M. Broeders and A.L.M. Verbeek

CONTENTS

1.1 Occurrence of Breast Cancer in Western Society ... 1
1.1.1 Breast Cancer Mortality ... 1
1.1.2 Risk of Developing Breast Cancer ... 1
1.1.3 Trends over Time ... 2
1.2 The Significance of Breast Complaints as Correlated with Age and Breast Cancer ... 3
1.3 Etiology of Breast Cancer: Current Hypotheses ... 4
1.4 Risk Factors for Breast Cancer ... 5
1.4.1 Established Risk Factors ... 5
1.4.2 Dubious Risk Factors ... 8
1.5 Primary Prevention of Breast Cancer ... 8
1.5.1 Modification of Exposure to Risk Factors ... 9
1.5.2 Prophylactic Mastectomy ... 9
1.5.3 Chemoprevention Trials ... 10
1.6 Early Diagnosis of Breast Cancer ... 10
1.6.1 Individual Counselling ... 10
1.6.2 Screening for Breast Cancer ... 10
1.6.3 Selection of High-Risk Groups for Screening ... 11
References ... 11

1.1 Occurrence of Breast Cancer in Western Society

1.1.1 Breast Cancer Mortality

Breast cancer is the most common malignancy among women in almost all of Europe, in North America, in much of Latin America, and in Australasia. In many of these populations, it is the leading cause of death for women between the ages of 35 and 54 years, and among women younger than 50 it is almost as common as all cancers combined among men (Miller 1987). The impact of breast cancer is magnified compared with other cancers because women are at risk beginning in their middle years rather than at more advanced ages. As a consequence, the average years of life lost by those with breast cancer (20 years) is higher than the average for all cancers combined (16 years) (Colditz 1993).

When comparing the cancer mortality or incidence rates at different places or at different times, conclusions might be drawn that are highly misleading. One of the potential causes of differences between recorded rates is the difference in age distribution of the populations that are to be compared. The most commonly used method of summarizing observations of a wide range of ages is to calculate standardized rates using an external reference population (most often the world population) (Smith 1992). For many years, age-standardized breast cancer mortality rates have been highest in North America and (Northern) Europe. However, some variation also exists in the these areas, as shown in Fig. 1.1.

1.1.2 Risk of Developing Breast Cancer

When assessing the impact of breast cancer in the general population, the incidence rate, i.e., the number of new cases per year per 100 000 women, is of vital importance. The incidence per year increases progressively with advancing age. The steepest increase is around the menopause and the increase slows in the postmenopausal period (McDermott 1991).

Wide geographic variation is observed for both incidence and mortality. The populations with the lowest risk for breast cancer are found in Asia, whereas the risks in Western Europe and in North America can be as much as fivefold greater. In addition, variation exists within these continents: in Western Europe, there is almost a twofold difference between the highest incidence rate, seen in Geneva (Switzerland), and the lowest, in Spain. A similar difference is seen in North America between white females in the San Francisco Bay Area, USA (highest incidence) and those in Newfoundland, Canada (Coleman et al. 1993). Age-standardized breast cancer incidence rates for various countries in North

M.J.M. Broeders, MSc, Department of Medical Informatics, Epidemiology and Statistics, Katholieke Universiteit Nijmegen, P.O. Box 9101, 6500 HB Nijmegen, The Netherlands
A.L.M. Verbeek, MD, PhD, Professor, Department of Medical Informatics, Epidemiology and Statistics, Katholieke Universiteit Nijmegen, P.O. Box 9101, 6500 HB Nijmegen, The Netherlands

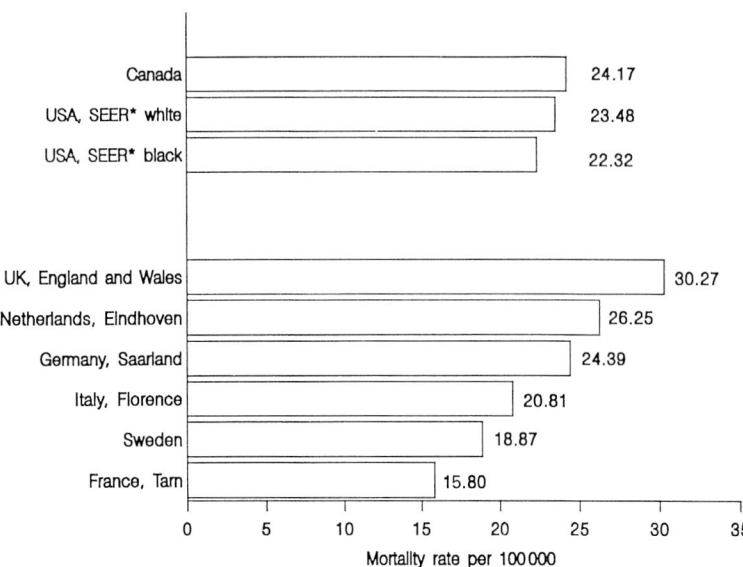

Fig. 1.1. Mortality from breast cancer per 100 000 women in North America and Europe (age-standardized to world population, 1983–1987). *SEER-Surveillance, Epidemiology, and End Results Program. (From PARKIN et al. 1992)

America and Europe also vary considerably, as shown in Fig. 1.2.

The probability of developing breast cancer is widely used for increasing awareness among the general population and in counselling individuals about their risk of developing the disease. The often-quoted risk of a woman developing breast cancer of "1 in 9" or, more recently, "1 in 8" is the lifetime risk of developing the disease among the general population (HELZLSOUER 1994). Using the life table method to adjust for competing causes of death, SCHOUTEN et al. (1994) recently published breast cancer risk estimates reflecting the probability of developing breast cancer from birth. In addition, estimates were given for the probability of developing breast cancer from a given age onwards (for women free of the disease at the beginning of the given interval). The results in Tabel 1.1, based on cancer incidence data from a regional cancer registry in the Netherlands, show that the ongoing lifetime risk of breast cancer starts to decline beginning at the age of 25. The risk of developing breast cancer from birth until age of death in this population is estimated to be 10.9%.

1.1.3 Trends over Time

1.1.3.1 Incidence

The rates of breast cancer have risen slowly but steadily in the United States since formal tracking of the cases through registries began in the 1930s (HARRIS et al. 1992a). Similar results have been reported by the Nordic countries in Europe, where, for instance, in Denmark the incidence remained almost constant up to around 1960, whereafter it rose steadily (EWERTZ and CARSTENSEN 1988). The age-specific incidence patterns, however, seem to differ between the United States and the Nordic countries. Whereas statistics from Portland, Oregon, showed the greatest rise in incidence among those 60+ years old and no change among those 20–44 years old, data from the Nordic countries indicated the greatest proportional increase to have occurred in age groups below 50 (EWERTZ and CARSTENSEN 1988; PERSSON et al. 1993).

The increase in the probability of developing breast cancer was studied extensively using incidence, mortality, and population data, representing the various geographic areas of the U.S. National Cancer Institute's Surveillance, Epidemiology, and End Results (SEER) Program. A large portion of the

Table 1.1. Probability of developing breast cancer (cancer incidence data from Comprehensive Cancer Centre East, the Netherlands, 1989–1990)

Probability (%) of developing breast cancer from birth until:			
Age 25	Age 50	Age 75	Age of death
0.0%	1.8%	8.2%	10.9%

Probability (%) of developing breast cancer in the remaining lifetime from:			
Birth	Age 25	Age 50	Age 75
10.9%	11.1%	9.6%	3.9%

Fig. 1.2. New cases of breast cancer per 100 000 women in North America and Europe (age-standardized to world population, 1983–1987). *SEER-Surveillance, Epidemiology, and End Results Program. (From PARKIN et al. 1992)

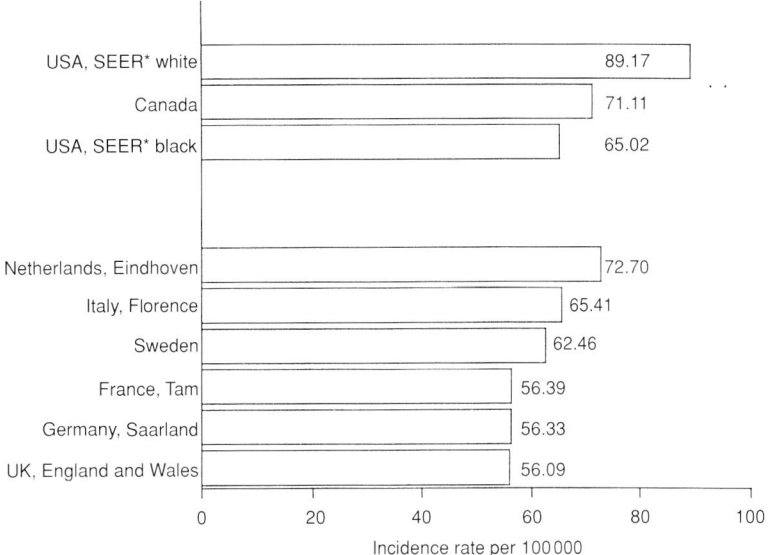

rise in estimated lifetime risk of breast cancer comparing 1975–1977 data (1 in 10.6) with 1987–1988 data (1 in 8) may be attributed to: (a) early detection of prevalent cases due to increased use of mammographic screening and (b) lower mortality due to causes other than breast cancer (FEUER et al. 1993). Putting these components together (and assuming independence between breast cancer incidence and mortality due to other causes), FEUER et al. (1993) partitioned the increase in the lifetime risk of breast cancer into three categories: 9% of the new cases are attributable to women living longer (lower mortality due to causes other than breast cancer); 31% of the new cases are attributable to the secular trend towards an increase in incidence (cause unknown); and 60% of the new cases are attributable to the rise in incidence above the secular trend (evidence points to early detection of prevalent cases, and some possible overdiagnosis, through screening).

1.1.3.2 Mortality

In contrast to the observed changes in incidence, age-adjusted breast cancer mortality rates have been relatively constant both in the United States and in Europe (see, e.g., EWERTZ and CARSTENSEN 1988; KELSEY and HORN-ROSS 1933). The stability of age-adjusted breast cancer mortality in the United States is striking since it has occurred during a period of dramatic change with respect to other diseases, notably large decreases in mortality due to heart disease and changes in mortality due to other cancers, especially recent large increases in female lung cancer mortality (KESSLER et al. 1991).

The relatively constant increase in the incidence of breast cancer compared with the relatively flat trend in mortality may be explained by a variety of hypotheses: (a) that improvements in treatment have kept pace with the rising incidence; (b) that cancers detected by screening are more readily cured; (c) that cancers are being identified which will not result in mortality; or (d) a combination of the three hypotheses (SONDIK 1994).

Looking at trends over time, one might wonder what the possible magnitude of the problem of breast cancer will be in the near future. The simplest approach is to assume that the latest observed (or estimated) incidence or mortality rates will apply to the world population at, for example, the year 2000, using the population projection of the United Nations. Assuming further a 2%–3% overall rate of continued increase in the incidence of breast cancer, the annual number of new cases diagnosed in the year 2000 in the world will probably be between 1.1 and 1.4 million (MILLER 1987).

1.2 The Significance of Breast Complaints as Correlated with Age and Breast Cancer

Information through the media on the rising number of new breast cancer cases has not only increased breast health awareness, but has also introduced anxiety in the female population. Women have been

Table 1.2. The significance of breast complaints as correlated with age and breast cancer (based on SELTZER 1992)

Primary complaint	<50 ($n = 1364$)		>50 ($n = 636$)	
	% of women presenting the complaint	% of women ultimately proven to have breast cancer	% of women presenting the complaint	% of women ultimately proven to have breast cancer
Lump	58.9	4.8	30.8	22.9
Pain	7.1	2.1	5.0	3.1
Nipple discharge	4.0	2.0	2.8	17.6
Abnormal mammogram	21.7	3.0	53.8	14.4
Other symptoms	8.3	2.9	7.6	10.9

urged to have periodic breast evaluation by a physician, to practice breast self-examination, and to have mammography for the purpose of early detection of breast cancer (SELTZER 1992). Due to the heightened awareness about breast cancer, women will present at the general practitioner with a great variety of breast complaints. Naturally, the greatest fear of both the patient and her physician is that the complaint may herald a breast cancer. Although the physician will very often suspect a minor, benign condition, he will not take the risk of overlooking breast cancer and will often refer the woman for further diagnosis (MEISCHKE-DE JONGH et al. 1983).

To properly evaluate a breast complaint, there must be an understanding of the risks for breast cancer associated with a given complaint at the time of patient referral. While there are many variables that are important in the evaluation of a breast complaint, the patient's age is most important (SELTZER 1992). In Table 1.2, based on data published by SELTZER (1992), a number of complaints are listed with which new patients, either under or above the age of 50, may present to the general practitioner or a breast clinic. This table is useful in presenting the percentage of patients among all women presenting with a given symptom who were proven to have breast cancer after further diagnostic workup.

No one particular breast complaint serves to signal breast cancer under the age of 50. In this age category, a breast lump is associated with cancer in only 5% of the approximately 60% of women who present with this symptom. Other symptoms are even less likely to be associated with breast cancer. The significance of breast complaints changes considerably with age. A complaint of a lump is almost 5 times more likely to represent cancer in a woman 50 years or older than in younger women; abnormal mammography is also 5 times more likely to herald breast cancer in older women. In both age categories, however, only 2%–3% of women presenting with pain as a primary complaint will be diagnosed with breast cancer.

1.3 Etiology of Breast Cancer: Current Hypotheses

The concepts of the etiology of breast cancer are changing rapidly, and physicians need to be aware of these changes. This is particularly important for the physician who is called upon to offer preventive advice to patients and their families (MANSFIELD 1993).

Breast cancer does not appear to be a single disease. The very fact that some breast cancers may be aggressive while others are less so, that some may depend strongly on estrogen for growth while others may not, and that breast cancer may well arise from cells at different points down the differentiation pathway clearly indicates the heterogeneity of the disease. It is a logical conclusion that each type of breast cancer may have a different "cause" or, at least, a specific etiologic factor may have more influence on one form of breast cancer than another (BOYLE and LEAKE 1988).

Carcinogenesis is believed to occur in a series of steps which have been variously described as a multistage process or as the occurrence of a number of "hits" which lead to irreversible cellular transformations progressing eventually to full malignancy (KNUDSON 1993).

In every country with adequate incidence data, the age-specific incidence curves for different birth cohorts have an identical shape, showing a steep increase in incidence with advancing age before menopause and a much shallower rise afterwards. This phenomenon, often referred to as Clemmesen's hook, is unique for breast cancer in females and is absent in male breast cancer (CLEMMESEN 1948). The shape of the aforementioned age curve is compatible with a two-stage carcinogenesis model. The model predicts that susceptibility to the first stage is proportional to the number of dividing mammary cells, with initiated, or potentially malignant, cells proliferating in response to a stimulus that largely ceases to exist at the menopause (in the same manner that the risk of lung cancer declines with cessation of smoking). The risk during the second stage is proportional to the number of initiated cells (MILLER and BULBROOK 1980).

The majority of breast tumors result from transformation of ductal or lobular epithelial cells. Once the tumor is established, it continues to grow as carcinoma in situ, i.e., a confined group of cells still linked by cell–cell contact and contained within a basement membrane. At some stage, usually prior to the tumor being detectable at clinical breast examination (palpation), cell–cell interactions begin to break down. At the same time the tumor cells secrete digestive enzymes and the invasive process begins, eventually resulting in metastasis (BOYLE and LEAKE 1988).

Precancerous lesions which are generated during the perimenarcheal years and adolescence may be promoted to clinical breast cancer in subsequent years under the influence of a number of factors, among which estrogens appear to play a major role. Several risk factors can be brought together within a concept of pathogenesis and carcinogenesis. They include nutritional factors as well as reproductive factors, both acting through endocrine mechanisms (DE WAARD and TRICHOPOULOS 1988). Breast tumors are usually slow growing. It takes about 10 years (by extrapolation) for a tumor to grow from the inital transformation event until the time that it becomes palpable. This means that the metabolic and hormonal conditions which may be related to the development of breast cancer are those in existence at the time of transformation, and that these may not be the same as those present at the time of diagnosis (BOYLE and LEAKE 1988).

1.4 Risk Factors for Breast Cancer

Large variations in the rates of breast cancer among countries and over time within countries, and large increases in the rates of breast cancer among populations migrating from nations with a low cancer incidence to those with a high incidence, indicate the existence of major nongenetic determinants of breast

Table 1.3. Risk factors for breast cancer

Established	Dubious
Age	Alcohol
Demographic characteristics	Oral contraceptives
Previous breast cancer	Hormone replacement therapy
Previous benign breast disease	Diet
Family history	Breast feeding
Radiation	Physical activity
Factors related to menses	
Factors related to pregnancy	
Mammographic parenchymal pattern	
Obesity	

cancer and the potential for prevention. The strength of a risk factor is typically indicated by its relative risk – the incidence among persons possessing a characteristic in question divided by the incidence among otherwise similar persons without the characteristic (HARRIS et al. 1992a). While results from epidemiologic studies regarding a number of risk factors remain fairly reproducible, other associations are not consistently found. In the following sections, an attempt will therefore be made to distinguish between established and dubious risk factors (Table 1.3).

1.4.1 Established Risk Factors

1.4.1.1 Age

The most prominent risk factor for breast cancer is age. The incidence of breast cancer increases steeply with age, doubling about every 10 years until the menopause. As described previously, the rise slows in the postmenopausal period and in some countries there is a flattening or even a (temporal) decrease of the age incidence curve after menopause (CLEMMESEN 1948; McPHERSON et al. 1994).

1.4.1.2 Demographic Characteristics

Breast cancer incidence rates are more than 100 times higher in females than in males (KELSEY and HORN-ROSS 1993). Age-adjusted incidence and mortality for breast cancer vary by at least a factor of 7 between countries. The difference between Far Eastern and Western countries is diminishing but is still about fivefold. Studies of migrants from Japan to Hawaii show that the rate of breast cancer in migrants assumes the rate in the host country within one or two generations, suggesting that environmental factors are of greater importance than genetic factors (MCPHERSON et al. 1994). Considerable variation in incidence rates occurs among major racial/ethnic groups in the United States. Above 40–45 years of age, white women have the highest rates, followed in order by blacks, Hispanics, and Asians. At younger ages, black women have slightly higher rates than white women, while Hispanic and Asian women again have the lowest rates (KELSEY 1993). Urban residents have an increased risk of breast cancer compared with rural residents, irrespective of whether the region is in a high- or a low-risk continent (MCDERMOTT 1991). Although lower socioeconomic characteristics of populations are usually related to a higher general cancer risk, the opposite is true for breast cancer. In general, the greater rates of breast cancer in women of higher socioeconomic status are thought to reflect differing reproductive patterns, such as parity, age at first birth, and age at menarche (KELSEY and HORN-ROSS 1993).

1.4.1.3 Previous Breast Cancer

In women with breast cancer the risk of developing a new primary lesion in the opposite breast or conserved ipsilateral breast is increased threefold (MCDERMOTT 1991).

1.4.1.4 Previous Benign Breast Disease

Women who have had "fibrocystic disease" are found to have a two- to threefold increased risk of breast cancer. Risk varies according to the type of benign breast disease diagnosed and is greatest in lesions characterized by atypical hyperplasia (BOYLE and LEAKE 1988; MCDERMOTT 1991). Women with severe atypical epithelial hyperplasia have a 4–5 times higher risk than women who do not have any proliferative changes in their breasts. A ninefold increase in risk is found in women with these changes as well as a family history of breast cancer (first-degree relative) (MCPHERSON et al. 1994).

The relationship between fibroadenoma and breast cancer remains unclear. On balance, fibroadenoma occurring alone is associated with, at most, a modest increase in risk, but fibroadenoma in the presence of epithelial hyperplasia may be an independent risk factor for breast cancer (BODIAN 1993).

1.4.1.5 Family History

A family history of breast cancer, particularly when the diagnosis was made in the mother or a sister at a young age, can be an important risk factor for breast cancer (HARRIS et al. 1992a). Studies have shown the relative risk to first-degree female relatives of patients with premenopausal breast cancer to be 3.1, while no increase in risk is observed among relatives of postmenopausal patients. When a patient has bilateral breast cancer, the risk to her first-degree relatives increases fivefold. If both conditions apply (i.e., the patient is premenopausal and has bilateral disease), the risk to first-degree relatives increases ninefold (MANSFIELD 1993).

There clearly is a familial component to breast cancer that is due to genetic predisposition, accounting for about 5% of the incidence of the disease in the population. Breast cancer susceptibility is generally inherited as an autosomal dominant with limited penetrance. This means that it can be transmitted through either sex and that some family members may transmit the abnormal gene without developing cancer themselves. It is not yet known how many breast cancer genes there may be (MCPHERSON et al. 1994). Familial breast cancer can be distinguished from hereditary breast cancer based on the proposition that at least two mutational events are required for the development of cancer derived from a single cell. In nonhereditary cases, normal cells undergo mutation to produce cells in an intermediate state. A second mutational event is required to transform this cell into a cancer cell. Individuals with a hereditary form of the disease, on the other hand, receive the first mutational event from a parental germ cell. Consequently only a second mutational event is needed for such cells to become cancer cells (WILLIAMS and OSBORNE 1987). Many families affected by hereditary breast cancer show an excess of ovarian, colon, prostatic, and other cancers attributable to the same inherited mutation. Patients with bilateral breast cancer, those who develop a combination of breast cancer and another epithelial cancer, and women who get the disease at an early age are most likely to be carrying a genetic mutation that has predisposed them to developing breast cancer (MCPHERSON et al. 1994). If an autosomal dominant mode of inheritance is assumed for a given family, the sisters and daughters of a woman with breast cancer may have a lifetime probability as high as 30%–50% of developing this cancer (VASEN 1994).

Recently, genetic linkage studies have established that a gene predisposing to breast and ovarian cancer

(BRCA1) is situated on the long arm of chromosome 17 (FORD et al. 1994). BRCA1 is found in many tissues in the body and almost certainly plays a vital role in normal cell function. In women who inherit a defective copy of this gene, the breast cancer risk has been estimated to be 51% by age 50 and 85% by age 70, and the ovarian cancer risk to be 23% by age 50 and 63% by age 70. Women in BRCA1 families who have breast cancer are subsequently at high risk of both a second primary breast cancer and ovarian cancer (EASTON et al. 1994).

1.4.1.6 Radiation

The importance of exposure to ionizing irradiation in carcinogenesis depends on age at the time of exposure (MANSFIELD 1993). The greatest risk has been found among women exposed to radiation around menarche. This suggests that breast tissue is particularly vulnerable at this time either because the breasts are developing rapidly or because these women have not given birth. The best explanation could be the former, since exposure to radiation prior to the age of 10 has consistently been shown to carry no increased risk while the greatest risk has been associated with exposure during the first pregnancy (BOYLE and LEAKE 1988). Increased risk is observed principally in women exposed to moderate to high levels of radiation (>100 cGy). Radiation risk at the extremely low-dose level imparted by modern mammography is estimated by extrapolation from higher dose data and is widely believed to be negligible, especially when viewed in the context of the observed benefits of mammography (FEIG 1995).

1.4.1.7 Factors Related to Menses

The risk of breast cancer may be modified according to the duration and the strength of breast tissue exposure to estrogens and prolactin (McDERMOTT 1991). Thus, the younger a woman's age at menarche and/or the later a woman's age at menopause, the higher her risk of breast cancer (KELSEY et al. 1993).

Early menarche is a well-established but weak risk factor. Women in whom menarche occurs before the age of 12 have a 20% increase in risk compared with women in whom it occurs at the age of at least 14. Even though the strength of the association is weak, this variable may account for a substantial part of the observed international differences in breast cancer incidence. For example, in China the average age at menarche is 17 years as compared with 12.8 years in the United States (HARRIS et al. 1992a).

Women who have a natural menopause after the age of 55 are twice as likely to develop breast cancer as women who experience the menopause before the age of 45 (McPHERSON et al. 1994). Artificial menopause through oophorectomy is associated with a reduction in breast cancer risk if the procedure is done before the age of 40 (MANSFIELD 1993).

1.4.1.8 Factors Related to Pregnancy

An early age at first birth is associated with a substantial reduction in risk of breast cancer. Women who have a child before the age of 18 have about one-third the risk of women whose first children are born after the age of 30 (BOYLE and LEAKE 1988). Having children in itself reduces the risk of breast cancer: the reduction in risk associated with five or more full-term pregnancies has been found in several studies to be 50% in comparison with women with no full-term pregnancies (KELSEY et al. 1993). It has been shown that the decreasing risk of breast cancer with increasing parity is an effect independent of age at first birth (BOYLE and LEAKE 1988).

The highest risk is found in women who have a first child after the age of 35; these women appear to be at even higher risk than nulliparous women (McPHERSON et al. 1994). A possible explanation for this phenomenon is that a full-term pregnancy at an early age may reduce the likelihood of tumor initiation while a full-term pregnancy at a later age may promote the growth of existing tumor cells (KELSEY et al. 1993).

1.4.1.9 Mammographic Parenchymal Pattern

An increased risk of breast cancer is found among women in whom the mammograms show abundant dense fibroglandular tissue. The risk estimates associated with these parenchymal patterns vary but in most studies they are comparable to most other known risk factors (SAFTLAS and SZKLO 1987).

1.4.1.10 Obesity

Data from several studies indicate that the association between obesity and breast cancer is dependent on menopausal status. Among postmenopausal women, the body of the evidence points to an increased risk of breast cancer in obese women (BOYLE and LEAKE 1988). However, there is a stronger association with mortality from breast cancer, due in part to delayed diagnosis among more obese women and to a worse prognosis that is independent of the stage of cancer (HARRIS et al. 1992a).

Heavy body weight appears to be associated with a slightly decreased risk of breast cancer in premenopausal women (KELSEY 1993).

1.4.2 Dubious Risk Factors

1.4.2.1 Oral Contraceptives

Several studies suggest a slightly increased risk of premenopausal breast cancer with prolonged use of oral contraceptives before first birth and with long-term use at an early age – irrespective of whether before or after first birth (MCDERMOTT 1991; MCPHERSON et al. 1994). Little evidence exists to indicate that the use or oral contraceptives affects risk for breast cancer diagnosed after the age of 45, but this needs to be closely monitored as substantial numbers of women with a history of long-term use are now entering this age group (KELSEY 1993).

1.4.2.2 Hormone Replacement Therapy

Most evidence from studies that have included large enough numbers of long-term users of estrogen replacement therapy indicates a slight (less than two-fold) elevation in risk associated with 10–15 years or more of use (KELSEY 1993). Fewer data are available on the use of combined estrogen and progesterone preparations, but the only large study to date shows a greater risk for the combined treatment than for estrogen therapy alone (MCPHERSON et al. 1994).

1.4.2.3 Diet

A role for diet in the etiology of breast cancer, particularly a diet high in fat, is thought to exist on the basis of results from animal studies, international variations in incidence rates, and underlying biologic principles. Results from direct studies on humans provide conflicting and weak evidence of an association, although results from some studies are so internally consistent that they cannot be ignored (BOYLE and LEAKE 1988; KELSEY 1993). High vegetable and fruit intake appear to be protective (MCDERMOTT 1991).

1.4.2.4 Alcohol

A number of studies of the effects of alcohol indicate an association between increased risk of breast cancer and drinking wine or hard liquor. The relationship, however, is inconsistent and the moderate association found may be due to other dietary factors rather than alcohol (MCPHERSON et al. 1994).

1.4.2.5 Breast Feeding

Breast feeding may play a modest or indirect part in reducing the risk of breast cancer, especially for premenopausal women. However, current evidence for a protective effect in Western countries is inconclusive. Data from China, where several years of breast feeding is common practice, suggest that very long-term breast feeding is protective (KELSEY et al. 1993).

1.4.2.6 Physical Activity

Epidemiologic studies provide some indication that strenuous physical activity, especially those sports that require intense training, may delay the onset of menses and promote anovulation, thereby reducing breast cancer risk (GAMMON and JOHN 1993).

1.5 Primary Prevention of Breast Cancer

Attempts to identify ways to reduce the frequency of breast cancer through primary prevention have been discouraging. Despite the fact that breast cancer has been one of the most investigated tumors, it is estimated that only half of the incidence of the disease is explained by established risk factors (BRINTON 1994). No single risk factor is common to a large proportion of disease, and many patients with breast cancer have none of the recognized risk factors (METTLIN 1994). However, it should be recognized that the potential benefit is great: the ability to prevent even 1% of breast cancer would mean a reduction of more than 5000 cases per year worldwide (BOYLE and LEAKE 1988). Current knowledge on primary prevention through modification of exposure to risk factors, prophylactic mastectomy, and chemoprevention trials is summarized in the following sections.

1.5.1 Modification of Exposure to Risk Factors

The extent to which prevention of breast cancer is feasible depends on, first, the proportion of breast cancers attributable to various factors and, second, the extent to which women are able and willing to modify their exposure to these factors (MILLER 1987). Although most of the generally accepted risk factors are not readily modifiable through either behavioral or environmental changes, the risk factors discussed below could be considered for primary prevention.

1.5.1.1 Diet

A number of studies provide supportive evidence of the association of diet, especially high fat in diet, with breast cancer. This would make the reduction of dietary fat an effective way of primary prevention of breast cancer (MANSFIELD 1993). However, reduction of intake of fat, or other possibly associated dietary factors, in whole communities may well be difficult to achieve without major social and cultural changes (MCPHERSON et al. 1994). In spite of the uncertainties, the National Institutes of Health in the United States is supporting a major prospective trial (the Women's Health Initiative) to determine whether a low-fat diet and an increased intake of vegetables, fruits, and grain products reduce the incidence of breast and colorectal cancer as well as mortality from coronary heart disease. Results from this multicenter study, which started accrual in 1994, are not expected for another decade (GREENWALD 1993).

1.5.1.2 Obesity

There is a measure of consistency about findings of increased breast cancer risk in postmenopausal obese women which, perhaps, offers some prospect for prevention (BOYLE and LEAKE 1988). However, in contrast to dietary fat interventions, little attention has so far been paid to weight loss as a specific intervention for lowering breast cancer risk (BRINTON 1994).

1.5.1.3 Nulliparity and Age at First Birth

It seems unlikely that all women who plan to have children could be induced to have their first birth before the age of 25 years. Nevertheless, providing information on degree of risk to permit women to make informed choices seems appropriate (MILLER 1987).

1.5.1.4 Alcohol

Restriction of alcoholic beverage intake is generally viewed as beneficial, although the levels of consumption that are associated with breast cancer risk as well as the biologic means of the action of alcohol remain to be clarified (BRINTON 1994).

1.5.1.5 Physical Activity

Recent research has suggested that high levels of physical activity during a woman's reproductive years can lead to substantial reductions in breast cancer risk, thereby offering a modifiable life-style characteristic for primary prevention (BERNSTEIN et al. 1994).

1.5.2 Prophylactic Mastectomy

Prophylactic mastectomy is the only known means by which breast cancer can be prevented; however, it is a drastic solution to the problem for which indications are not standardized and efficacy is unproved (HOUN et al. 1995). Only very few women (extremely strong family history) have a lifetime risk of breast cancer that exceeds 50%. In addition, it is useful to understand that a woman's risk of breast cancer over a more limited time span (e.g., from the age of 35 to the age of 70) or of dying of the disease may be considerably smaller than her lifetime risk of having the disease (HARRIS et al. 1992b). Prophylactic total mastectomy should therefore be reserved for those rare individuals with a definite major risk factor that is unacceptable to the patient. In the absence of a phenotypic marker other than cancer, it has been proposed that this procedure be considered only for women with either (a) hereditary breast cancer or (b) carcinoma in situ (OSBORNE 1987).

1.5.3 Chemoprevention Trials

There has been increasing interest in the development of "chemoprevention" or "chemosuppression," i.e., interventions directed at inhibiting neoplastic development through pharmacologic measures (HARRIS et al. 1992b). The feasibility and acceptability of using any drug for the primary prevention of breast cancer are dependent on two factors. The first is the ability to identify accurately women at elevated risk of breast cancer among whom most of the cases would occur; these are the women who would benefit from such an intervention. The second requirement is the availability of an agent which can block the carcinogenic process and which has low toxicity (BUSH and HELZLSOUER 1993).

The pursuit of effective chemopreventive agents for breast cancer will require unusually long and costly research commitments (HARRIS et al. 1992b). Because of the uncertainty of net risks and benefits, close monitoring for adverse side-effects should be incorporated into ongoing prevention trials (HELZLSOUER 1994).

Three types of agents being studied in research on breast cancer chemoprevention are tamoxifen, retinoids, and gonadotropin-releasing hormone agonists.

1.5.3.1 Tamoxifen

During trials of tamoxifen as an adjuvant treatment for breast cancer, the number of contralateral breast cancers was less than expected, suggesting that this drug might have a role in preventing breast cancer (MCPHERSON et al. 1994). On the basis of these findings, randomized trials have been started in several countries to evaluate the potential of tamoxifen for preventing breast cancer in high-risk women (HARRIS et al. 1992b). However, the reasonabless of exposing large numbers of healthy women, who are at low absolute risk of developing breast cancer, to a drug which has been shown to increase the risk of serious conditions such as thromboembolic disease and endometrial cancer has been questioned (BUSH and HELZLSOUER 1993).

1.5.3.2 Retinoids

The term "retinoids" applies to vitamin A (retinol) and its isomers, derivatives, and synthetic analogues (HARRIS et al. 1992b). Retinoids affect the growth and differentiation of epithelial cells. Experiments suggest that through this mechanism, they may have a role in preventing breast cancer (MCPHERSON et al. 1994).

1.5.3.3 Gonadotropin-Releasing Hormone Agonist

Another approach to chemoprevention of breast cancer involves the total blockage of ovarian steroid production through the use of a luteinizing hormone-releasing hormone agonist. A pilot trial study of gonadotropin hormone agonist with replacement hormones is underway (HELZLSOUER 1994).

1.6 Early Diagnosis of Breast Cancer

Acknowledging the difficulties encountered in primary prevention of breast cancer, an important strategy to try to reduce breast cancer mortality is early detection through individual counselling or mass breast screening programs.

1.6.1 Individual Counselling

Individualized probabilities based on risk factors such as family history alone or family history and other risk factors have been developed and used to counsel individuals regarding their risk of developing breast cancer (HELZLSOUER 1994). It is important that this information is conveyed to the woman and her relatives in a manner that enables them to have a clear understanding of their risk as well as knowledge of the various options for medical treatment to which they have access (WILLIAMS and OSBORNE 1987). Caution must be exercised since for the individual woman, the risk of breast cancer is all or none. The individualized probability should only be a guide as to whether she is a member of a group of women who are more or less likely to develop breast cancer than members of other groups of women with different risk profiles (HELZLSOUER 1994). Recently, results from a prospective randomized trial comparing individualized breast cancer risk counselling to general health counselling became available. The authors concluded that efforts to counsel women about their breast cancer risks are not likely to be effective unless their breast cancer anxieties are also addressed (LERMAN et al. 1995).

1.6.2 Screening for Breast Cancer

The pattern of breast cancer occurrence according to age bears directly on the determination of advisable screening guidelines because age is the most important determinant of a woman's risk for breast cancer (METTLIN 1994). Randomized controlled trials have shown that screening women over the age of 50 by mammography can significantly reduce mortality from breast cancer, regardless of screening interval or number of mammographic views per screen. A recently published meta-analysis showed an overall relative risk estimate of 0.74 (95% confidence interval 0.66–0.83) for breast cancer mortality among women aged 50–74 years who underwent screening mammography, as compared with those who did not (KERLIKOWSKE et al. 1995).

Population-based screening for women aged 40–49 has not been shown to be as effective, although after at least 10 years of follow-up, a substantial trend toward reduced mortality with borderline statistical significance ranging from 13% to 24% has been observed in two meta-analyses (KERLIKOWSKE et al. 1995; SMART et al. 1995). Although there is no direct evidence on the value of screening at ages older than 74 years, the findings in women aged 60–74 imply that screening might be effective among women over age 74 years in reducing deaths from breast cancer (MORRISON 1993; FAULK et al. 1995).

A number of countries have adopted national or regional mammography screening programs, including Sweden, Finland, the Netherlands, Canada, the United Kingdom, and Australia. All such programs include the screening of women in their 50s and 60s. Some programs also include the screening of women aged 40–49. At this time, the United States is not actively considering a national program (HARRIS et al. 1992a), but routine mammography is widely performed at the local-regional level among women aged 40 and older.

1.6.3 Selection of High-Risk Groups for Screening

Using risk factors for selective screening has been proposed as one means of improving the efficiency of breast cancer screening programs. While intuitively attractive, this approach has never been implemented in a prospective study to demonstrate its practicality and value (METTLIN 1994). Screening targeted at high-risk groups within the population is attractive for a number of reasons. First, the yield of screening will be much higher, a more invasive test may be justifiable, and compliance will be greater if an individual perceives herself to be at high risk. This holds particularly for individuals belonging to a family in which a number of members have died from the disease (VASEN 1994).

References

Bernstein L, Henderson BE, Hanisch R, Sullivan-Halley J, Ross RK (1994) Physical exercise and reduced risk of breast cancer in young women. J Natl Cancer Inst 86:1403–1408

Bodian CA (1993) Benign breast diseases, carcinoma in situ, and breast cancer risk. Epidemiol Rev 15:177–195

Boyle P, Leake R (1988) Progress in understanding breast cancer: epidemiological and biological interactions. Breast Cancer Res Treat 11:91–112

Brinton LA (1994) Ways that women may possibly reduce their risk of breast cancer. J Natl Cancer Inst 68:1371–1372

Bush TL, Helzlsouer KJ (1993) Tamoxifen for the primary prevention of breast cancer: a review and critique of the concept and trial. Epidemiol Rev 15:233–243

Clemmesen J (1948) Carcinoma of the breast. I. Results from statistical research. Br J Radiol 21:583–590

Colditz AC (1993) Epidemiology of breast cancer. Findings from the Nurses' Health Study. Cancer 71:1480–1489

Coleman MP, Esteve J, Damiecki P, Arslan A, Renard H (1993) Trends in cancer incidence and mortality. IARC Scientific Publications no. 121. IARC, Lyon, pp 411–432

De Waard F, Trichopoulos D (1988) A unifying concept of the aetiology of breast cancer. Int J Cancer 41:666–669

Easton DF, Narod SA, Ford D, Steel M, on behalf of the Breast Cancer Linkage Consortium (1994) The genetic epidemiology of BRCA1 (letter). Lancet 344:761

Ewertz M, Carstensen B (1988) Trends in breast cancer incidence and mortality in Denmark, 1943–1982. Int J Cancer 41:46–51

Faulk RM, Sickles EA, Sollitto RA, Ominsky SH, Galvin HB, Frankel SD (1995) Clinical efficacy of mammography screening in the elderly. Radiology 194:193–197

Feig SA (1995) Estimation of currently attainable benefit from mammographic screening of women aged 40–49 years. Cancer 75:2412–2419

Feuer EJ, Lap-Ming W, Boring CC, Flanders WD, Timmel MJ, Tong T (1993) The lifetime risk of developing breast cancer. J Natl Cancer Inst 88:892–897

Ford D, Easton DF, Bishop DT, Narod SA, Goldgar DE, and the Breast Cancer Linkage Consortium (1994) Risks of cancer in BRCA1-mutation carriers. Lancet 343:692–695

Gammon MD, John EM (1993) Recent etiologic hypotheses concerning breast cancer. Epidemiol Rev 15:163–168

Greenwald P (1993) NCI cancer prevention and control research. Prev Med 22:642–660

Harris JR, Lippman ME, Veronesi U, Wilett W (1992a) Breast cancer. I. N Engl J Med 327:319–328

Harris JR, Lippman ME, Veronesi U, Wilett W (1992b) Breast cancer. III. N Engl J Med 327:473–480

Helzlsouer KJ (1994) Epidemiology, prevention, and early detection of breast cancer. Cur Opin Oncol 6:541–548

Houn F, Helzlsouer KJ, Friedman NB, Stefanek ME (1995) The practice of prophylactic mastectomy: a survey of Maryland surgeons. Am J Public Health 85:801–805

Kelsey JL (1993) Breast cancer epidemiology: summary and future directions. Epidemiol Rev 15:256–263

Kelsey JL, Horn-Ross PL (1993) Breast cancer: magnitude of the problem and descriptive epidemiology. Epidemiol Rev 15:7–16

Kelsey JL, Gammon MD, John EM (1993) Reproductive factors and breast cancer. Epidemiol Rev 15:36–47

Kerlikowske K, Grady D, Rubin SM, Sandrock C, Ernster VL (1995) Efficacy of screening mammography. A meta-analysis. JAMA 273:149-154

Kessler LG, Feuer EJ, Brown ML (1991) Projections of the breast cancer burden to U.S. women: 1990-2000. Prev Med 20:170-182

Knudson AG (1993) All in the (cancer) family. Nature Genet 5:103-104

Lerman C, Lustbader E, Rimer B, Daly M, Miller S, Sands C, Balshem A (1995) Effects of individualized breast cancer risk counseling: a randomized trial. J Natl Cancer Inst 87:286-292

Mansfield CM (1993) A review of the etiology of breast cancer. J Natl Med Assoc 85:217-221

McDermott F (1991) Risk factors in breast cancer. Aust Fam Physician 20:1455-1460

McPherson K, Steel CM, Dixon JM (1994) Breast cancer – epidemiology, risk factors and genetics. BMJ 309:1003-1006

Meischke-de Jongh ML, Blonk DI, Gan-Siauw IN, Den Hoed-Sijtsema S, Ter Laag M (1983) Breast symptoms and their significance for the diagnosis of breast cancer (Dutch). Ned Tijdschr Geneeskd 127:2361-2367

Mettlin C (1994) The relationship of breast cancer epidemiology to screening recommendations. Cancer 74:228-230

Miller AB (1987) Breast cancer epidemiology, etiology, and prevention. In: Harris JR, Hellman S, Henderson IC, Kinne DW (eds) Breast diseases. Lippincott, Philadelphia, pp 87-102

Miller AB, Bulbrook RD (1980) The epidemiology and etiology of breast cancer. N Engl J Med 303:1246-1248

Morrison AS (1993) Screening for cancer of the breast. Epidemiol Rev 15:244-255

Osborne MP (1987) Prophylactic mastectomy. In: Harris JR, Hellman S, Henderson IC, Kinne DW (eds) Breast diseases. Lippincott, Philadelphia, pp 120-121

Parkin DM, Muir CS, Whelan SL, Gao Y-T, Ferlay J, Powell J (eds) (1992) Cancer incidence in five continents, vol VI. IARC Scientific Publications no. 120. IARC, Lyon

Persson I, Bergström R, Sparén P, Thörn M, Adami H-O (1993) Trends in breast cancer incidence in Sweden 1958-1988 by time period and birth cohort. Br J Cancer 68:1247-1253

Saftlas AF, Szklo M (1987) Mammographic parenchymal patterns and breast cancer risk. Epidemiol Rev 9:146-174

Schouten LJ, Straatman H, Kiemeney LALM, Verbeek ALM (1994) Cancer incidence: life table risk versus cumulative risk. J Epidemiol Community Health 48:596-600

Seltzer MH (1992) The significance of breast complaints as correlated with age and breast cancer. Am Surg 58:413-417

Smart CR, Hendrick RE, Rutledge JH, Smith RA (1995) Benefit of mammography screening in women aged 40-49: current evidence from randomized, controlled trials. Cancer 75:1619-1626

Smith PG (1992) Comparison between registries: age-standardized rates. In: Parkin DM, Muir CS, Whelan SL, Gao Y-T, Ferlay J, Powell J (eds) Cancer incidence in five continents, vol VI. IARC Scientific Publications no 120. IARC, Lyon, pp 865-870

Sondik EJ (1994) Breast cancer trends. Incidence, mortality, and survival. Cancer 74:995-999

Vasen HFA (1994) Screening in breast cancer families: is it useful? Ann Med 26:185-190

Williams WR, Osborne MP (1987) Familial aspects of breast cancer: an overview. In: Harris JR, Hellman S, Henderson IC, Kinne DW (eds) Breast diseases. Lippincott, Philadelphia, pp 109-120

2 Mammographic-Pathological Correlations

A.H. Tulusan

CONTENTS

2.1	Introduction	13
2.2	Pathology	16
2.2.1	Invasive Carcinomas	16
2.2.2	Noninvasive Carcinoma (Carcinoma In Situ)	18
2.3	Mammography	22
2.3.1	Areas of Increased Density	22
2.3.2	Microcalcifications	23
2.3.3	Galactography	24
	References	30

2.1 Introduction

The branching ductal system and its lobular units constitute the *functional components of the mature breast*. Between 15 and 20 components arranged in segments converge radially towards the nipple. This can be demonstrated clearly through galactography (Fig. 2.1). The ductal and lobular system is surrounded by fat and connective tissue, which make up the bulk of the breast tissue. These structures, together with the Cooper's ligaments extending from the pectoralis fascia to the skin, give the breast its typical hemispherical shape. The *prepubertal* mammary gland consists of simple epithelial-lined ducts. As a result of hormonal stimulation after the menarche these ducts branch out to form lobules. These lobules, each made up of 100 or more acini with the corresponding terminal ducts, the so-called terminal-ductal lobular units, are the basic structural unit of the mammary gland.

The entire lobular-ductal system is lined by epithelial and myoecpithelial cells with varying numbers of cell layers in different parts of the system. The lumen is separated from the surrounding connective and fat tissue by the epithelial lining and the basement membrane. The ductal system is a complex irregularly branching structure. The whole ductal-lobular system is surrounded by a capillary network which is richer than that seen in the connective and fat tissue.

Although complete *functional and structural development* of the breast is not reached until pregnancy and lactation, cyclic changes do occur which are related to the reproductive system. Many women experience slight enlargement of the breast accompanied by nodularity or tenderness in the premenstrual phase. This premenstrual hypersensitivity is usually bilateral and often concentrated in the upper quadrants of the breast. According to Haagensen, breast enlargement is more severe in nulliparous women or in those who have never breast-fed. It often increases in the fourth decade and is most severe just before menopause, unless this is artificially postponed by estrogen replacement therapy. Histological studies have not confirmed any significant change in the lobules and acini during the various *phases of the menstrual cycle*. Only a slight increase in acinar epithelial proliferation, vacuolization of the cells of the basal layers, secretion into the acinar lumen, and intralobular edema have been observed in the gestagen phase. It must be presumed that the premenstrual increase in size and density of the breast is the result of an overall increase in the extracellular fluid content. As all these changes usually regress by the end of the menstrual flow, it is recommended to examine the breast in this phase.

On completion of the *menopause*, the breasts normally decrease in size and the tissue becomes less dense. Histologically seen, atrophic lobules in a dense fibrous matrix with an increase in the elastic tissue component are a prominent feature of the aging process. This is probably due to the reduction in estrogen production. As hormonal replacement therapy in post-menopausal women is not uncommon today, many have less pronounced atrophic changes of the breast after menopause.

The main *blood supply* of the breast is delivered by the perforating branches of the internal mammary artery. Several branches of the axillary and subclavian artery also share in supplying blood to the

---

A.H. Tulusan, MD, Professor, Direktor der Frauenklinik, Klinikum Bayreuth, Preuschwitzstraße 101, 95445 Bayreuth, Germany

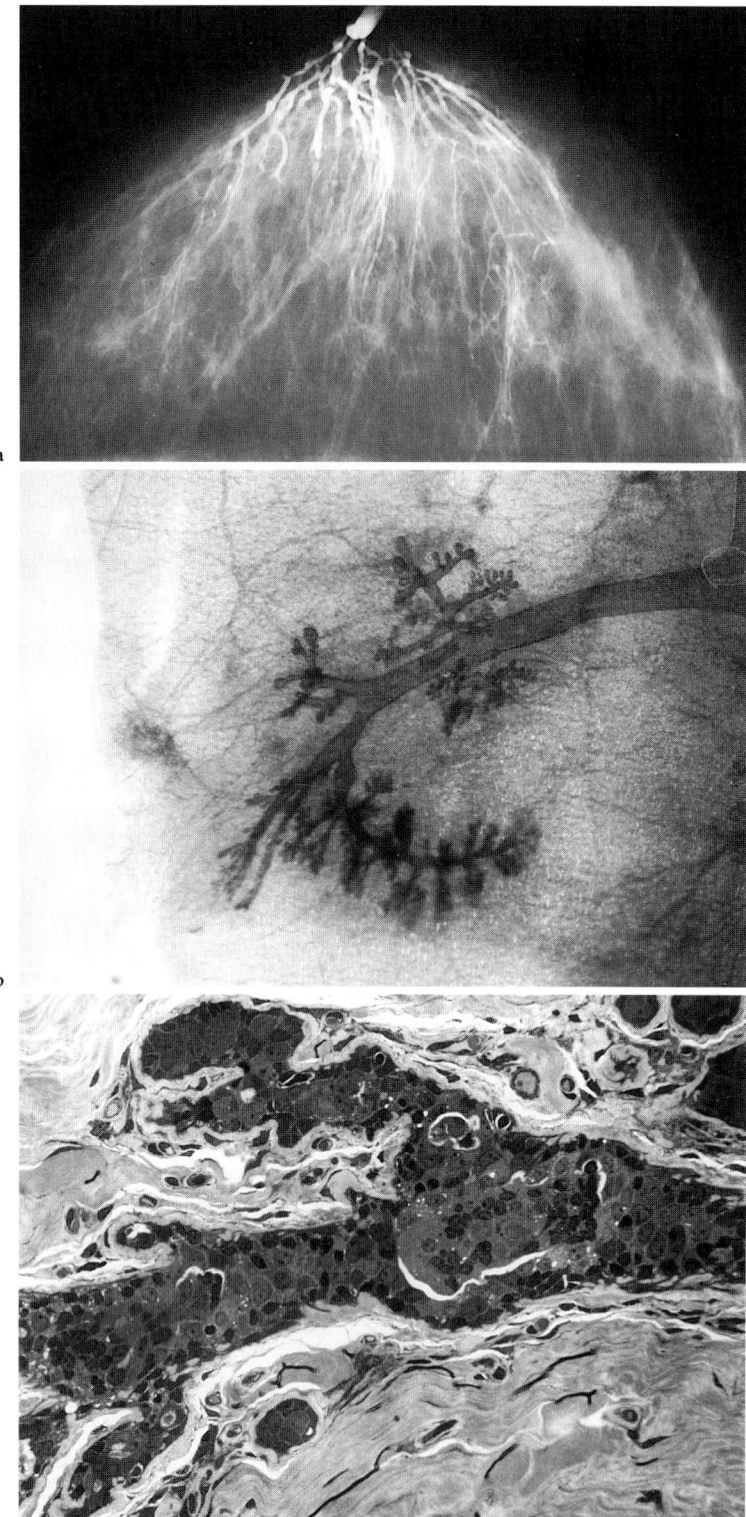

Fig. 2.1. a Galactogram demonstrating the converging radial structure of the ductal system (sinus lactiferi). **b** Terminal ductular-lobular branch of the ductal system (translucent system). **c** Histological longitudinal section of a branching duct showing the epithelial and myoepithelial cells lining the ductal lumen. The surrounding stroma shows fibrous tissue with small blood and lymph vessels

Mammographic-Pathological Correlations

breast (lateral thoracic artery) and another source of lesser importance are the intercostal arteries. In general the venous drainage of the gland is analogous to the arterial supply.

The *lymphatic drainage* of the breast is similar to that of other parts of the body, the lymph vessels accompanying blood supply. The importance of the lymphatic drainage lies in the possibility of regional spread of carcinoma. Most of the lymph is drained along the lateral thoracic and thoracodorsal vessels. The axillary lymph nodes are the main drainage centers for mammary lymph fluid, except for that of the lower inner quadrants, where the lymph has a greater tendency to flow to the internal mammary lymph node chain. Normally there is no significant drainage of the lymph vessels to the contralateral breast, contralateral internal mammary nodes, or the axilla. The subcutaneous lymphatic plexus of the breast lies in the same plane as the superficial venous plexus and is connected to the skin surrounding the breast. This lymph network of the corium is dilated in cases of inflammatory breast diseases. There is also usually edema and thickening of the skin. In a particular type of breast cancer, the *inflammatory breast carcinoma*, the dilated lymph vessels are filled with carcinoma cells and there is extensive reddening of the skin. This thickening and reddening of the skin, however, is not only typical for inflammatory carcinoma. Similar thickening and reddening of the skin is evident in all other cases of lymph vessel blockage. These clinical signs have a characteristic appearance on a mammogram.

Definite diagnosis of a benign or malignant breast disease can only be made by histological examination of a tissue sample (fine-needle aspiration biopsy, core-biopsy or open biopsy). Fortunately most patients referred for diagnosis suffer from complaints which are not cancer related. On the other hand, as the signs and symptoms relating to breast cancer are in no way restricted or exclusive to malignancy, and indeed are often present in benign conditions, the possibility of malignancy must always be considered.

Assessment of the medical and family history, thorough physical examination of the breast, and the application of various breast imaging methods (mammography, ultrasonography and magnetic resonance imaging) all contribute to successful diagnosis.

The presence of a palpable mass or retraction of the skin is the most common *physical sign* of breast cancer (Fig. 2.2). Histologically, retraction of the skin

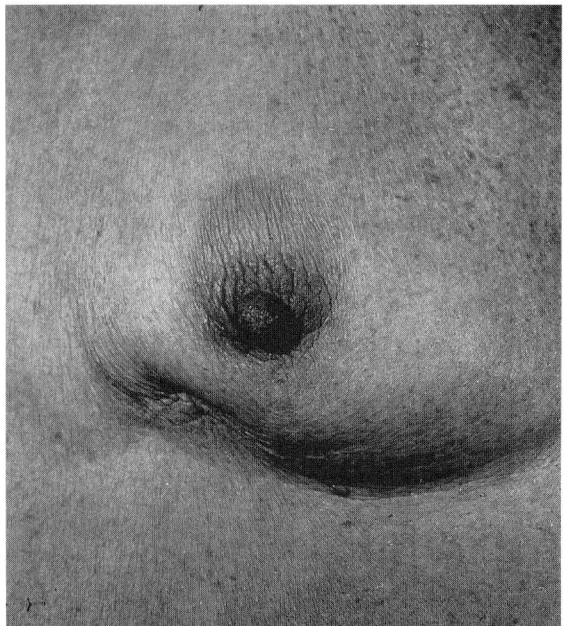

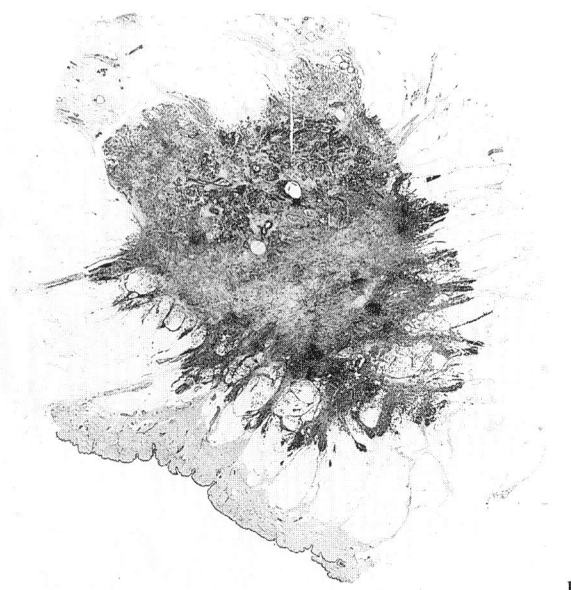

Fig. 2.2. a Palpable mass with skin retraction. b Skin retraction or dimpling caused by a shortening of the Cooper's ligaments due to infiltration by cancer cells and fibrosis

above the carcinoma is due to fixation and retraction of the Cooper's ligaments caused by the fibrosis surrounding the tumor. Where fibrosis of the larger mammary ducts is involved, the nipple may also appear flattened or in some cases retracted.

2.2 Pathology

2.2.1 Invasive Carcinomas

Eight-five percent of all invasive carcinomas of the breast are ductal, 12% are lobular, and the remaining 3% are special forms of differentiation, i.e., metaplastic carcinoma, apocrine carcinoma, lipid-rich carcinoma, etc. Apart from the generally accepted WHO classification there are other suggested morphological classifications of invasive breast carcinoma (HERMANEK et al. 1987). All current pathological classifications are based almost exclusively on histological architectural features. Of the 4000 invasive breast carcinomas treated at the Frauenklinik of the University of Erlangen between 1975 and 1993, about 60% were ductal (scirrhous, not other specified, NOS), 8% were medullary, 1% tubular, 1% papillary, 3% mucinous, 10% lobular, and 16% a combination of different subtypes.

2.2.1.1 Invasive Ductal Carcinoma

Invasive ductal carcinoma is the most common form of breast cancer. WHO defined this as an invasive carcinoma excluding special forms of other invasive carcinomas (1981). The gross pathology of invasive ductal carcinoma, especially those containing a large amount of fibrotic stroma (scirrhous), shows an extremely hard solid tumor, with a gray to white surface. Thus the terms "scirrhous" or "not other specified" are often used synonymously for invasive ductal carcinoma. The gross tumor configuration is typically irregular spiculated or radial (Fig. 2.3). Approximately 15% of invasive ductal carcinomas have a circumscribed rounded margin. Generally the gross configuration of invasive ductal carcinoma is analogous to that visualized by mammography.

2.2.1.2 Tubular Carcinoma

A small number (1%–2%) of invasive ductal cancers have a very distinctive well-differentiated form. These so-called tubular carcinomas are characterized by tubular or ovoid invasive glands that closely resemble nonneoplastic mammary ductules (Fig. 2.4). Typically a radial arrangement of the glandular elements and sclerosing stroma is found. Histologically and mammographically they can mimic a radial scar or a benign proliferative sclerosing lesion with stroma elastosis (HAMPERL 1975; LINNEL and LJUNGBERG 1980). The presence of "naked" tubular elements within the fatty tissue without the surrounding stroma mantle is always indicative of pure/

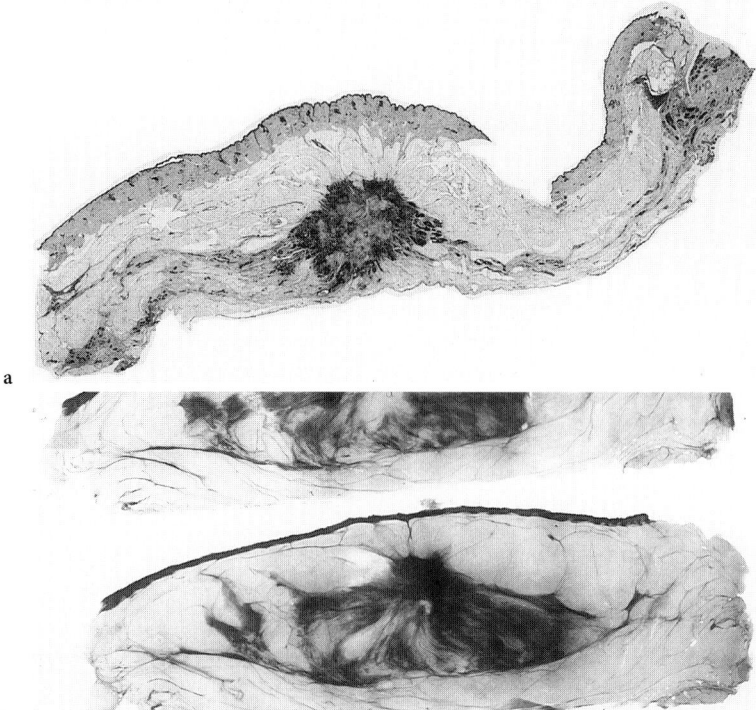

Fig. 2.3a,b. Large-area histological section and slide specimen of a typical scirrhous carcinoma with stellate configuration of the tumor border

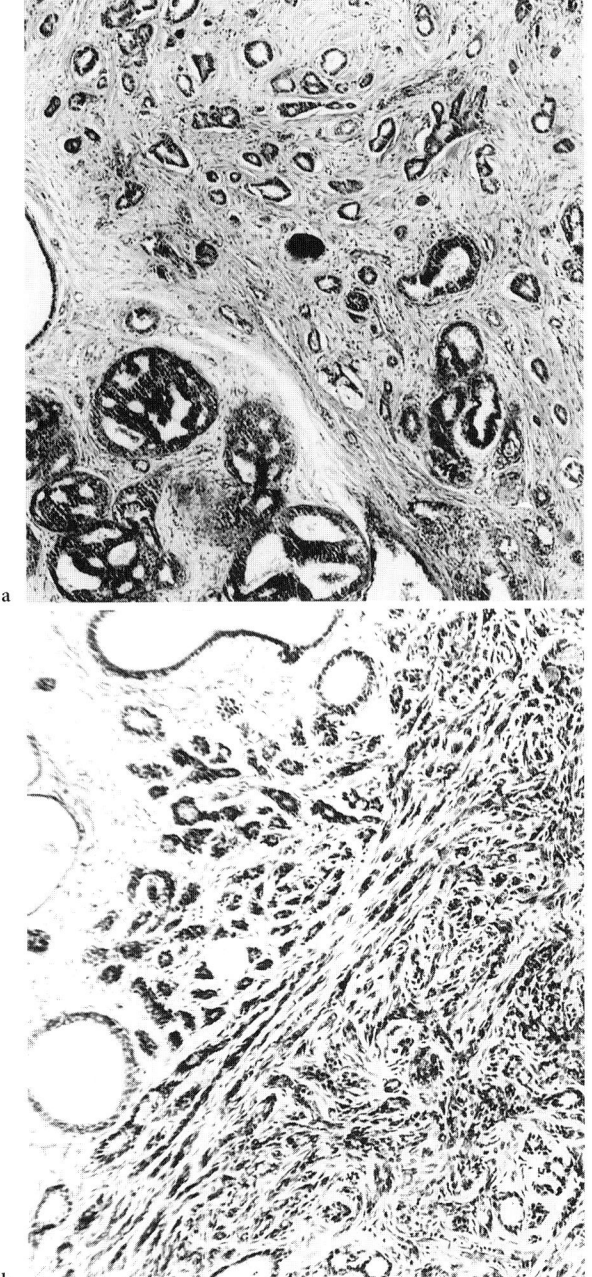

Fig. 2.4. a Typical tubular carcinoma with ovoid structure. Note the similarity with the ductal structure of (nonmalignant) sclerosing adenosis (b)

true invasive carcinoma (BÄSSLER 1978; TULUSAN et al. 1982). The favorable prognosis of most tubular carcinomas is explained by their high degree of differentiation and the low grade of malignancy for tubular carcinoma with at least 75% tubular elements.

2.2.1.3 Mucinous Carcinoma

Pure mucinous carcinomas constitute about 2% of breast carcinomas (Fig. 2.5). Mammographically they present as a round or lobulated circumscribed mass and may lack several radiological criteria of malignancy. Coarse calcifications may be present. Clinically there is no retraction and the mass may be too soft to be palpated. Sometimes patients present with a large bulky tumor which manifests itself clinically as a lump or bulge on the breast. Mucinous carcinoma is more common in older women, and 7% of all breast carcinomas in women over the age of 75 fall into this category (ROSEN et al. 1985). In its pure form, mucinous carcinoma is regarded as a prognostically favorable variant of invasive ductal carcinoma. Histologically it consists of well-differentiated neoplastic cells arranged in small groups that are surrounded by acellular mucus which mainly constitutes the tissue content.

2.2.1.4 Medullary Carcinoma

Medullary carcinoma presents on mammograms as a fairly well-defined spherical mass. However, at spot compression magnification mammography subtle border irregularities often are seen, as are areas where the tumor margins are indistinct and even subtly spiculated. Medullary carcinoma cells have a high mitotic rate and a poorly differentiated nuclear grade, with bizarre giant tumor cells. These cytological characteristics as well as an intense lymphoplasmatic infiltration around the clusters of tumor cells and a sharp demarcation from the surrounding stroma are essential in discriminating between medullary carcinoma and other types of invasive ductal carcinoma which can also have lymphocytic infiltration (especially at the advancing edge of the carcinoma) (Fig. 2.6). Medullary carcinoma is more common in younger patients and accounts for about 5%–9% of carcinomas in most series. In contrast to its low histological grading, it is also a carcinoma with a favorable prognosis.

2.2.1.5 Papillary Carcinoma

Papillary carcinoma is a rare carcinoma whose invasive pattern is predominantly in the form of papillary structures (WHO 1992) (Fig. 2.7). Invasive papillary carcinoma represents 2% of all breast carcinomas (FISHER et al. 1980). In cases with lymph node

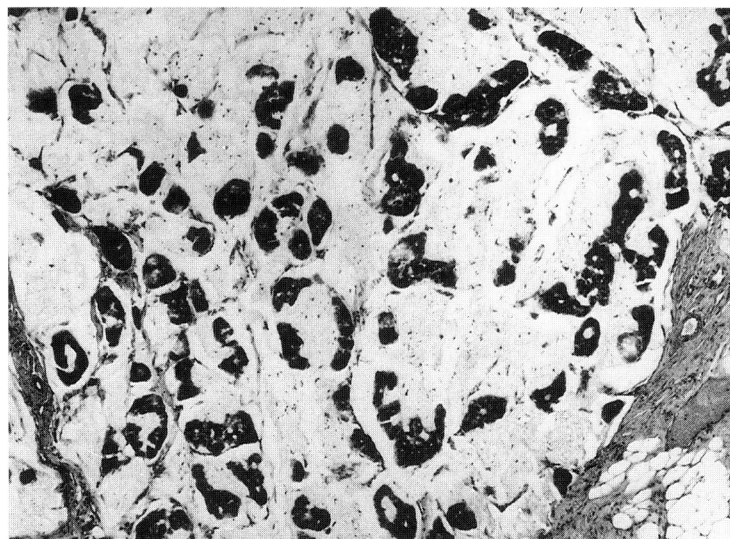

Fig. 2.5. Mucinous carcinoma with carcinomatous structures within a mucinous mass

involvement the metastases also have an obvious papillary pattern. In most cases this papillary growth pattern is also found in the intraductal component. Bloody nipple discharge is a frequent symptom; this is reflected in galactography as a ductal filling defect.

2.2.1.6 Invasive Lobular Carcinoma

Invasive lobular carcinoma originates from the lobules and constitutes another special type of invasive breast cancer. The frequency of invasive lobular carcinoma varies from 8% to 15% (FISHER et al. 1985). Since the study carried out by FOOTE and STEWART in 1941, the origin of this type of carcinoma and its relation to lobular carcinoma in situ have been debated. Microscopically the pure form of invasive lobular carcinoma is recognized by the characteristic "Indian file" alignment or target-like arrangement of individual neoplastic cells (Fig. 2.8). These neoplastic cells can infiltrate the surrounding tissue diffusely without any distortion of the original breast parenchyma. Therefore, gross pathological distinction, clinical diagnosis, or mammographic visualization of invasive lobular carcinoma can be difficult. As calcification is usually not found in this type of carcinoma, the neoplasm is often missed on the mammogram. In contrast to invasive ductal carcinoma, the extension and size of the invasive lobular carcinoma do not correlate closely with its mammographic appearance (EGAN 1988).

2.2.1.7 Other Unusual Types of Invasive Carcinoma

Rare types of breast cancer such as adenocystic carcinoma, secretory carcinoma, metaplastic carcinoma, apocrine carcinoma, and lipid-rich carcinoma constitute only about 2% of diagnosed breast cancers (FISHER et al. 1975; BÄSSLER 1978).

As the biological features of invasive ductal carcinomas are not represented clearly in the pathological classification of the subtypes of invasive breast carcinoma, further classificaton has been suggested. Subclassification according to *their cytonuclear and histological malignancy grades* was suggested by several study groups: BLOOM and RICHARDSON (1975), BLACK et al. (1975), and ROSEN et al. (1985). Nuclear and histological grading has been shown to be of prognostic importance, especially for patients without axillary lymph node involvement. The *TNM classification* has endeavored to take all these prognostic parameters (tumor size, lymph node status, local and distant tumor spread, metastases) into account (HERMANEK et al. 1987) (Table 2.1).

2.2.2 Noninvasive Carcinoma (Carcinoma In Situ)

The characteristic feature of breast carcinoma in situ is the proliferation of malignant epithelial cells within the ducts or lobular acini with no microscopic evidence of stromal invasion. In most cases *lobular carcinoma in situ* is a microscopic carcinoma. As only 3%–5% of palpable breast cancers are in situ,

Fig. 2.6a–c. Small medullary carcinoma with well-defined rounded tumor border. **a** Mammography. **b** Large-area cross-section. **c** Histological pattern of the tumor cells and their pleomorphic nuclei with extensive lymphocytic and plasmocytic infiltration

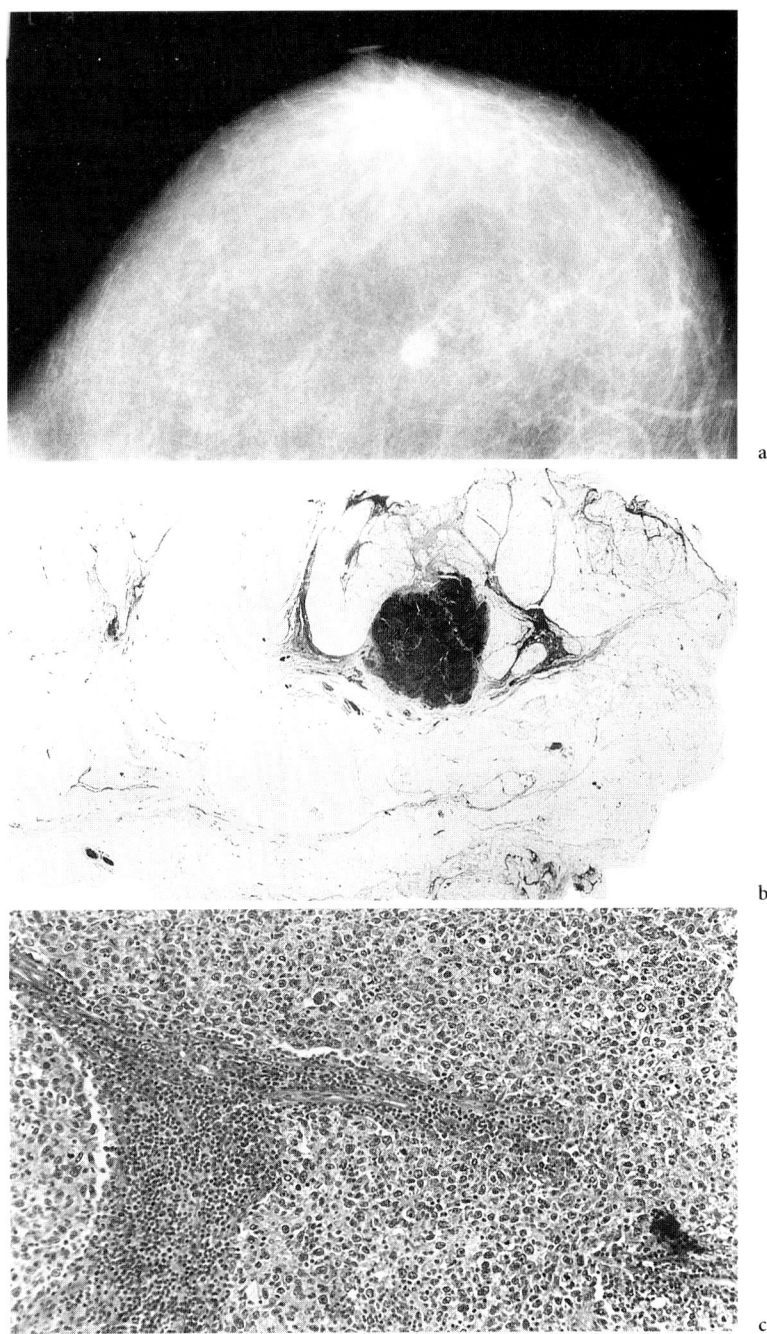

until the widespread availability of mammography the disease was usually an unexpected finding in breast tissue that had been removed because of a lump or density. Most in situ breast cancers are now detected on mammography through evidence of clustered microcalcifications or on the basis of alterations observed during galactography.

2.2.2.1 Ductal Carcinoma In Situ (DCIS)

Current pathological classification of DCIS is based almost exclusively on histological architectural features: comedo, cribriform, micropapillary and solid subtypes (Fig. 2.9a). Usually more than one subtype will be present in a given case, except in very small in

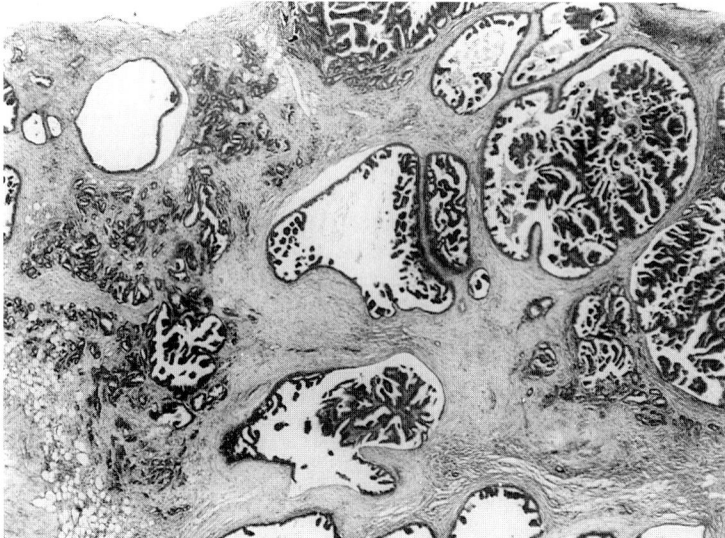

Fig. 2.7. Papillary carcinoma with intraductal and invasive papillary components

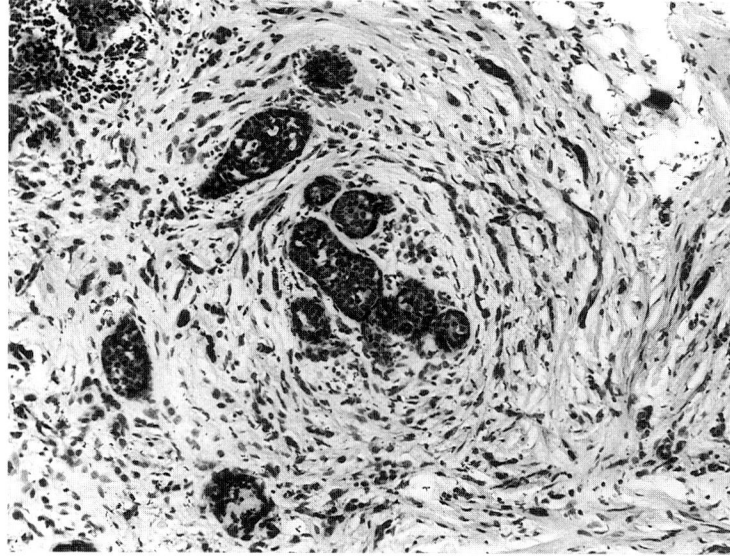

Fig. 2.8. Invasive lobular carcinoma with target-like arrangement of small rounded cancer cells around lobular carcinoma in situ components

situ foci. The size of the DCIS can be estimated by the extent of microcalcifications as seen on the mammogram or specimen radiograph. Though this is an easy and convenient method, it does not always mirror the pathological extent of the disease. Even in cases of comedo DCIS, more than 15% of the carcinomas may extend 2 cm beyond the area of microcalcifications seen on the mammogram. Complete microscopic evaluation of the surgical specimen is required in order to determine the extent of the DCIS lesion. Evidence of microinvasive foci or suspicion of multifocality or multicentricity in DCIS larger than 2.5 cm in diameter is of vital importance when the decision against or in favor of breast-conserving treatment is being made (LAGIOS et al. 1981; TULUSAN et al. 1989).

2.2.2.2 Lobular Carcinoma In Situ (LCIS)

The term lobular carcinoma in situ was first used by FOOTE and STEWART (1941). LCIS is almost always a clinically asymptomatic and mammographically occult lesion. The diagnosis is usually an incidental microscopic finding in the surrounding of proliferative benign or malignant breast disorders that may produce clinical or mammographic abnormalities that lead to a biopsy. Microcalcifications are rarely

Mammographic-Pathological Correlations

Table 2.1

Tis	In situ			
T1	≤2 cm			
T1a	≤0.5 cm			
T1b	>0.5 to 1 cm			
T1c	>1 to 2 cm			
T2	>2 to 5 cm			
T3	>5 cm			
T4	Chest wall/skin			
T4a	Chest wall			
T4b	Skin edema/ulceration, satellite skin nodules			
T4c	Both 4a and 4b			
T4d	Inflammatory carcinoma			
N1	Movable axillary	pN1		
		pN1a	Micrometastasis only ≤0.2 cm	
		pN1b	Gross metastasis	
			i) 1–3 nodes/>0.2 to <2 cm	
			ii) ≤4 nodes/>0.2 to <2 cm	
			iii) through capsulc/<2 cm	
			iv) ≥2 cm	
N2	Fixed axillary	pN2		
N3	Internal mammary	pN3		

pT – Primary Tumor

The pathological classification requires the examination of the primary carcinoma with no gross tumor at the margins of respection. A case can be classified pT if there is only microscopic tumor in a margin.

The pT categories correspond to the T categories.

pN – Regional Lymph Nodes

The pathological classification requires the resection and examination of at least the low axillary lymph nodes (level I). Such a resection will ordinarily include six or more lymph nodes.

pNX   Regional lymph nodes cannot be assessed (not removed for study or previously removed)
pN0   No regional lymph node metastasis
pN1   Metastasis to movable ipsilatreal axillary node(s)
    pN1a   Only micrometastasis (none larger than 0.2 cm)
    pN1b   Metastasis to lymph node(s), any larger than 0.2 cm
        pN1bi   Metastasis in one to three lymph nodes, any more than 0.2 cm and all less than 2.0 cm in greatest dimension
        pN1bii   Metastasis to four or more lymph nodes, any more than 0.2 cm and all less than 2.0 cm in greatest dimension
        pN1biii   Extension of tumor beyond the capsule of a lymph node metastasis less than 2.0 cm in greatest dimension
        pN1biv   Metastasis to a lymph node 2.0 cm or more in greatest dimension
pN2   Metastasis to ipsilateral axillary lymph nodes that are fixed to one another or to other structures
pN3   Metastasis to ipsilateral internal mammary lymph node(s)

pM – Distant Metastasis

The pM categories correspond to the M categories.

produced by LCIS. The classic LCIS shows distension of the acini and terminal ductules filled with small round cells with round nuclei demonstrating a lack of cellular cohesion and orientation (Fig. 2.9b). Commonly intracytoplasmatic vacuoles can be seen in each cell. Multicentricity and bilaterality are frequent in LCIS. Depending on the extension of the primary LCIS lesion, the size of contralateral biopsy, and the type of surgical procedure for further diagnosis or therapy, multicentricity has been reported in up to 80% and bilaterality in 15%–70% of cases. When patients with LCIS are treated by biopsy alone, the risk of development of invasive carcinoma can be expected to be 30% within 30 years of follow-up time either in the affected or the contralateral breast. These figures have been used as arguments for bilateral mastectomy after LCIS diagnosis. However, the great majority of physicians recommend local excision and close mammographic and clinical follow-up of the patients with LCIS for the rest of their life time.

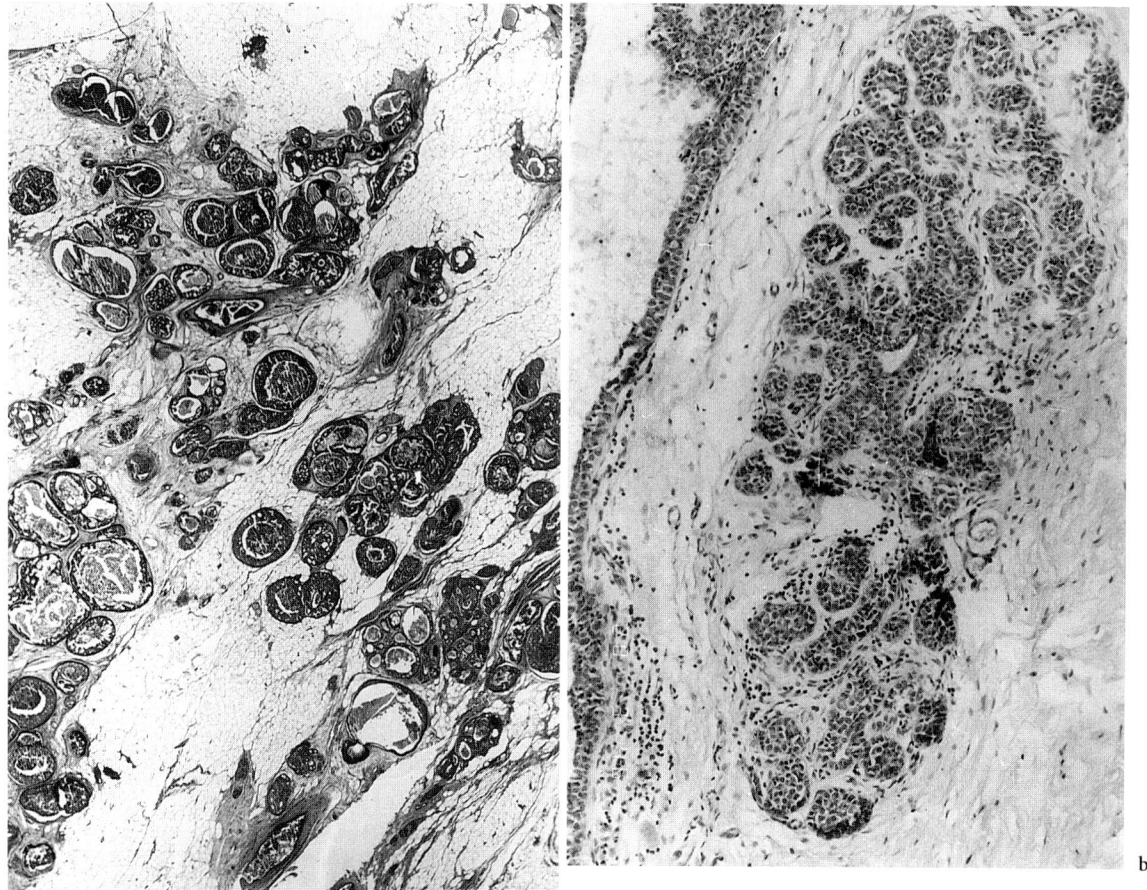

Fig. 2.9. a Typical DCIS comedo type with necrosis and microcalcifications within the lumen. **b** LCIS with distended acini and terminal ductules filled with round tumor cells

Thus, management of LCIS is still controversial and at this time it is obvious that none of the several alternatives for therapy is entirely satisfactory.

2.3 Mammography

Mammography is still the most widespread and important method of breast diagnosis. There are several mammographic characteristics which have a clear histological correlation that are invaluable tools in the differential diagnosis of breast disease. The most important of these characteristics are:

1. Areas of increased density (mass)
2. Clustered microcalcification
3. Filling defect or irregularity of ductal filling in galactography

2.3.1 Areas of Increased Density

By the time cancer presents as a palpable mass, it is visible on a mammogram in about 80%–90% of cases. This represents the sensitivity of mammography. The diagnosis of benign or malignant lesions is largely dependent on the visualization of increased density which is due to the contrast between a lesion and its background. The fatty breast parenchyma in postmenopausal women is usually radiolucent and thus provides the best background against which radiodense tumors can be detected on mammograms (Fig. 2.10). In contrast, mammograms of younger women more often show extremely dense parenchyma, rendering detection of lesions more difficult. Consequently, failure to detect tumors through mammography occurs some what more frequently often in premenopausal women than in patients who are over 50 years old. However, mammography routinely identifies most breast cancers months to years before they grow large enough to be palpable, both in premenopausal and postmenopansal women. This important observation supports the use of mammography as a screening test for asymptomatic women, beginning at age 40.

Typically carcinomatous tissue appears on a mammogram as a spiculated mass or as a mass with irregular borders and indistinct margins. Some types of breast cancer, however, such as mucinous or medullary carcinoma, can have well-defined borders with a corresponding appearance on the mammogram. It is sometimes difficult to distinguish between these mucinous or medullary carcinomas and degenerating fibroadenomas or cysts. Spot compression magnification mammography and ultrasonography can be very helpful in making the distinction.

Another possible mammographic characteristic of malignancy is an asymmetric density of the breast. As both breasts generally are similar in density, substantial areas of asymmetry in the mammogram is to be viewed with suspicion. In the absence of a palpable mass, however, asymmetry alone is not a criterion of malignancy.

2.3.2 Microcalcifications

Microcalcifications which are due to calcium deposits occurring in various breast tissue changes have for a long time been visible in microscopic sections. However, the exact morphological analysis of microcalcifications and their diagnostic significance in breast cancer detection have been emphasized in the last several decades. The size of the microcalcifications on the mammogram is often so minute that they can only be fully detected and evaluated by use of a magnifying lens, or by using magnification mammographic technique with modern mammographic equipment (Fig. 2.11a,b).

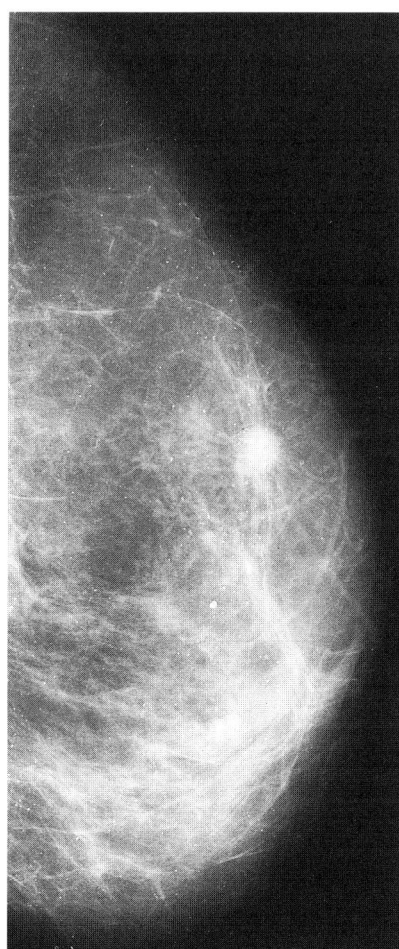
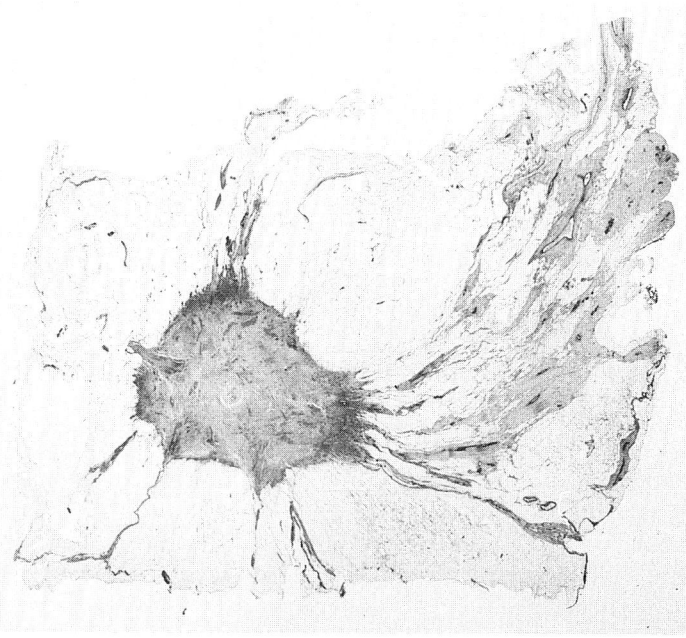

Fig. 2.10. a Radiolucent mammogram of a 78-year-old patient with a small carcinoma displaying a spiculated tumor border. b Large-area section of the tumor showing fatty parenchyma surrounding the tumor and the spiculae of fibrous tissue radiating from its borders

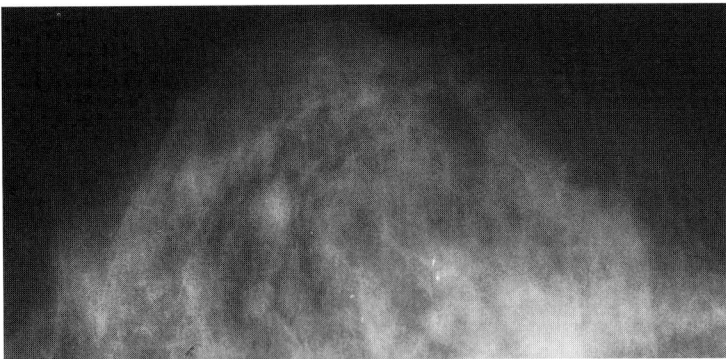
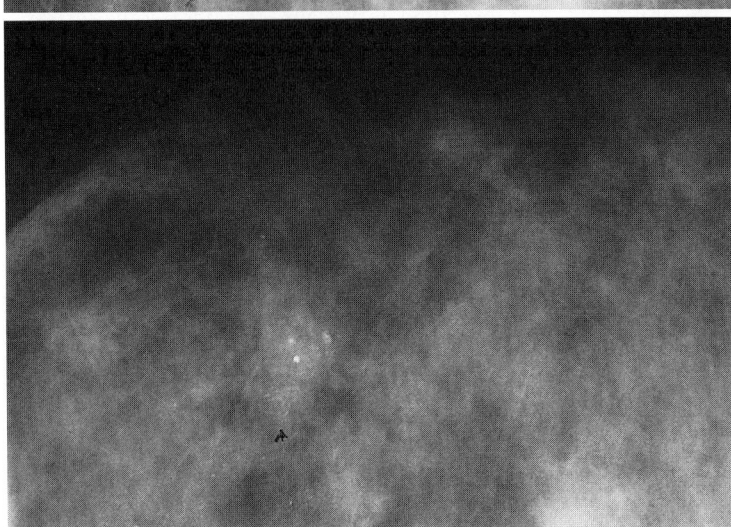

Fig. 2.11. a Cluster of fine microcalcifications in the mammogram of a nonpalpable mass. b Magnification mammogram of the same area depicting the microcalcifications in the surrounding area more clearly

As the calcium deposits themselves are not palpable, their exact localization prior to surgical excision is essential. The presence of the microcalcifications in the biopsy specimen must be verified by specimen radiography, preferably during surgery, in order to enable the surgeon to excise a second sample (Fig. 2.11c,d), if necessary.

Sometimes, there is no clear-cut differentiation between benign and malignant microcalcifications. *Benign-type* calcifications are typically uniformly round, facetted, lucent-centered, or tea-cup shaped. However calcium deposits are produced in adenosis, papillomatosis, duct ectasia, cysts, degenerating fatty tissue, or fibroadenoma as well as in other benign proliferating and degenerating alterations of breast tissue (mastopathic or fibrocystic disease, Fig. 2.12).

Malignant-type calcifications, on the other hand, are generally pleomorphic, clustered, irregularly linear, or branched according to the ductular structure, and are of varying density (Fig. 2.13) (see chapter on microcalcifications).

Microcalcifications can be detected in about 50% of breast cancers. The calcium is deposited in the necrotic carcinoma cells filling the central lumina of the ducts in comedo or papillary type ductal carcinoma (Fig. 2.14). In asymptomatic women with no palpable mass, microcalcifications are a very important sign of malignancy. Out of a total of about 50 000 mammographic studies performed in our clinic, clustered microcalcifications were found in 2% and were subsequently biopsied. Among these cases, occult breast carcinoma was diagnosed in 21% (12% invasive and 9% in situ carcinoma) (PATEROK et al. 1983). On the other hand, in the great majority of noninvasive breast carcinomas (ductal carcinoma in situ), microcalcifications were the earliest sign of malignancy detectable on the mammogram (Table 2.2).

Five or more microcalcifications clustered within an area of 1 square cm are considered to be suspicious, and the risk of malignancy increases with the number of calcium deposits (see Chap. 7).

2.3.3 Galactography

Nipple discharge may be the only symptom indicating the presence of breast disease. It is neither a fre-

Fig. 2.11. c Specimen radiograph with localizer hook wire showing the full extent of the microcalcifications. **d** Histological section showing regressive microcalcifications within the ductal system with mastopathic changes in the absence of malignancy

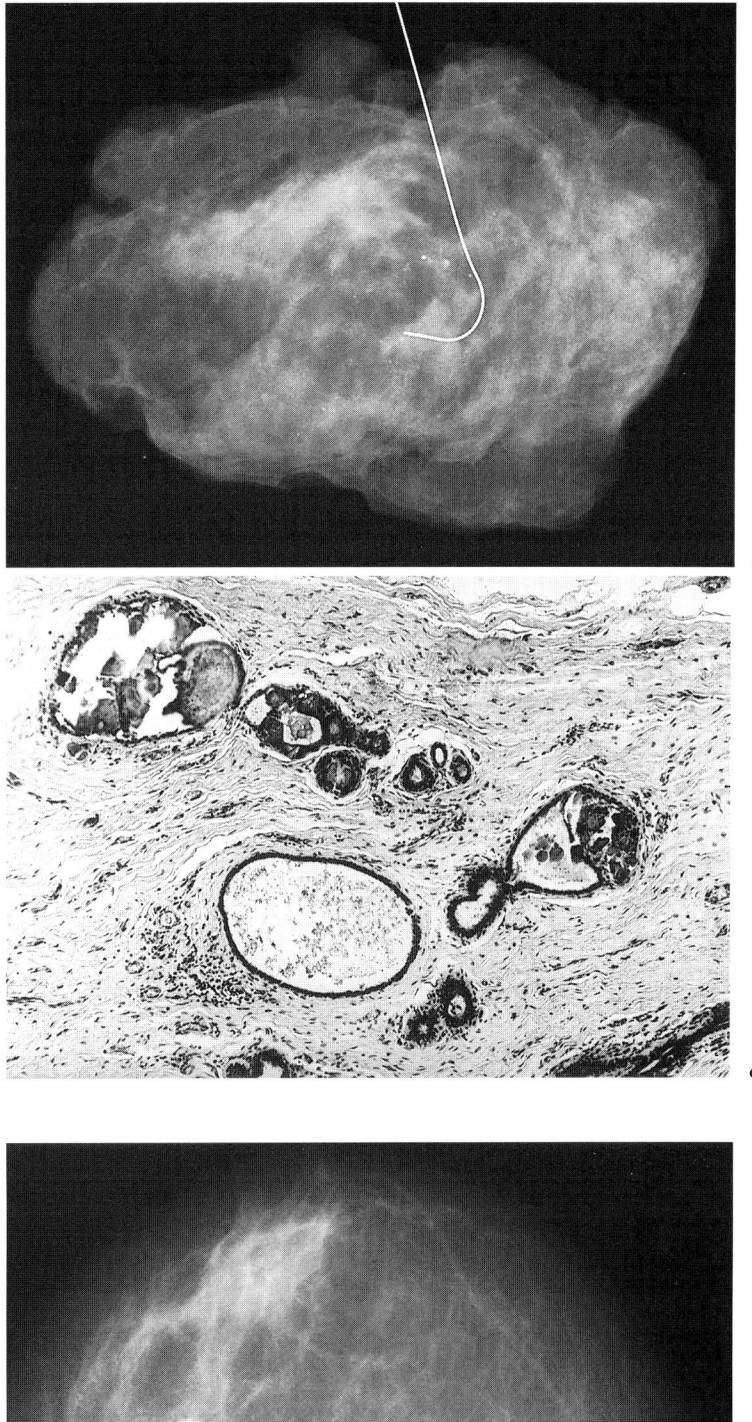

Fig. 2.12. Mammogram of a well-defined rounded fibroadenoma with coarse calcifications due to hyaline degeneration. In this older patient the soft tissue component of the fibroadenoma is not so apparent as in younger women

quent complaint, nor is it a frequent indicator of malignancy. Surgery on patients presenting with nipple discharge and pathological galactograms accounts for less than 10% of all breast operations.

Galactography is usually only performed in cases of unilateral spontaneous discharge from a single duct orifice. Discharge from both breasts is generally endocrine in nature (hyperprolactinaemia, hypo-

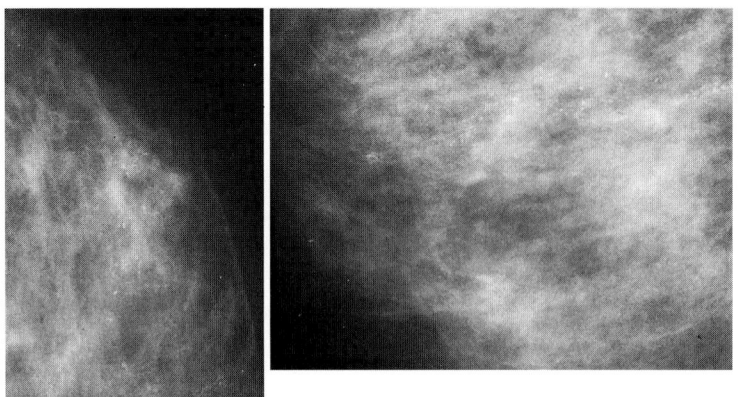

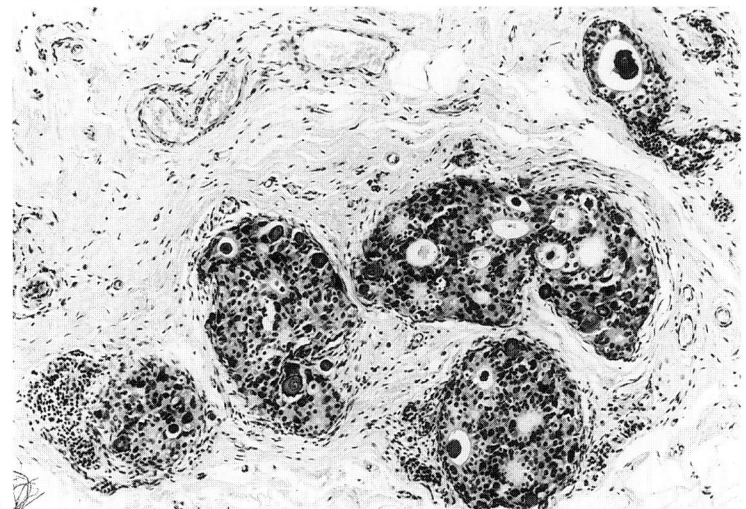

Fig. 2.13. a Clusters of pleomorphic microcalcifications in a barely palpable ductal carcinoma. b Magnification mammogram with clearer depiction of the microcalcifications. c Histological section showing distribution of the microcalcifications within the lumina of the carcinomatous ducts (cribriform subtype)

Table 2.2. Mammographic findings of in situ breast carcinoma (n = 163) (Women's Hospital, University of Erlangen, 1970–1988)

Microcalcification	85 (53%)
Increase or asymmetric density	36 (22%)
Tumor	8 (5%)
No mammographic sign	34 (21%)

Table 2.3. Histological findings of 566 breast biopsies because of nipple discharge and pathological galactography (from a series of 2215 galactographic studies at the Women's Hospital, University of Erlangen)

No pathological finding	14 (2.5%)
Fibrocystic mastopathy	152 (26.8%)
Papilloma	246 (43.5%)
Papillomatosis	85 (14.8%)
Ductal in situ carcinoma	17 (3.0%)
Invasive carcinoma	53 (9.4%)

thyroidism), drug induced (antidepressants), or, much more rarely, due to diffuse mastopathic disease. The galactogram can demonstrate filling defects, blocking of the ductal passage, or irregularity in the size or shape of the ductal structure. This corresponds to intraductal changes in a distinct segmental area of the breast (Figs. 2.15, 2.16).

In a series of 2215 galactographic studies in our institution, the diagnosis of papilloma or papillomatosis was established in more than 50% of the cases. Another 25% yielded the diagnosis of fibrocystic mastopathy and blunt duct adenosis. Invasive carcinoma was diagnosed in 10% and ductal carcinoma in situ in 3%, whereby there were no palpable nodules (Table 2.3).

Nipple discharge can vary in color and consistency. Although discharge associated with malignancy usually contains blood, it can present in varying forms. Thick, pasty discharge bluish in color is indicative of mastopathy or blunt duct disease.

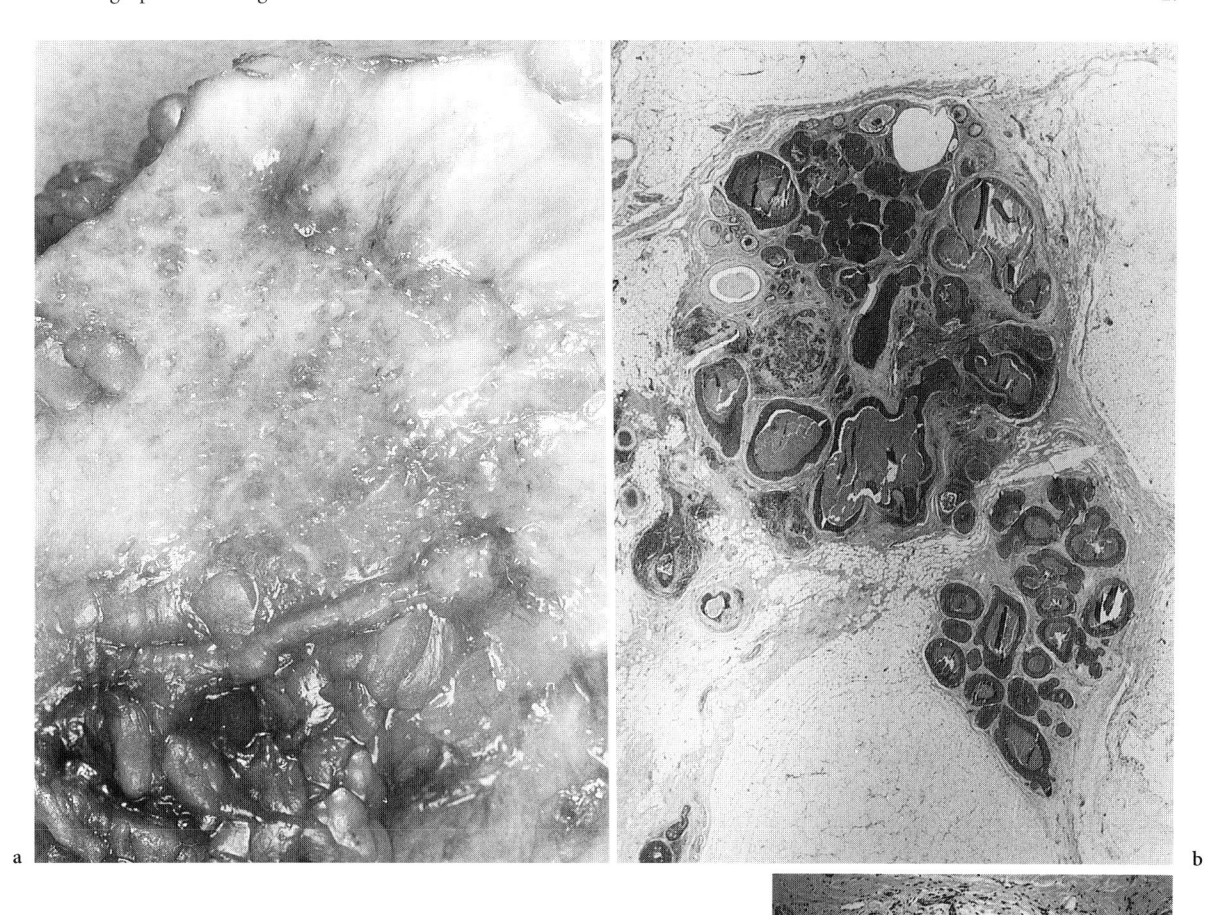

Fig. 2.14. Cross-section of a ductal comedo carcinoma with typical appearance of the cross-section of the ducts filled with comedo-like debris. **b** Histological section of a comedo-type ductal carcinoma with a distended ductal system containing calcified necrotic cancer cells. **c** Necrotic cancer cells with microcalcifications in the lumen of a micropapillary ductal carcinoma in situ

That associated with papilloma or papillomatosis is often serous or serosanguinous.

Mammography is an essential complement to the physical examination of patients with clinical symptoms of breast disease. Since the routine introduction of mammography, biopsy of the breast is increasingly being performed for the pathological assessment of abnormalities detected on mammograms. It is evident today that most cancers smaller than 1 cm in diameter can only be detected by mammography. In our institution the detection rate of invasive cancers smaller than 1 cm in diameter

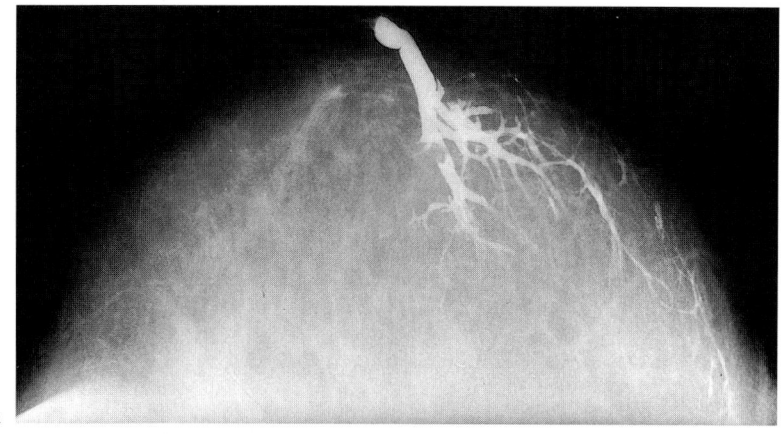

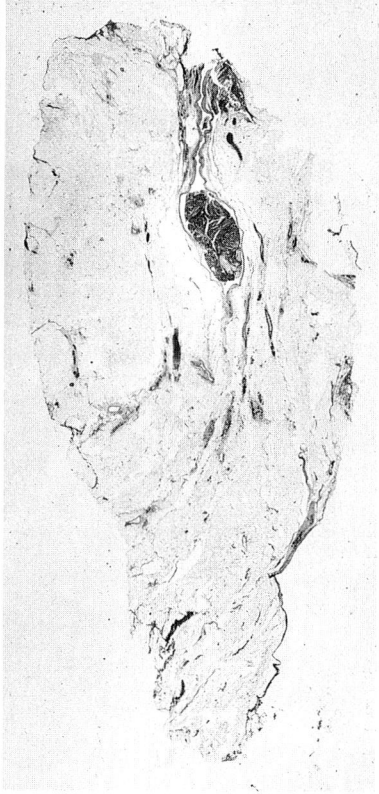

Fig. 2.15. a Galactogram of a patient with nipple discharge showing a filling defect in a distinct area in one of the ductal branches. **b** The histological section of the same area shows an intraductal papilloma

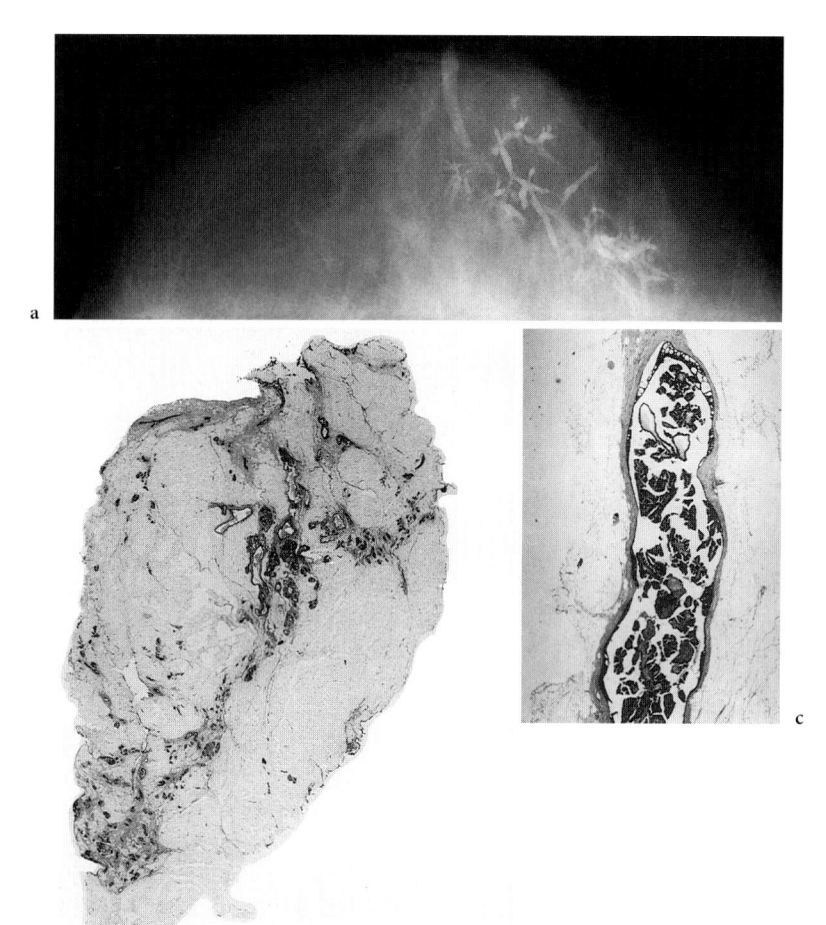

Fig. 2.16. a Galactogram of a patient with nipple discharge reveals a filling defect combined with duct ectasia about 2.5 cm behind the nipple (*arrow*). There is also some distal irregularity in the ductal filling. **b** The corresponding histological section shows intraductal proliferations. This is a combination of intraductal papillomatosis with ductal carcinoma of cribriform and micropapillary type (**c**) with distension of the ductal segment

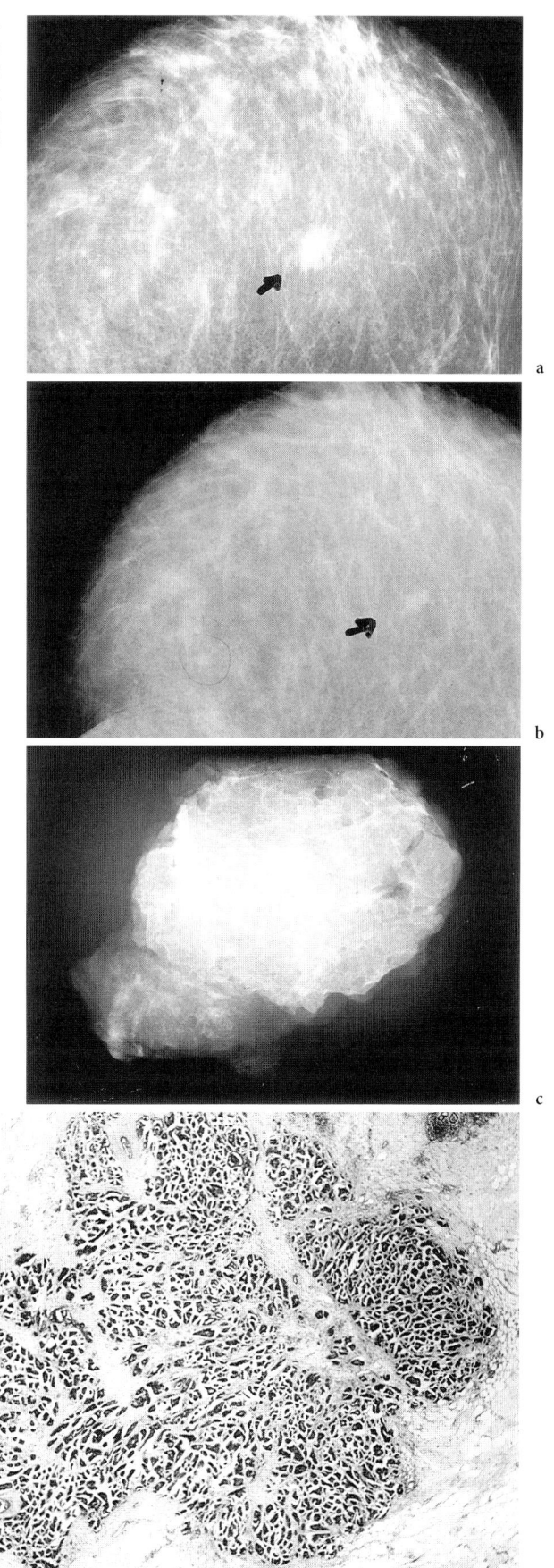

Fig. 2.17a–d. Inferior quality of a mammogram often contributes to false-negative results due to misinterpretation of the image. The nonpalpable carcinoma was easily detected on a mammogram of adequate image quality (**a**: *arrow*) but was not diagnosed because of the poor image quality of a previous mammogram (**b**). **c** Radiograph of the surgical specimen. **d** Histological appearance

rose significantly from 1% in the early 1970s to almost 20% in the late 1980s (TULUSAN 1993). The most dramatic impact of mammography has been in the detection of DCIS, and smaller invasive cancers. Prior to widespread application of this technology only 3%–5% of all new cancers diagnosed were in situ compared to 22% of all new cancer cases in the years 1985/1986, and compared to 40% of all new breast cancer cases detected in screening programs (LAGIOS 1995). The average size of these cancers is 8 mm in diameter.

Because of the increasing number of mammographically detected small lesions, breast conservation therapy could be selected in an increasing number of cases over the last 10 years. However, as mammographic characteristics of malignancy are never completely reliable there is still a high rate of false-positive and false-negative results. There is considerable variation among radiologists regarding the interpretation of mammograms. Interpretation of the mammograms varies in accordance with the radiologists experience and the quality of the image (Fig. 2.17). Clinically suspect masses which show up as "benign" on mammograms may subsequently proven to be malignant in 6% of cases. This is particularly true of invasive lobular carcinoma (TULUSAN et al. 1982; EGAN 1988), because in invasive lobular carcinoma there is no marked change in the surrounding fibrous tissue, there is often an absence of calcification, and the pattern of invasion is diffuse without well-defined borders. A normal mammogram is of no consequence when signs of malignancy are evident on clinical examination and further diagnostic steps such as ultrasonography and cytological or histological evaluation must be taken. Apart from open biopsy there are various techniques suitable for obtaining histological evaluation such as fine-needle aspiration biopsy, drill biopsy or core biopsy (Tru-Cut needle, see Chap. 16). Image-guided high-speed core biopsy is one of the most effective methods for lesions that can be visualized by mammography or ultrasonography. Even small targets can be sampled accurately without false-positive diagnosis (BAUER et al. 1994). Used preoperatively (usually 1 or 2 days prior to definitive surgery), in combination with frozen sections (ADAM et al. 1989; SCHULZ-WENDTLAND et al. 1995), needle or drill biopsy has several advantages: waiting for the results of the frozen section during surgery is no longer necessary and, with the definitive histological diagnosis before surgery, the patient can be informed and advised on the individually planned surgical procedure and therapeutic scheme.

Mammography may also help in the staging and the evaluation of the extent of the disease (multifocality, multicentricity). This can be important in selecting patients for breast conservation therapy (TULUSAN 1993).

References

Adam R, Falter E, Düll W, Reitzenstein M, Tulusan AH (1989) Erfahrungen mit der Drillbiospie in der Diagnostik von Mammatumoren. Geburtsh u Frauenheilk 49:442–447

Adler OB, Engel A (1990) Invasive lobular carcinoma: mammographic pattern. RÖFO 152(4):460

Bässler R (1978) Pathologie der Brustdrüse. In: Spezielle Pathologische Anatomie, vol 11. Springer, Berlin Heidelberg New York

Bauer M, Schulz-Wendtland R, Krämer S, Bühner M, Lang N, Tulusan AH (1994) Indikationen, Technik und Ergebnisse der sonographisch gezielten Stanzbiopsie in der Mammadiagnostik (n = 307). Geburtsh u Frauenheilk 54:311–317

Black MM, Barclay THC, Hankey BF (1975) Prognosis in breast cancer utilising histologic characteristics of the primary tumor. Cancer 36:2048–2055

Bloom HJG, Richardson WW (1957) Histologic grading and prognosis in breast cancer. A study of 1409 cases of which 359 have been followed for 15 years. Br J Cancer II:359–363

Egan RL (1988) Breast imaging: diagnosis and morphology of breast diseases. W.B. Saunders, Philadelphia

Egan RL, McSweeney MB (1984) Multicentric breast carcinoma. In: Brunner S (ed) Recent results in cancer research. Springer, Berlin Heidelberg New York, pp 28–35

Fisher ER (1985) What is early breast cancer? In: Zander J, Baltzer J (eds) Early breast cancer. Histopathology, diagnosis, treatment. Springer, Berlin Heidelberg New York, pp 1–13

Fisher ER, Gregorio RM, Fisher B (1975) The pathology of invasive breast cancer. A syllabus derived from the findings of the National Surgical Adjuvant Breast Project (protocol 4). Cancer 36:1–85

Fisher ER, Palekar AS, Redmond C, Barton B, Fisher B (1980) Pathologic findings from the National Surgical Adjuvant Breast Project (protocol no. 4). VI. Invasive papillary cancer. Am J Clin Pathol 73:313–322

Foote FW Jr, Stewart FW (1941) Lobular carcinoma in situ: a rare form of mammary cancer. Am J Pathol 17:491

Gallager HS, Martin JE (1969) Early phases in the development of breast cancer. Cancer 243:1170–1178

Gallager HS, Martin JE (1969) The study of mammary carcinoma by correlated mammography and subserial whole organ sectioning: early observations. Cancer 23:855–873

Haagensen CD (1986) Diseases of the breast. W.B. Saunders, Philadelphia

Haagensen CD, Nane N, Lattes R, Bodian C (1978) Lobular neoplasia (so-called lobular carcinoma in situ) of the breast. Cancer 42:737–769

Hilleren DJ, Anderson TT, Lindholmn K et al (1991) Invasive lobular carcinoma: mammographic findings in a 10 year experience. Radiology 178:149

Hamperl H (1975) Strahlige Narben und obliterierende Mastopathie. Beiträge zur pathologischen Histologie der Mamma. XI. Virchows Arch Pathol Anat 369:55–68

Helvie MA, Paramagul C, Oberman HA, Adler DD (1993) Invasive lobular carcinoma: imaging features and clinical detection. Invest Radiol 28:202

Hermanek P, Sobin LH, UICC (International Union Against Cancer) (1987) TNM classification of malignant tumours. Springer, Berlin Heidelberg New York

Holland R, Connoly J, Gelman R et al (1990) The presence of an extensive intraductal component (EIC) following a limited excision correlates with prominent residual disease in the remainder of the breast. J Clin Oncol 8:113

Holland R, Hendriks JHCL (1994) Microcalcifications associated with ductal carcinoma in situ: mammographic pathologic correlation. Sem Diagn Pathol 11:181

Lagios MD (1995) Ductal carcinoma in situ: controversies in diagnosis, biology, and treatment. Breast J 1:68–78

Lagios MD, Westdahl PR, Rose MR (1981) The concepts and implications of multicentricity in breast carcinoma. Pathol Annu 16:83–102

Lagios MD, Westdahl PR, Margolin FR, Roses MR (1982) Duct carcinoma in situ. Cancer 50:1309–1314

LeGal M, Oliver L, Asselein B et al (1992) Mammographic features of 455 invasive lobular carcinomas. Radiology 185:705

Linnel F, Ljungberg O (1980) Breast carcinoma. Progression of tubular cancer and a new classification. Acta Pathol Microbiol Scand 88:59–60

Mendelsohn EB, Harris KM, Doshi N et al (1989) Infiltrating lobular carcinoma: mammographic pattern with pathologic correlation. Am J Roentgenol 153:265

Newstead GM, Baute PB, Toth HK (1992) Invasive lobular and ductal carcinoma: mammographic findings and stage at diagnosis. Radiology 184:623

Paterok EM, Egger H, Willgeroth F (1983) Mehr als 1500 radiologisch indizierte Mammabiopsien. Mikrokalk und pathologisches Galaktogramm, 1964–1982. Geburtsh Frauenheilk 43:721–725

Ridolfi RL, Rosen PP, Post A, Kinne DW (1977) Medullary carcinoma of the breast. A clinical pathological study with 10 years' follow up. Cancer 40:1365–1385

Rosen PP (1987) The pathology of breast carcinoma. In: Harris JR, Hellman S, Henderson IC, Kinne DW (eds) Breast diseases. J.B. Lippincott, Philadelphia, pp 147–209

Rosen PP (1996) Invasive mammary carcinoma. In: Harris JR, Lippman ME, Morrow M, Hallman S (eds) Diseases of the Breast. Lippincot-Raven, Philadelphia, New York

Rosen PP, Lesser ML, Kinne DW (1985) Breast carcinoma at the extremes of age: a comparison of patients younger than 35 years and older than 75 years. J Surg Oncol 28:90–96

Schulz-Wendtland R, Bauer M, Krämer S, Büttner A, Lang N (1995) Stereotaxie. Eine Methode zur Punktion, Stanzbiopsie und Markierung kleinster mammographischer Herdbefunde. Chir Praxis 49:123–136

Sickles FA (1991) The subtle and atypical mammographic features of invasive lobular carcinoma. Radiology 178:25

Sickles EA (1994) Nonpalpable, circumscribed, noncalcified solid breast masses: likelihood of malignancy based on lesion size and age of patient. Radiology 192:439

Silverstein MJ, Lagios MD, Craig PH et al (1996) A prognostic index for ductal carcinoma in situ of the breast. Cancer 77:2267–2274

Stomper PC, Davis SP, Weidner N et al (1988) Clinically occult, noncalcified breast cancer: serial radiologic-pathologic correlation in 27 cases. Radiology 169:621

Tabar L, Fagerberg N, Day E et al (1992) Breast cancer treatment and natural history: new insights from the results of screening. Lancer 339:412

Tulusan AH (1993) Breast cancer pathology. In: Burghardt E, Webb MJ, Monaghan JM, Kindermann G (eds) Surgical gynecologic oncology. Thieme, Stuttgart New York, pp 542–560

Tulusan AH, Egger H, Schneider ML, Willgeroth F (1982) A contribution to the natural history of breast cancer. IV. Lobular carcinoma in situ and its relation to breast cancer. Arch Gynecol 231:219–226

Tulusan AH, Ronay G, Egger H, Willgeroth F (1985) A contribution to the natural history of breast cancer. V. Bilateral primary breast cancer: incidence, risks and diagnosis of simultaneous primary cancer in the opposite breast. Arch Gynecol 237:85–91

Tulusan AH, Reitzenstein M, Ronay G, Schmidt C, Adam R, Lang N (1989) Pathologic-anatomical aspects of breast cancer with therapeutic considerations. In: Bohmert HH, Leis HP, Jackson IT (eds) Breast cancer: conservative and reconstructive surgery. Thieme Medical, New York, pp 35–38

Wellings SR, Jensen HM, Marcum RG (1975) An atlas of subgross pathology of the human breast with special reference to possible precancerous lesions. JNCI 55:231–273

3 Technical Aspects of Screen-Film Mammography*

A.G. Haus

CONTENTS

3.1 Introduction 33
3.2 Dedicated X-ray Equipment 33
3.2.1 X-ray Tube Target Filtration and kVp Setting 33
3.2.2 Breast Compression 36
3.2.3 Grids for Mammography 36
3.2.4 Exposure Time 36
3.2.5 Focal Spot Size and Geometry (Magnification) ... 36
3.2.6 Magnification Techniques for Mammography 37
3.2.7 Automatic Exposure Control 38
3.3 Cassette-Screen-Film Processing Systems 39
3.3.1 Cassettes 39
3.3.2 Screen-Film Combinations 39
3.3.3 Screens 39
3.3.4 Films 39
3.3.5 Film Processing System 39
3.3.6 Process Verification and Quality Control 46
3.3.7 Film Contrast 46
3.3.8 Screen-Film Blurring 46
3.3.9 Radiographic Noise 50
3.3.10 Film Speed 51
3.4 Radiation Dose 54
References 54

3.1 Introduction

In mammography, it is most important to consistently produce high-contrast, high-resolution images at the lowest radiation dose possible. During the past 20 years, there have been many significant technologic improvements in mammographic x-ray equipment and in screen-film recording systems (Haus 1990, 1991, 1994). Twenty years ago, many x-ray units were used that were not dedicated for mammography. These x-ray units had tungsten target tubes which were originally designed for general-purpose medical imaging procedures, such as chest radiography. Some of these units had compression devices that were homemade; therefore, breast compression was less than optimal by today's standards. Many of these units had very large focal spots and/or short focal spot-to-breast surface distances

---

A.G. Haus, 195 Crossroads Lane, Rochester, NY 14612, USA
*Portions of this chapter are based on the following references: Haus 1987, 1990a,b, 1994

which could result in significant geometric blur (unsharpness). Direct exposure (industrial type) x-ray films were being used, which often required long exposure times (causing blur due to motion) and which resulted in high radiation exposure.

Today, mammography is performed with dedicated mammographic x-ray equipment. These units have specially designed tube targets, smaller focal spots, and significantly improved breast compression devices, among other features. Cassettes and screen-film combinations are designed specifically for mammography. Film processing has also improved significantly over the years. Today it is possible to obtain mammograms with higher image quality which require significantly lower radiation dose compared to mammograms dating back about 20 years (Fig. 3.1). In this chapter, some of the important technologic improvements that have led to today's high-quality screen-film mammographic imaging will be discussed. Table 3.1 summarizes factors that affect mammographic screen-film image quality.

3.2 Dedicated X-ray Equipment

Approximately 30 companies provide dedicated mammographic x-ray units (Haus 1990). Inherent in the design of all dedicated mammographic x-ray equipment are: (a) appropriate beam quality, (b) breast compression device, (c) grid capability, and (d) automatic exposure control. Some of the differences that distinguish these units from each other are: (a) focal spot size, (b) geometry (focal spot-to-object and object-to-receptor distances), (c) magnification capability, (d) x-ray output (mA), (e) design of compression device, and (f) price of unit.

3.2.1 X-ray Tube Target Filtration and kVp Setting

Selection and use of the appropriate tube target material, added beam filtration, and kVp setting are

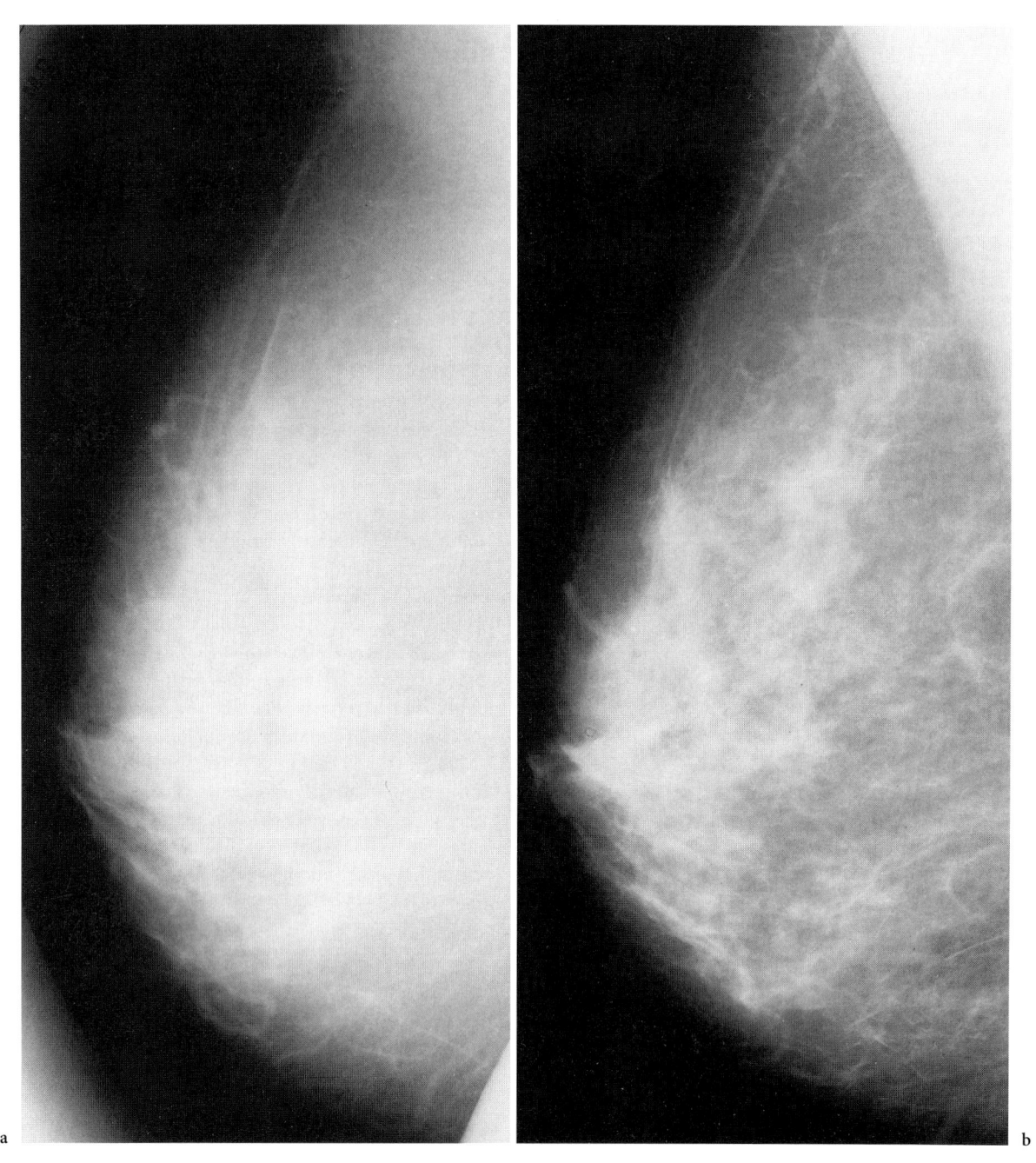

Fig. 3.1. Mammograms demonstrating (**a**) best quality possible in 1981 and (**b**) quality possible today. The mammograms are of the same patient taken 10 years apart. (Images courtesy of Wende Logan-Young, MD)

factors controlling radiation quality that are important in achieving the high subject contrast necessary for screen-film mammography.

Subject contrast is determined by the ratio of the x-ray intensity transmitted through one part of the object (breast) to that transmitted through a more or less absorbing adjacent part (NCRP 1986). Subject contrast is especially important in mammography because of the subtle differences in the soft-tissue density of normal and pathologic structures of the breast, and also because of the importance of detecting minute details such as microcalcifications and the marginal structural characteristics of soft-tissue masses.

The majority of dedicated mammographic x-ray units have a molybdenum target tube and a 0.03-mm molybdenum filter. Tungsten target tubes designed for conventional screen-film radiography should not

Table 3.1. Factors affecting mammographic image quality (HAUS 1991)

Radiographic sharpness		Radiographic noise	
Radiographic contrast	Radiographic blurring ("unsharpness")	Radiographic mottle	Radiographic artifacts
Subject contrast	*Motion blurring*	*Receptor graininess*	*Handling*
Absorption differences	Breast immobilization (compression)		Crimp marks
Thickness		*Quantum mottle*	Finger marks
Density	Exposure time	Film speed	Scratches
Atomic number		Film contrast	Static
Radiation quality	*Geometric blurring*	Screen absorption	Exposure
Target material (e.g., Mo, W. Rh)	Focal spot size	Screen conversion efficiency	Fog
Kilovoltage (kVp)	Focal spot-object distance	Light diffusion	
Filtration (e.g., Mo, Rh)	Object-image receptor distance	Radiation quality	*Processing*
Scatter radiation			Streaks
Beam collimation		*Structure mottle*	Spots
Compression	*Screen-film blurring*		Scratches
Air gap	Phosphor thickness		Dirt
Grid	Light absorbing dyes and pigments		Stains
Film contrast	Phosphor particle size		
Film type	Screen-film contact		
Processing			
Chemistry			
Temperature			
Time			
Agitation			
Photographic density			
Fog			
Storage			
Safelight			
Light leaks			

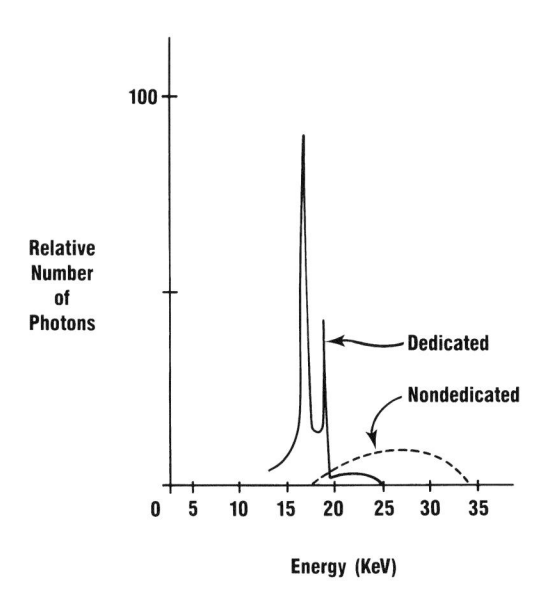

Fig. 3.2. Typical x-ray emission spectra (normalized to unit area) using dedicated and nondedicated x-ray units for screen-film mammography. The graph shows spectra from a dedicated unit using a molybdenum (Mo) target, 0.03-mm Mo filter, and 25 kVp setting and from a nondedicated unit using a tungsten target tube, aluminum filtration, and 35 kVp setting. (From HAUS 1990)

be used for screen-film mammography because the resulting subject contrast is too low due to the radiation quality characteristics of these tubes (Fig. 3.2) (HAUS et al. 1976; FEWELL and SHUPING 1978; JENNINGS et al. 1981; NCRP 1986). Dedicated molybdenum target x-ray units are widely used, and settings of less than 28 kVp are generally recommended with these units (NCRP 1986). The use of low-energy photons, such as those produced by the 17.9- and 19.5-keV characteristic lines from the molybdenum target, provide high subject contrast for breasts of average thickness. When a 0.03-mm molybdenum filter is used, the spectrum is strongly suppressed at photon energies greater than 20 keV because of the k-shell absorption edge of molybdenum at that energy. This allows more radiation from the characteristic lines to be used in image formation. Other tube target and filter combinations used in dedicated mammographic units include (a) a tungsten target with an approximately 0.06-mm molybdenum filter, (b) a tungsten target with an approximately 0.05-mm rhodium filter, and (c) a rhodium target with an approximately 0.025-mm rhodium filter.

3.2.2 Breast Compression

Good breast compression is a very important factor in reducing scattered radiation in screen-film mammography. Scattered radiation can significantly reduce subject contrast in screen-film mammography (BARNES and BREZOVICH 1978; NIELSON and FAGERBERG 1986; YESTER et al. 1981). By reducing the ratio of scattered to primary radiation, subject contrast is improved (Table 3.2). In addition to contributing to a reduction in scattered radiation, compression can provide several other technical improvements in image quality, which can be achieved without compromising other image quality factors. These improvements include: (a) immobilization of the breast, which reduces blurring caused by motion; (b) location of structures in the breast closer to the image receptor, which reduces geometric blurring; (c) production of a more uniformly thick breast, which, in turn, results in more even penetration by x-radiation and less difference in radiographic density in the area between the chest wall and the nipple; and (d) reduction of radiation dose. An added benefit is the spreading of breast tissue, enabling suspicious lesions to be more easily identified.

3.2.3 Grids for Mammography

The use of specifically designed grids for mammography can further reduce scattered radiation and improve subject contrast, which is especially significant when imaging thick, dense breasts (BARNES and BREZOVICH 1978; CHAN et al. 1985; SICKLES and WEBER 1986). Grids are now included with dedicated mammographic x-ray units. Grids used for mammography consist of lead strips separated by spacers of radiolucent material such as carbon fiber. Most of these grids are of the moving type, which blur the grid lines. Moving-type grids are preferred for mammography. Focused stationary grids for mammography with ultra-high-strip density (80 lines per cm) are also commercially available.

Grids designed for mammography require exposure increases of approximately 2–2.5 times the exposure required for non-grid techniques. This exposure increase can be accomplished by increasing the mAs setting. It may be possible to offset the increased radiation dose required with grids by using a higher kilovoltage setting or a recording system that provides a higher speed or a combination of several factors.

3.2.4 Exposure Time

The use of long exposure time can result in image blurring due to motion. In mammography, motion blurring is caused by movement of the breast during exposure. It can be minimized by using a short exposure time of less than 1 s and by firmly compressing the breast.

3.2.5 Focal Spot Size and Geometry (Magnification)

The size, shape, and intensity distribution of the x-ray tube focal spot in combination with focal spot-to-object and object-to-image receptor distances affect geometric blurring (Fig. 3.3). To minimize geometric blurring, the focal spot size and object-to-image receptor distance should be minimized, whereas focal spot-to-object distance should be maximized. Focal spot sizes and shapes for the dedicated and general-purpose x-ray units used for mammography vary considerably (HAUS 1983, 1985; HAUS et al. 1978; KIMME-SMITH et al. 1988). Likewise, the focal spot-to-breast surface distances for different mammographic units vary.

Several years ago it was common to compress the breast directly on top of the mammographic cassette. The distance between the edge of the breast and the screen-film combination was very small. Today many mammographic procedures are performed with a moving Bucky type grid. With the grid in place, a gap of 1–2 cm between the edge of the breast and the screen-film combination may occur. The size of the focal spot, therefore, needs to be smaller in terms of limiting geometric resolution for a given focal spot-to-breast surface distance (HAUS 1987).

The limit of geometric resolution corresponding to various planes in the breast can be calculated using the focal spot size, the distance from the focal

Table 3.2. Ratio of scattered to primary radiation for 6-cm- and 3-cm-thick breast and for no-grid and grid techniques (3-cm-thick breast) (from BARNES and BREGOVICH 1978)

	Technique	Ratio of scattered to primary radiation
6-cm-thick breast phantom	No grid	0.8
3-cm-thick breast phantom	No grid	0.4
3-cm-thick breast phantom	Grid	0.14

Data for a plastic breast phantom at 30 kVp

Technical Aspects of Screen-Film Mammography

the breast surface distance should exceed 15 cycles per mm (line pairs per mm) (Figs. 3.4, 3.5).

3.2.6 Magnification Techniques for Mammography

The use of a magnification techniques is often very helpful in diagnosis. There are several technical advantages associated with magnification radiography, including (a) improvement in the effective spatial resolution of the recording system, (b) reduction of the effective noise, (c) reduction of scatter, and (d) improvement in the visual appearance of the magnified image (DOI 1977; SICKLES et al. 1977; HAUS et al. 1979; TABÁR and DEAN 1983). Improvement in effective spatial resolution can be obtained due to the enlargement of the x-ray pattern relative to the inherent unsharpness of the recording system. Therefore, given the situation where an x-ray tube with a very small focal spot is used, the effective spatial resolution capability of the recording system will improve with the magnification technique (Fig. 3.6).

Reduction in effective noise is obtained because the recording system noise remains the same with either magnification or nonmagnification technique, but the size of the x-ray pattern is enlarged with magnification.

As discussed previously, the effect of scattered radiation is an important factor contributing to the total mammographic exposure. Using magnification technique with its inherent air gap, significant reduction of scattered radiation can be accomplished for some diagnostic procedures. In mammography, however, several studies have indicated that the scatter reduction is minimal when a magnification factor

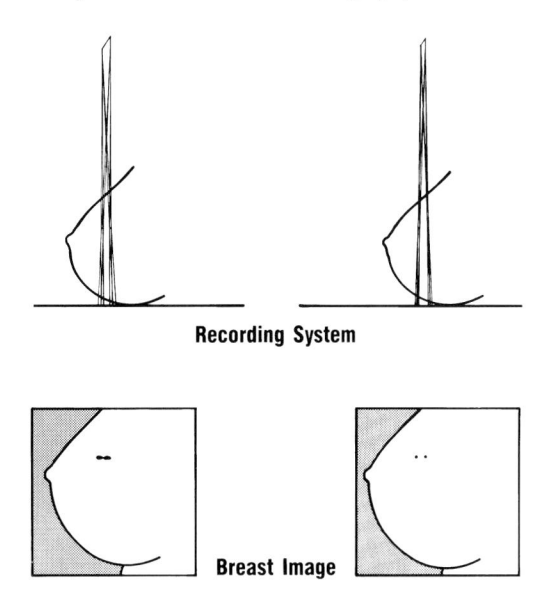

Fig. 3.3. Illustration of the effect of geometric blurring. The focal spot size in the drawing at the *upper left* limits the imaging of the two microcalcifications shown in the image of the breast at the *lower left*. The microcalcifications are unsharp and one is indistinguishable from the other. The focal spot size in the *upper right* drawing is smaller. The microscalcifications are sharp and clearly distinguishable. (From HAUS 1990)

spot to the receptor, and the distance from the object to the receptor (HAUS et al. 1978). These values can be compared with a calculation of the limit of resolution for the screen-film combination. Limiting resolution data can be obtained from modulation transfer function (MTF) data or from bar-pattern resolution test objects. Most mammographic screen-film combinations have resolutions of at least 15 cycles per mm. In order to make the recording system the limiting factor, the geometric resolution at

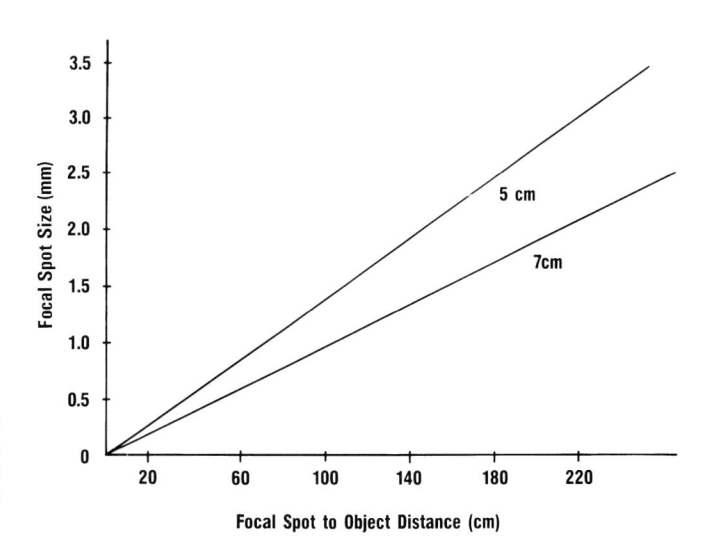

Fig. 3.4. Graph of equivalent focal spot size versus focal spot-to-object distance for 5-cm and 7-cm object-to-recording system distances to achieve 15 cycles per mm limiting resolution. (From HAUS 1990)

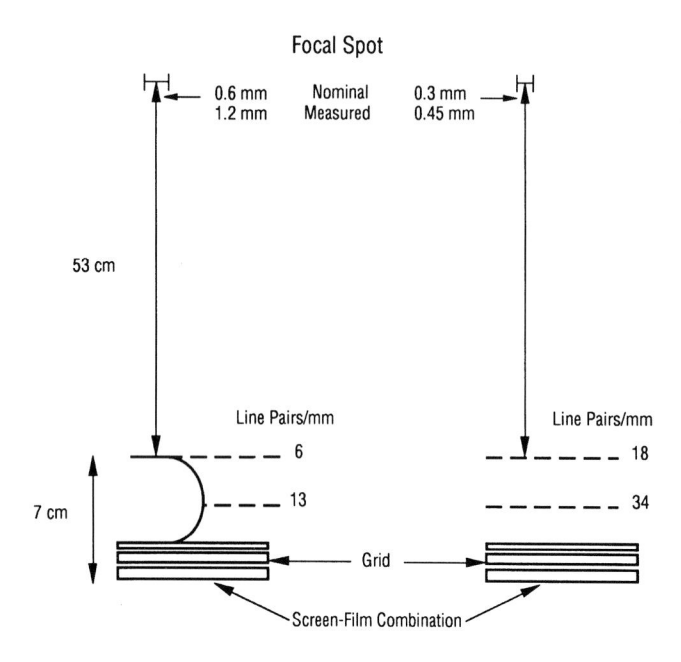

Fig. 3.5. Diagram comparing mammographic x-ray unit geometric resolutions (line pairs per mm) for two focal spot sizes. Note improved limiting resolution and, therefore, reduced geometric blurring when the smaller (0.45 mm measured) focal spot is used

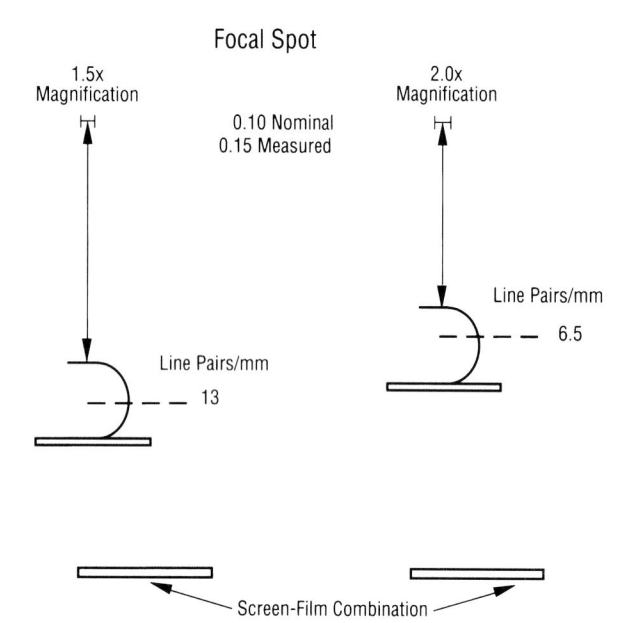

Fig. 3.6. Diagram comparing mammographic x-ray unit geometric resolution (line pairs per mm) for 1.5× and 2.0× magnification techniques using a 0.15 measured focal spot size. If the measured focal spot is 0.3 mm, then the limiting resolution would be 6.5 line pairs per mm for 1.5× magnification, and 3.3 line pairs for 2.0× magnification techniques

of 1.5 is used due to the small air gap (approximately 11 cm) (BARNES and BREZOVICH 1978; NEILSON and FAGERBERG 1986; YESTER et al. 1981). Significant reductions in scatter cannot be obtained unless the air gap exceeds 25 cm, which can be achieved with greater (approximately 2×) magnification. The advantages of magnification techniques are achieved at the expense of increased radiation exposure.

The use of a very small focal spot to minimize geometric blurring is important in any magnification technique. When a very small focal spot is used, x-ray tube output is reduced significantly. This, in turn, requires longer exposure times (1–4 s). Two important factors must be considered when long exposure times are used: (a) blurring due to patient motion, and (b) additional radiation dose necessitated by reciprocity law failure when screen-film combinations are used (HAUS 1991). Higher-speed screen-film combinations designed for mammography may be especially appropriate for use with magnification techniques in order to reduce exposure time and radiation dose, and to minimize the effect of reciprocity law failure without compromising resolution (HAUS 1987).

3.2.7 Automatic Exposure Control

Automatic exposure control systems, also referred to as phototimers, are designed to automatically provide the radiation exposure needed to produce a mammogram with an acceptable (and consistent) optical density. Most dedicated mammographic x-ray units have automatic exposure control devices. New circuit modifications and developments in detector arrangements which take into account changes in breast tissue thickness and composition can provide more consistent film optical density (LaFrance et al. 1988; Aichinger et al. 1988).

3.3 Cassette-Screen-Film Processing Systems

3.3.1 Cassettes

Cassettes designed for mammography have front panels which provide both low x-ray absorption and intimate screen-film contact (which also reduces blur).

3.3.2 Screen-Film Combinations

For many years, direct exposure with medical x-ray film or industrial film was used for mammography (Fig. 3.7) (Egan 1976). In the early 1970s, the first screen-film combination designed for mammography utilizing a single-screen, single-emulsion film became commercially available (Fig. 3.7) (Ostrum et al. 1973; Wayrynen 1979). Most single-screen, single-emulsion film combinations commonly used today have higher film contrast and require significantly lower radiation exposure than those used a few years ago. It is interesting to note that today's screen-film combinations require approximately 50–100 times less radiation than direct-exposure films.

3.3.3 Screens

The great majority of mammographic images are produced with a single intensifying screen used as a back screen in combination with a single-emulsion film (Fig. 3.8). Many mammographic screens incorporate phosphors containing metals from the lanthanide series of elements such as terbium-activated gadolinium oxysulfide (Gd_2O_2S:Tb). Screens may incorporate light absorbers in the phosphor which are used to increase sharpness. Intensifying screens have a protective overcoat to resist surface abrasion, are edge-sealed to minimize edge wear, and the base includes a backing layer to eliminate screen curl. Mammographic screens consisting of terbium-activated gadolinium oxysulfide material emit light in the visible spectral region from 382 nm to 622 nm, although the primary emission peak is in the green spectral region (545 nm) (Fig. 3.9) (Eastman Kodak Company Technical Report 1986).

3.3.4 Films

Films used in mammography usually have a single emulsion and are used in combination with a single back screen (Barnes 1982; Haus 1987; Kimme-Smith 1991; Yaffe 1990; Vyborny and Schmidt 1990; Schueler et al. 1992; NCRP 1986; AAPM 1990). Conventional three-dimensional (3-D) silver halide grains are widely used for mammography rather than tabular-grain film emulsions (Fig. 3.10). The lower degree of light crossover afforded by tabular-grain films results in improved sharpness in conventional double screen-double emulsion combinations. Because single screen-single emulsion combinations are used in mammography, there is no light crossover and, therefore, use of tabular grains would not offer increased sharpness. The single-emulsion side of films used for mammography is coated with larger amounts of silver halide and gelatin than are coated on double-emulsion films used in conventional radiography (Fig. 3.8).

3.3.5 Film Processing System

Film processing must be considered as part of a system which includes the automatic film processor (Fig. 3.11), film type, and chemicals (Haus et al. 1994). These components must be considered together as a system and must be properly optimized in order to obtain appropriate image quality in terms of film contrast of the processed radiography. The resulting film speed affects radiation dose to the patient. Automatic film processor variables include: (a)

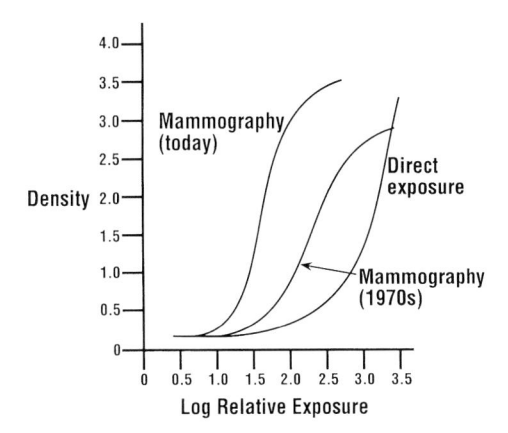

Fig. 3.7. Characteristic curves for (a) a direct-exposure film, (b) a single-screen, single-emulsion film used in the 1970s and early 1980s, and (c) a single-screen, single-emulsion film combination used for mammography today. (From Haus 1994)

Fig. 3.8. Diagrams comparing physical configurations for a single-emulsion film in contact with a single (back) intensifying screen (as used for mammography) and a double-emulsion film sandwiched between two intensifying screens (used for other radiologic procedures). (From Haus 1994)

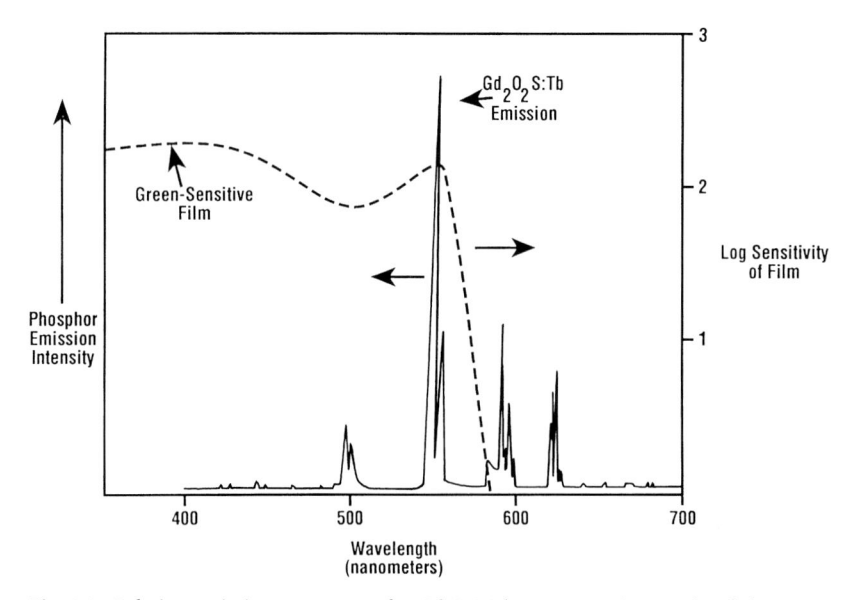

Fig. 3.9. Relative emission spectrum of a Gd_2O_2S:Tb screen superimposed on a graph showing the spectral sensitivity of a commonly used mammographic film. The high spectral emission peak of the green-emitting screen coincides with the film's high sensitivity to green light. (From Haus 1994)

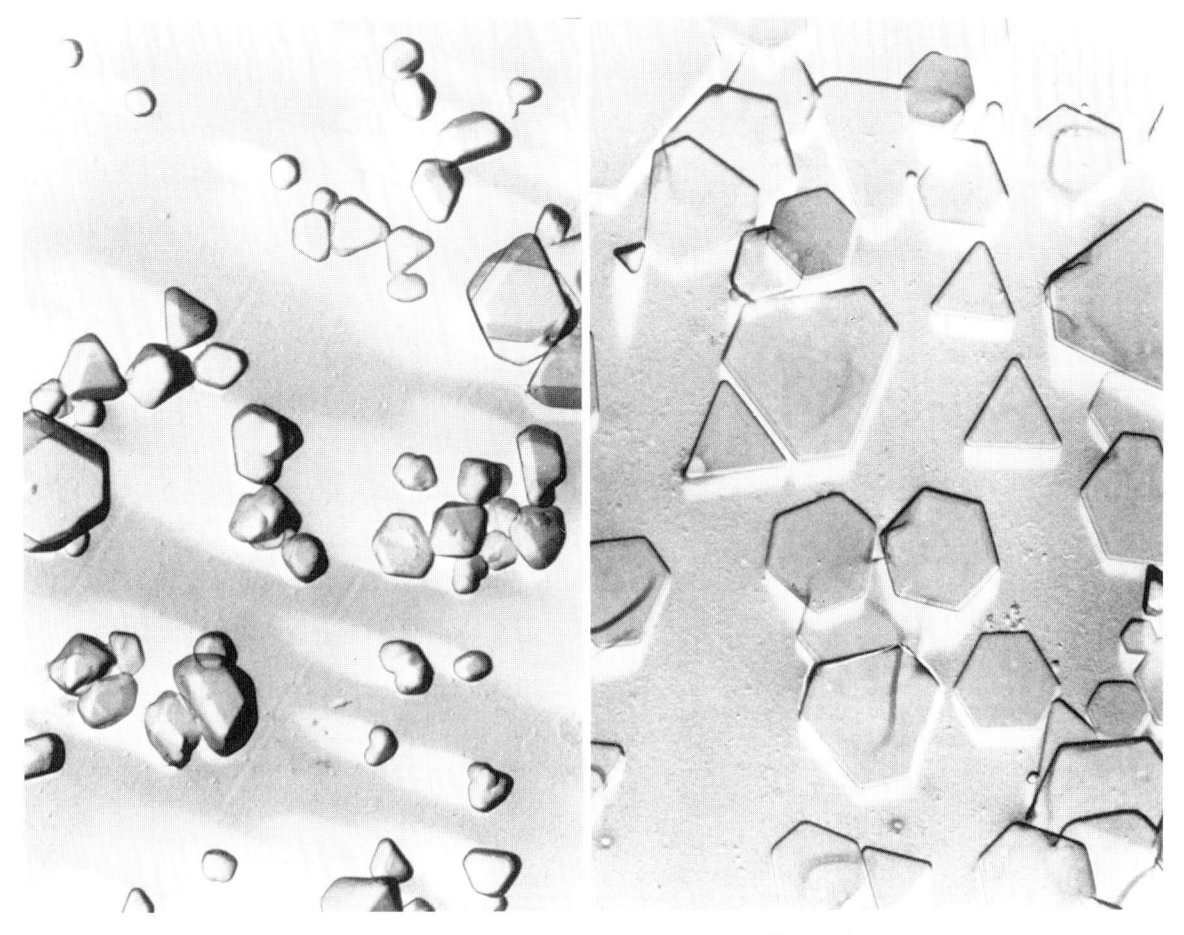

Fig. 3.10. Microphotographs of three-dimensional (*left*) and tabular-grain (*right*) film emulsions

processing cycle time, (b) temperature, (c) chemicals, (d) replenishment, (e) agitation, and (f) drying.

3.3.5.1 Processing Cycle Time

Processing cycle time is usually defined as the time it takes for (a) the leading edge of the film to enter and exit the processor, or (b) the leading edge of the film to enter and the trailing edge of the film to exit the processor. The latter definition will be used here. Processing cycles range from approximately 90 to 210 s, depending on whether standard- or extended-cycle processing is used. Standard processing cycles are between 90 and 150 s (Table 3.3). Developer temperature and replenishment rates are determined by the processing cycle in order to achieve the desired sensitometric characteristics (contrast, speed, base plus fog) for the type of film being used.

Extended-cycle processing can be used for some single-emulsion films (KIMME-SMITH et al. 1989; TABÁR and HAUS 1989). In extended-cycle processing (Table 3.3), the film remains in the developer longer. Developer temperature is not altered significantly. For some single-emulsion films, the film contrast is higher and the film speed is increased, resulting in an approximate 35% reduction in radiation dose when extended-cycle processing is used (Fig. 3.12). For double-emulsion films, the extended-cycle process does not significantly affect film contrast and film speed and is, therefore, not recommended (Fig. 3.13).

3.3.5.2 Developer Temperature

Developer temperatures in automatic film processors range from 91°F (33°C) to 103°F (39°C) (HAUS 1983). The developer temperature depends on film type, transport speed, and the manufacturers' recommendations. Developer temperature affects film speed, film contrast, and fog levels (Fig. 3.14). These variables can be expected to change in similar fashion as a function of development time.

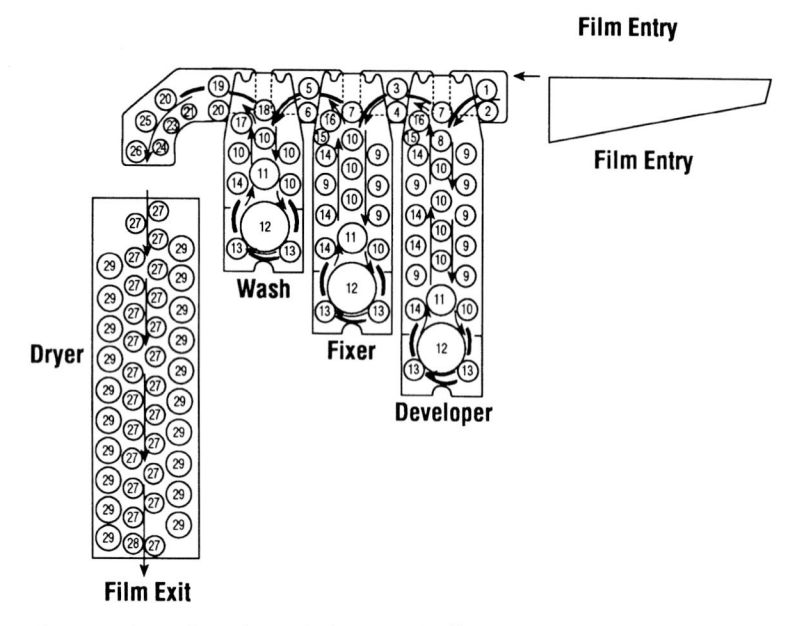

Fig. 3.11. Operation of a typical automatic film processor. Typically, film is manually inserted into the processor transport system from the feed tray. The film is transported through (a) the developer rack, (b) the fixer rack, (c) the wash rack, (d) the dryer section, and (e) exits dry and ready to read. The film path is a "serpentine" route. This enables proper emulsion agitation as well as maximum chemical-to-emulsion "coupling," which produces the optimum development for speed and contrast. Developer makes the latent image visible. Fixer essentially "stops" the development process and makes the resultant image "permanent" for keeping purposes. Washing removes chemicals to promote uniform drying and long-term, archival keeping of the radiograph

Table 3.3. Processing conditions for Kodak mammographic film

Film/processing cycle	Kodak X-Omat processors					
	M35 M35A M35A-M M20	M6B M6-N M6A-N M6AW	M7 M7A M7B	M8	270 RA	460 RA 480 RA
MIN-R E/extended cycle processing						
Processing time (s)	207	172	192	N/A	201	170
Developer time (s)	47	47	43		53.2	46.2
°F	95	95	96		94	95
°C	35	35	35.6		34.4	35
MIN-R H or MIN-R M/standard cycle processing						
Processing time (s)	140	90	122	90	100	88
Developer time (s)	32	24	27	21.5	26.6	23.8
°F	92	95	94	96	94	95
°C	33.5	35	34.4	35.6	34.4	35

Note that when the developer temperature is lower than the manufacturer's recommendation, film speed is reduced. This may dictate an unnecessary increase in radiation dose in order to produce mammograms of proper optical density. Similarly, film contrast is reduced when developer temperature is lowered. Conversely, if the developer temperature is higher or development time longer (extended-cycle process) than the manufacturer's recommendation, film speed is increased. This may permit a reduction in radiation dose, and film contrast may also be increased. However, these changes can be expected to cause an increase in quantum mottle and radiographic noise. In addition, film fog may increase with increased developer temperature. Developer stability may also be affected adversely when

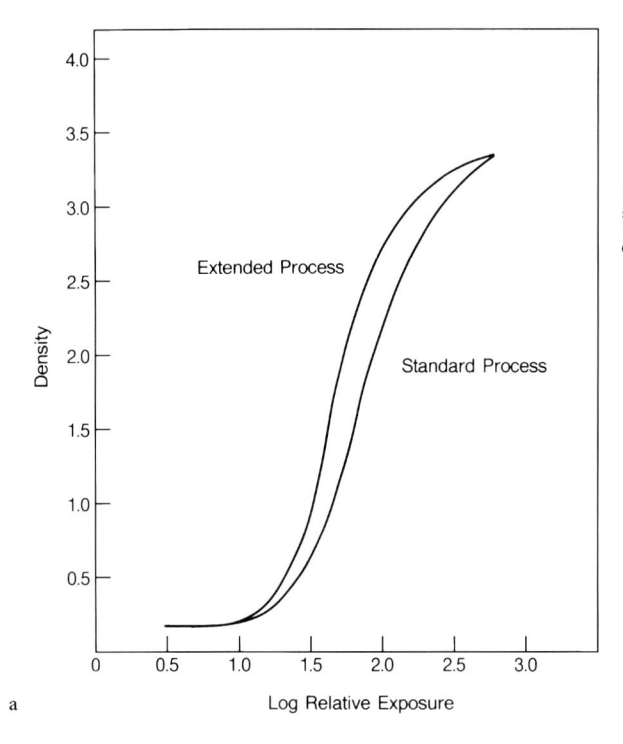

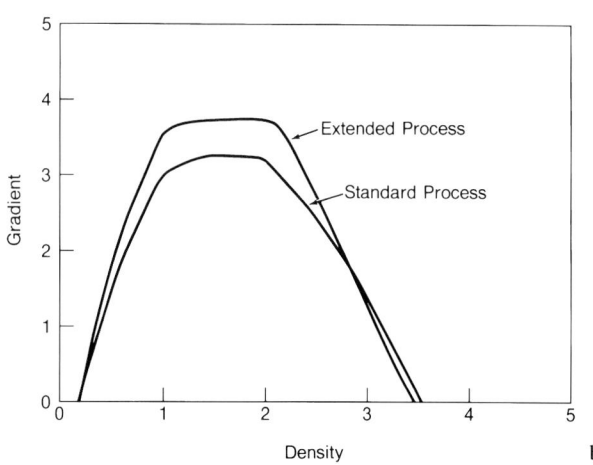

Fig. 3.12.a Characteristic curves for a single-emulsion mammographic film in the standard- and extended-cycle processes. There is approximately a 35% exposure reduction for the extended-cycle process without an increase in film fog. **b** Gradient versus optical density curves taken from the data in **a**. Note that film contrast (gradient) is higher for optical densities from 0.30 to 2.70 for the extended-cycle process. The gradient is defined as the slope of the characteristic curve at a specified optical density. (From Tabár and Haus 1989)

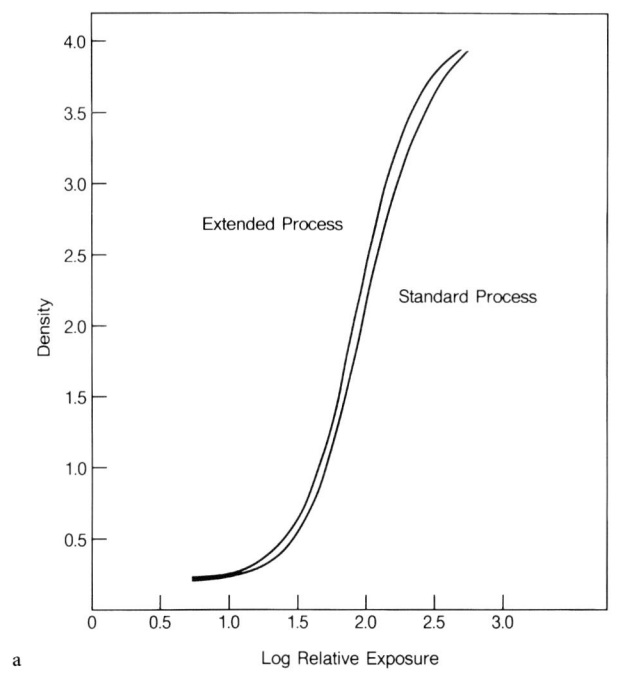

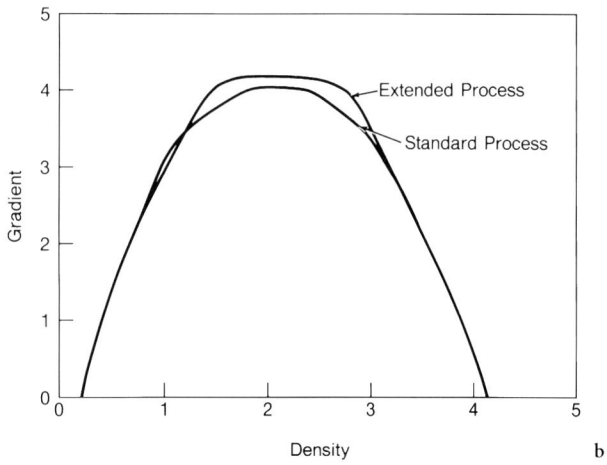

Fig. 3.13. a Characteristic curves for double-emulsion, tabular-grain film in the standard- and extended-cycle processes. There is approximately an 8% exposure reduction for the extended-cycle process. **b** Gradient versus optical density curves taken from the data in **a**. Note that film contrast is increased very slightly for optical densities from 1.20 to 2.70 for the extended-cycle process. (From Tabár and Haus 1989)

developer temperatures higher than recommended are used.

The American College of Radiology (ACR) *Mammography Quality Control Manual for Radiologic Technologists* indicates that the developer temperature should be within ±0.5°F (±30°C) of that recommended by the manufacturer for the specific film-developer combination being used (Mount and Gray 1990). The measurement accuracy, precision, and repeatability of the thermometer used to monitor developer temperature is most important. The thermometer should have an accuracy at least equal

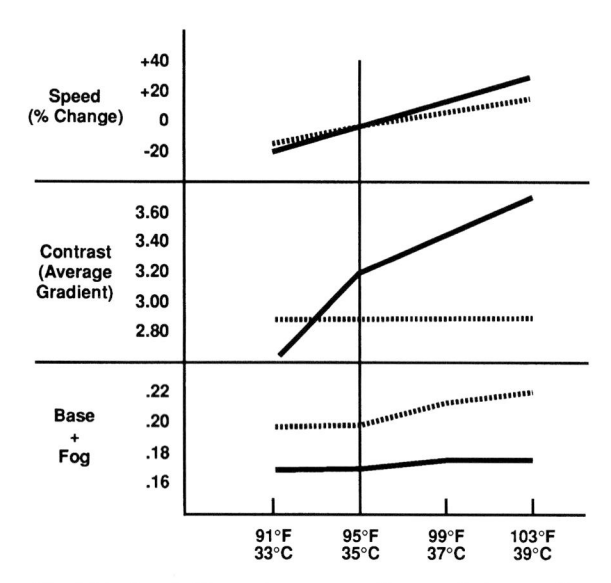

Fig. 3.14. Graph illustrating percent film-speed change, film contrast, and film base plus fog plotted versus developer temperature for a single-emulsion mammographic film (*solid line*) and a double-emulsion, tabular-grain film (*dotted line*) using the film manufacturer's recommended processor and chemicals. The *vertical line* represents the recommendation for a standard processing cycle

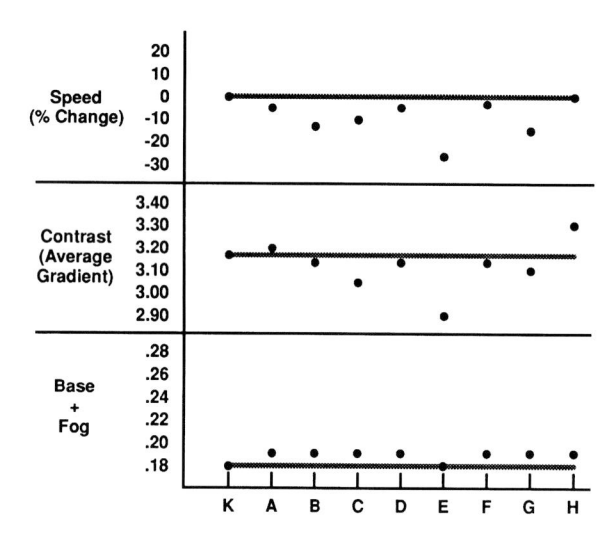

Fig. 3.15. Chart produced from film processing survey data which shows film processing variations due to use of different chemicals for single-emulsion mammographic film. The letter K indicates processing data (and expected values) using the film manufacturer's processor and chemicals (SPRAWLS 1987). A *horizontal line* is drawn at the letter *K* data point. Letters A–H are data for different brands of chemicals. Data were obtained using film strips which were sensitometrically preexposed to light that simulates the light spextrum from a mammographic screen. Film speed differences, film contrast (average gradient), and base plus fog values were determined from the sensitometry data (SPRAWLS 1987)

to, and preferably better than, the tolerance allowed in the NCRP and ACR documents. In the radiology or medical imaging department, a variety of thermometers are used to measure developer temperature. These thermometers vary in accuracy, precision, ease of reading, and cost. A recent study suggests that clinical digital thermometers which are available in pharmacies and supermarkets are inexpensive but accurate devices for measuring the temperature of the developer solution (Fig. 3.15). It is also recommended that the thermometers used to measure developer temperature be evaluated against a thermometer that has a calibration traceable to the National Institute of Standards and Technology.

It is important to confirm that proper film contrast, film speed, and base plus fog values are being obtained for each film type used (according to the manufacturer's specifications and tolerances). This information should be requested from the film manufacturer (HAUS et al. 1994). In order to maintain consistent film contrast, film speed, and base plus fog values, it is important to implement a processor quality control program.

3.3.5.3 Chemicals

All film manufacturers recommend specific chemicals for processing their films (HAUS et al. 1994). Many users consider chemicals from various manufacturers to be interchangeable. However, surveys have documented that film speed, film contrast, and base plus fog respond differently to various types of chemicals (Fig. 3.15). These effects also depend on the type of film being processed.

Chemical manufacturers distribute chemicals as concentrates. Solution service providers add water locally to complete the mixture. In some cases, chemicals are not mixed to the appropriate concentration in accordance with the manufactuer's recommendations.

Processing chemical variability can occur in medical imaging due to a number of factors. Although most manufactuers use similar processing chemicals to achieve development and fixing, the concentration of these chemicals can vary, either initially or after being mixed by solution service providers. This concentration variation can result in changes in film response of differing magnituders, depending on the film type. In addition, variability can also result from improper replenishment. Either overdevelopment or underdevelopment can occur, depending on the degree of replenishment or initial chemical concentration.

For the initial start-up and/or when fresh chemicals are used, it is important to follow the manufacturer's recommendations by (a) using the proper chemicals, (b) mixing to the correct concentration, and (c) adding the appropriate amount of starter solution. Adding starter solution begins the seasoning process. The developer solution becomes more completely seasoned as more films are processed. This additional seasoning may continue to cause slight changes in film speed and contrast; at some point, film speed and contrast will stabilize. Seasoning effects depend on film type, chemical formulation, and replenishment.

Since both the concentration and the composition of chemicals used in film processing can impact the contrast, speed, base plus fog, and long-term keeping of films used in medical imaging, it is sometimes of interest to attempt to analyze the chemicals used. There are several approaches that are being used to accomplish this. They include pH measurement, specific gravity measurement, laboratory component analysis, and process control sensitometry.

Measurement of pH can be used as a measure of activity of process chemistry because development generally decreases in activity as pH decreases. This measurement, however, is not very accurate and is useful only for finding trends or large changes in developer concentration. pH measurements, or detection of hydrogen ion concentration, are difficult to achieve in high salt solutions (such as developers) unless carefully calibrated electrodes are used.

Specific gravity measurements can also be used to determine relatively large changes in concentration. Measurement of specific gravity involves determining the ion and salt concentration of a solution. This type of measurement is the same as is used to measure the acid content of a car battery and is not accurate or specific with respect to any particular chemical. Again, although information as to large changes in concentration can be determined, it is not specific enough to determine whether critical components such as developer antifoggants are missing from the developer solution.

Analysis of samples of developer solution by an analytical laboratory is, of course, the most accurate and predictive approach. However, this approach is costly and time consuming.

The last approach and probably the most widely used is to do process control sensitometry. By monitoring changes in sensitometry of a process control film strip, changes due to process chemistry can be detected. If variations in process control values (speed, contrast, and base plus fog) exceed operating tolerances, the chemicals should be changed to assure appropriate and consistent results. Although this approach does not identify the actual cause of sensitometry change, it is probably the most cost-effective and time-effective approach. The cost of changing chemistry is small compared to the total cost of doing medical radiography; the down time and investigative time required to identify the cause of a specific change in process chemistry may not be justified.

3.3.5.4 Replenishment

Replenishment is important to maintain stable developer and fixer activity (Haus et al. 1994). Proper replenishment (a) provides stable sensitometric results (film contrast, film speed, and base plus fog), (b) reduces or eliminates artifacts, and (c) enables long-term keeping. Replenishment rates are sometimes divided into groups based on daily film

Table 3.4. Replenishment rates based on film volume for mammography films (standard or extended cycle) for Kodak RP X-Omat processors, models M35, M6, and M7

Film type and feeding	Use condition	Average amount 18 × 24 cm films per 8 h of processor operation	Replenishment rates (ml per 18 × 24 cm) Developer	Fixer
MIN-R E double film feeding	High	150 sheets or more	40	60
	Medium	60–150 sheets	54	70
	Low	60 sheets or less[a]	70	80

[a] If sensitometry does not stay within controls limits, flooded replenishment may be needed

volumes (Table 3.4). Low film use per day requires higher replenishment per sheet. Processors with very low film volume throughput (such as surgery rooms) are very difficult to stabilize in order to maintain consistency. Flooded replenishment is recommended under these conditions. A starter solution is added to the developer replenisher holding tank; the processor is replenished at specific time intervals in addition to replenishment per sheet of film processed – independent of film volume. Flooded replenishment provides a stable fresh process. High film use per day requires a lower replenishment per sheet.

For extended-cycle processing (mammography), film processors require even closer monitoring of replenishment. Film throughput (film sheets per day) is the basis for determining replenishment volumes; however, since the typical film sizes for mammography are 18 × 24 cm and 24 × 30 cm, the actual area of the film is less than for larger films. One should consult with the manufacturer to correctly adjust and set up the film processor and replenishment rates to obtain the desired results and to obtain consistency in those results.

3.3.5.5 Agitation

Agitation maintains processing uniformity and temperature control. Agitation is provided by roller contact as well as chemical recirculation pumps. Film surface agitation is caused by roller contact. Tank solution agitation is caused by recirculation pumps.

3.3.5.6 Drying

The adjustable range of drying temperatures is from 38°C (100°F) to 71°C (160°F). Drying conditions depend on the environment. These may range from cool/dry to hot/humid. Many users tend to over-dry films. This may cause surface-pattern artifacts on the film (water spotting, etc.) that may impact the radiologist's ability to read films. The dryer temperature should, therefore, be adjusted to as low as possible while still providing dry film as it exits the processor. This will also result in energy savings for the processor operations.

3.3.6 Process Verification and Quality Control

For good film processing, it is important to confirm and verify that film contrast, film speed, and base plus fog values are being obtained for each film in use, according to the manufacturer's specifications and tolerances. This information should be requested from the film manufacturer. When proper processing has been established, it is necessary to implement a processor quality control program for routine monitoring of the film processor (Fig. 3.16).

3.3.7 Film Contrast

Film contrast characteristics determine how the x-ray intensity pattern will be related to optical density in the mammogram. Film contrast is affected by (a) film type, (b) processing conditions (solutions, temperature, time, agitation), (c) fog level (storage, safelight, light leaks), and (d) the optical density level. Low film contrast can be the result of using a film with inherently low contrast and processing the film as recommended, or using a film with inherently high-contrast capability and processing the film less than optimally.

Film gradient is defined as the slope of the curve of optical density versus log (exposure) (Haus 1983; Yaffe 1990; Ncrp 1986; Aapm 1990). Gradient determines how change in the optical density in the mammogram will result from the variations in x-ray intensity across the breast. The trend is to use mammographic films with high film gradient, i.e., with the maximum slope of the characteristic curve between 2.8 and 3.5 Maximum gradient occurs at different optical densities for different film types (Fig. 3.17), which may affect the optimum exposure for that film.

It is important to note that overall radiographic contrast is influenced by both subject contrast and film gradient. Therefore, a mammogram of acceptable contrast is best obtained by (a) use of appropriate beam quality, (b) breast compression, (c) use of a grid when necessary, and (d) properly processed high-contrast film.

3.3.8 Screen-Film Blurring

For screen-film radiography, light diffusion (spreading of the light emitted by the intensifying screen before it is recorded by the film) causes blurring (Fig. 3.18) (Haus 1985, 1990, 1991, 1994; Kimme-Smith 1991; Yaffe 1990; Vyborny and Schmidt 1990; Ncrp 1986; Aapm 1990). Factors involved include: (a) phosphor layer thickness in the screen, (b) phosphor particle size, (c) light-absorbing dyes and pig-

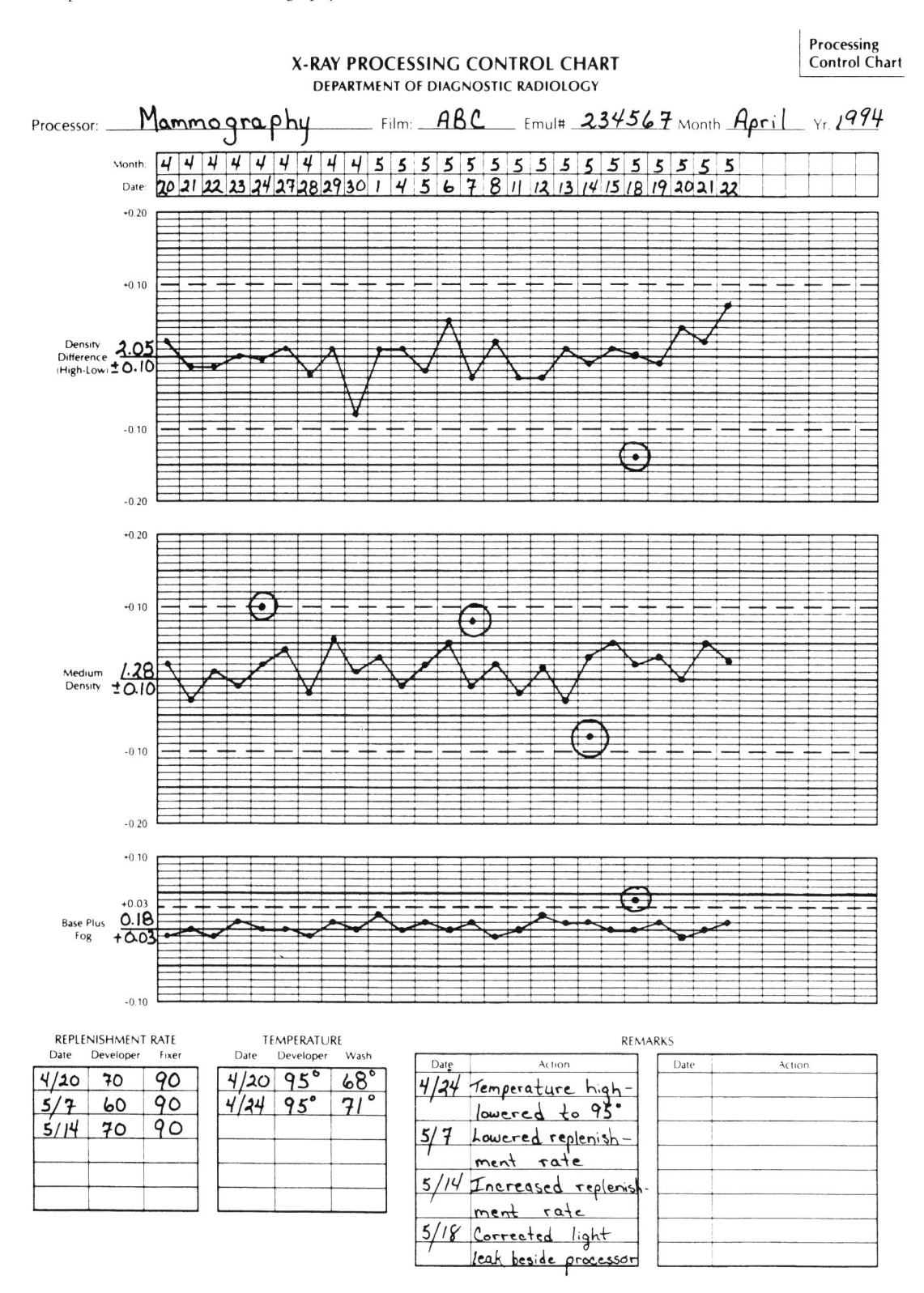

Fig. 3.16. Processor quality control form used as part of the ACR Mammography Accreditation Program. The chart shows typical data

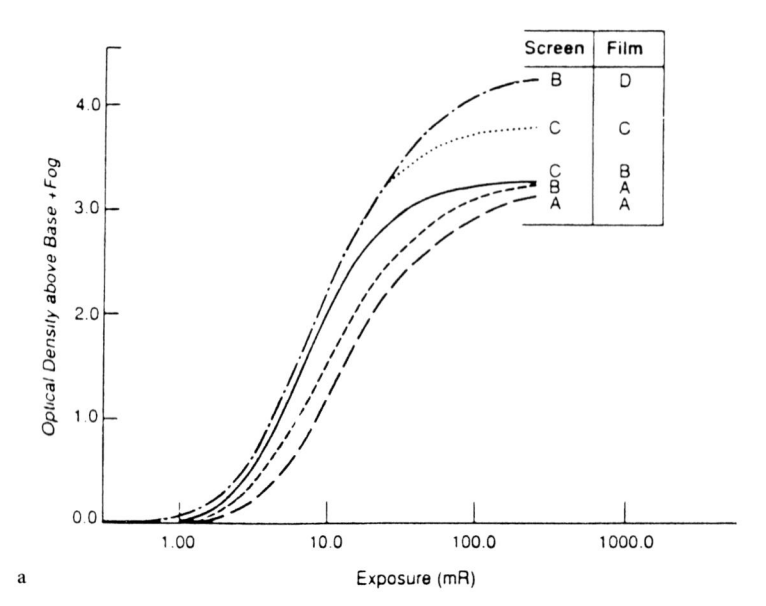

Fig. 3.17. a Typical characteristic curves of combinations of screens and films available for mammography. **b** Gradient vs optical density for the characteristic curves in a. (From AAPM 1990)

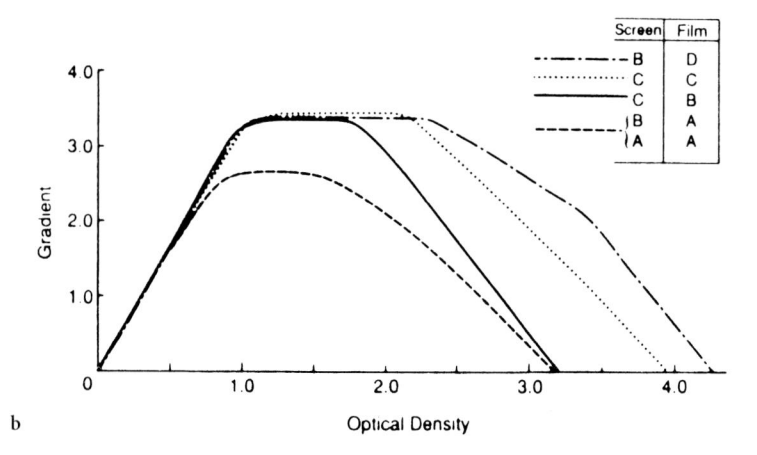

ments in the screen, and (d) screen-film contact (HAUS 1991). In recent years, screen-film combinations for mammography have utilized a single high-definition screen in contact with a single-emulsion film.

The single screen is used as a back screen for mammography because x-ray absorption (and emission of screen light) is highest on the side of the screen where the x-rays enter. If the screen were used as a front screen, x-ray absorption would be higher in the plane of the screen that is the farthest distance from the screen-emulsion contact surface (HAUS 1991, 1994). This causes greater light spread (blur) than when x-ray absorption is highest near the screen-emulsion contact surface, as is the case when it is used as a back screen. Both parallax and crossover are eliminated in a single-backscreen configuration.

Figure 3.18 shows MTF curves for a direct-exposure film and five mammographic screen-film combinations. Also shown is an MTF curve for a screen-film combination used for conventional diagnostic radiology procedures. These curves show that screen-film combinations used for mammography have much higher spatial resolution than do those used for conventional diagnostic procedures (SICKLES and WEBER 1986).

Analysis of the MTFs of the system components is helpful in determining which is the limiting factor controlling spatial resolution. In some situations the x-ray unit may be the major cause of image blur resulting from motion blur due to long exposure times, or geometric blur due to focal spot size and magnification (HAUS 1990, 1991, 1994; NCRP 1986). In these situations the higher speed, slightly less sharp mammographic screen-film combination may

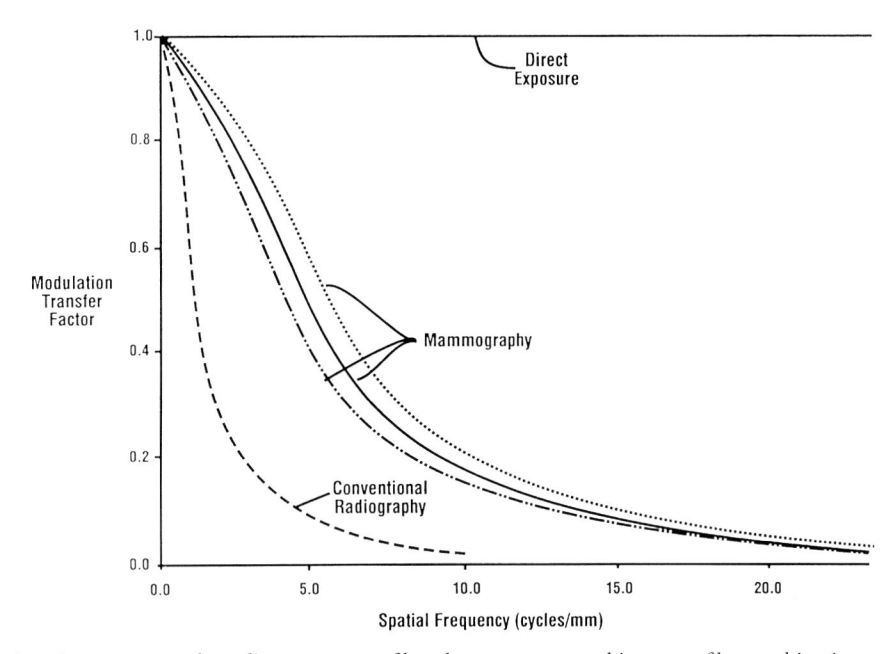

Fig. 3.18. Modulation transfer function curves are for a direct-exposure film, three mammographic screen-film combinations, and a two-screen, double-emulsion film combination commonly used for conventional radiography

Table 3.5. Typical mammographic screen-film characteristic

Screen	Film	Process	Relative speed[a]	Relative average glandular dose[b]	Contrast[c] (average gradient)	Typical limiting resolution[d] (cycles/mm)	Noise
1	1	Standard	100	0.10	2.9	21	Low
1	2	Extended	150	0.07	3.2	21	
2	1	Standard	160	0.06	2.9	19	
1	3	Standard	170	0.06	3.2	21	
2[e]	2	Extended	240	0.04	3.2	19	
2[e]	3	Standard	270	0.03	3.2	19	High

[a] Relative speed determined from matched-density radiographs. Kodak Min-R M film arbitrarily assigned a relative speed of 100
[b] Technique based on average-sized breast, craniocaudal view, molybdenum target tube, 0.03-mm molybdenum filter, 28 kVp setting
[c] Contrast measured as the average gradient between densities 0.25 and 2.00 above gross fog
[d] Limiting resolution based on 5% value of modulation transfer function
[e] Screen-film combination recommended for special applications such as magnification

produce mammograms with less overall image blur because shorter exposure times and/or a smaller focal spot size can be selected than is possible with lower speed high-resolution combinations. For example, a higher speed screen-film combination may be appropriate for magnification techniques (with which geometric blurring may be more limiting) to reduce exposure time (minimize motion blur) and to reduce radiation dose. Resolution has sometimes been specified in terms of the spatial frequency (line pairs per mm or cycles per mm) at which the MTF equals a certain value (e.g., 4% or 5% level) (Haus et al. 1979). Resolution values for several mammographic screen-film combinations determined from the 5% MTF level were between 19 and 21 cycles per mm (Table 3.5).

A simple method of demonstrating and evaluating blur in screen-film mammography is with a metal bar test object (Nuclear Associates, Carle Place, N.Y., USA) (Fig. 3.19) (HAUS 1985, 1994). Metal bar test objects are constructed in a linear array or in a star pattern array.

A line pair consists of one lead strip and one adjacent space of the same width. For example, 20 line pairs per mm (lp/mm) means that is each millimeter there are 20 metal strips (each one 0.025 mm wide) and 20 spaces (each one 0.025 mm wide) so that each line pair is 0.05 mm wide. It takes 20 of these pairs to fill a millimeter, so there are 20 lp/mm. A photograph of a metal bar resolution test object is shown in Fig. 3.19. Limiting resolution can be defined as the number of line pairs per mm, which can be visually identified in an image of a bar test object (Table 3.5) (HAUS 1985, 1994).

Limiting resolution is strongly affected by factors such as film contrast, noise, and blur. Experimental factors that can affect limiting resolution values for screen-film images of metal bar test objects include bar pattern thickness, kVp setting, and film contrast. Typical limiting values for mammographic screen-film combinations may range from approximately 15 to 20 line pairs per mm (Table 3.5).

Good screen-film contact is very important in screen-film mammography in order to minimize image blur across the mammographic image. A wire mesh test object is commonly used to evaluate screen-film contact. A recent study demonstrated that a wire mesh test object with approximately 40 wires per inch was more sensitive for detecting screen-film blur in mammographic cassettes than wire mesh test objects that are commonly used for checking conventional radiographic cassette-screen-film systems (MOUNT and GRAY 1990).

3.3.9 Radiographic Noise

Radiographic noise or mottle is the unwanted variation in random optical density in a radiograph that has been given a uniform x-ray exposure (HAUS 1991, 1994; NCRP 1986) (Fig. 3.20). Major sources of radiographic noise include: (a) quantum mottle, (b) screen structure, (c) film grain, (d) film processing artifacts, and (e) x-ray-to-light conversion noise (HAUS 1990, 1991, 1994; YAFFE 1990; BARNES 1982; AAPM 1990; NCRP 1986). Screen mottle is usually of negligible magnitude (HAUS 1976; NCRP 1986). Film granularity is caused by the random distribution of the finite number of developed silver halide grains (SCHUELFR et al. 1992; YAFFE 1990; BARNES 1982; AAPM 1990).

Quantum mottle is caused by the random spatial variation of the x-ray quanta absorbed in the image receptor. In general radiography, quantum mottle is usually the principal contributor to the optical density fluctuation seen in a uniformly exposed radiography. Factors affecting the perception of quantum mottle include: (a) film speed and contrast, (b) screen absorption and conversion efficiency, (c) light diffusion, and (d) radiation quality. When speed is increased due to increased x-ray absorption by the screen for a given film optical density, quantum mottle is not increased. When speed is increased due to increased light output of the screen per absorbed x-ray or increased film speed (faster film or increased developer temperature or time), fewer x-rays are used to form the image and, therefore, quantum mottle is increased.

In mammography, quantum mottle may not be the limiting factor governing noise because of the

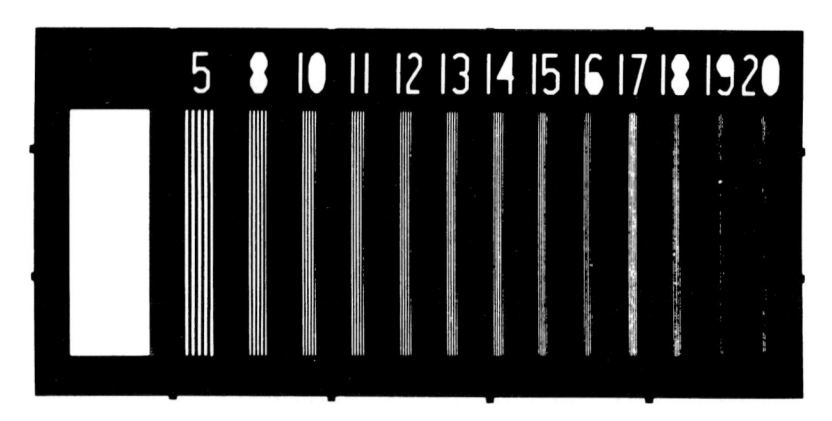

Fig. 3.19. X-ray resolution test pattern to determine limiting resolution value. This test pattern is capable of 20 lp/mm limiting resolution

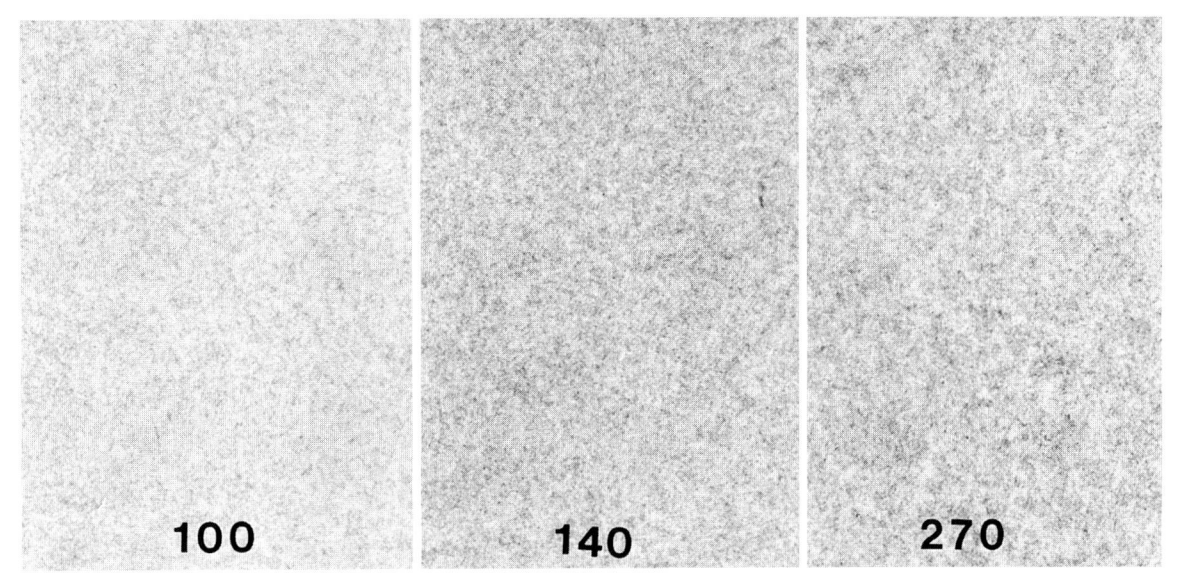

Fig. 3.20. Uniformly exposed radiographs using a 28-kVp setting demonstrate radiographic noise differences for mammographic screen-film combinations with relative speeds of 100, 140, and 270. The average gradients of these films are approximately 2.9, 3.2, and 3.21 respectively. These images were photographically magnified ×10. Note the appearance of increased noise as system speed increases. This noise increase is primarily due to quantum mottle; as the speed of the screen-film combination increases (and radiation dose decreases), fewer x-ray photons are involved in producing the mammographic image

high quantum efficiency (approximately 70%) of the screen, the low average energy of the photons, and the relatively low light emission in the screen (HAUS 1987, 1994; YAFFE 1990, AAPM 1990). In many cases, film granularity is a major noise source (BARNES 1982) and this is always the case at spatial frequencies higher than a few cycles per mm. This suggests that image quality might be improved by the use of finer grained film.

Higher speed mammographic screen-film combinations resulting in reduced radiation dose can be obtained by employing a higher speed screen and/or high speed film. Assuming all other factors are optimized, high speed systems are generally less sharp and/or present more noise than images produced using a conventional lower speed single-screen, single-emulsion combination (Table 3.5).

A limited number of publications include discussions on noise contributions for the many mammographic screen-film combinations available today. The basic description of system noise properties of screen-film combinations is the noise power spectrum (NPS). Figure 3.21 shows NPS data for two mammographic systems at simulated low kilovoltage conditions and for a general-purpose system at high kilovoltage.

3.3.10 Film Speed

The speed or sensitivity of a radiographic material is inversely related to the exposure required to produce a given effect (HAUS 1991, 1994; YAFFE 1990; SPRAWLS 1987; AAPM 1990). Speeds of radiographic films are often determined in terms of the reciprocal of the exposures required to produce a density of 1.0 above the base plus fog. Mammographic films have different sensitivities or relative speeds, as illustrated in Fig. 3.17 and Table 3.5.

Factors which influence film speed include: film type, type of screen light, film processing conditions, ambient conditions, reciprocity law failure, and latent image fading. Relative speeds and relative average glandular doses for several screen-film combinations for mammography are shown in Table 3.5.

3.3.10.1 Film Type

The compoisition of the film and the way it is manufactured affect film speed. The ingredients used in making the emulsion, the mammer in which they are treated and combined, and the technique by which

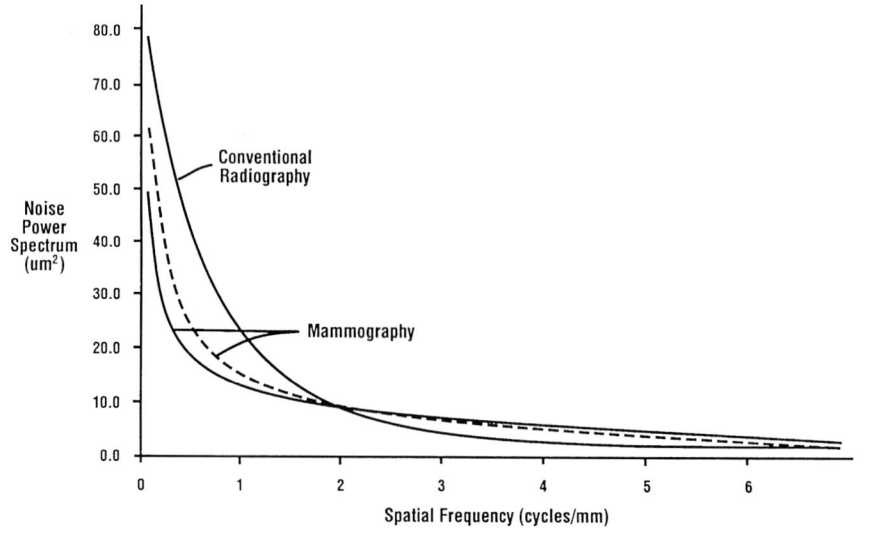

Fig. 3.21. Noise power spectrum data at an optical density of 1.0 for two screen-film combinations used for mammography (measured at 28 kVp) and a screen-film combination used in conventional radiography (measured at 70 kVp) (From HAUS 1990)

they are coated on the support all play a part in determining the sensitivity of the film.

3.3.10.2 Screen Type

Film emulsions are optically sensitized to cover the spectral emission range of the emitted screen light. It is most important that the spectral sensitivity of the film match the spectral emission of the screen in order to obtain appropriate film speed (Fig. 3.9). As an additional note, the color of light transmitted by safelight filters is selected to provide only wavelengths for which the film has little sensitivity.

3.3.10.3 Processing Conditions

Among the most important factors affectint film speed are the conditions used in processing the film after exposure. The chemical formulation of the solutions used, the way in which they are mixed and replenished, their temperatures, the manner in which they are agitated, the film's time of immersion in each, and washing and drying conditions all contribute to the film's speed and appearance.

3.3.10.4 Ambient Conditions

The film's sensitivity may also be affected by such factors as temperature, humidity, age, chemical fumes, and storage conditions. High temperatures, high humidity, and chemical contaminants in the atmosphere should be avoided insofar as possible. Protection from light leaks, exceesive safelight exposure, and x- and gamma radiation must also be provided.

3.3.10.5 Reciprocity Law Failure

The effect of reciprocity law failure can be important in screen-film mammography when long exposure times are used, because additional exposure may be required to compensate for reduced film speed. The definition given for exposure (Exposure = Intensity × Time) states that the response of the film to radiation of a given quality will be unchanged if the product of intensity and time remains the same. It is implied that this relationship remains constant, regardless of whether long or short exposure times are used, provided that time changes are compensated for by a proportional change in intensity. This relationship, also known as the reciprocity law, applies to direct exposure of film by x-rays; however, for exposure by screen-produced light, the law fails (JAMES 1977).

Reciprocity failure can be either high intensity or low intensity. High-intensity failure occurs when a large number of elextrons are produced in a short period of time. This can result in the formation of a greater number of initial latent image specks than would normally occur. Each individual center would be of smaller size than if fewer centers were formed.

These centers (greater in number but smaller in size) are less stable and the probability of their growing to a size suitable for developement is reduced. The result is the formation of less density as a function of exposure than might otherwise occur.

Low-intensity failure is a result of too small a number of light photons over an exposure time period. If the time period between two subsequently absorbed light photons is too long in the earliest stages of latent image formation, then the resulting metallic silver speck is of subcritical size and can regress back to a smaller than optimum size for growth and amplification by the developer. Again, less density is achieved than would normally occur as a function of exposure. Consideration of reciprocity law failure becomes increasingly important because techniques in screen-film mammography may necessitate the use of long exposure times due to: (a) use of grids, (b) use of small focal spots for conventional and magnification techniques (low mA settings), and (c) use of low-powered x-ray units with limited mA output settings. In mammography, reciprocity law failure may affect film density when long exposure times (approximately 1.0 s or longer) are used (HAUS 1994; HAUS et al. 1979; ARNOLD et al. 1978; ROSSI and HENDRICK 1985). When reciprocity law failure effects occur, additional exposure may be required in order to provide the proper optical density on the mammogram (Table 3.6). Some mammographic units have built-in features which compensate for loss of film speed due to reciprocity law failure using data (Table 3.6). There is very little change in film contrast due to film reciprocity law failure.

3.3.10.6 Latent Image Fading

If an exposure has been made on a film and processing is postponed for a relatively long time, the optical density obtained may be lower than if processing had immediately followed the exposure (HAUS 1994). This effect is called "latent image fading" (Table 3.7).

In screen-film mammography, film speed loss due to latent image fading can occur if the time between exposure and processing is delayed due to (a) transporting film from a van or mammography facility to a central location for film processing, or (b) batch processing films at the end of the day. In order to minimize latent image fading in the clinical environment, it is important that the time interval between exposure and processing be as consistent as possible from day to day. Ideally, films should be consistently processed as soon as possible after exposure. To minimize time interval differences, films should be processed in the order in which they are exposed. If films with slightly greater speed losses (due to latent image fading) are created and the time between exposure and processing is relatively long, the exposure technique can be adjusted on a one-time basis to obtain and maintain the appropriate density. If it is known in advance that processing will be delayed (for example, by more than 8 h), it may be advisable to increase exposure time (AEC setting) in order to obtain proper optical density in the mammogram. There is very little change in film contrast due to latent image fading.

For film processor quality control, it is recommended that film strips be processed immediately after exposure by the sensitometer to minimize the effects of latent image fading.

A recent study has shown that latent image fading is not accompanied by clinical impairment of mammographic interpretation if films are processed at the end of the workday (SICKLES 1995). Therefore, latent image fading should not deter the use of batch film processing.

Table 3.6. Example of reciprocity law failure data for a medical x-ray film[a]

Exposure time (s)	0.001	0.01	0.1	1	5	10
Percent film speed loss	6	0	0	12	30	38
Percent contrast change (average gradient)	0	0	0	2	3	4

[a] Speed: determined at a density of 1.00 above base plus fog
Average gradient: determined from the slope of the characteristic curve between densities of 0.25 and 2.00 above base plus fog

Table 3.7. Example of latent image keeping data for a medical x-ray film[a]

Time delay exposure for film processing (h)	0	4	8	24	48
Percent film speed loss	0	10	12	18	23
Optical density difference	0	0.12	0.15	0.21	0.27
Percent contrast change (average gradient)	0	2	3	3	5

[a] Speed: determined at a density of 1.00 above base plus fog
Average gradient: determined from the slope of the characteristic curve between densities of 0.25 and 2.00 above base plus fog

3.4 Radiation Dose

Factors which affect radiation dose include: (a) breast tissue composition and thickness; (b) x-ray tube target material, filtration, and kVp setting; (c) grid; (d) magnification; (e) screen-film combination, film processing; and (f) optical density level. In order to calculate the dose received during mammography using a specific technique, the exposure at the entrance surface of the breast must be known (ROTHENBERG et al. 1975; STANTON et al. 1984; NCRP 1986; AAPM 1990). The most straightforward measurement that can be made is that of the exposure (roentgens) received at the bottom of the cone or the compression device employed.

This exposure measurement can be made with an ionization chamber or with a thermoluminescent dosimeter. However, the importance of proper calibration to assure accurate results with either method cannot be overemphasized. The tube output for typical exposure conditions should be measured periodically for quality assurance and whenever significant changes are made in the mammographic unit (ROTHENBERG et al. 1975; HAMMERSTEIN et al. 1979; NCRP 1986; AAPM 1990). This measurement should be made by a qualified medical physicist or engineer.

Several years ago, it was common to use the exposure at the breast surface for comparison of various techniques (for example, changes in kilovoltage and filtration of the beam) and image receptors. Recent studies have shown that exposure at the surface of the breast is not the most appropriate parameter for comparison of such factors, or for comparison of the radiation risk associated with various mammographic x-ray techniques (HAMMERSTEIN et al. 1979; ROSENSTEIN et al. 1985; NCRP 1986). Absorbed dose (in rads) received by the glandular tissue below the skin surface is more pertinent than surface exposure because this is presumably the tissue at risk for the future development of cancer. Radiation dosage at a given depth depends on many factors: (a) the ratio of glandular to fatty tissue (b) the quality of the x-ray beam, (c) the area of the breast irradiated (port size), and (d) the exposure at the entrance surface of the breast. Several articles containing depth doses for the low-energy x-ray beams used in mammography have been published (STANTON et al. 1984; HAMMERSTEIN et al. 1979; ROSENSTEIN et al. 1985; WU et al. 1991; WHITE et al. 1977).

Midbreast dose has been used in several studies to estimate the risk of mammography. In these studies, the surface exposure was derived without consideration of beam quality or breast composition. More recently, mean and integral doses have been considered better estimates of risk from mammography because they include the effects of beam quality and breast composition (ROTHENBERG et al. 1975; HAMMERSTEIN et al. 1979; ROSENSTEIN et al. 1985; WU et al. 1991; WHITE et al. 1977; AAPM 1990).

The entrance skin exposure (in air) is measured using an ionization chamber. Average glandular dose per unit exposure in air for a 5-cm-thick average breast is calculated using the appropriate conversion factors (Table 3.8) (ROTHENBERG et al. 1975; STANTON et al. 1984; HAMMERSTEIN et al. 1979; ROSENSTEIN et al. 1985; WU et al. 1991; NCRP 1986; AAPM 1990).

The ACR Mammography Accreditation Program requires that the mean glandular dose for a 4.5-cm-thick breast phantom image for screen-film mammography be less than 3 mGy (0.3 rads). The average mean glandulr dose for a screen-film image with grid is 1.27 mGy (0.127 rads). It is important to note that if the radiation dose is too low, mammographic image quality may be compromised.

Table 3.8. Example of average glandular dose calculation for screen-film combination

Half-value layer (mm aluminum)	Average glandular dose/radiation in air (rad/R)	Radiation in air (R)	Average glandular dose (rad)[a]
0.31	0.14	0.80	0.112

Note: Dose calculation based on recommendations in HAUS (1994) and VYBORNY and SCHMIDT (1990). Data based on breast phantom that is 5 cm thick (ROTHENBERG et al. 1975)
[a] Calculated as (average glandular dose/radiation in air) × radiation in air. Data also presented in centigrays

References

AAPM (1990) AAPM report no. 29. Equipment requirements and quality control for mammography. American Institute of Physics, New York

Aichinger H, Arnann E, Joite S (1988) Automatic exposure control system in mammography: a new answer to the NCRP report 85 (abstract). Radiology 169:158–159

Arnold BA, Eisenberg H, Bjarngard BE (1978) Measurement of reciprocity law failure in green sensitive x-ray films. Radiology 126:493–498

Barnes GT (1982) Radiographic mottle: a comprehensive theory. Med Phys 56:667

Barnes GT, Brezovich IA (1978) The intensity of scattered radiation in mammography. Radiology 126:243–247

Chan HP, Frank PH, Doi K, Iida N, Higashida Y (1985) Development of ultra-high strip density (UHSD) grids: a new anti-scatter technique for mammography. Radiology 154:807–815

Doi K (1977) Advantages of magnification radiography. In: Logan WW (ed) Breast carcinoma: the radiologist's expanded role. Wiley, New York, pp 93–108

Eastman Kodak Company Technical Report 0997 (1986) Eastman Kodak Company, Rochester, NY

Egan RL (1976) Mammographic image quality and exposure levels using conventional generator and type m film. In: Application of optical instrumentation in medicine IV. Proc Soc Photo-Opt Instrum Engineers 70:393–397

Fewell TR, Shuping RE (1978) Handbook of mammographic x-ray spectra. HEW Publication (FDA) 79–8071

Hammerstein GR, Miller DW, White DR, et al. (1979) Absorbed radiation dose in mammography. Radiology 130:485–491

Haus AG (1983) Physical principles and radiation dose in mammography. In: Feig SA, McLelland R (eds) Breast carcinoma: current diagnosis and treatment. Masson, New York, pp 9–114

Haus AG (1985) Evaluation of image blur (unsharpness) in medical imaging. Med Radiogr Photogr 61:42–53

Haus AG (1978) Recent advances in screen-film mammography. Radiol Clin North Am 25:913–928

Haus AG (1990) Technologic improvements in screen-film mammography. Radiology 174:628–637

Haus AG (1991) State of the art screen-film mammography: a technical overview. In: Barnes GT, Frey DG (eds) Screen-film mammography: imaging considerations and medical physics responsibilities. Medical Physics Publishing, Madison, Wis., pp 1–46

Haus AG (1994) Screen-film image receptors and film processing. In: Haus AG, Yaffe MJ (eds) A categorical course in physics: technical aspects of breast imaging syllabus. Radiological Society of North America, Oak Brook, Ill., pp 85–101

Haus AG, Metz CE, Chiles JY, et al. (1976) The effects of x-ray spectra from molybdenum and tungsten target tubes on image quality in mammography. Radiology 118:705

Haus AG, Cowart RW, Dodd GD, et al. (1978) A method of evaluation and minimizing geometric unsharpness for mammographic x-ray units. Radiology 128:775–778

Haus AG, Paulus DD, Dodd GD, et al. (1979) Magnification mammography: evaluation of screen film and xeroradiographic techniques. Radiology 133:223–226

Haus AG, Batz TA, Dickerson RE, et al. (1993) Automatic film processing in medical imaging. In: Siebert JA, Barnes GT, Gould RG (eds) Specification acceptance testing and quality control of diagnostic x-ray imaging equipment. American Institute of Physics, New York, pp 383–412

James TH (ed) (1977) The theory of the photographic process, 4th edn. Macmillan, New York

Jennings RJ, Eastgate RJ, Sieband MP (1981) Optimal x-ray spectra for screen-film mammography. Med Phys 8:629–639

Kimme-Smith C (1991) Mammography screen-film selection, film exposure and processing. In: Barnes GT, Frey DG (eds) Screen film mammography: imaging considerations and medical physics responsibilities. Madison, Wis: Medical Physics Publishing, Madison, Wis., pp 135–158

Kimme-Smith C, Bassett LW, Gold RH (1988) Focal spot measurements with pin hold and slit for microfocus mammography units. Med Phys 15:293–298

Kimme-Smith C, Rothchild PA, Bassett LW, Gold RH, Moler C (1989) Mammographic film processor temperature, development time, and chemistry: effect on dose, contrast and noise. AJR 152:35–40

LaFrance RL, Gelskey DE, Barnes GT (1988) A circuit modification that improves mammographic phototimer performance. Radiology 166:773–776

Mount CJ, Gray JE (1990) Mammography screen-film contact: problems with conventional screen-film contact setting. Radiographcs 10:1049–1054

NCRP (1986) NCRP Report 85. Mammography – a user's guide. National Council of Radiation Protection and Measurements, Bethesda, Md

Nielson B, Fagerberg G (1986) Image quality in mammography with special reference to anti scatter grids and the magnification technique. Acta Radiol 27:467–479

Ostrum BJ, Becker W, Isard HJ (1973) Low-dose mammography. Radiology 109:323–326

Rosenstein M, Andersen LW, Warner GG (1985) Handbook of glandular tissue doses in mammography. HHS publication FFDA 85-8239. US Department of Health and Human Services, Rockville, Md

Rossi RP, Hendrick RE (1985) Performance evaluation of a new dedicated mammographic system. Medical Imaging and Instrumentation 85 Proc SPIE 555:116–126

Rothenberg LN, Kirch RLA, Snyder RE (1975) Patient exposures from film and xeroradiographic mammographic techniques. Radiology 117:701–703

Schueler BA, Gray JE, Gisvold JJ (1992) A comparison of mammographic screen-film combinations. Radiology 184:629–634

Sickles EA (1995) Latent image fading is screen-film mammography: lack of clinical relevance for batch-processed films. Radiology 194:389–392

Sickles EA, Weber WN (1986) High-contrast mammography with a moving grid: assessment of clinical utility. AJR 146:1137–1139

Sickles EA, Doi K, Genant HK (1977) Magnification film mammography: image quality and clinical studies. Radiology 125:69–76

Sprawls P (1987) The physical principles of medical imaging. Aspen, Rockville, Md

Stanton L, Villafana T, Day JL, et al. (1984) Dose evaluation in mammography. Radiology 150:577–584

Tabár L, Dean PB (1984) Teaching atlas of mammography. Thieme, Stuttgart

Tabár L, Haus AG (1989) Processing mammographic films: technical and clinical considerations. Radiogy 173:65–69

Vyborny C, Schmidt RA (1990) Mammography as a radiographic examination an overview. Radiographics 9:723–764

Wayrynen RE (1979) Fundamental aspects of mammographic receptors. Film process. In: Logan WW, Muntz EP (eds) Reduced dose mammography. Masson, New York, pp 521–528

White DR, Martin RJ, Darlison R (1977) Epoxy resin based tissue substitutes. Br J Radiol 50:814–821

Wu X, Barnes GT, Tucker DM (1991) Spectral dependence of glandular tissue dose in screen film mammography. Radiology 179:143–148

Yaffe MJ (1990) Physics of mammography: image recording process. Radiographics 10:341–363

Yester MV, Barnes GT, King MA (1981) Experimental measuremnts of the scatter reduction obtained in mammography with a scanning multiple slit assembly. Med Phys 8:158–162

4 Current Legislation on Mammography Quality Assurance

R.E. Hendrick

CONTENTS

4.1 Introduction 57
4.2 Quality Legislation 57
4.3 MQSA Requirements 59
4.4 MQSA Interim Rules 60
4.4.1 Personnel Requirements 60
4.4.2 Equipment Requirements 61
4.4.3 Dose Requirements 61
4.4.4 Quality Assurance 61
4.4.5 Medical Records 62
4.4.6 Accrediting Body Requirements 62
4.5 The Impact of MQSA 62
 References 63

4.1 Introduction

Legislation on mammography in the United States has taken two forms: legislation on reimbursement for mammography and legislation on the quality of mammography. Legislation has been passed federally and in most states on these two issues (Fintor et al. 1995; McKinney et al. 1992).

The purpose of legislation on reimbursement is to ensure that age-eligible women have access to screening mammography. Most legislation requires third-party payors to cover screening mammography, or to offer mammography coverage as an optional benefit to age-appropriate asymptomatic women (McKinney and Marconi 1992). Such legislation began with the state of Maryland requiring Medicare Supplementary Insurers to cover screening mammography. Table 4.1 summarizes legislative activity through the end of 1993 on mandated coverage of screening mammography. By the end of 1993, 44 states and the District of Columbia had passed such legislation.

Prior to 1991, the Medicare federal health insurance program provided coverage to Medicare-eligible women for diagnostic, but not screening, mammography. Beginning 1 January 1991, the Omnibus Budget Reconciliation Act of 1990 (Public Law 101-508) extended Medicare coverage to screening mammography of asymptomatic Medicare-eligible women: the 17 million women aged 65 and over were covered for biennial screening and approximately 1.5 million disabled women aged 35–64 were covered for biennial screening (under age 50) or annual screening (ages 50–64), with reimbursement of up to $55 for each screening mammography (Medicare Coverage of Screening Mammography 1990).

The Breast and Cervical Cancer Mortality Prevention Act (Public Law 101-354) was also passed in 1990, providing federal funding for qualifying states to provide screening services to low-income women for the early detection of breast and cervical cancer. To qualify, states had to match federal contributions to the screening programs. Four states were funded under the program in 1991, ten states in 1992. In 1995, 35 states were providing screening services to low-income women through this federally funded program, with all 15 other states receiving funding to provide screening services in the future.

4.2 Quality Legislation

Legislation on the quality of mammography began with quality standards accompanying the Maryland reimbursement legislation in 1986 (Table 4.2). Other states enacted quality standards following Maryland, most standards being based largely on the technical requirements of the American College of Radiology's Mammography Accreditation Program (ACR MAP), which was established in 1987 (Hendrick et al. 1987; McLelland et al. 1991). By the end of 1993, 41 states and the District of Columbia had passed legislation or established regulations on the quality of mammography (Fintor et al. 1995). Figure 4.1 summarizes the requirements established in each state in the general categories of equipment specifications (E), radiation exposure or dose limits (R), facility

---

R.E. Hendrick, PhD, Associate Professor and Chief, Division of Radiological Sciences, Department of Radiology, C278, University of Colorado Health Sciences Center, 4200 E. 9th Avenue, Denver, CO 80262, USA

Table 4.1. Legislation on reimbursement for mammography

1986 – State of Maryland passes legislation mandating inclusion of screening mammography as a health benefit to women covered by Medicare Supplemental Insurance
1990 – Federal Omnibus Budget Reconciliation Act provides Medicare coverage of screening mammography for women 65 and over and for disabled women over 35
   – Federal Breast and Cervical Cancer Mortality Prevention Act of 1990 provides funding for mammography screening of age-eligible indigent women
1993 – 44 states and the District of Columbia have passed legislation mandating insurance coverage of screening mammography

Table 4.2. Legislation on quality of mammography

1986 – State of Maryland passes legislation requiring mammography x-ray equipment to be dedicated
1990 – Quality standards mandated for Medicare screening sites and published as Interim Final Rules for screening mammography
1992 – Mammography Quality Standards Act passed requiring all mammography in the United States to meet minimum quality standards
1993 – Forty-one states and the District of Columbia have passed legislation mandating quality standards for mammography

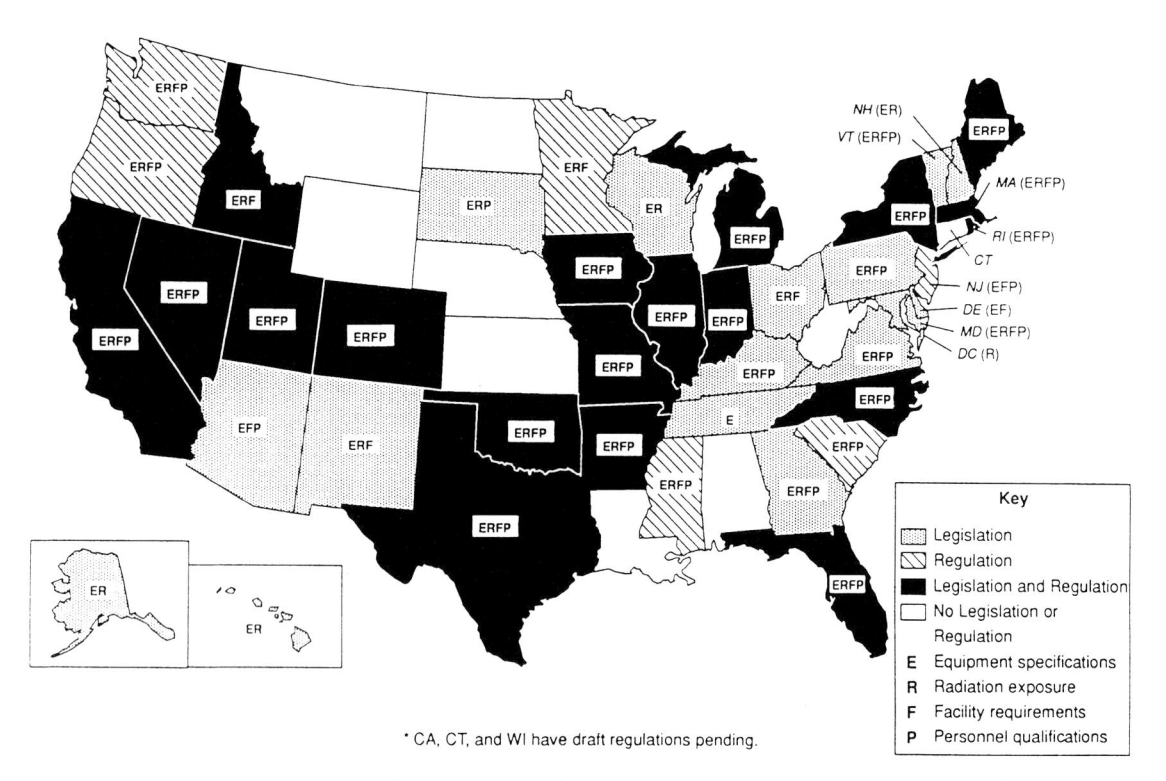

Fig. 4.1. States with mammography quality assurance legislation and/or regulation (as of December 1993). (From FINTOR et al. 1995)

requirements (F), and personnel requirements (P).

All 41 states with equipment requirements specify that only dedicated equipment should be used for mammography, but most differ on specific additional requirements (FINTOR et al. 1995). State-legislated equipment requirements range from simply requiring dedicated equipment (in eight states) to specifying most aspects of the x-ray system, including the tube target material, filter material, focal spot size, collimation, compression device, grid capability, and automatic exposure control.

Dose requirements vary considerably among the 38 states that have breast exposure or dose limits (FINTOR et al. 1995). The most common dose requirement is that average glandular dose to a 4.5-cm breast be less than or equal to 1 mGy for nongrid screen-film image receptors, less than or equal to 3 mGy for grid screen-film image receptors, and less than or equal to 4 mGy for xeromammographic image receptors.

Thirty-eight states have facility requirements consisting primarily of quality assurance measures such as maintaining an ongoing quality control (QC) program, evaluating clinical images, and monitoring repeat mammograms. Specific requirements, however, vary considerably among states (FINTOR et al. 1995).

Personnel requirements also vary considerably among states, with 36 states requiring licensure or certification of radiologic technologists performing mammography (FINTOR et al. 1995). Twenty-one states have interpreting physician qualification requirements, and approximately one-third of states have medical physicist requirements for mammography, although requirements differ from state to state.

National mammography quality requirements were first defined through the voluntary ACR MAP (HENDRICK et al. 1987). These quality standards served as the model for the quality standards required of Medicare screening sites in Medicare's Interim Final Rules (MCKINNEY and MARCONI 1992), published in late 1990, and the Mammography Quality Standards Act (MQSA) Interim Rules (21 CFR Part 900 1993), published in early 1993 (Table 4.2). MQSA Interim Rules have now superseded Medicare quality standards and Medicare inspections of mammography facilities have been replaced by MQSA inspections. Medicare recognizes MQSA certification as demonstration that a facility meets quality standards and qualifies to receive Medicare reimbursement for screening mammography performed on Medicare-eligible women. Because MQSA requirements have superseded other national quality standards, attention in this chapter will be focused on MQSA Interim Rule requirements.

4.3 MQSA Requirements

The cornerstone of the Mammography Quality Standards Act of 1992 (Public Law 102-539) is that every mammography facility must become accredited by an approved accrediting body within 6 months of entry into the program. The process of MQSA certification begins when a facility applies for accreditation from an FDA-approved accrediting body. The name of the applicant facility is transmitted by the accrediting body to the FDA and, while the facility is in the application process, the FDA grants provisional certification to the facility for a period of up to 6 months. Once accreditation is granted to a facility, the FDA confers full certification for a period of 3 years, with FDA certification expiring 30 days after the facility's accreditation expires. A provisionally certified facility that fails to become accredited within the provisional 6-month period must cease performance of mammography. While no mechanism was written into MQSA legislation to allow facilities to reapply for certification after initial failure, the FDA has developed a process for facilities that are proceeding in good faith to correct deficiencies. Facilities that fail must cease performance of mammography and must submit a plan of corrective action to their accrediting body. If the accrediting body finds the plan of corrective action acceptable, the facility may resume performing mammography for another 6-month period of provisional certification.

Currently, the American College of Radiology is the only organization approved by the FDA to accredit mammography facilities nationally. Three states (Arkansas, California, and Iowa) also have been approved to accredit facilities within their own states. California has passed a state law that requires facilities to pass the California accreditation program. In Arkansas and Iowa, facilities may apply either to the state or to the American College of Radiology for accreditation.

A second key element of MQSA is that each facility performing mammography must meet MQSA quality standards. Quality standards include performance of regular QC testing by a radiologic technologist and a medical physicist according to either the 1992 or the 1994 version of the ACR Mammography QC Manuals, which have been adopted by reference in the Interim Rules. Quality standards also include requirements on equipment, personnel film retention, and follow-up of positive mammograms (21 CFR Part 900 1993).

MQSA Interim Rules were published in the *Federal Register* in December 1993, were adopted on 22 February 1994, and went into effect as minimum standards for mammography on 1 October 1994. It will be at least 1997 before Final Rules for MQSA, which will supersede the Interim Rules, are put into effect. Proposed Final Rules have not yet been published, but are likely to appear in the *Federal Register* in late 1995.

A third key element of MQSA is that each mammography facility must undergo annual inspection by an MQSA inspector. Inspections consist of physical testing performed on each mammography unit (Table 4.3) and an extensive review of records, including the facilities' records on the quality assurance (QA) program (including assigned QA/QC responsibilities), radiologic technologist's QC results, medical physicist's QC report, personnel qualifications, medical records and

Table 4.3. Physical tests performed by MQSA inspectors

Collimation assessment:
  Alignment of x-ray field with image receptor
  Compression paddle alignment
Entrance skin exposure
Exposure reproducibility test
Exposure linearity test
Half-value layer (HVL) measurement
Processing Speed (S.T.E.P.) Test
Darkroom fog test
Phantom image quality evaluation

report policies, and the medical audit and outcome analysis.

MQSA inspectors are employed by their state's radiation control program. The FDA contracts with each state radiation control program to conduct inspections on behalf of MQSA, providing up to 6 weeks' training for inspectors. If the state has inspection requirements that go beyond MQSA requirements, the inspector will conduct both state and MQSA inspections on the same visit. One of the goals of MQSA was to unify state and federal inspections of mammography facilities to minimize repeated inspections of the same facility.

Unlike Medicare, where inspections were federally funded, MQSA inspections are funded through fees charged to inspected facilities. The FDA has determined that uniform fees will be charged throughout the United States for MQSA inspections. Current fees are set at $1178 for a mammography facility with a single unit, plus $152 for each additional mammography unit (21 CFR Part 900 1993). If reinspection is required, an additional fee of $670 is charged to the facility.

For purposes of inspection fees under MQSA, a "facility" is defined as a single address. Practices owning units at different addresses will have to pay separate inspection fees (of at least $1178 for each facility). Although all government entities except Veterans Health Administration facilities are required to meet MQSA requirements and undergo annual inspections, MQSA exempts *all government entities* from payment of inspection fees. Government entities exempt from paying inspection fees include facilities "operated by any Federal department, State, district, territory, possession, Federally-recognized Indian tribe, city, county, town, village, municipal corporation, or similar political organization or subpart thereof" (Inspection Fees to be Assessed During FY '95 1995). Also exempt from inspection fees are nongovernment facilities that provide screening under the Breast and Cervical Cancer Mortality Prevention Act of 1990, where at least 50% of the mammography screening examinations provided during the previous 12 months were funded under that statute.

4.4 MQSA Interim Rules

MQSA Interim Rules include facility requirements for personnel, equipment, radiation dose, quality assurance (including quality control), and medical records. Interim Rules also specify requirements for accrediting bodies. Below is a summary of MQSA requirements adapted from the Interim Rules (21 CFR 900 1993).

4.4.1 Personnel Requirements

Personnel requirements include qualifications, experience, and continuing medical education requirements for interpreting physicians, radiologic technologists, and medical physicists in mammography.

Interpreting physicians are required to be licensed to practice medicine in the state or facility and to be board certified by an FDA-approved certifying body or to have had at least 2 months of documented full-time training in the interpretation of mammograms, including instruction in radiation physics, radiation effects, and radiation protection. Currently, the American Board of Radiology, the American Osteopathic Board of Radiology, and the Canadian Royal College of Physicians and Surgeons are approved certification bodies. In addition, physicians interpreting mammograms must have at least 40 h of continuing medical education in mammography (time spent in residency specifically in mammography will be accepted if documented in writing by the radiologist), must have interpreted the mammograms of at least 240 patients in the 6 months preceding application, must continue to interpret the mammograms of at least 40 patients per month over 24 months, and must teach or complete an average of at least 5 h of continuing medical education in mammography per year. The requirements of a medical license and board certification or demonstration of meeting alternative criteria must be documented at the mammography site. The additional requirements of education and experience, if obtained before 1 October 1994, may be documented by self-attestation of the interpreting physician. Specific forms are provided by the FDA for self-attestation.

Radiologic technologists performing mammography are required to have a license to perform radiographic procedures in the state or facility where they are practicing or to have certification by one of the bodies approved by the FDA to certify radiologic technologists (currently, the American Registry of Radiologic Technologists is the only approved certifying body for radiologic technologists). In addition, radiologic technologists associated with facilities applying for accreditation before 1 October 1996 must have undergone training specific to mammography, through either a training curriculum or special mammography course, or have at least 1 year of experience in mammography and obtain special training by 1 October 1996. For facilities applying for accreditation on or after 1 October 1996, radiologic technologists must have undergone specific training in mammography through documented curriculum and on-the-job training under the direct supervision of experienced mammographers. All radiologic technologists performing mammography must also accumulate an average of at least five continuing education units (CEUs) in mammography per year.

Medical physicists performing mammography surveys and overseeing QC programs at mammography facilities must either (1) have a license or approval by a state to conduct evaluations of mammography equipment, or (2) have certification in an accepted specialty area by one of the bodies approved by the FDA to certify medical physicists (currently the American Board of Radiology in Radiological Physics or Diagnostic Radiological Physics or the American Board of Medical Physics in Medical Imaging Physics), or (3), for medical physicists associated with facilities applying for accreditation before 27 October 1997, meet each of the following criteria: (a) have a masters or higher degree in physics, radiological physics, applied physics, biophysics, health physics, medical physics, engineering, radiation science, or public health with a bachelor's degree in the physical sciences, (b) have at least 1 year of training in medical physics specific to diagnostic radiologic physics, and (c) have at least 2 years of experience in performing evaluations of mammography equipment. Medical physicists performing mammography surveys must teach or complete an average of at least 5h of CME in mammography per year.

4.4.2 Equipment Requirements

X-ray equipment used for mammography shall be specifically designed for mammography, have a breast compression device, and be able to operate with a removable grid (except for xeromammography systems).

4.4.3 Dose Requirements

The average glandular dose due to a single craniocaudal view of an accepted phantom (the RMI-156 or Nuclear Associates 18-220 Mammographic Phantom) simulating a 4.5-cm-thick, 50% glandular, 50% adipose compressed breast shall not exceed 3.0 mGy (0.3 rad) per exposure for screen-film and 4.0 mGy (0.4 rad) per exposure for xeromammography image receptors.

4.4.4 Quality Assurance

Each facility is required to establish and maintain a quality assurance (QA) program to assure adequate performance of equipment, assuring "reliability and clarity of mammograms" and periodic monitoring of dose (21 CFR Part 900 1993). For screen-film systems, the quality assurance program should be substantially the same as that described in the ACR Mammography QC Manuals 1992 or 1994 edition (American College of Radiology 1994). For alternate image receptor systems (xerography or digital, for example), the facility should follow the quality assurance program recommended by the image receptor manufacturer. Log books should be maintained documenting compliance with quality assurance (QA) requirements and corrective actions taken.

Phantom images should be taken and assessed using a phantom approved by the ACR or an equivalent type accepted by the FDA. Although a minimum frequency is not stated in the Interim Rules, the ACR Mammography QC Manuals call for at least monthly phantom images. The phantom images must meet at least the minimum score required by the accrediting body.

A quality assurance program for clinical images must be established to monitor mammograms repeated due to poor image quality and to maintain results and remedial actions taken.

Clinical image interpretation must be monitored by establishing a system for collection and review of outcome data, including follow-up on the disposition of positive mammograms and correlation of surgical biopsy results with mammography results.

Each facility shall have a medical physicist establish, monitor, and direct the quality assurance procedures described above and perform a survey of the facility to assure that it meets equipment and QC standards. Such surveys shall be performed at least annually, with a copy of the survey report transmitted to the accrediting body and another copy retained by the facility until receipt of the next annual survey report.

4.4.5 Medical Records

Each facility shall retain mammograms and associated records for a period of not less than 5 years, or not less than 10 years if no additional mammograms of the examinee are performed at the facility, or longer if mandated by state or local law, or until requested by the examinee to permanently transfer the records to a medical institution, the examinee's physician, or the examinee herself, and the records are so transferred.

Each facility shall prepare a written report of the results of any mammography examination, completed as soon as possible, and signed by the interpreting physician. The report must be provided to the examinee's physician, if any. If the examinee does not have a physician or the physician is not available, the report shall be sent directly to the examinee, and shall include a summary written in language easily understood by a lay person. The report and communications shall be maintained in the patient's record for at least the time periods stated above.

4.4.6 Accrediting Body Requirements

Under MQSA, potential accrediting bodies are limited to private, nonprofit organizations or state agencies. To receive FDA approval, accrediting bodies must require each facility they accredit to meet the standards stated in Sects. 4.4.1–4.4.5 above. In addition, accrediting bodies must be updated annually by accredited facilities on the information listed above.

Accrediting bodies must review clinical images from each facility they accredit at least once every 3 years, along with a random sample of clinical images from accredited facilities in each 3-year period. No conflict of interest may exist between qualified physicians conducting clinical image reviews and reviewed facilities.

The FDA requires fees charged by accrediting bodies to be reasonable, usually limiting fees to actual costs plus overhead expenses.

Accrediting bodies must receive and review an annual medical physicist's report and QC records from each facility they accredit. If the results of the survey create doubt as to the quality of clinical images produced by the facility, the accrediting body is required to investigate by examining recent clinical images from the facility.

The accrediting body shall conduct on-site inspections of a sufficient number of its accredited facilities to assess overall compliance with accrediting body standards and to assess the quality of mammography at accredited facilities.

The accrediting body shall require all facilities it accredits to publish an address where complaints about the facility can be filed with the accrediting body. The accrediting body is required to investigate each complaint within 90 days of receipt, and shall maintain records of all complaints for a period of 3 years from completion of the investigation.

The accrediting body is required to report to the FDA names of any facilities for which the accrediting body denies, suspends, or revokes accreditation, and the basis for the action, within 48 h of the action. The accrediting body must also report to the FDA receipts of applications for accreditation, successful completion of accreditation, and other requested information within 5 working days.

The FDA will evaluate annually the performance of each approved accrediting body by inspecting a sample of facilities accredited by the body, by evaluating inspection reports, and by evaluating a sample of the accrediting body's clinical and phantom image reviews, examining speed and efficiency in accrediting facilities, filing reports, and keeping records.

4.5 The Impact of MQSA

While it may be too soon to assess the full impact of MQSA, it may be possible to predict some of the impact of this legislation.

In passing MQSA, the clear intention of Congress was, as the bill Report states, to establish "uniform quality standards for mammography." That goal is not likely to be achieved. While the bill establishes uniform *minimum* requirements, it permits states to maintain or add to MQSA whatever requirements they see fit. Fox example, California has added the requirements that facilities be accredited by the California accreditation program, pass tighter dose standards for film-screen mammography with a grid (<2 mGy per view) than those of MQSA, and meet additional on-site inspection and documentation requirements beyond those of MQSA.

It also remains to be seen whether accreditation standards will be "substantially equivalent" among different approved accrediting bodies. For example, among facilities undergoing review by the ACR MAP between 1 October 1994 and 1 August 1995, the first-round failure rate was 35% and the final overall failure rate was approximately 5%. Among facilities applying to the Iowa accreditation program, the first-round failure rate was 15% and the final failure rate 0%, and among facilities applying to the Arkansas accreditation program, the initial failure rate was 69% and the final failure rate 2.5%. These figures suggest that standards may vary among accreditation bodies.

Two likely effects of MQSA are to increase the overall cost of mammography and to decrease the number of facilities providing mammography. The addition of an annual $1178 inspection fee per facility having a single mammography unit, plus additional fees for additional units and reinspections, if needed, is likely to cause some facilities to discontinue mammography, while other facilities are likely to try to increase charges to women undergoing mammography to cover the added costs of inspections. Most facilities, however, operate with fixed reimbursement for mammography by Medicare, HMOs, and other third-party payors, making the recovery of added costs difficult or impossible. There are also additional costs to facilities in preparing for, undergoing, and responding to MQSA inspections, which may have an additional impact on the ability of mammography sites to remain cost-effective.

It is hoped that MQSA will improve the overall quality of mammography. That, in turn, should lead to earlier detection, fewer missed breast cancers, and improved outcomes for women who have breast cancer. It should also lead to fewer false-positives and fewer additional procedures triggered by mammography among women who do not have breast cancer.

Data to monitor the effect of MQSA on the quality of mammography will not be collected under MQSA, but will have to come from individual facilities that voluntarily collect and present mammography outcome data. Such data may also come from the National Breast Cancer Consortium, a collection of mammography surveillance programs funded by the NCI as stipulated by MQSA legislation. Even with such data, it will be a difficult task to accurately assess the beneficial effects of MQSA on mammography, separating improvements due to the program from the improvements in mammography that would have occurred without MQSA. Only time and good data collection will tell whether MQSA has had its intended effect of improving the quality of mammography, without adversely affecting the cost and availability of mammography in the United States.

References

American College of Radiology mammography quality control manual (revised edition) (1994) American College of Radiology, Reston, VA
21 CFR Part 900 (1993) Mammography facilities – requirements for accrediting bodies and quality standards and certification requirements; interim rules. Federal Register 58 (no. 243):67558–67572
Fintor L, Haenlein M, Fischer R (1995) Legislative and regulatory mandates for mammography quality assurance. J Public Health Policy 16:81–107
Hendrick RE, Haus AG, Hubbard LB, et al. (1987) American College of Radiology accreditation program for mammographic screening sites: physical evaluation criteria. Radiology 165(P):209
Inspection fees to be assessed during FY '95 (1995) Federal Register 60 (no. 52):14585–14586
McKinney MM, Marconi KM (1992) Legislative interventions to increase access to screening mammography. J Community Health 17:333–349
McLelland R, Hendrick RE, Zinninger MD, Wilcox PW (1991) The American College of Radiology mammography accreditation program. Am J Roentgenol 157:473–479
Medicare Coverage of Screening Mammography, Interim Final Rules with Comment (1990) Federal Register 55:53510–53525

5 Digital Mammography

J.-W. Oestmann

CONTENTS

5.1 Introduction 65
5.2 Basic Principles of Digital X-ray Mammography ... 66
5.3 The Issue of Spatial Resolution 66
5.4 The Potential of Image Postprocessing 67
5.5 Computer-Assisted Detection 68
5.6 Commercial Digital Mammography Systems 69
5.6.1 Storage Phosphor Systems 70
5.6.2 Charge Coupled Device-Based Systems 70
5.7 Conclusion and Outlook 72
      References 72

5.1 Introduction

The prognosis for patients with breast cancer is closely related to the size and stage of the lesion at the time of diagnosis. For this reason, any technological improvement that holds promise to detect breast cancers of smaller size and at an earlier stage must be closely scrutinized. Despite improvements in ultrasound and contrast-enhanced magnetic resonance imaging of the breast, x-ray mammography maintains its role as the method of choice to screen asymptomatic women to detect early-stage breast cancer (Feig 1994; Vogel 1994). The effectiveness of mammography in detecting early disease correlates closely with the image quality achieved with the specific system. Digital systems intended for mammography must thus equal the quality requirements established for conventional film-screen systems and offer significant advantages that alleviate existing shortcomings. The rapid retrieval of archived images in a digital picture archival and communications system (PACS) could be one of these improvements. The most important potential advantage, however, promises to be the implementation of computer-assisted detection (CAD) algorithms which are specifically intended for a screening situation. It is the continuous improvement of CAD techniques for mammography screening that has increased interest in digital mammography more than a decade after the first commercial systems became available (Sonoda et al. 1983).

With microcalcifications as small as 200–300 μm in diameter frequently being the earliest detectable sign of breast cancer, high spatial resolution is mandatory (Kimme-Smith et al. 1987; Oestmann et al. 1988b; Sickles 1982). State of the art film-screen mammography offers a spatial resolution of up to 15–20 lp/mm. An even higher spatial resolution, however, could theoretically be of value since about 60% of breast cancers contain microscopically visible calcium undetectable with current high-resolution mammographic methods (Oestmann et al. 1988a; Millis et al. 1976). Apart from being necessary for the detection of lesions, good spatial resolution is also essential for sophisticated morphological analysis of calcifications and soft tissue lesions.

The radiographic density of the breast shows great intra- and interindividual variations. The maximum density of a breast may be very high while those structures indicative of malignant disease may show very low contrast in relation to surrounding tissues. The distribution of tissue elements within the breast also may be very heterogeneous. In about 30% of women, the breast parenchyma shows a high percentage of dense fibroglandular elements, which may easily obscure small tumor masses (Moskowitz 1982; Page and Windfield 1986; Egan and Sweeney 1979). In addition, subtle calcium deposits may be lost to detection due to the density and the heterogeneity of surrounding breast tissues (Oestmann et al. 1988a). Mammography must thus offer a wide dynamic range, i.e., demonstrate low- and high-density areas of the breast with good quality, while at the same time providing excellent contrast in these same regions.

The mammographic dose to the breast should be as low as possible, but diagnostic image quality, i.e., maintaining the ability to detect early breast cancers,

---

J.-W. Oestmann, MD, Professor, Klinikum der Georg-August-Universität, Röntgendiagnostik I, Robert-Koch-Straße 40, 37075 Göttingen, Germany

should not be impaired. With film-screen recording systems the conspicuousness of breast lesions decreases if dose is lowered substantially (OESTMANN et al. 1988b). Although digital systems permit dose reductions without changing the image receptor, the same physical restrictions with regard to lesion conspicuousness should apply.

5.2 Basic Principles of Digital X-ray Mammography

Digital radiography systems are characterized by two main principles: (a) the translation of the continuous or *analog* signal of the detected radiation into a discontinuous or *digital* data format, and (b) the segmentation of the imaging process into *image acquisition*, *image display*, and *data communication and storage*, involving separate and dedicated components for each task.

The anatomic information in mammography is contained in the three-dimensional pattern of X-ray attenuation that exits the breast. This information is either digitized at once or after temporary storage in an analog image receptor. The process of digitization consists in the segmentation of the image into discrete picture elements ("pixels") that make up the image matrix. The number of pixels per unit area determines the spatial resolution of the system. Doubling the spatial resolution quadruples the number of pixels required. The contrast resolution of each pixel is determined by its bit depth. A typical bit depth of 12 encodes 2^{12} or 4096 gray-scale levels. A high gray-scale resolution is of particular value when image receptors have a very wide dynamic range, to capture wide variations in tissue attenuation. Every increase in spatial and contrast resolution in digital systems has to be paid for in terms of hardware costs, data processing and transfer times, and data storage requirements. For this reason, digital mammography systems must meet but not greatly exceed resolution requirements. A digital format is the precondition for processing and communication of pictorial and other information without data loss or damage due to noise. It is also the prerequisite for any system of CAD.

The separate tasks of radiation detection, image display, and data storage are performed by highly specialized and optimized modular components. For digital mammography, storage phosphors, diode arrays, charge coupled devices, and conventional film have been used as image receptors. Image display components are video display monitors, transparency film hard copy, and paper hard copy. For image data storage, magnetic hard disks, optical disks, and film hard copies are frequently used. For image communication, high-speed, high-capacity networks have been developed within the context of PACSs.

All hardware components of a digital mammography system must be joined into a compatible and functional system for optimal performance. Spatial and contrast resolution capabilities of the detector, for example, must be matched by the system's capability to process the resulting huge amount of data with adequate processing and communication speed. The display modalities must be able to communicate the spatial and contrast resolution provided by the system. This is a special problem for current video display monitors. For technical reasons they fail to match the large dynamic range (PIZER et al. 1982) and high spatial resolution (FROST and STAAB 1989) needed for digital mammography. Systems will therefore continue to rely on hard copy for image display in the foreseeable future.

Optimal performance and coordination of the equipment hardware must be matched by adequate software components for image processing and data management. Image processing algorithms are supposed to enhance the information content of the original image data set, but the opposite may occur if algorithms are not optimized. Post-processing image enhancement can only partially compensate for potential shortcomings of the hardware components.

Digital mammography constitutes an extreme challenge for existing digital imaging technologies because of the requirements outlined above. The required spatial resolution constitutes the greatest hurdle for a digital system.

5.3 The Issue of Spatial Resolution

A high spatial resolution at good contrast is the prerequisite for the detection and analysis of microcalcifications. Optimized conventional screen-film systems offer spatial resolutions in excess of 15 lp/mm. Digital equipment approaches 5 lp/mm with a system pixel matrix of 2000^2 (pixel size of 0.1 mm) and 10 lp/mm with a matrix of 4000^2 (pixel size of 0.5 mm). As already pointed out, any increase in spatial resolution in digital radiography is paid for with higher hardware expenses and increased processing and data transfer times.

The detectability of microcalcifications is the most important parameter for definition of the minimum requirement for spatial resolution. Even with film-screen systems under optimized conditions, breast calcifications smaller than 0.1 mm cannot be reliably documented (SICKLES 1982; KARSSEMEIJER et al. 1993). Most (KARSSEMEIJER et al. 1993; DE MAESENEER et al. 1992; OESTMANN et al. 1988c) but not all (CHAN et al. 1987a) systematic comparisons between film-screen systems and either digitally acquired or digitized conventional mammography have shown that the detection of microcalcification clusters is not significantly decreased with a system matrix of 2000^2. In some studies, however, this matrix was found to be suboptimal for a closer morphological analysis of detected clusters (LAMBRUSCHI et al. 1993; OESTMANN et al. 1988c). Only one study found equivalence of film-screen mammography and 2000^2 matrix digitized images for both detection and analysis of microcalcifications (KARSSEMEIJER et al. 1993).

For the detection and analysis of soft tissue lesions the spatial resolution is of less importance, with 2000^2 matrix images having been found to be equivalent to film-screen mammography (KARSSEMEIJER et al. 1993; LAMBRUSCHI et al. 1993; BRETTLE et al. 1994; NAB et al. 1992).

In conclusion, doubts remain as to whether a 2000^2 matrix is sufficient for digital mammography. Most workers in the field would probably agree that a 4000^2 matrix would fulfill the requirements for screening. As it turns out, advanced CAD projects start out with image matrices in excess of 2000^2 (KEGELMEYER et al. 1994).

5.4 The Potential of Image Postprocessing

Image postprocessing in digital mammography includes all those operations that are intended to optimize the image data for viewing. This can be as simple as manually changing the *window* and *level*. Different look-up tables may be chosen to modify the image in ways similar to the effects of changing the H&D curve for film-screen systems. The risks of these operations are identical to those in analog systems: In regions outside the optimal range of optical density and/or areas of suboptimal contrast, pathology may be overlooked or misinterpreted. The higher contrast resolution possible with narrow window settings can improve the conspicuousness of soft tissue lesions and has also been felt to be responsible for the equivalent detectability of microcalcifications in comparison to higher resolution film-screen systems (BRETTLE et al. 1994). *Grayscale reversal* is easily performed with appropriate look-up tables, but has not shown any advantages over traditional image presentation (OESTMANN et al. 1988d).

Edge enhancement is a more complex type of image postprocessing that was initially felt to hold great promise (ISHIDA et al. 1983). It is achieved in most systems with the help of an unsharp masking technique (Fig. 5.1) which has long been used in analog systems (ST. JOHN and CRAIG 1957). As a first step, an unsharp copy (mask) of the original image is subtracted from the original to produce a pure "edge image." The spatial frequencies in the "edge image"

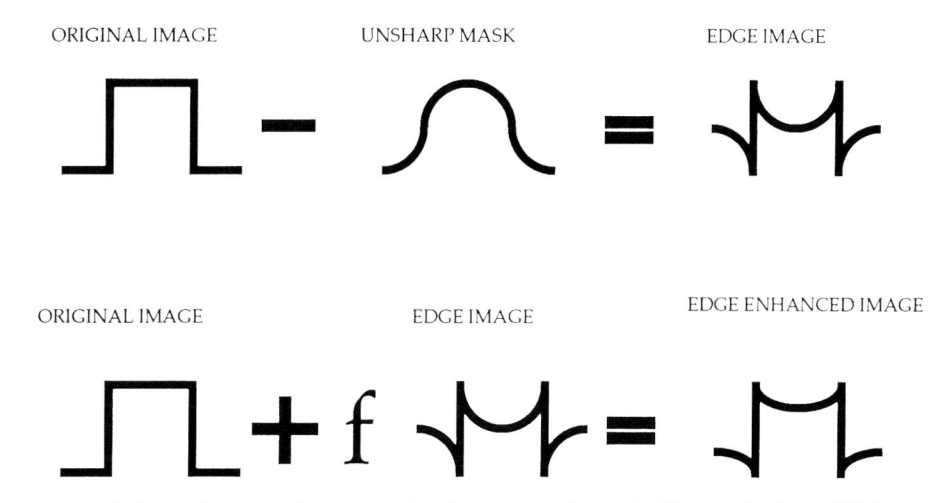

Fig. 5.1. Graphic representation of the unsharp masking process. An "edge image" is generated by subtracting the unsharp mask from the original. All wide-area contrasts are suppressed in this image. The final image is produced by adding the edge image to the original image. The factor "f" determines the amount of edge enhancement in the final image version

depend on the degree of unsharpness of the mask. In the second step, the "edge image" is added to the original image, after modification by an enhancement factor, to establish the degree of enhancement in the final image. High-frequency edge enhancement sharpens the edges of small details. Low-frequency edge enhancement accentuates intensity differences between larger regions. Unsharp masking may produce "halo" artifacts due to overshoot at the abrupt transitions between high- and low-intensity regions in the image (OESTMANN et al. 1991). To many mammographers the resultant images will look familiar, since high-frequency edge enhancement is also inherent to xeromammography (SICKLES 1982). High-frequency enhancement, however, has resulted in a decreased detectability of microcalcification clusters (OESTMANN et al. 1988d). This is probably at least partially due to (a) the increase in image noise seen with this technique and (b) the simultaneous enhancement of very small details that belong to the anatomic background and are mistaken for pathology. Enhancement of low spatial frequencies, on the other hand, has been found to improve somewhat the detectability of aluminum or bone specks and pathologically verified breast microcalcifications on digitized film (CHAN et al. 1986, 1987a; SMATHERS et al. 1986).

Adaptive histogram equalization is a postprocessing procedure that is not normally available in most commercial systems. It serves to "equalize" the image by locally spreading the used gray levels over the whole available dynamic range of the display. Contrasts are thus optimized.

Dual-energy subtraction is inherently more than a postprocessing procedure because special requirements also have to be met during image acquisition. The technique, however, is practically feasible only with digital processing. Differences in attenuation between soft tissue and calcium at two levels of exposure energy [i.e., two exposures at different kV or one exposure with a beam hardening filter between two image receptors (CHAKRABORTY and BARNES 1989)] are used to calculate separate "calcium" (where the soft tissue components of the image have been subtracted) and "soft tissue" images (where the calcium components of the image have been subtracted). In digital dual-energy mammography, the conspicuousness of calcifications could thus theoretically be increased by selectively looking at a calcium image without interference from overlying soft tissue structures (JOHNS et al. 1985). This positive effect appears to be offset, however, by the significant increase in image noise seen with the technique (PROKOP et al. 1990). Initial clinical studies were not able to prove any diagnostic advantage of dual-energy subtraction in mammography (ASAGA et al. 1987) and its impact has consequently remained low.

5.5 Computer-Assisted Detection

A digital data format is the precondition for automatic lesion detection and computerized image analysis routines. These are of special interest for large-volume screening programs in which the mammographic projections are highly standardized, the degree of image magnification is predictable, breast contours are regular, and landmarks are easily detected. Mammographic screening thus is a perfect candidate for CAD, with considerable potential diagnostic and economic impact.

Computer-assisted detection techniques for mammography have been under development for almost a decade (CHAN et al. 1987b). Their complexity has grown immensely (PRIEBE et al. 1994), making a "black box" type of approach inevitable for most radiologists. The basic techniques, however, are straightforward and give some insight into how CAD procedures work. The individual techniques are almost always combined for improved overall performance.

The detection of parenchymal asymmetries, which can be due to malignant masses, is possible by subtracting identical views of both breasts from one another (YIN et al. 1993). A digital alignment of both views prior to the subtraction procedure increases the diagnostic yield (YIN et al. 1994).

In one microcalcification detection algorithm, the image is searched for pixel values within a previously defined range typical of microcalcifications. After recognition of such a pixel, the absolute and relative offset in comparison to the surrounding tissue is tested, and it is marked as a calcium pixel if the offset meets a predetermined standard. A "region growing technique" (i.e., decreasing the threshold of the image histogram) is then applied and the complete microcalcification is outlined. The size of the calcification is checked against predetermined values. In these schemes, when a threshold number of single calcifications are located in an area of a given size, they are considered to be a cluster which needs to be indicated to the radiologist (FAM et al. 1988).

The detection of masses or microcalcifications is possible with a "matched" filter subtraction algo-

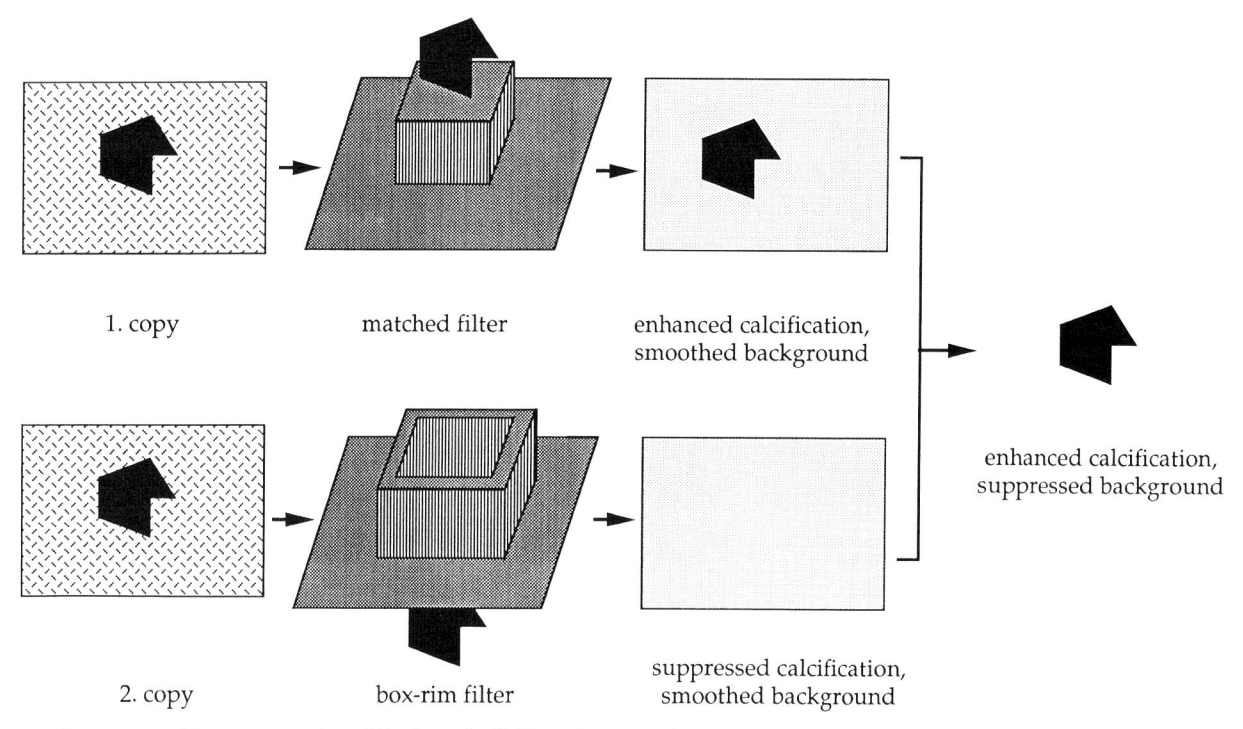

Fig. 5.2. Graphic representation of the "matched" filter algorithm in calcification detection. An enhancing filter that fits the size and approximate contour of the calcification is run over the first copy of the original image pixel by pixel, thus enhancing the calcification and smoothing the background (*top row*). A suppressing or smoothing filter of equivalent size and contour is run over the second copy of the original image pixel by pixel, now suppressing the calcification but also smoothing the background (*bottom row*). When both resulting images are subtracted, the calcification is maximally enhanced while the background is subtracted out

rithm (CHAN et al. 1987b, 1988). Two copies of the original image are created (Fig. 5.2). In a first step, the lesion in the first copy is enhanced and the background is smoothed by passing a two-dimensional matched filter over the image. This matched filter is tailored to the expected lesion size and shape (HERMAN 1988). In a second step, the second copy is smoothed with a "box-rim" (for microcalcifications) or "ring" (for masses) averaging filter of equivalent size in order to maximally suppress the lesion while achieving a background structure similar to the first algorithm. The subtraction of both processed copies results in a "difference" image in which the lesion should be maximally enhanced if the matched filter is properly chosen. Detected microcalcifications are then subjected to further analysis as outlined above.

For detected masses, the differentiation between benign and malignant lesions can be improved by quantitating the degree of margin spiculation in a two-step procedure (Fig. 5.3) (GIGER et al. 1989).

Sophisticated CAD techniques have been quite successful in detecting malignant lesions in mammography (VYBORNY 1994). In fact, the number of clinically missed lesions has been shown to decrease by up to 50% if radiologists are given computer prompts (KEGELMEYER et al. 1994; CHAN et al. 1990). The diagnostic and economic advantages of CAD schemes for breast screening programs are becoming increasingly attractive with every further improvement. Currently, most CAD projects rely on the digitization of film mammograms for their raw image data input. The incorporation of CAD techniques into genuine digital mammography systems promises to increase further the radiologist's performance in the detection and differentiation of breast lesions.

5.6 Commercial Digital Mammography Systems

A considerable number of digital mammography prototypes have been presented in the past (FRITZ et al. 1986; HOLDSWORTH et al. 1990; KIMME-SMITH et al. 1989; NISHIKAWA et al. 1987; YAFFE 1993; OESTMANN et al. 1988e), but only two systems with digital image acquisition are currently available commercially. While storage phosphors have been studied extensively for more than a decade now,

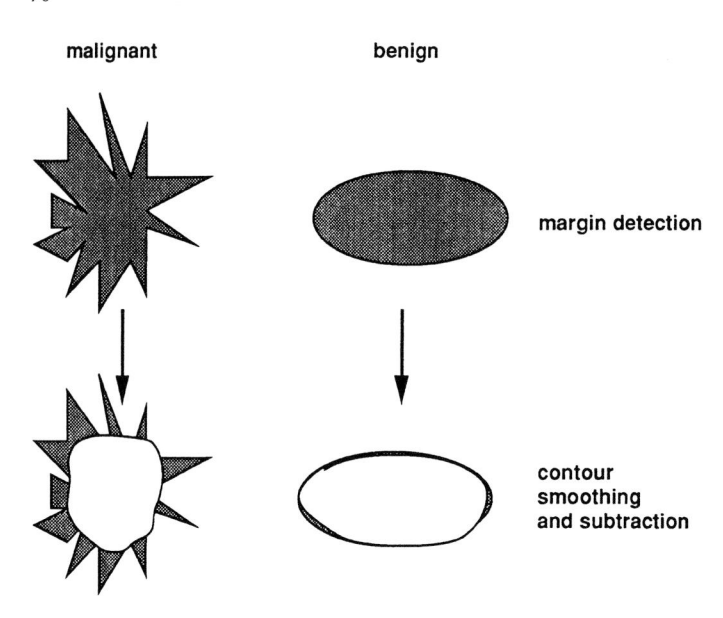

Fig. 5.3. Graphic representation of the quantification of lesion spiculation. As a first step, the margins of the lesion are determined. The lesion contour is then smoothed. The difference in area between the smoothed lesion and the original lesion can be used as a parameter of degree of spiculation – and potential malignancy

charge coupled devices have only recently become accessible to the greater scientific community.

5.6.1 Storage Phosphor Systems

Storage phosphor imaging plates (SONODA et al. 1983) were introduced in the early 1980s. The imaging plates consist of a thin layer of $BaFBr:Eu^{2+}$ on a carrier base. They differ from traditional radiographic intensifying screens in that they temporarily retain the absorbed energy until the latent image in the phosphor is excited by a laser beam of specific wavelength. In most systems, an He-Ne laser scans the image plate optoelectronically with a 100-μm pitch beam. During a preliminary low-energy scan, a histogram of the range and strength of the image signal is calculated in order to optimize the final data read-out. The light emitted from the storage phosphor is collected by an optic fiber, transferred to a photomultiplier, and subsequently converted to a digital format. High spatial resolution phosphors (e.g., FUJI HR plates) intended for mammography yield 2000 × 2510 pixels of 100 μm, and a nominal spatial resolution of 5 lp/mm for plates of 18 × 24 cm. The relation between the quantity of absorbed radiation and the eventual amount of emitted light is linear over an extraordinarily wide range (approximately 1:10000). This is about two orders of magnitude greater than that normally attained with film radiography. The quantum absorption efficiency tends to be slightly lower than that of a standard film radiographic system. After the plate has been scanned to obtain an image, it can be erased for subsequent reuse by exposure to a large amount of visible light. The processed images are printed out on hard copy.

This system's usefulness for mammography is compromised by its low spatial resolution, which – as has been stated above – seems to be just short of the requirements for breast screening. Standard postprocessing procedures and dual-energy techniques have failed to produce significant gains in diagnostic information. Dose reductions have resulted in significant loss of diagnostic performance (OESTMANN et al. 1989). Artifacts have been found to be another major problem (OESTMANN et al. 1991), with some of them simulating clustered calcifications (BRETTLE et al. 1994; JARLMAN et al. 1991).

5.6.2 Charge Coupled Device-Based Systems

Charge coupled devices (CCDs), such as those used in popular video cameras, can be used as detectors for digital imaging. They offer a high signal-to-noise ratio (KARELLAS et al. 1992), wide latitude (HOLDSWORTH et al. 1990), good wide-area contrast and spatial resolution (pixel size of less than 50 μm (NISHIKAWA et al. 1987), and an almost real-time operation. Their small size (the largest being 6 × 6 cm) prevents use in standard mammography (KRUPINSKI E, personal communication, 1995). For stereotaxic mammography, however, this

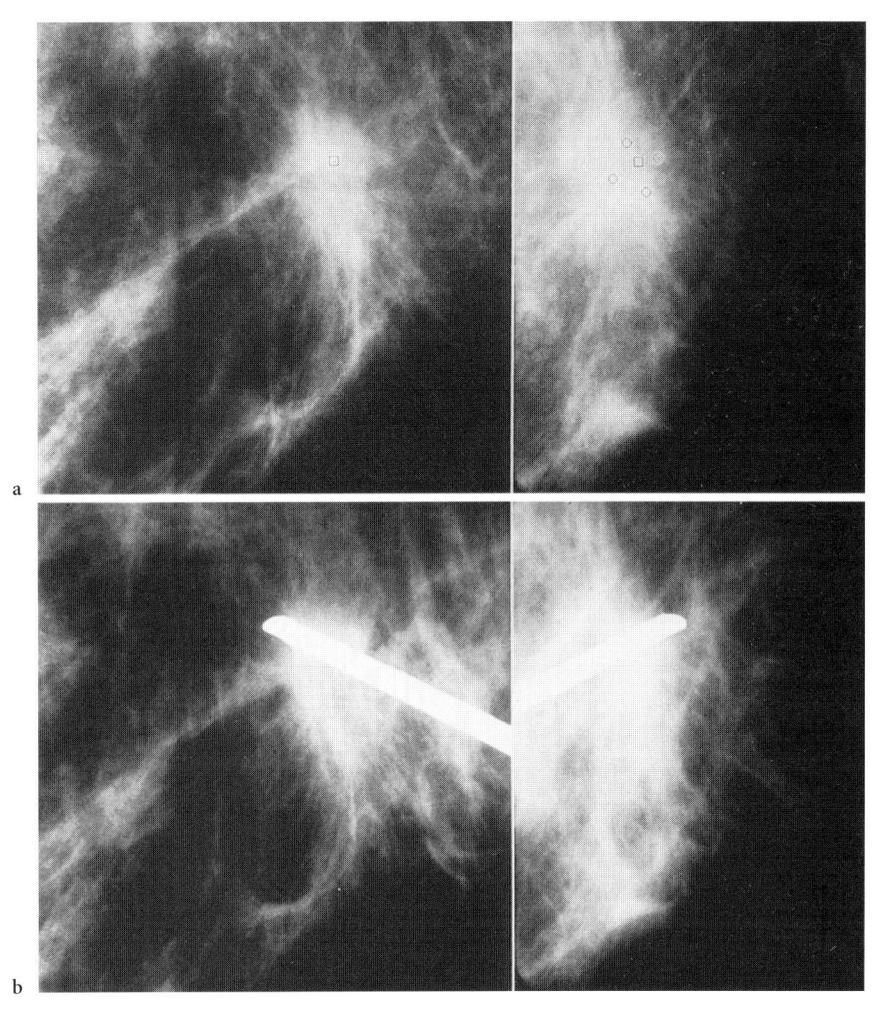

Fig. 5.4a,b. Stereotaxic images of a suspicious stellate lesion to be biopsied. **a** The initial images show the lesion with good spatial and contrast resolution. **b** The control images after puncture show the biopsy needle in situ. The stereotaxic views are available only seconds after the exposure. (Images courtesy of Fischer Imaging, Denver, Colo.)

limited filed of view is adequate. For stereotaxic localization, CCD-based systems offer unique opportunities.

Two systems are currently marketed. Both use intensifying screens as primary radiation detectors. In one unit (LoRad Imaging, Danbury, Conn.), the CCD is coupled to the screen with a lens, while in the other (Fischer Imaging, Denver, Colo.) fiberoptic coupling is used. A comparison of both systems with physical phantoms has shown a significantly better observer performance with the lens-coupled system (KRUPINSKI 1994). Further improvements of both technologies, however, are probable. For sterotaxic use, both systems offer good image quality and an almost immediate image display thereby significantly shortening the procedure (Fig. 5.4). This near-immediate image availability constitutes such a major advantage that these CCD systems may eventually replace analog stereotaxic equipment despite their very high cost.

The described CCD technology has been modified for standard size mammographic imaging in prototype systems (PICCARO 1994; BIRD et al. 1994; ANDRE et al. 1994). The small size of the CCDs has been overcome by electronically stitching together multiple adjacent images. The resulting mammograms have a 4000×6000 matrix capable of delivering the spatial resolution needed for breast screening. If data processors, data networks, and display modalities can be found that handle the enormous amount of information (>30 Mbyte per image) with adequate speed, these systems could be the most promising candidates for standard-use digital mammography in the near future.

5.7 Conclusion and Outlook

Although digital systems for mammography were introduced more than a decade ago, so far they have not achieved either diagnostic or economic success. The initial systems were unable to fulfill the minimum image quality requirements for breast imaging, mostly due to limited spatial resolution. The digital format provided little if any advantage over sophisticated and well-maintained analog mammographic equipment. The advantages of data management within a PACS system remained hypothetical because systems adequate for mammographic use were not available.

The development of CAD algorithms and their potential impact on large-scale breast screening programs constitutes the main reason for reconsidering digital mammography techniques at the present time. While current storage phosphor technology will probably continue to provide suboptimal image quality, CCD-based techniques promise to offer the spatial resolution, the dynamic range, and the detection efficiency needed for mammography. For stereotaxic procedures, digital systems such as those outlined above may soon become the modalities of choice.

References

André, Olson L, Spivey B, Ysreal M, Tran J (1994) Full-view digital mammography with a small-field image-stitching approach: image quality and initial clinical results. Radiology 193(P):476

Asaga T, Chiyasu S, Mastuda S, et al. (1987) Breast imaging: dual-energy projection radiography with digital radiography. Radiology 164:869–870

Bird R, André M, Spivey B, Horton S, Neff B, Storm J (1994) Full breast digital imaging receptor utilizing advanced optics design. Radiology 193(P):476

Brettle DS, Ward SC, Parkin GJ, Cowen AR, Sumsion HJ (1994) A clinical comparison between conventional and digital mammography utilizing computed radiography. Br J Radiol 67:464–468

Chakraborty DP, Barnes GT (1989) An energy sensitive cassette for dual-energy mammography. Med Phys 16:7–13

Chan H, Vyborny C, MacMahon H, Metz C, Doi K, Sickles E (1986) Evaluation of digital unsharp-mask filtering for the detection of subtle mammographic microcalcifications. SPIE medicine XIV/Pacs IV 626

Chan HP, Vyborny CJ, MacMahon H, Metz CE, Doi K, Sickles EA (1987a) Digital mammography. ROC studies of the effects of pixel size and unsharp-mask filtering on the detection of subtle microcalcifications. Invest Radiol 22:581–589

Chan HP, Doi K, Galhotra S, Vyborny CJ, MacMahon H, Jokich PM (1987b) Image feature analysis and computer-aided diagnosis in digital radiography. I. Automated detection of microcalcifications in mammography. Med Phys 14:538–548

Chan H, Doi K, Vyborny C, Lam K, Schmidt R (1988) Computer-aided detection of microcalcifications in mammograms: methodology and preliminary clinical study. Invest Radiol 23:664–671

Chan H, Doi K, Vyborny C, et al. (1990) Improvement in radiologist's detection of clustered microcalcifications on mammograms: the potential of computer-aided diagnosis. Invest Radiol 25:1102–1110

De Maeseneer M, Beeckman P, Osteaux M, et al. (1992) Detecting clustered microcalcifications in the female breast: secondary digitized images versus mammograms. J Belge Radiol 75:173–178

Egan RL, Sweeney MB (1979) Mammographic parenchymal patterns and risk of breast cancer. Radiology 133:65–76

Fam BW, Olson SL, Winter PF, Scholz FJ (1988) Algorithm for the detection of fine clustered calcifications on film mammograms. Radiology 169:333–337

Feig SA (1994) Mammographic screening of women aged 40 to 49 years. Is it justified? Obstet Gynecol Clin North Am 21:587–606

Fritz SL, Chang CH, Gupta NK, et al. (1986) A digital radiographic imaging system for mammography. Invest Radiol 21:581–583

Frost M, Staab E (1989) Displays: contrast and spatial requirements. Invest Radiol 24:95–98

Giger M, Doi K, Yin F, Schmidt R, Vyborny C (1989) Computerized classification of mass lesions in digital mammograms: lesion spiculation in analysis of malignancy. Radiology 173(P):394

Herman S (1988) Feature-size dependent selective edge enhancement of X-ray images. SPIE medical imaging II(914):654–659

Holdsworth DW, Gerson RK, Fenster A (1990) A time-delay integration charge-coupled device camera for slot-scanned digital radiography. Med Phys 17:876–886

Ishida M, Frank P, Doi K, Lehr J (1983) High quality digital radiographic images: improved detection of low contrast objects and preliminary clinical studies. Radiographics 3:325–338

Jarlman O, Samuelsson L, Braw M (1991) Digital luminescence mammography. Early clinical experience. Acta Radiol 32:110–113

Johns PC, Drost DJ, Yaffe MJ, Fenster A (1985) Dual-energy mammography: initial experimental results. Med Phys 12:297–304

Karellas A, Harris LJ, Liu H, Davis MA, D'Orsi CJ (1992) Charge-coupled device detector: performance considerations and potential for small-field mammographic imaging applications. Med Phys 19:1015–1023

Karssemeijer N, Frieling JT, Hendriks JH (1993) Spatial resolution in digital mammography. Invest Radiol 28:413–419

Kegelmeyer W Jr, Pruneda JM, Bourland PD, Hillis A, Riggs MW, Nipper ML (1994) Computer-aided mammographic screening for spiculated lesions. Radiology 191:331–337

Kimme-Smith C, Bassett L, Gold RH, Roe D, Orr R (1987) Mammographic dual-screen-dual-emulsion-film combination: visibility of simulated microcalcifications and effect on image contrast. Radiology 165:313–318

Kimme-Smith C, Bassett LW, Gold RH, Gormley L (1989) Digital mammography. A comparison of two digitization methods. Invest Radiol 24:869–875

Krupinski E (1994) Observer performance using lens-coupled vs fiberoptic-coupled digital X-ray cameras for stereotaxic breast imaging. Radiology 193(P):476

Lambruschi G, Tagliagambe A, Palla L, et al. (1993) A comparison between traditional mammography and digital with storage phosphors. Radiol Med 85:59–64

Millis R, Davis R, Stacey A (1976) The detection and significance of calcifications in the breast. A radiological and pathological study. Br J Radiol 49:12–26

Moskowitz M (1982) Mammographic parenchymal patterns: more controversy. JAMA 247:210

Nab HW, Karssemeijer N, Van Erning LJ, Hendriks JH (1992) Comparison of digital and conventional mammography: a ROC study of 270 mammograms. Med Inf 17:125–131

Nishikawa RM, Mawdsley GE, Fenster A, Yaffe MJ (1987) Scanned-projection digital mammography. Med Phys 14:717–727

Oestmann J, Kopans D, Schaefer C, et al. (1988a) Visibility of individual microcalcifications in the breast-what percentage can we expect to see? Radiology 169(P):352

Oestmann J, Kopans D, Linetsky L, et al. (1988b) Comparison of two screen film combinations for mammographic studies. Radiology 168:657–659

Oestmann J, Kopans D, Hall DA, McCarthy KA, Rubens JR, Greene R (1988c) A comparison of digitized storage phosphors and conventional mammography in the detection of malignant microcalcifications. Invest Radiol 23:725–728

Oestmann J, Kopans D, Hall D, McCarthy K, Rubens J, Greene R (1988d) Digitale Mammographie mit Speicher-Phosphoren: Einfluß der Bildnachverarbeitung auf die Erkennung von malignen Mikroverkalkungen. Zentralbl Rad 136:615

Oestmann J, Kopans D, Greene R (1988e) Digitale mammographie. In: Riemann H, Kollath J, Rienhoff O (eds) 3. Frankfurter Gespräche über Digitale Radiographie. Schnetztor, Konstanz, pp 133–137

Oestmann J, Reichelt S, Rosenthal H, et al. (1989) Digital mammography with storage phosphors: substantial reductions in photon flux or voltage impair detectability of microcalcifications. Radiology 173(P):394

Oestmann J, Prokop M, Schaefer C, Galanski M (1991) Hardware and software artefacts in storage phosphor radiography. Radiographics 11:795–805

Page DL, Windfield AC (1986) The dense mammogram. AJR 147:487–489

Piccaro M (1994) Digital mammography: a step up in image quality through high resolution and scatter rejection. Radiology 193(P):474

Pizer S, Johnston E, Zimmermann J, Chan F (1982) Contrast perception with video displays. SPIE Medical Applications 318:223–230

Priebe CE, Solka JL, Lorey RA, et al. (1994) The application of fractal analysis to mammographic tissue classification. Cancer Lett 77:183–189

Prokop M, Schaefer C, Oestmann J, Galanski M (1990) Isodose dual-energy radiography with storage phosphors: fast non-linear subtraction and noise suppression with standard equipment. Radiology 177(P):328

Sickles E (1982) Mammographic detectability of breast calcifications. AJR 139:913–918

Smathers RL, Bush E, Drace J, et al. (1986) Mammographic microcalcifications: detection with xerography, screen-film, and digitized film display. Radiology 159:673–677

Sonoda M, Takano M, Miyahara J, Kato H (1983) Computed radiography utilizing scanning laser stimulated luminescence. Radiology 148:833–838

St. John E, Craig D (1957) Logetronography. AJR 78:123–133

Vogel VG (1994) Screening younger women at risk for breast cancer. Monogr Natl Cancer Inst 16:55–60

Vyborny C (1994) Can computers help radiologists read mammograms? Radiology 191:315–317

Yaffe MJ (1993) Direct digital mammography using a scanned-slot CCD imaging system. Med Prog Technol 19:13–21

Yin FF, Giger ML, Vyborny CJ, Doi K, Schmidt RA (1993) Comparison of bilateral-subtraction and single-image processing techniques in the computerized detection of mammographic masses. Invest Radiol 28:473–481

Yin FF, Giger ML, Doi K, Vyborny CJ, Schmidt RA (1994) Computerized detection of masses in digital mammograms: automated alignment of breast images and its effect on bilateral-subtraction technique. Med Phys 21:445–452

6 The Art of Mammographic Positioning

G.W. Eklund

CONTENTS

6.1	Introduction	75
6.2	Breast Anatomy: Effects on Mammographic Positioning	75
6.2.1	Mobility	75
6.2.2	Amount and Distribution of Glandular Tissue	76
6.2.3	Breast Size and Patient Habitus	78
6.3	The Mammographic Unit	80
6.4	Basic or "Routine" Views for Screening Mammography	80
6.5	The Craniocaudal View	80
6.6	The Mediolateral Oblique View	81
6.7	The Exaggerated Craniocaudal View	82
6.8	Diagnostic Mammography	83
6.8.1	The Exaggerated CC (XCC) View	84
6.8.2	The Spot Compression View	84
6.8.3	The Magnification View	84
6.8.4	The Tangential Spot View	84
6.8.5	The Anterior Compression View	85
6.8.6	The Change of Angle View	85
6.8.7	The 90° Lateral View	85
6.8.8	The Cleavage View	86
6.8.9	The Caudocranial View	86
6.8.10	The Modified Compression View for the Augmented Breast	86
6.9	Summary	88
	References	88

6.1 Introduction

It is difficult to obtain high-quality mammograms. Features uniquely inherent to the breast, such as shape, size, density, and low contrast, combine with patient factors such as anxiety, tenderness, and fear of radiation to challenge the skills of the best-trained technologist. The science of breast imaging has helped overcome the inherent low contrast of fat and parenchyma and the disease processes that affect both. Special film screen combinations, use of low kVp techniques, and extended processing have made possible the acquisition of high-contrast breast radiographs. Strict adherence to basic principles of mammographic imaging and quality assurance monitoring have made it possible for any facility, using appropriate equipment, to obtain technically adequate images. However, mammographic positioning does not lend itself to a set of rigid, precisely defined techniques; rather it depends heavily on the technologist's understanding of the variability of breast anatomy and morphology and the capabilities and limitations of available mammographic equipment. Recognizing the factors which influence optimal tissue visualization is an art. Not all x-ray technologists are sufficiently talented to develop the skills or to perform the procedures required for optimal mammographic imaging. No technologist with the required talent can produce optimal mammographic images without specialized training and supervised experience. This chapter is directed to technologists with an interest in high-quality mammography. It is also directed to radiologists, who must understand the art of mammographic positioning in order to recognize high-quality images and to direct corrective measures for deficient images.

6.2. Breast Anatomy: Effects on Mammographic Positioning

6.2.1 Mobility

The breast is a conical skin appendage protruding from the chest wall, with its broad base positioned on the pectoral fascia. Most breast diseases develop in the glandular parenchyma, separated from the underlying muscle fascia by fat (the retroglandular fat). To achieve maximum and optimal visualization of tissue, the breast must be pulled away from the chest wall, appropriately compressed, and stabilized before obtaining an image. The most neglected anatomic principle in breast imaging is the breast's natural mobility on the chest wall (EKLUND and CARDENOSA 1992). Failure to take advantage of this mobility when performing mammography inevitably

---

G.W. EKLUND, MD, 15251 SE 58th Street, Bellevue, WA 98006, USA

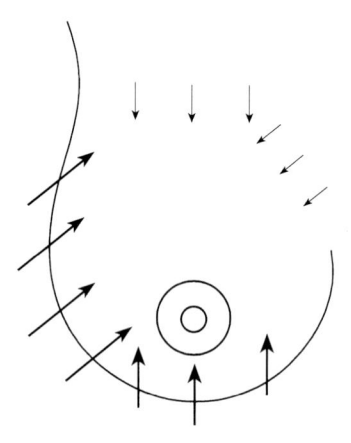

Fig. 6.1. Illustration of the right breast showing the mobile margins (*large arrows*) and the relatively immobile margins (*small arrows*). The film holder is placed at the mobile margin for both craniocaudal (CC) and mediolateral oblique (MLO) views. To minimize the distance the compression must move across the immobile medial or upper breast, the mammographer must move the breast cephalad for the CC view and medially for the MLO view

leads to exclusion of breast tissue from the final recorded mammographic image.

The breast has two mobile margins and two relatively fixed or immobile margins (Fig. 6.1). The mobile margins are the inferior margin, represented by the inframammary fold (IMF), and the lateral margin, which parallels the lateral margin of the pectoralis major muscle. The upper and medial margins of the breast are relatively fixed or immobile. The IMF, and the breast above it, can be elevated from 1.5 to 7 cm along the pectoral fascia (Fig. 6.2). Breast size, ptosis, and patient habitus contribute to this variability in achievable elevation. The lateral margin of the pectoral muscle is unattached to the chest wall, enhancing the ability to move the breast and pectoral muscle medially.

Like skin, the breast can be pulled away from the underlying muscle more easily when pulled parallel to the underlying muscle fibers. This principle is nicely illustrated by grasping skin on the forearm and pulling it away from the muscle, first by pinching the skin parallel, then perpendicular to the underlying muscle. It is therefore the breast's oblique orientation on the pectoral muscle which enables visualization of more breast tissue with the mediolateral oblique (MLO) view than with the 90° lateral view. The MLO and craniocaudal (CC) views are thus preferred for routine imaging (BASSETT and GOLD 1983; BASSETT et al. 1987; EKLUND et al. 1994; EKLUND and CARDENOSA 1992; MUIR et al. 1984; SICKLES 1986).

6.2.2 Amount and Distribution of Glandular Tissue

Glandular tissue within the breast is variable in amount and distribution (Fig. 6.3). Some breasts have very little glandular tissue, being composed pri-

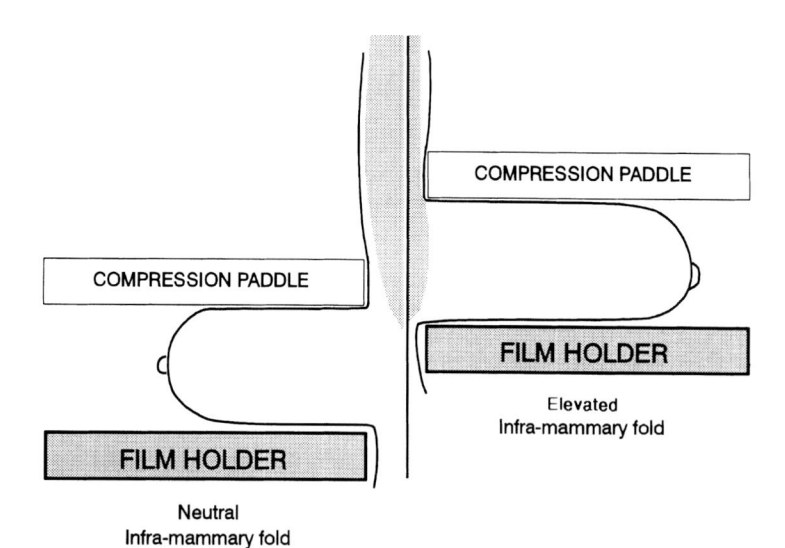

Fig. 6.2. Illustration on the *left* shows positioning for a CC view with the film holder at the inframammary fold (IMF). In order to compress the breast, the compression paddle must come down over upper posterior breast tissue, which will be excluded from the image. Illustration on the *right* shows the breast and IMF elevated with the film holder maintaining the breast in this elevated position as compression is applied. Upper posterior tissue is retained in the field of view by first elevating the IMF

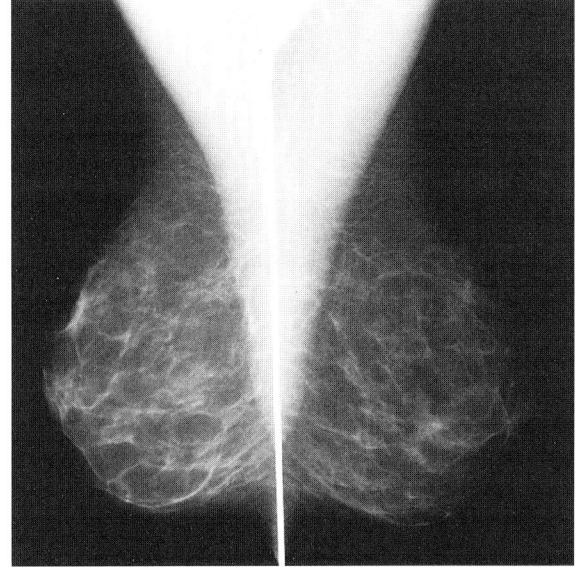

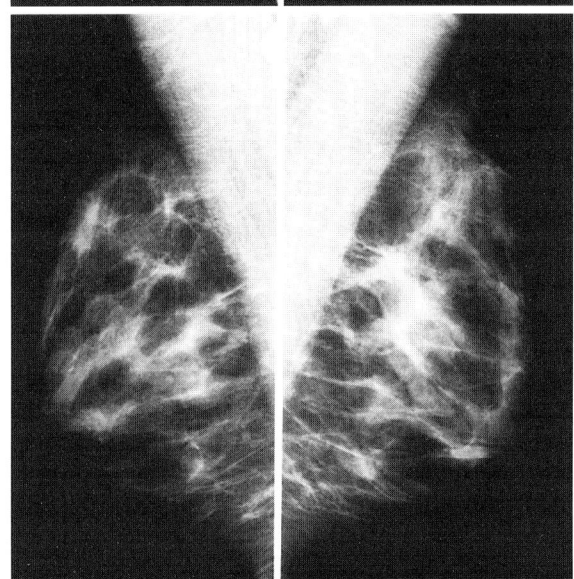

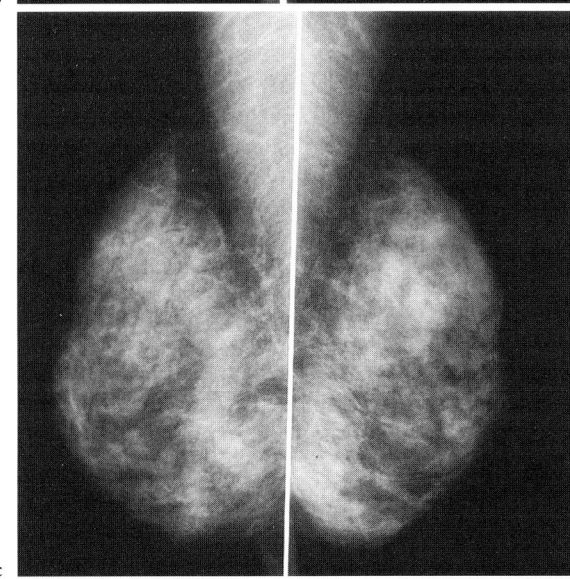

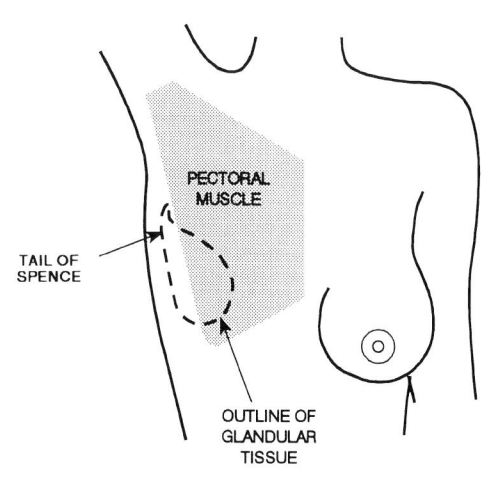

Fig. 6.4. Relationship of the glandular component of the breast to the pectoral muscle. The axillary extension of breast tissue (tail of Spence, seen in approximately 11% of women) is shown wrapping around the lateral margin of the pectoral muscle

marily of fat. Other breasts are predominantly glandular with variable amounts of adipose tissue. Glandular tissue tends to predominate in the anterior third and upper/outer quadrant of the breast. In order to provide the appropriate mAs for proper exposure of the glandular elements, it is important to understand the amount and distribution of glandular tissue when using phototimed techniques. Ideally, the photocell should be positioned under the more dense parenchyma. However, if previous films are not available to make this determination, it is prudent to select the anterior third of the breast as the location for the photocell until the first images are available for review (EKLUND et al. 1994). The technologist can then adjust the photocell position to ensure a technique that adequately exposes dense tissue.

Approximately 11% of women will have prominent extension of glandular tissue (tail of Spence) into the lower axilla, extending lateral to (and occasionally tucking in behind) the lateral margin of the pectoral muscle (Fig. 6.4) (EKLUND and CARDENOSA 1992). Frequently, it is impossible to image this lateral breast tissue in the CC projection without sacrificing medial breast tissue. Techniques for reducing the amount of lateral tissue exclusion and special additional views for its proper visualization

◀

Fig. 6.3a–c. Examples of normal breast parenchymal patterns. **a** Almost total fatty replacement of glandular parenchyma. **b** Fibroglandular pattern with prominent areas of fatty lobulation **c** Dense parenchymal pattern with very little fatty tissue

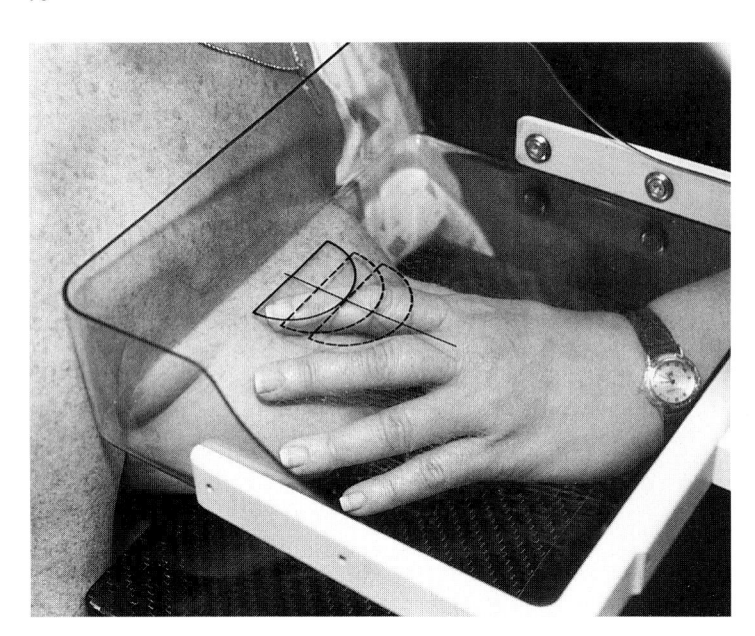

Fig. 6.5. A large compression paddle engages the knuckles of the technologist as she tries to maintain control of the breast with her fingers

will be discussed later. Breasts containing dense parenchyma anteriorly may require additional anterior compression views to achieve proper exposure and/or compression of the anterior portion (EKLUND and CARDENOSA 1992).

6.2.3 Breast Size and Patient Habitus

Small breasts can be very difficult to maintain in proper position when using standard compression paddles: The technologist may be unable to keep her hand in control of a small breast as the compression paddle is engaged. The large paddle engages the technologist's knuckles before engaging the breast (Fig. 6.5), forcing the technologist to release her hold on the breast, allowing it to retreat out from under the paddle (EKLUND and CARDENOSA 1992). The same problem arises when imaging the male breast and when performing modified compression views on augmented breasts. Several manufacturers have overcome this problem with the design of narrow compression paddles (10–12 cm in the anterior/posterior dimension) (Fig. 6.6). These narrow paddles allow the technologist to maintain control of the breast using only her fingers as the paddle engages the breast.

Large breasts present several challenges for the mammographer, including limiting the amount of tissue included in a single image, even when using the larger 24-cm × 30-cm cassettes. Very large breasts may not fit between the compression paddle and the taller magnification stands supplied with some units. The need for higher radiation doses to expose the parenchyma adequately may exceed the limits of a mammographic unit, especially one with a 400-mAs tube limit. With the demand for more radiation, the resulting longer exposures will increase the risk of motion "unsharpness" or "blur" (EKLUND and CARDENOSA 1992). Higher kVp levels are needed to assure short enough exposures to avoid the effects of motion. Although an inevitable loss of contrast occurs with use of higher kVp, the effects of motion, caused by a long exposure time, can be more compromising. The technologist should routinely use the larger 24-cm × 30-cm cassette size if the entire breast will not fit on an 18-cm × 24-cm film (EKLUND and CARDENOSA 1992). However, in patients with obese upper arms and a protuberant abdomen, it may not be possible to get the larger cassette holder back against the chest wall. It may be easier to include lower axillary tissue or posterior breast tissue when using the smaller cassette size in some obese women.

Although we rightly stress the importance of including as much of the pectoral muscle as possible on the MLO view, there are some women in whome *very prominent pectoral muscles* limit the ability to compress the anterior portion of the breast adequately. These women will also require an anterior compression view to assure adequate compression and exposure or to limit the effects of motion resulting from suboptimal compression.

The Art of Mammographic Positioning

Fig. 6.6. A narrow compression paddle (12 cm anterior-posterior measurement, Instrumentarium, Finland) enables the technologist to maintain control of the breast as the compression paddle is applied

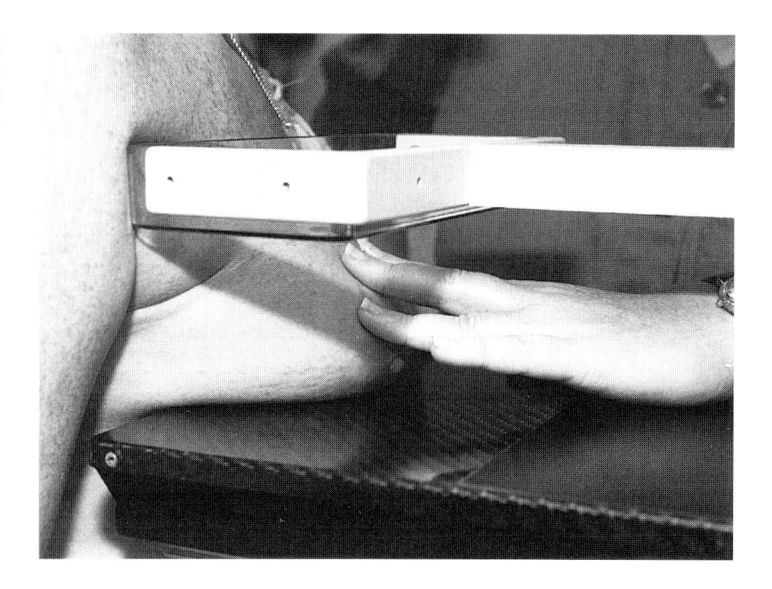

The *kyphotic patient* may require creative positioning techniques to assure adequate visualization of breast tissue in the CC projection (EKLUND and CARDENOSA 1992). The MLO view is less of a problem for these women. If the mammographic unit allows for 180° gantry rotation and the patient can straddle the x-ray tube (Fig. 6.7), a *caudo*cranial view may enable better tissue inclusion than would be possible with the standard CC view. One manufacturer (Bennett) has developed a mammographic unit that allows the gantry to tilt toward or away from the patient. Kyphotic patients can lean into the unit, allowing the x-ray tube to be positioned away from the patient's head.

Patients with *pectus excavatum* risk exclusion of medial breast tissue on the CC and MLO views. A 90° *latero*medial view, obtained with the cassette holder positioned against the sternum, will generally include more medial tissue than the conventional oblique view or the 90° *medio*lateral view. A CC view, taken with medial exaggeration (XCCM) to include more medial breast tissue, is a supplemental view to the standard CC view.

Congenital absence of the pectoral muscle (Poland's syndrome) can create a humbling experience for the conscientious technologist who takes pride in being able to achieve optimal pectoral inclusion on MLO views. This congenital variant should always be suspected when no pectoral muscles is seen on the MLO view.

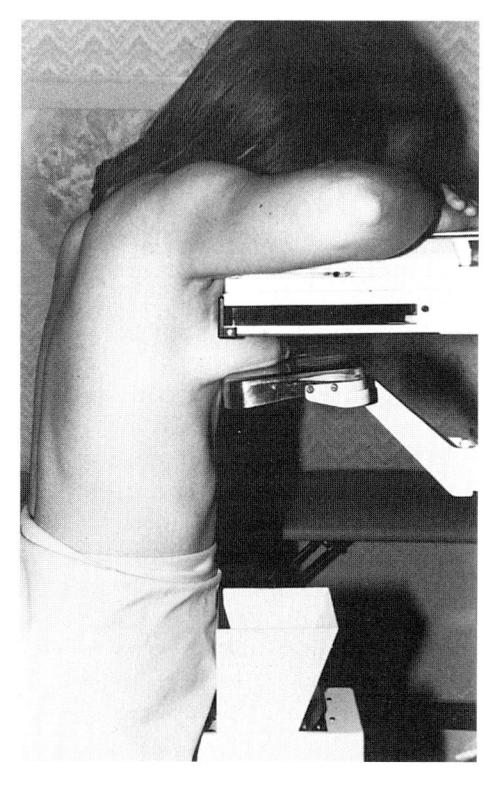

Fig. 6.7. Patient positioned for a *caudo*cranial view, which is only possible if the gantry of the mammographic unit can be roated 180°. This view is especially useful if the patient is kyphotic and unable to turn her hear away from the tube housing for the standard craniocaudal view. Lesions located in the upper half of the breast will be more sharply seen with this view, which positions lesions in the upper half of the breast closer to the film

6.3 The Mammographic Unit

The mammographic unit is a machine that provides a source of x-rays and a mechanism for securing and compressing the breast between the x-ray source and a recording device. A latent image of the breast is formed on the recording device, cast by the differential in photon absorption of various parenchymal elements as an x-ray beam passes through the tissue. To ensure preservation of optimal image detail, the breast tissue is placed as close to the recording device as possible. Compression is achieved by moving a radiolucent paddle against the breast which has been positioned on the fixed recording device. Compression is essential to immobilize the breast and separate overlapping structures within the breast and to reduce scatter radiation that degrades image sharpness and contrast (EKLUND 1991; HALL 1989; TABAR and DEAN 1989). The added benefit of reducing radiation dose is a welcome advantage of breast compression. Much has been written about the advantages of mammographic compression and the variability in patient tolerance for the procedure (DE PARADES 1989; HAUS 1984; SULLIVAN et al. 1991). We stress the importance of compression and the need to limit compression to what is necessary to achieve "tautness" of the skin or to "just less than painful," *whichever comes first* (EKLUND 1991).

When selecting equipment, it is important to consider how various functions are controlled. Seemingly minor tasks, such as raising and lowering the gantry, can be made simple or complex by the machine's control devices. In usual practice the technologist maintains the breast in position with one hand, while releasing the breast with her other hand to activate the switch that raises or lowers the gantry. By limiting control of the breast to only one hand, she may be unable to maintain the breast in proper position for optimal imaging. A foot control to activate the function of raising or lowering the gantry overcomes this problem. Manufacturers recognized the need for foot control of the compression paddle years ago; the need for foot control of the gantry movement is also important. Most mammographic units can be equipped with such a foot switch for a modest cost. The task of the mammographer in performing each step of positioning deserves constant reevaluation, with simplification and time saving as primary goals for improvement.

6.4 Basic or "Routine" Views for Screening Mammography

Screening mammography involves the search for clinically unsuspected breast cancer. The success of a screening program depends on the threshold sensitivity of the screening procedure, the growth rate of a given breast cancer, and the time between screening intervals. Adequate image quality, including such technical factors as exposure of dense parenchymal elements, contrast, and image detail, is important to the success of a screening program. Optimal positioning to avoid excluding tissue that might contain significant pathology is essential. The CC and the MLO views are the two basic views for routine mammographic screening (BASSETT and GOLD 1983; BASSETT et al. 1987; EKLUND et al. 1994; EKLUND and CARDENOSA 1992; MUIR et al. 1984; SICKLES 1986). It has been our practice to have the technologist include a modified CC view, exaggerated to include lateral breast tissue (XCCL) if there is any concern that lateral breast tissue is being excluded from view on the standard CC image (EKLUND and CARDENOSA 1992). Determining the need for an additional XCCL view is easily accomplished by reviewing the previous study. If the patient has no previous studies, initial images should be reviewed to determine the need for an XCCL view.

6.5 The Craniocaudal View

Properly performed, the CC image should include all but the lateral or "axillary" portion of the breast. The

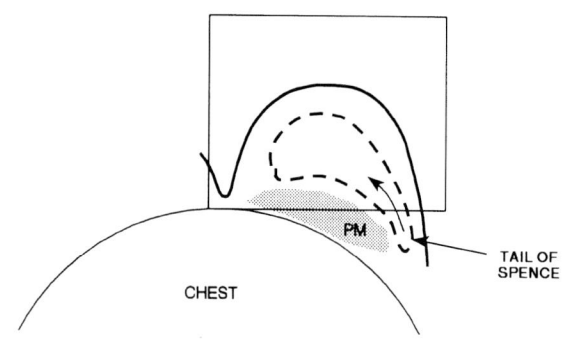

Fig. 6.8. Illustration of the right breast positioned on the film holder for a CC image. Exclusion of lateral glandular tissue is minimized if the technologist pulls lateral breast into view before applying the compression paddle. The contralateral breast is draped over the corner of the film holder to avoid interposition of the breast between the chest wall and the film holder. Such interposition prevents the film holder from being positioned against the chest wall, resulting in exclusion of medial tissue of the breast being examined. *PM*, pectoral muscle

Fig. 6.9. Technologist standing on the contralateral side to the breast being examined. Lateral breast tissue is being pulled into the field of view to minimize exclusion of glandular tissue

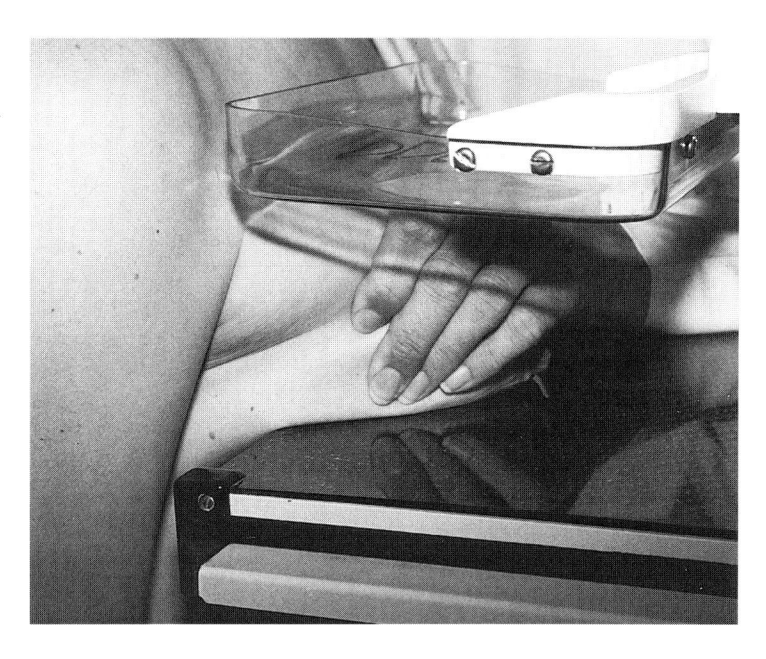

CC image must be obtained with proper elevation of the inframammary fold to ensure inclusion of upper posterior breast tissue (EKLUND and CARDENOSA 1992). The breast must be maintained in this elevated position by the film holder before applying compression (Fig. 6.2). Just before engaging the compression paddle, the technologist should pull lateral breast tissue into the field, to avoid sacrificing medial breast tissue (Figs. 6.8, 6.9) (EKLUND and CARDENOSA 1992). Pulling lateral breast into the field significantly diminishes the need for adding an XCCL view. To properly position the breast, the technologist must stand on the side of the patient that is contralateral to the breast being examined (Fig. 6.9). A common pitfall in CC positioning is the interposition of the contralateral breast between the film holder and the chest wall. This pitfall is avoided by bringing the contralateral breast up and over the corner of the film holder (Fig. 6.8).

6.6 The Mediolateral Oblique View

The MLO view, properly performed, should be regarded as a view of nearly all of the breast. To ensure maximum inclusion of breast tissue, full use of breast mobility must occur (EKLUND and CARDENOSA 1992). The mobile lateral margins of the breast and pectoral muscle are moved medially to reduce the distance the compression paddle must move across medial breast, thereby decreasing the amount of medial tissue excluded from view (Fig. 6.10). Again, it is important that the technologist stand on the contralateral side of the breast being imaged.

Assessing the adequacy of mammographic images, as related to tissue inclusion, requires experience and a presumption that the technologist is competent, complete, and consistent in her positioning techniques. Although not a guarantee of optimal positioning, there are several helpful landmarks that help ensure that images are adequate (Fig. 6.11).

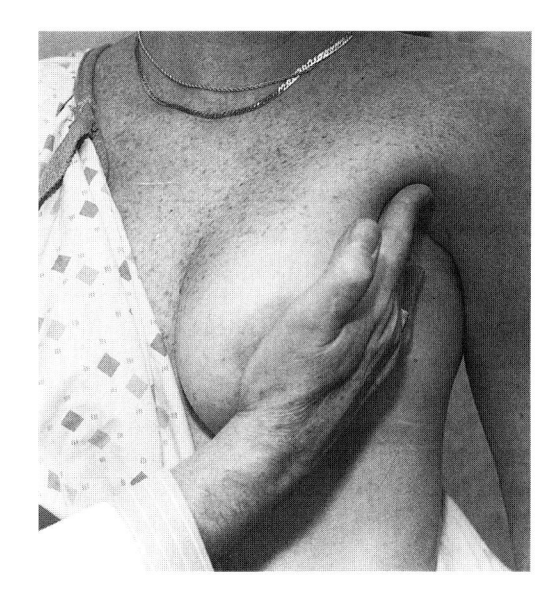

Fig. 6.10. Lateral margin of the breast being moved medially. By first moving the lateral aspect of the breast medially, there is less risk of excluding medial tissue as compression is applied

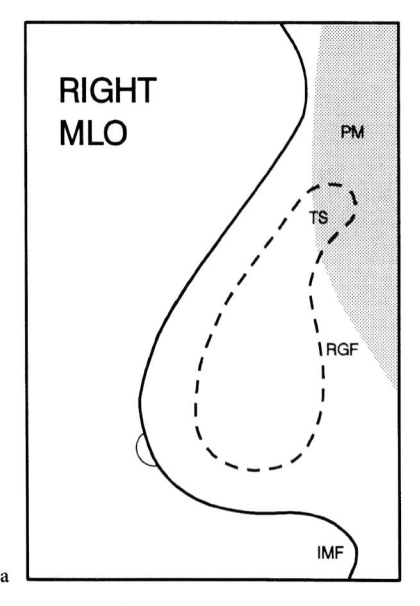

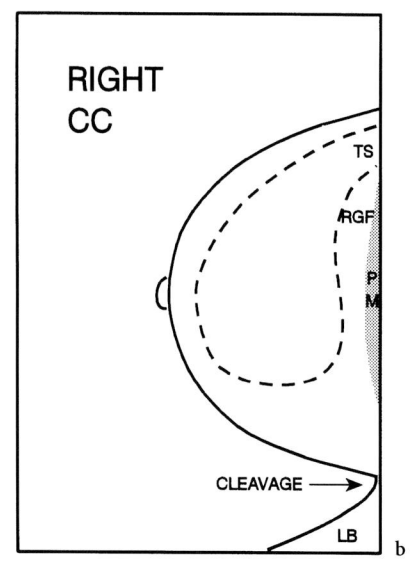

Fig. 6.11a,b. Landmarks for evaluating adequacy of mammographic images. **a** MLO view of the right breast. Ideally, the pectoral muscle (*PM*) should be seen to the level of the nipple. The wedge-shaped pectoral muscle has an anterior convexity. The tail of Spence (*TS*), projecting over the pectoral muscle, is not excluded from the back of the film. Retroglandular fat (*RGF*) is well seen, assuring that posterior glandular tissue is not excluded. *IMF*, inframammary fold. **b** CC image showing some cutoff of the tail of Spence (*TS*). Although efforts to pull lateral breast into the field of view may have been used, if the tail of Spence is prominent, it is not possible to see all of this tissue in some patients, thus requiring the addition of an exaggerated CC view (XCCL). Visualization of retroglandular fat (*RGF*) assures that posterior glandular tissue is included. Visualization of the pectoral muscle on the CC view is possible in only about 30%–40% of patients; when it is seen, the mammographer can be assured that posterior breast tissue is included. Although not possible in all patients, inclusion of the cleavage assure optimal visualization of posterior-medial breast tissue. If a portion of the contralateral breast (*LB*) is seen on the corner of the film, the mammographer can be assured that interposition of breast tissue between the chest wall and the film holder has not caused exclusion of posterior medial tissue of the breast being examined

6.7 The Exaggerated Craniocaudal View

The XCCL view, emphasizing the lateral aspect of the breast, is the most frequently used supplemental view in our practice (EKLUND and CARDENOSA 1992). Because adequate inclusion of all breast tissue in at last two projections is essential for proper screening, the technologist may selectively add this view if it is perceived that a significant amount of lateral breast tissue is excluded from the CC view. If the patient has previous films available for comparison, the need to include an XCCL view is decided by reviewing the adequacy of lateral tissue inclusion on the previous films. To perform the XCCL view, the technologist rotates the patient to bring the anterior axillary line in contact with the leading edge of the film holder (Fig. 6.12). The gantry is angled 5° for all XCCL images to allow the compression paddle to clear the humeral head. The most common errors in performing XCCL views are: (a) failure to angle the gantry 5° as described above, (b) simply centering

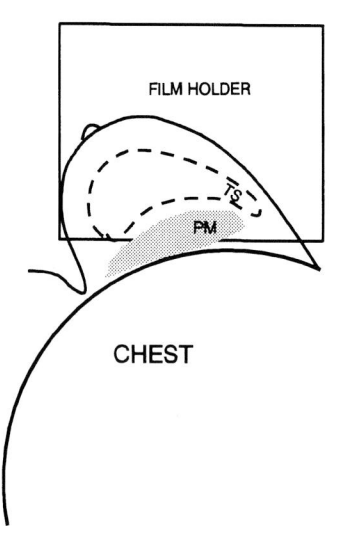

Fig. 6.12. Illustration of the right breast positioned for an XCCL image. The patient has been rotated to bring the anterior axillary line into contact with the film holder. The axiallary extension of breast tissue will be included. Some pectoral muscle (*PM*) should be included on all XCCL views

the x-ray tube over the lateral breast, and (c) failure to rotate the patient. Pectoral muscle should be included on all properly performed XCCL images (Fig. 6.13).

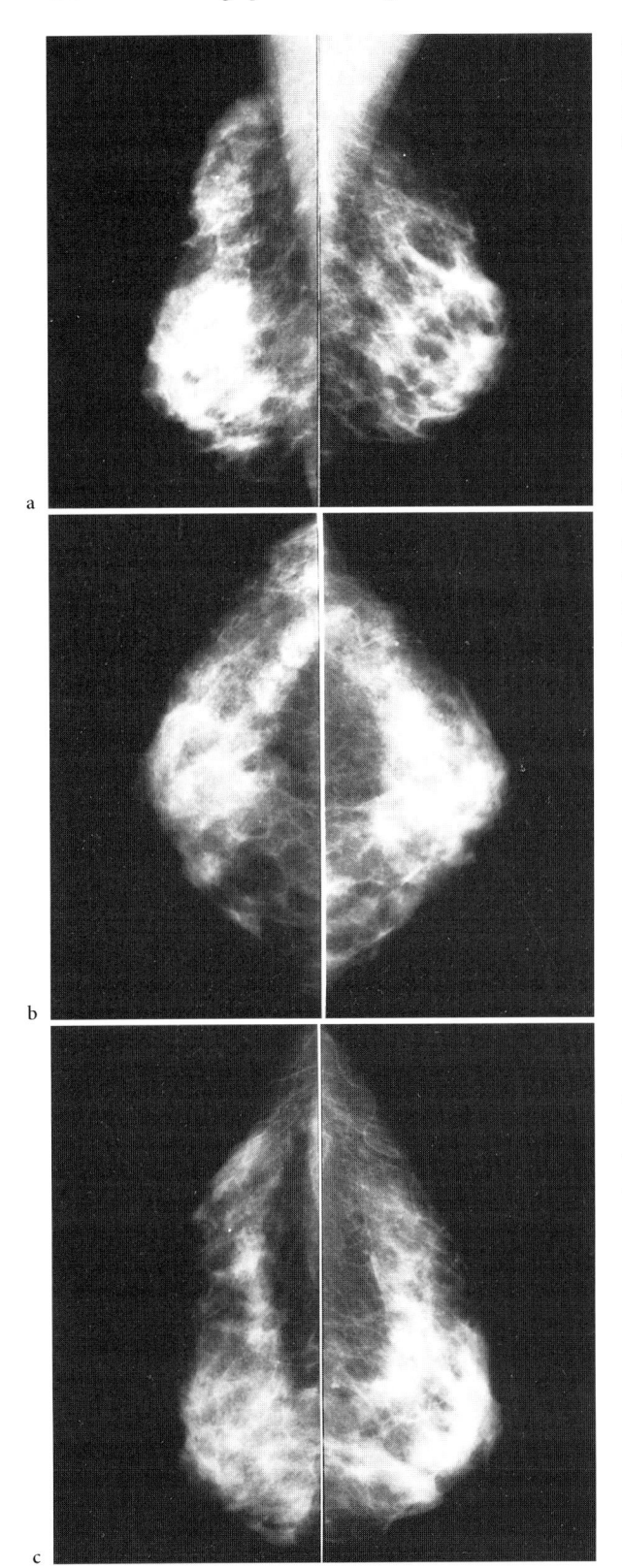

6.8 Diagnostic Mammography

Diagnostic mammography involves the workup of clinical concerns or radiographic findings detected on screening mammography. One or more supplemental views or special tailored views may be required to properly characterize the area in question (Bassett and Axelrod 1979; Bassett et al. 1987; Berkowitz et al. 1989; de Parades 1988; Eklund et al. 1988, 1994; Eklund and Cardenosa 1992). Although not a subject of this chapter, selected use of ultrasonography should be considered an essential component of diagnostic mammography.

Frequently used supplemental views include:

1. Exaggerated CC view
2. Spot compression view
3. Magnification view
4. Tangential spot view
5. Anterior compression view
6. Change of angle view
7. 90° lateral view
8. Cleavage view
9. Caudocranial view
10. Modified compression view (for the augmented breast)

Occasionally it is necessary to perform a modified view, specifically tailored to an area of concern. We refer to these as "tailored" views. Tailored views may be slight modifications of the routine supplemental views or creative images unique to the area being investigated.

Fig. 6.13a–c. MLO, CC, and XCCL images showing a prominent tail of Spence on the right (**a**). In spite of efforts to pull lateral breast tissue into the field of view, much of the lateral breast tissue has been excluded on the CC views (**b**). The addition of the XCCL view (**c**) provides an excellent look at this axillary extension of breast tissue. Note the inclusion of some pectoral muscle on the XCCL views

6.8.1 The Exaggerated CC (XCC) View

(See above, under Sect. 6.4.) Because of the common extension of breast tissue laterally and toward the axilla, the standard CC view will often exclude lateral breast tissue as discussed above. Although the XCCL view is included under our routine views, there are times when it is added as a "change of angle" view. By angling the tube 5° and centering over the lateral aspect of the breast, a slightly different orientation of parenchymal elements may reveal a lesion or improve its visualization.

6.8.2 The Spot Compression View

Spot compression can separate overlapping structures through better compression than is possible with whole-breast compression (BERKOWITZ et al. 1989; EKLUND and CARDENOSA 1992; SICKLES 1989). Spot compression over an island of asymmetrical density may enable the definite classification of the finding as a real mass or benign breast parenchyma. When a real mass is revealed, spot compression may be critical for careful evaluation of its marginal characteristics. Spot compression, combined with magnification, is often essential for characterization of a group of calcifications. Enhanced image detail is achieved by creating greater contrast between relatively compressible fat and normal breast parenchyma and relatively noncompressible pathologic lesions.

6.8.3 The Magnification View

Magnification, performed with microfocal spot technique, is essential for optimal characterization of microcalcifications or the finite features of the margins of masses (EKLUND and CARDENOSA 1992; SICKLES 1987). Degradation of image sharpness results from the widening penumbra effect as an object is moved away from the image receptor to obtain magnification. The use of a smaller focal spot is essential to overcome this disadvantage. Magnification should be performed only with a focal spot size of 0.1 mm or smaller. CC and MLO views with spot magnification images of the biopsy site and subareolar region constitute our routine views for patients who have undergone breast-conserving surgery. Rarely are magnified images performed with full-field exposure. Full-field magnification images, in the CC and 90° lateral projections, are obtained with ductography. Occasionally we have used full-field magnification to aid in the identification of calcifications that cannot be located on one of the standard views.

6.8.4 The Tangential Spot View

The tangential spot view is performed with the x-ray beam directed tangentially to the skin that overlies an area of radiographic concern or over a palpable finding (EKLUND and CARDENOSA 1992). When a patient presents with a palpable "lump" or area of

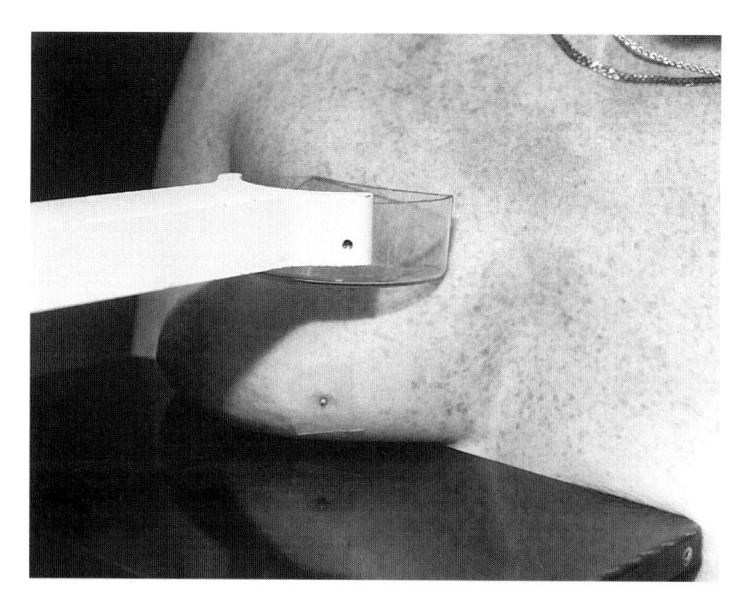

Fig. 6.14. Tangential spot compression image over a palpable nodule (marked with a lead "BB") enhances visualization of its margins

focal point tenderness, the technologist places a lead "BB" on the skin directly over the area of concern (Fig. 6.14). Performing a tangential image to the area under the "BB" enables visualization of the area in closest promimity to the subcutaneous fat. The fine marginal characteristics of masses are best seen with optimal contrast to the surrounding parenchyma. The radiolucency of fat (here, subcutaneous fat) compared to the higher density of pathologic lesions enhances contrast when tangential positioning juxtaposes a lesion against the subcutaneous fat. This is facilitated by the use of spot compression as discussed previously.

6.8.5 The Anterior Compression View

In some patients, dense parenchyma is found primarily in the anterior breast, especially if there is a bulbous anterior portion of the breast. With this anatomic pattern, it is often impossible to obtain adequate exposure of the dense areas without "burning out" the more fatty posterior breast. In such cases, an anterior compression view (limiting compression to the anterior half or third of the breast), enable better separation and exposure of parenchymal tissue (EKLUND and CARDENOSA 1992).

6.8.6 The Change of Angle View

Every density or "shadow" created on a mammographic film represents a summation of all objects or structures between the points of entry and exit of the x-ray beam (EKLUND and CARDENOSA 1992; SICKLES 1989). Superimposition of stromal elements can create two serious dilemmas for the mammographer. The most dangerous of these is the masking of a malignancy by superimposed densities. Less dangerous to the patient, but very frustrating nonetheless, is the creation of a "pseudo lesion" or "imaginoma" that leads to additional views, needless anxiety, and, occasionally, unnecessary biopsies. Changing the orientation of these superimposed parenchymal densities to the x-ray beam can uncover masked lesions and make pseudo lesions disappear. By angling the gantry or the the x-ray beam in relation to the breast, a reorientation of parenchymal densities is achieved. This occurs when using a 90° lateral view in combination with a 45° oblique view, or by adding an XCC view with its slightly different angle compared to the perpendicular CC view. Alternatively, the technologist can roll or angle the breast in relation to the x-ray beam (Fig. 6.15). An effective angled view can be obtained by simply altering the tissue/x-ray beam orientation by 5°–30°.

6.8.7 The 90° Lateral View

The 90° lateral view has been replaced by the MLO view for standard imaging due to its inability to include as much posterior tissue in the field of view and because of some limitation in compression. The most

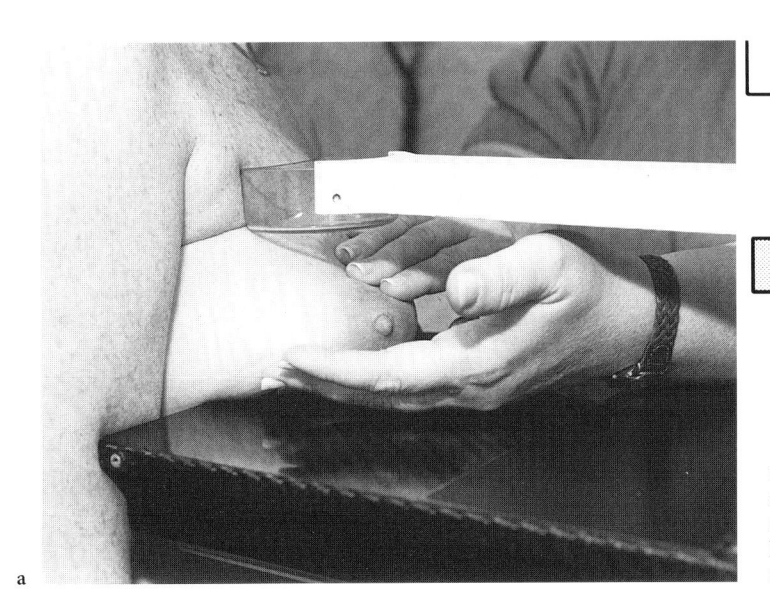

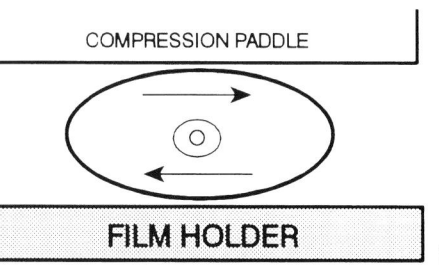

Fig. 6.15. a Technologist rolling the breast before applying compression. b Illustration showing upper breast tissue being rolled to the left; lower breast tissue is being rolled to the right

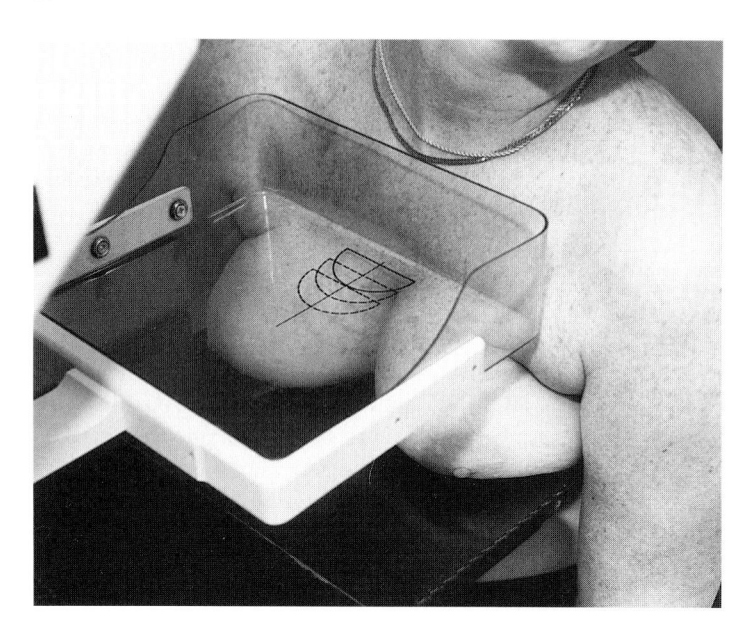

Fig. 6.16. Cleavage view is obtained by placing both breasts on the film holder and centering the x-ray beam between the breasts or on the medial side of the breast containing the area of concern. This view enables the film to be placed closer to the chest than with the standard CC view

popular use of the 90° lateral view is to provide a true orthogonal view to the CC view when triangulating the position of a lesion for preoperative localization. Another important use for this view (true of any two images taken at different angles) is to enable triangulation of the location of a lesion seen on the MLO view and not on a CC view, or vice versa. The 90° lateral view can also be used as "change of angle" view described above (EKLUND and CARDENOSA 1992). A 90° lateral image can be obtained in either a *medio*lateral or *latero*medial projection. To better visualize a lesion localized to the lateral half of the breast, a mediolateral projection places the lesion closer to the film and provides the sharpest image of the lesion. If a lesion is in the medial half of the breast, a lateromedial projection places the lesion closest to the film, making it appear more sharply defined.

6.8.8 The Cleavage View

Lesions located posteriorly against the pectoral fascia and in the medial aspect of the breast may be better visualized in the CC projection by bringing both breasts onto the film and centering the x-ray beam over the cleavage between the breasts (Fig. 6.16) (EKLUND and CARDENOSA 1992). It is sometimes possible to include slightly more posterior medial breast tissue with this view. Use of the spot compression paddle often provides the same advantage of "seeing" slightly more posterior tissue. Manual techniques must be used when the x-ray beam is centered between the breasts. With no breast tissue between the x-ray source and the automatic exposure control (AEC), exposure time will be prematurely terminated by the AEC, resulting in an underexposed film. By positioning the medial portion of the breast being examined over the AEC, phototiming is feasible.

6.8.9 The Caudocranial View

Use of the caudocranial view has been described earlier in the text dealing with imaging a patient with severe kyphosis who may have difficulty turning her head away from the x-ray tube housing during performance of the CC view (Fig. 6.7) (EKLUND and CARDENOSA 1992). By keeping the lesion closer to the film, this view will also improve the image sharpness of a lesion located in the upper portion of the breast.

6.8.10 The Modified Compression View for the Augmented Breast

Routine imaging of the augmented breast consists of four views of each breast (EKLUND et al. 1988; EKLUND and CARDENOSA 1992). The two standard views (MLO and CC) include the implant in the field. The modified MLO and CC views are performed by bringing native tissue over and in front of the implant, limiting compression to those tissues anterior to the implant (Fig. 6.17). There are important limitations of the modified compression technique and important considerations relating to the compression used with standard, full-view mammographic

The Art of Mammographic Positioning

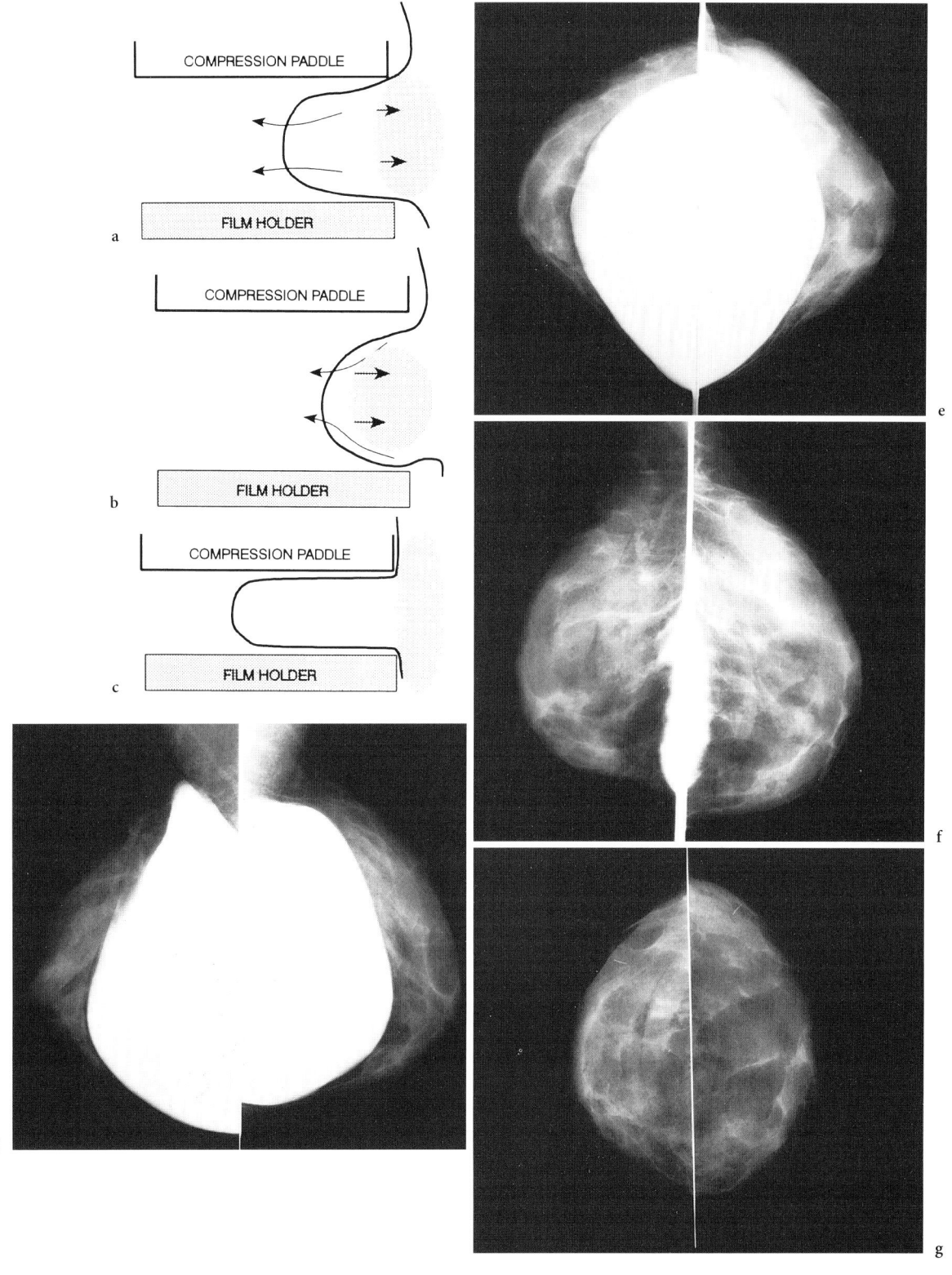

Fig. 6.17a–g. Modified compression views of the augmented breast obtained by pulling breast tissue out over the implant and limiting compression to native tissue free of the implant. **a** Breast containing implant. Native tissue will be pulled forward as the implant is pushed back against the chest. **b** Compression is increased as breast tissue is pulled anteriorly. **c** With the implant displaced posteriorly, more breast tissue will be seen and better compression achieved. **d,e** Standard MOL (**d**) and CC (**e**) views of a breast with augmentation implants. Much of the native tissue is obscured by the implants. **f,g** Modified MLO (**f**) and CC (**g**) views obtained after pulling native tissue anteriorly and displacing the implants posteriorly

images. When imaging the entire breast with implants included in the field of view, the only purpose of compression is to immobilize the breast; the implant absorbs compression while the breast tissue visualized around the implant remains uncompressed. Other than stabilizing the breast, compression contributes nothing to improved image quality when the full breast and implant are in the field. With the implant displaced and compression limited to the native tissue brought anterior to the implant, all of the usual benefits of compression accrue, with significant improvement in image quality.

The degree to which an implant can be displaced and breast tissue pulled forward is dependent on several factors:

1. *Fibrous encapsulation.* All implants in the breast are subject to the formation of fibrous encapsulation, which can cause the implant to feel very rigid and be resistant to displacement.

2. *Retropectoral vs subglandular placement.* Implants can be placed anterior to the pectoral muscle (retroglandular) or behind the pectoral muscle (subpectoral). The tendency to form firm encapsulation is reduced with subpectoral implants. Better modified compression views are obtainable with subpectoral placement of implants and when encapsulation is minimal.

3. *Amount of native breast tissue.* The greater the amount of native tissue, the more elastic the surrounding skin. When an augmentation implant is so relatively large that native tissue and skin must be stretched over the implant, the effect is the same as firm encapsulation – the implant is virtually fixed and very little tissue can be pulled forward over the implant.

4. *Patient anxiety and fear of implant damage.* An apprehensive patient, fearful of anything that might harm her implant, may not tolerate the procedure or may simply not cooperate with the technologist.

6.9 Summary

Suboptimal mammography has been shown to delay the diagnosis of early breast cancer. There is a growing body of evidence supporting the axiom that *success in reducing breast cancer mortality is more dependent on when breast cancer is found than on how it is treated.* Good mammography is complete mammography! Improper positioning, excluded tissue, and incompletely visualized or worked-up lesions represent suboptimal mammogrpahy. Such deficiencies contribute to the missed or delayed diagnosis of breast cancer. Mammographic positioning is an art that, combined with the science of imaging, can achieve the high-quality studies necessary for early breast cancer detection. Appropriately mastered and skillfully applied, the mammographic positioning techniques described in this chapter should enable the mammographer to obtain images with optimal tissue visualization.

References

Bassett LW, Axelrod SA (1979) A modification of the craniocaudal view in mammography radiology 132:222–224

Bassett LW, Gold RH (1983) Breast radiography using the oblique projection. Radiology 149:585–587

Bassett LW, Bunnell D, Jahanshahi R (1987) Breast cancer detection: one view versus two views. Radiology 165:95–97

Berkowitz JE, Gatewood OMB, Gayler BW (1989) Equivocal mammographic findings: evaluation with spot compression. Radiology 171:369–371

de Parades ES (1989) Atlas of film screen mammography. Urban & Schwarzenberg, Baltimore, p 17

Eklund GW (1991) Mammographic compression: science or art? Radiology 181:339–341

Eklund GW, Cardenosa G (1992) The art of mammographic positioning. Radiol Clin North Am 30:21–53

Eklund GW, Busby RC, Miller SH, Job JS (1988) Improved imaging of the augmented breast. Radiology 151:469–473

Eklund GW, et al. (1994) Assessing adequacy of mammographic image quality. Radiology 190:297–307

Feig SA (1988) Importance of supplementary mammographic views to diagnostic accuracy. AJR 151:40

Hall FM (1989) Magnification spot compression of the breast (letter). Radiology 173:284

Haus AG (1984) Screen-film mammography update: x-ray units, breast compression, grids, screen-film characteristics, and radiation dose. Proc SPIE p 486

Muir B, Kirkpatrick A, Roberts M (1984) Oblique-view mammography; adequacy for screening. Radiology 151:39–41

Sickles EA (1986) Baseline screening mammography. Am J Roentgenol 147:1149–1153

Sickles EA (1987) Magnification mammography In: Bassett LW, Gold RH (eds) Breast cancer detection: mammography and other methods in breast imaging, 2nd edn. Grune & Stratton, New York, pp 111–117

Sickles EA (1988) Practical solutions to common mammographic problems: tailoring the examination. AJR 151:31–39

Sickles EA (1989) Combining spot-compression and other special views to maximize mammographic information. Radiology 173:571

Sullivan DC, Beam CA, Goodman SM, Watt DR (1991) Measurement of force applied during mammography. Radiology 181:355–357

Tabár L (1984) Microfocal spot magnification mammography. In: Brünner S, Langfedt B, Anderson PE (eds) Early detection of breast cancer. Springer, Berlin Heidelberg New York, pp 62–68

Tabár L, Dean PB (1989) Optimum mammographic technique: the annotated cookbook approach. Administrative Radiology pp 54–56

7 Differential Diagnosis of Microcalcifications

M. Lanyi

CONTENTS

7.1 Introduction 89
7.2 Acinar Microcalcifications 92
7.2.1 Microcystic (Blunt Duct) Adenosis 92
7.2.2 Microcystic Mastopathy 94
7.2.3 Fibrosing (Sclerosing) Adenosis 100
7.2.4 Fibroadenoma 100
7.3 Microcalcifications of Ductal Origin 104
7.3.1 Intraductal Carcinoma 104
7.3.2 Secretory Calcifications 119
7.3.3 Microcalcifications in Papillomatosis
      and Papilloma 119
7.4 Simultaneous Occurrence of Acinar
    and Ductal Microcalcifications 124
7.5 Microcalcifications Outside of the Acini
    and Milk Ducts 125
7.5.1 Fat Necrosis 125
7.5.2 Arterial Calcifications 126
7.5.3 Calcifications in Axillary Lymph Nodes 127
7.5.4 Calcified Foreign Bodies 129
7.5.5 Calcified Sebaceous Glands 130
7.6 Calcium-like Artifacts 132
7.7 Conclusion 133
      References 134

7.1 Introduction

Leborgne, in 1951, was the first to point out that microcalcifications occur in 30% of breast carcinomas. He wrote: "With sufficient experience differential diagnosis between calcifications of malignant processes ... and ... in benign processes is generally easy." Egan (1964) also asserted: "The typical calcifications are pathognomonic of carcinoma. They are so specific, that in their presence, a histological diagnosis of benign disease usually indicates that either the surgeon has selected the wrong tissue for biopsy, or that the pathologist is in error." However, analysis of 23 articles on microcalcifications published between 1964 and 1994 shows that cancer was detected in only 27.5% of 5481 cases operated on for microcalcifications (Table 7.1). Similar results can be found in studies carried out by Rosen et al. (1974),

M. Lanyi, MD, Martinweg 8, 94072 Bad Füssing, Germany

Tinnemans et al. (1986), and Abbes et al. (1988), which yielded figures of 24%, 28.3%, and 29%, respectively.

The true rate of cancer detection is, however, even poorer because, except in studies by Abbes et al. (1988) and De Lafontan (1994), cases of lobular carcinoma in situ (LCIS) were counted as carcinomas. Apart from the controversy which still exists with regard to this histological diagnosis even after 25 years of discussion, other factors such as nonspecific radiographic features, acinus-localized microcalcifications, and detection by chance have a role to play in the diagnosis of LCIS (Snyder 1966; Lewison 1964; Rosen 1984; Lanyi 1986; Pope et al. 1988; Beute et al. 1991; Sonnenfeld et al. 1991; Rebner and Raju 1994). Therefore the detection of LCIS cannot logically be considered as a success in diagnosing microcalcification. As LCIS represents 5%–6% of all carcinomas listed in Table 7.1, the number of carcinomas is reduced to at least 22%–23%. Is this low rate of prediction – unacceptable in any diagnostic process – due to the complexity of the subject or are the diagnostic criteria inadequate?

Fourteen publications with analyses of the radiomorphological features of "benign" and "malignant" microcalcifications were evaluated (Abbes et al. 1988; Colbassini et al. 1982; Egan 1988; Hassler 1969; Kersschot et al. 1985; de Lafontan et al. 1994; Levitan et al. 1964; Martin et al. 1979; Millis et al. 1976; Muir et al. 1983; Murphy and de Schryver-Kecskemeti 1978; Powell et al. 1983; Rosen et al. 1974; Roselli del Turco 1986). The authors assessed the following items: shape, number (within a cluster and number per cm^2), size (and variations in size), homogeneity, intensity, borders of microcalcifications, and size and spatial arrangement of clusters (form of clusters). After statistical evaluation of the data, all authors reached a similar conclusion to that of Egan et al. (1980): "These signs are so nonspecific, that all radiographically demonstrable clusters of stippled calcifications require histopathological study" because "calcifications in benign and malignant disease were often similar"

Table 7.1. Detection of cancer in cases operated on due to microcalcifications

Author	No. of cases operated on due to microcalcifications	Carcinoma	Rate of detection of carcinoma (%)	LCIS	Carcinoma without LCIS	Detection rate without LCIS
Abbes et al. (1988)	112	56 (27 DCIS)	50	3[a]	–	–
Bauermeister et al. (1973)	54	14	26	–	–	–
Bjurstam (1978)	148	86 (15 occult)	58	–	–	–
Citoler (1978)	481	97	20	49	48 (21 DCIS)	10
Colbassini et al. (1982)	55	15 (7 DCIS)	27.2	–	–	–
De Lafontan et al. (1994)	400	98 (54 DCIS)	24.5	2[b]	–	–
Egan et al. (1980)	468	115	24.5	13	102 (52 DCIS)	21.7
Galkin et al. (1983)	100	42	42	–	–	–
Kindermann et al. (1979)	387	90	23.3	–	–	–
Le Gal et al. (1984)	227	101	44.5	6	95 (52 DCIS; 29 non-comedo)	41.8
Levitan et al. (1964)	240	78 (1 DCIS)	32.5	–	–	–
Menges et al. (1973)	67	13	19.4	–	–	–
Muir et al. (1983)	45	17 (12 DCIS)	37.7	–	–	–
Murphy and De Schryver-Kecskemeti (1978)	31	11 (5 DCIS)	35.5	–	–	–
Paterok et al. (1993)	1393	323	26.9	–	–	–
Powell et al. (1983)	282	47	17	10	37 (26 DCIS)	13.1
Prorok et al. (1983)	62	20	32	2	18 (3 DCIS)	29
Rogers and Powell (1972)	46	19	41	3	16	34.7
Rosen et al. (1974)	125	32	25	4	28 (18 DCIS)	22.4
Roses et al. (1980)	52	17	33	1	16	30.7
Schwartz et al. (1984)	320	96	30	–	–	–
Sigfusson et al. (1983)	213	70	32	10	60 (30 DCIS)	28.1
Tinnemans et al. (1986)	173	51	29.5	7	44 (22 DCIS)	25.4
Total	5481	1508	27.5	110	464[c]	21.8[c]

[a] Assigned to the "benign lesions"
[b] With 23 cases of atypical ductal hyperplasia assigned to the "borderline cases"
[c] From among 2129 cases biopsied due to microcalcifications

and "there is such a wide overlapping in fibrocystic disease and carcinoma, the mammographer cannot confidently exclude carcinoma." The reason for this uncertainty is deficiency in the design of the various studies: most of the parameters (number, size, homogeneity, border, and cluster size) are irrelevant for diagnosis, as has been repeatedly shown in the statistical results of the reviewed publications. The really important mammographic features, such as the shapes of individual microcalcifications and the form of the clusters, were removed from their histological context and usually not all or insufficiently investigated. It is characteristic that, for example, Egan, in his second book in 1988, listed the same "malignant" shapes of microcalcifications as 23 years previously: "sandlike," with the appearance of innumerable "grains of salt," "heterogeneous," with a resemblance to a "jumble of the alphabet," "coarse," "smooth," with the appearance of spilled droplets of mercury," "lacy," "wavy," "faint," and "rounded." The comparative term "grains of salt" was used by Leborgne as early as 1951 when, due to technical limitations, microcalcifications could not be imaged with great clarity. Even the so-called EGAN technique of the early 1960s was deficient compared with contemporary standards, particularly with regard to the assessment of fine details such as microcalcifications. Between 1965 and 1988, however, mammographic technique made enormous progress, e.g., film-screen systems, magnification mammography! What use are most of the above-mentioned or further comparisons such as "comets and tadpoles" (MUIR et al. 1983) or "a stone crushed by a hammer" (HOEFFKEN and LANYI 1973)?

LE GAL et al. (1976, 1984) described vermiform microcalcifications as highly suspicious of carcinoma. According to MOSKOWITZ (1979) and KERSSCHOT et al. (1985), linear microcalcifications are particularly alarming. SIGFUSSON et al. (1983) thought that the risk of cancer is greater in the presence of a few irregularly shaped calcifications than in the presence of a larger number.

Most of the above descriptions are contradictory, misleading, cannot be applied in practice, or are of only limited use. This is because assessment was made solely according to radiographic aspects without considering the histological correlation. Cluster shape is rarely mentioned in publications and, when it is, then only the linear branched form. According to the author's studies this linear branched shape accounts for only 4% of all cluster forms (GERSHON-COHEN et al. 1966; LEBORGNE 1951; MOSKOWITZ 1979; DE LAFONTAN et al. 1994).

LEVITAN et al. (1964), ROSELLI DEL TURCO (1984), and SIGFUSSON et al. (1983) maintain that irregularity in cluster shape is characteristic of carcinoma. However, SIGFUSSON et al. mention my own description of the triangular principle (1977) as a helpful sign/tool in diagnosis.

A further error in the design of the previously published studies was that microcalcifications in LCIS, and those found in ductal carcinomas, were grouped and analyzed together under the heading "carcinoma." LCIS is found in 5%–50% of the carcinomas detected at mammography by demonstration of microcalcifications (CITOLER 1978; EGAN et al. 1980; LE GAL et al. 1984; POWELL et al. 1983; ROSEN et al. 1974; EGAN 1988). As has already been mentioned, LCIS is usually detected histologically in cases operated on because of lobular microcalcifications, often at sites distant from the locations of the calcifications. The mammographic features of lobular microcalcifications are, however, completely different to those of intraductal carcinoma in its various forms. Consequently the profile of microcalcifications in intraductal carcinomas was distorted. The profile of benign microcalcifications was also distorted, as "benign" microcalcifications were not further specified. It is completely misleading to analyze the shape and spatial distribution of microcalcifications in small lobular cysts together with secretory microcalcifications just because they both happen to be benign!

There is another recently discussed and very important problem: Just how reliable is the histological diagnosis on which our findings on the shape of microcalcifications in ductal carcinoma are based? The most important question of all is: How frequently are borderline cases over- or underdiagnosed by pathologists? The histological diagnosis of atypical ductal hyperplasia and with it that of intraductal *noncomedocarcinoma* is subjective (HELVIE et al. 1991). Accordingly SCHNITT et al. (1992) reported that six experts conformed in carcinoma diagnosis in only 20% of cases of noncomedo ductal in situ carcinomas which were presented to them for analysis, based on mutually agreed criteria. In 80% of the cases the very same specimens were diagnosed as hyperplasia, atypical hyperplasia, and carcinoma! This uncertain histological assessment must have influenced the mammographic analysis of microcalcifications, especially since according to Table 7.1 almost 40% of the carcinomas were in situ ($n = 201/503$).

The ratio of *noncomedo-* to *comedocarcinoma* among the cases of ductal carcinoma in situ (DCIS) has been given as 56%:44% (LE GAL et al. 1984). On the basis of this information we can assume that in 5% of cases operated on for microcalcifications and in more than 20% of carcinomas, the verdict "still benign" or "already malignant" is solely dependent on an individual pathologist's interpretation. Thus the rate of accuracy not only of cancer diagnosis but also of the analysis of the shape of microcalcifications is greatly influenced.

Microcalcifications develop in microscopically small cavities within or outside of the lobular-ductal system. The radiologist must classify microcalcifications according to their localization and raise alarm if possible only in cases of intraductal microcalcifications. Microcalcifications which can be definitely localized in the lobule and can be easily recognized as microcystic adenosis or clustered milk of calcium cysts account for almost 60% of false-positive preoperative diagnoses (LANYI and NEUFANG 1984). The carcinoma yield can be almost doubled simply by winnowing out these cases!

Table 7.2. Accuracy of reported system of differential diagnosis, as tested by the author with respect to the case material of four large institutions in the early 1980s

	Catholic University, Nijmegen (Dr. Hendriks)	University of California (Dr. Sickles)	Institut Curie, Paris (Dr. Le Gal)	University of Cologne (Dr. Neufang)	Total[b]
No. of cases					
Malignant	46	41	54	42	183
Benign	54	44	99	255	452
True-pos.	42	39 (36[a])	53	41	175
False-neg.	4	2	1	1	8
True-neg.	22	38	63	187	310
False-pos.	32	6 (9[a])	36	68	142
Total	100	85	153	297	635

[a] Numbers prior to second biopsies (see text)
[b] Summary of author's diagnostic accuracy: 175 of 317 (55%) recommended biopsies yielded malignant samples; no. of unnecessary biopsies = 310/452 (68%); no. of undiscovered carcinomas = 8 (4.3%); sensitivity = 95.6%; specificity = 68.5%

To ascertain the anatomical position two parameters must be analyzed in two planes: the shape of the individual microcalcifications and the form of the cluster. With the aid of this system the author managed to improve his own rate of accuracy over a period of 11 years from 13.8% (1974) to 52% (1985). Note that the percentage of carcinomas detected solely through microcalcifications remained unchanged. This suggests that the 52% success rate was not achieved at the expense of undetected carcinomas. This success rate was further improved between 1985 and 1989 to 69.2%.

In the early 1980s the author was able to test the accuracy of this system of differential diagnosis on case material of four large institutions (Table 7.2). The malignant and benign cases selected by Dr. Hendriks (University of Nijmegen, Holland), Dr. Le Gal (Institut Curie, France) Dr. Neufang (Universitäts Frauenklinik, Cologne, Germany), and Dr. Sickles (University of California San Francisco, USA) were not consecutive. All cases were histologically proven. The histological diagnosis was unknown to the author. There were no cases of LCIS. A total of 635 cases were included in the study (183 carcinomas and 452 "benign" cases). Of the 317 biopsies recommended by the author, 175 yielded malignant samples (55%); eight carcinomas were not detected (4.37%). Of the 452 biopsies, 310 were unnecessary. The sensitivity was 95.6%, and the specificity, 68.5%. An interesting fact is that although the author originally diagnosed nine false-positive cases in the collection from the University of California, some months later the figure was reduced to six, because out of four second biopsies three were histologically proven to be carcinomas (personal communication, Dr. Sickles).

7.2 Acinar Microcalcifications

Clustered microcalcifications were detected in 87 of 1044 successive mammograms. Forty-two of these (48%) were acinar (LANYI 1986). Acini are finger-like tubes at the ends of the milk ducts. They have an epithelial lining, the outermost layer of which is covered by smooth muscle cells, so-called myoepithelial cells. These myoepithelial cells are responsible for the transport of the milk to the milk ducts. Roughly 20–40 acini, along with the intralobular connective tissue surrounding them, form a lobule 0.5 mm in size. The acini are separated from each other by collageneous *intra*lobular connective tissue.

Secretory microcalcifications within the acini can be found in the following histological diagnoses:

1. Microcystic (blunt duct) adenosis
2. Microcystic mastopathy
3. Fibrosing (sclerosing) adenosis
4. Fibroadenoma

7.2.1 Microcystic (Blunt Duct) Adenosis

The formation of lobular cysts is shown in Fig. 7.1. Initially there is lobular hypertrophy: The number of acini may be increased up to fourfold and they become elongated and somewhat serpentine. The lob-

Differential Diagnosis of Microcalcifications

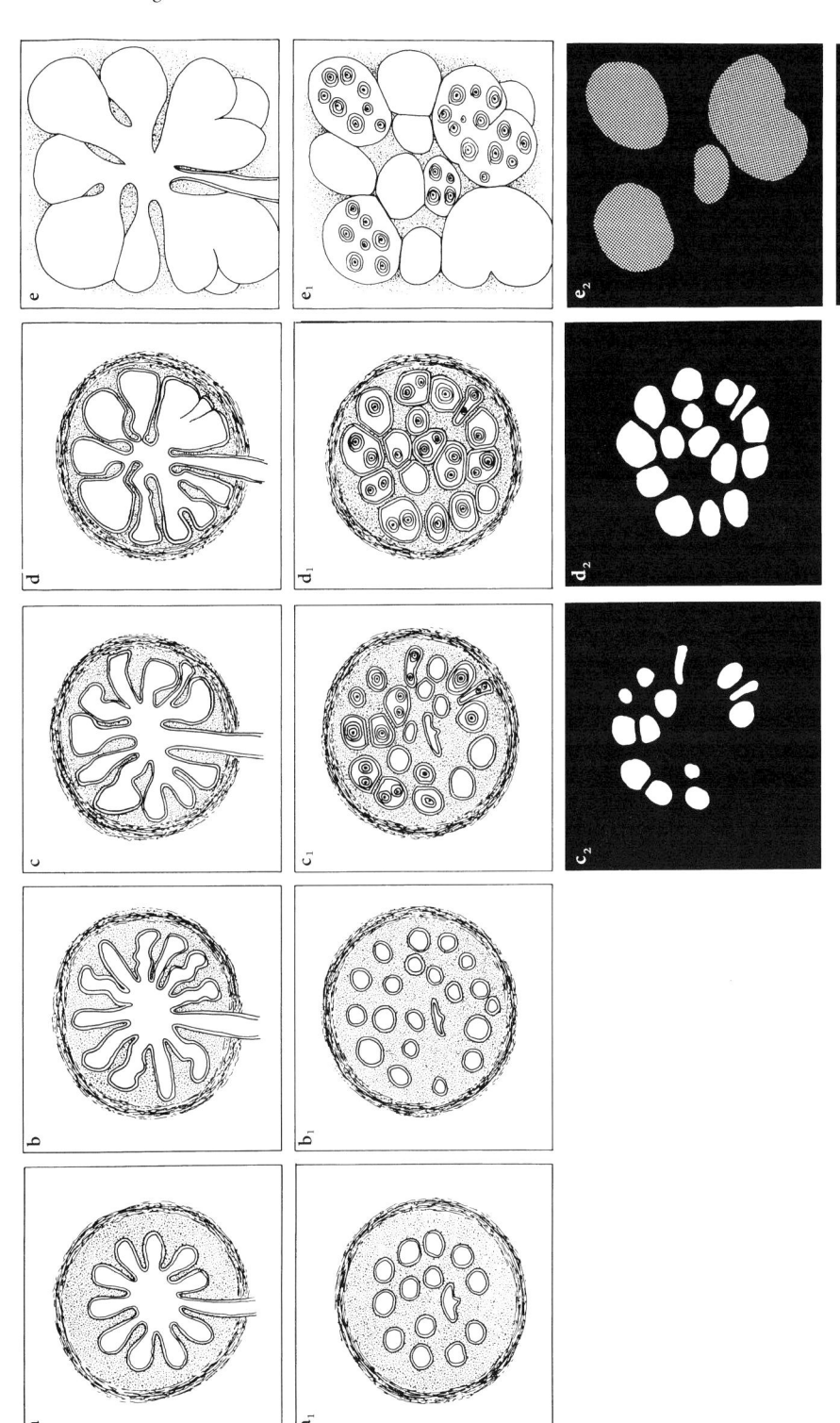

Fig. 7.1a–e. Schematic representation of development of cysts and cystic microcalcifications. *Top row:* vertical sections; *center row:* cross-sections; *bottom rows:* mammographic representation of the microcalcifications. **a,a₁** Normal lobule. **b,b₁** Lobular hypertrophy. **c** Blunt duct adenosis: **c₁** Blunt duct adenosis with psammoma bodies. **c₂** Mostly round (sometimes accompanied by border flattening) quasi-"facetted" microcalcifications with "septa." The linear microcalcifications correspond to psammoma bodies in flattened cysts. The cluster shape is round. **d** Microcystic adenosis; the septa are also visible here. **d₁** Psammoma bodies in acini which have become widened through cysts. **d₂** The microcalcifications are larger. There is flattening, septa are visible, and the cluster shape is round. **e** Microcystic mastopathy. The cysts have the borders of the lobule. **e₁** Numerous psammoma bodies in some cysts. **e₂,e₃** Teacup phenomenon

ule doubles in size to 1 mm in diameter. Later the acini lose their form and become coarse and blunt (blunt duct adenosis, Foote and Stewart 1945). The lobules may further increase to 2 mm in size. If these acini widen even more, the condition is called microcystic adenosis. The size of the lobules at this stage is about 4–5 mm. If, though further increase in size, these cysts (still contained within a lobule = microcystic adenosis), trespass the collagenous borders, the lobule no longer forms an anatomical unit; this condition is referred to by pathologists as microcystic mastopathy.

All these changes in the acinar dilatation can occur in combined forms. These histologically and clinically irrelevant changes become significant if they are (unfortunately) rendered visible through microcalcifications on the mammogram and thus cause problems in differential diagnosis. Based on comparative mammographic/histological correlation (Lanyi and Citoler 1981), the following mammographic criteria for microcalcifications in microcystic (blunt duct) adenosis were established:

1. *Cluster shape*: round/oval in all views
2. *Cluster size*: 2–5 mm
3. *Size and shape of individual microcalcifications*:
    a) 0.1–0.3 mm
    b) Monomorphous, round/punctate, sometimes accompanied by border flattening
    c) Quasi-facetted

If the microcalcifications are close together they are separated by fine lines, giving the cluster a morula-like appearance (Figs. 7.2, 7.3). Two microcalcifications side by side appear diplococcus-like. A similar appearance is extremely rare in intraductal calcifications.

Clusters of more than 5 mm in diameter are formed by several closely located foci of microcystic (blunt duct) adenosis with microcalcification. These are usually round/oval or rosette shaped (Fig. 7.4). Angled cluster shapes are rare. The disseminated, usually bilateral microcalcifications in microcystic (blunt duct) adenosis are similar in size, monomorphous, and round/punctate shaped. Border flattening as described above can also be observed in closely located microcalcifications (Fig. 7.5). In cases of microcystic (blunt duct) adenosis and in microcystic mastopathic disease, microcalcifications represent secretory calcifications with psammoma bodies. These psammoma bodies form as concretions in a way similar to the formation of pearls in oysters (Fig. 7.6).

7.2.2 Microcystic Mastopathy

Microcalcifications in microcystic mastopathy can be identified by their different shapes evident in two mammographic views. This so-called teacup phenomenon (Lanyi 1977; Sickles and Abele 1981; Homer et al. 1988; Linden and Sickles 1989) results from the fact that in a lateral view, the psammoma bodies because of their higher specific gravity are seen as dregs which have sedimented to the bottom. This is similar to the phenomenon observed in galactography when the denser contrast medium fails to mix with the thicker intraductal secretions. This layering of milk of calcium is not at all visible in the craniocaudal view and is less obvious in the mediolateral oblique view. Figures 7.7–7.9 show the varying shapes of the teacup phenomenon. The shape of the cluster is usually round/oval in two views, and rarely amorphous. Sedimented calcium in cysts usually occurs bilaterally, although not symmetrically, and is often diffusely distributed (Fig. 7.9).

Differential Diagnosis of Microcalcifications

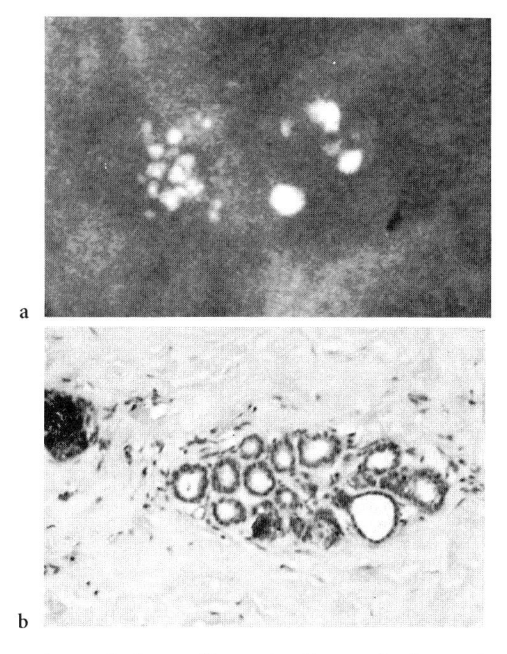

Fig. 7.2. a An oval cluster (4 mm in diameter) of round, sometimes facetted microcalcifications with septa. **b** Histology: microcystic (blunt duct) adenosis

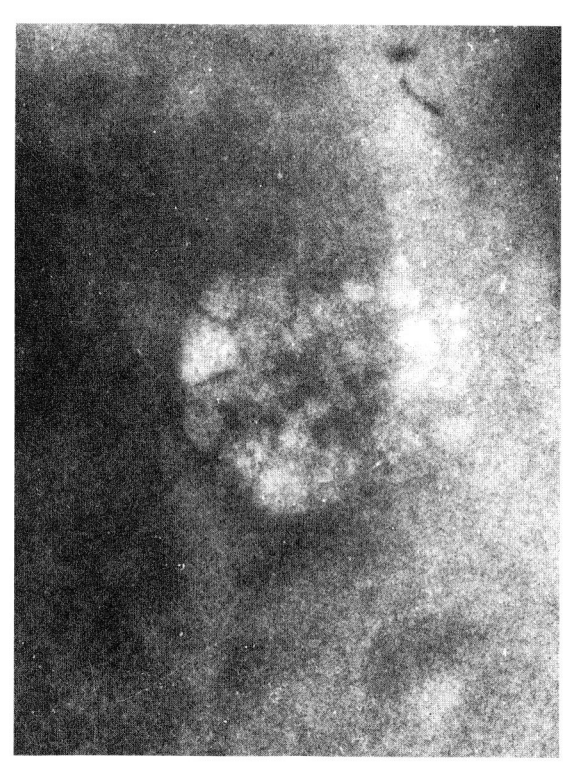

Fig. 7.3. A round cluster of microcalcifications. The cluster is 5 mm in diameter and morula-like in appearance. Some of the microcalcifications show contour flattening and septa are visible. The appearance represents microcystic (blunt duct) adenosis

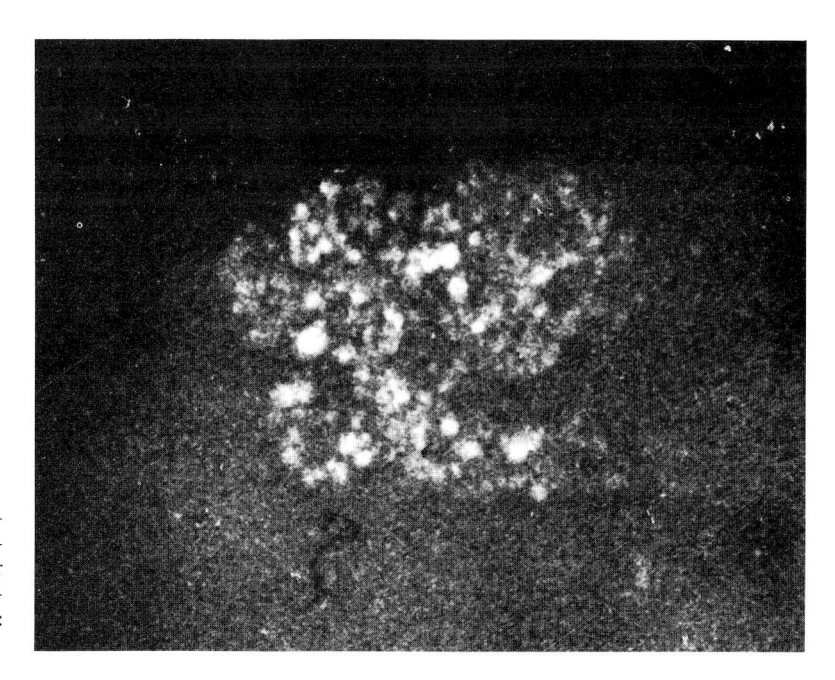

Fig. 7.4. Rosette-shaped cluster, 6–7 mm in diameter, of round microcalcifications, some with contour flattening, obviously located in several neighboring lobules. Histology: microcystic (blunt duct) adenosis

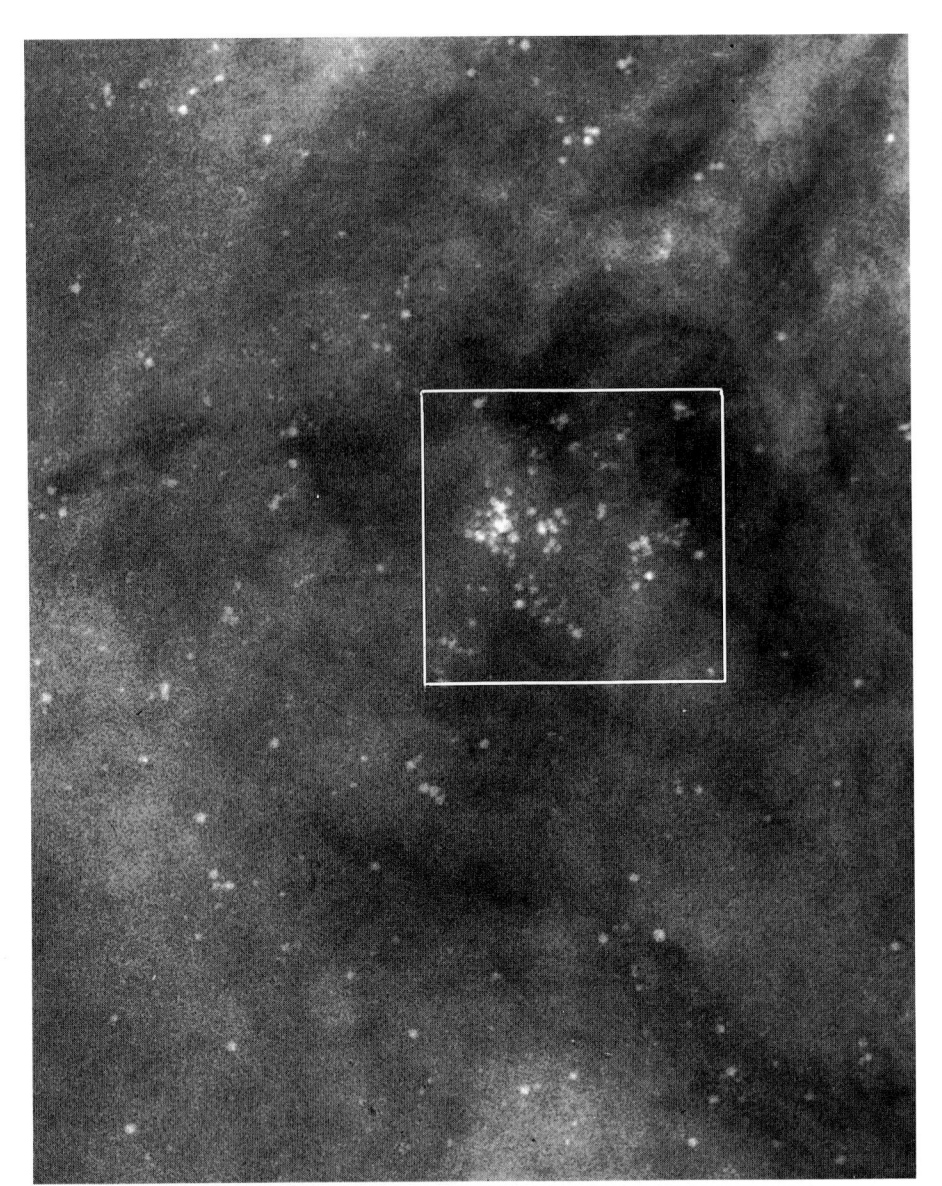

Fig. 7.5. Diffuse, disseminated microcalcifications that are similar in size; such microcalcifications often occur in a circumscribed area (pseudocluster!). Contour flattening and septa are seen. Histology: microcystic (blunt duct) adenosis

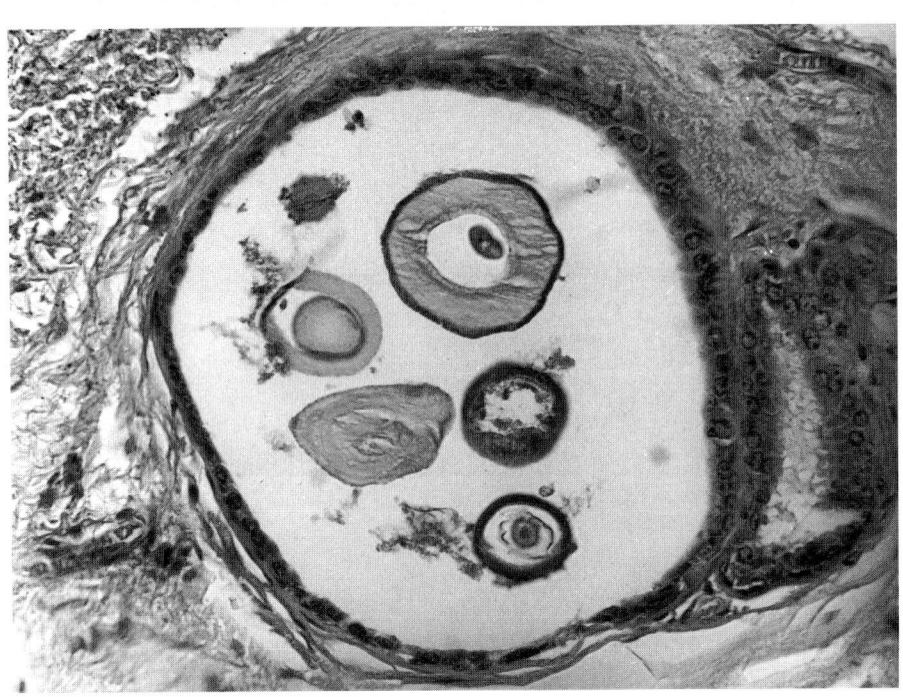

Fig. 7.6. Milk of calcium cyst with layering of psammoma bodies

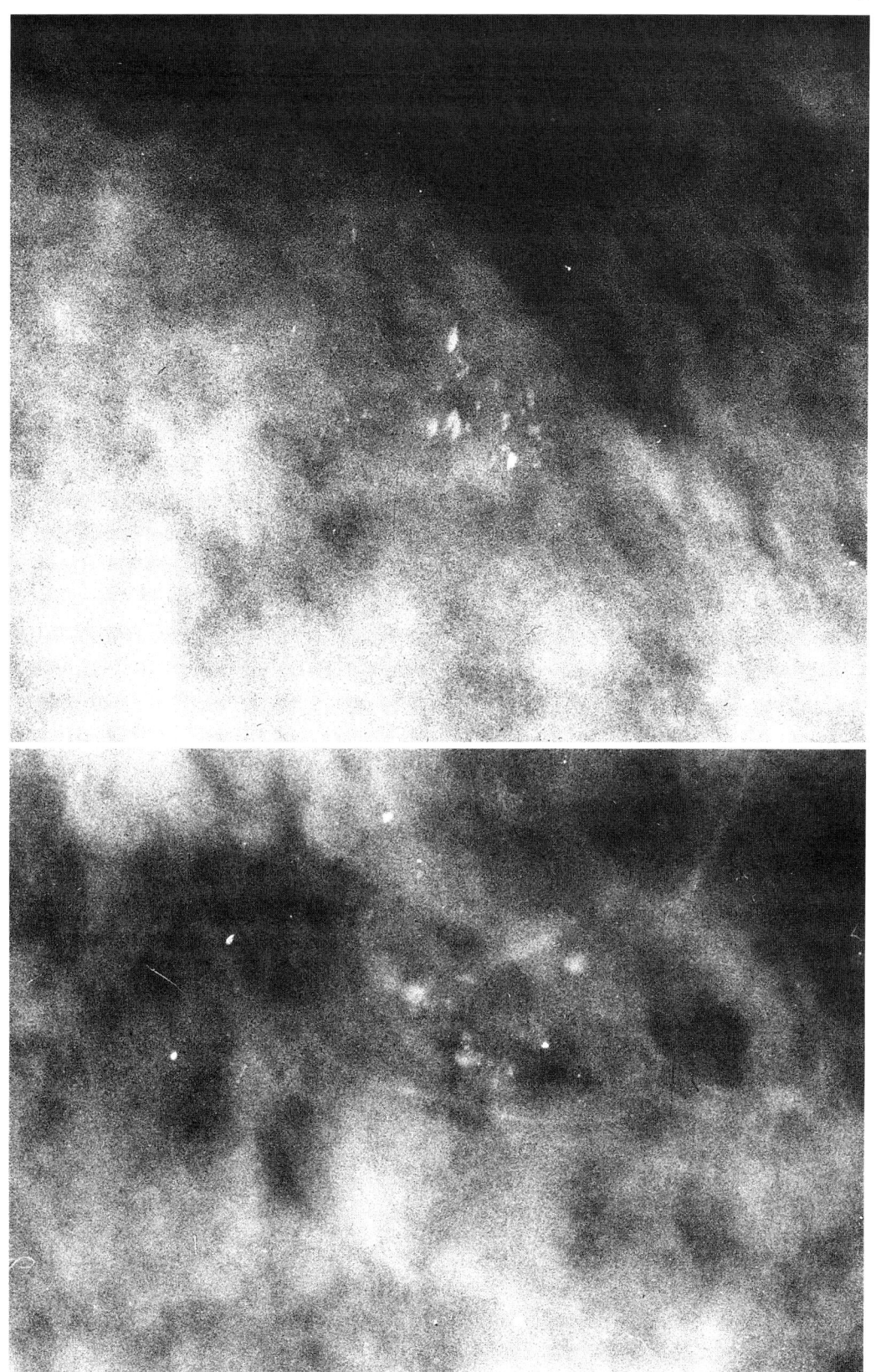

Differential Diagnosis of Microcalcifications

Fig. 7.7. a Craniocaudal view showing some faint round microcalcifications. **b** Lateral view. *Top:* faint, linear microcalcifications; *center:* spindle-shaped and teacup-like microcalcifications; *bottom* faint, round microcalcifications (no sedimentation). A septum is visible, indicating lobular localization

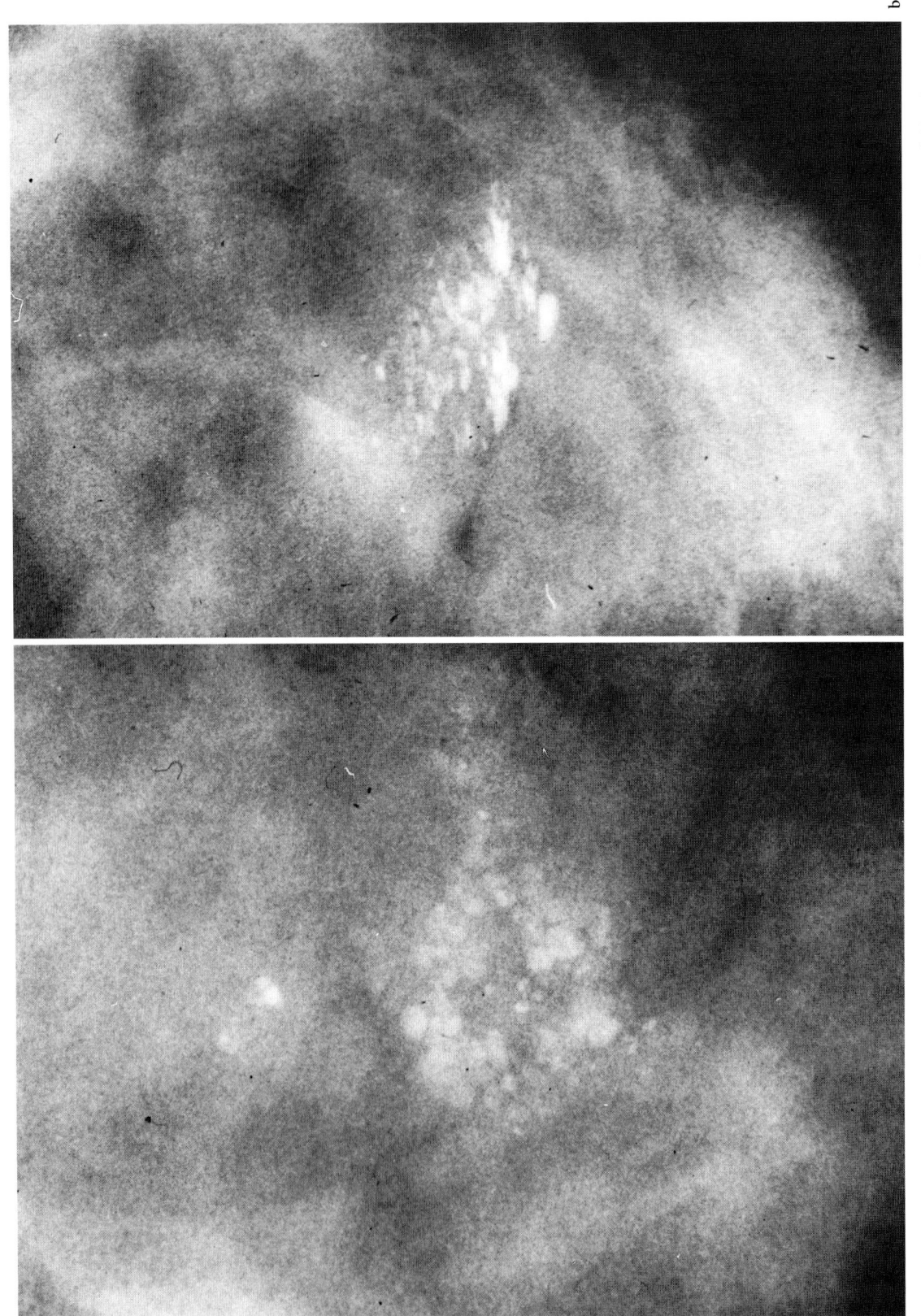

Fig. 7.8. a Craniocaudal view: highly contrasted, round microcalcifications with facetting and septa. b Lateral view: teacup and occasional linear microcalcifications

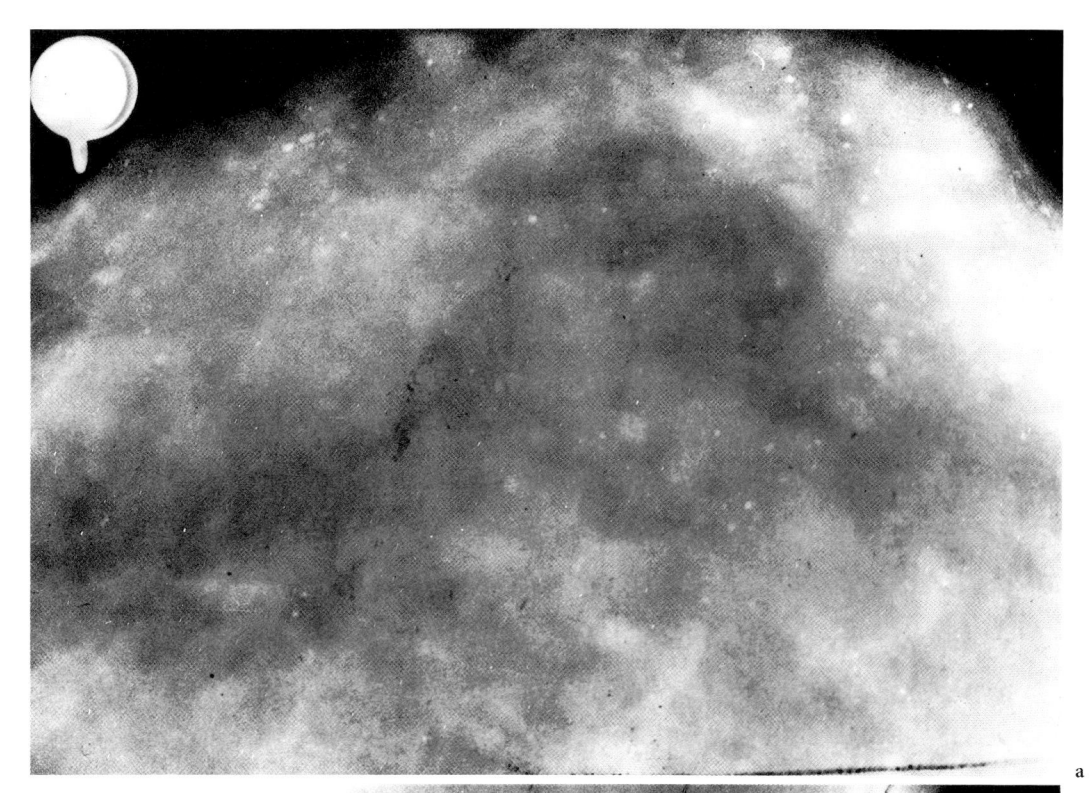

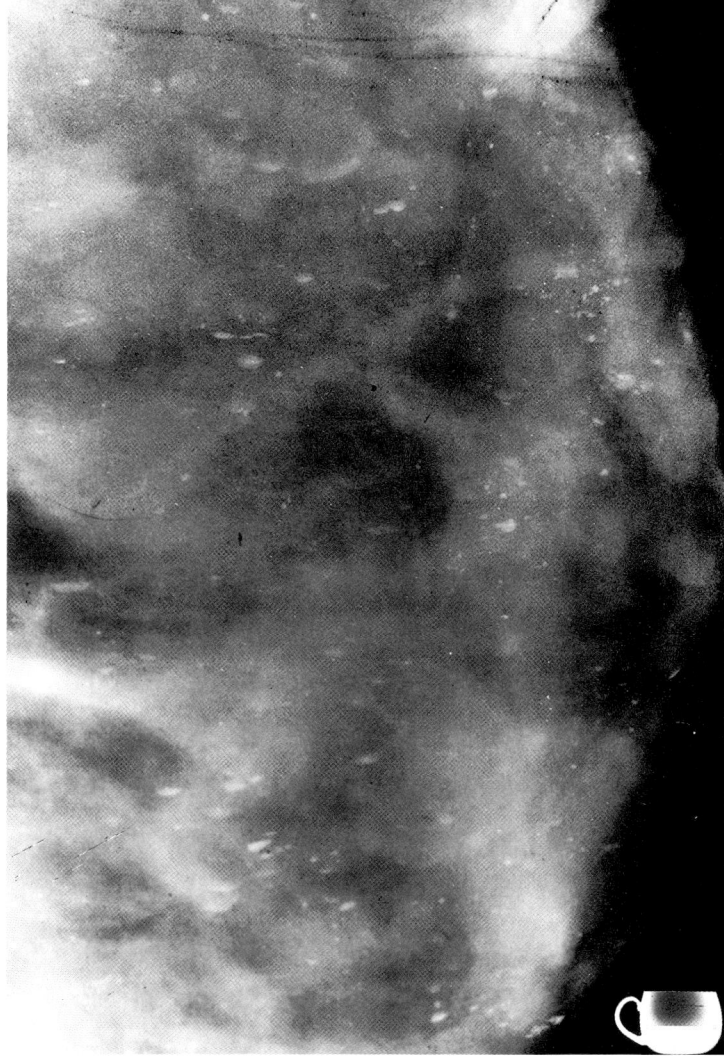

Fig. 7.9a,b. Diffuse, disseminated milk of calcium cysts. **a** Craniocaudal view: faint, round microcalcifications. **b** Lateral view: linear, spindle, and teacup-shaped microcalcifications; occasional granular appearance

7.2.3 Fibrosing (Sclerosing) Adenosis

Milk of calcium cysts used to be regarded as characteristic of fibrosing (sclerosing) adenosis (GERSHON-COHEN et al. 1966; HOEFFKEN and LANYI 1973). However, among 90 cases operated on for clustered microcalcifications in milk of calcium cysts, fibrosing (sclerosing) adenosis was histologically detected in the vicinity of only 39.4% (see below). In 5%–27% of other "benign" calcification forms and in 6.8%–26.6% of "malignant" microcalcifications, fibrosing (slerosing) adenosis was found histologically. Obviously, sclerosing adenosis is a ubiquitous histological finding.

Fibrosing (sclerosing) adenosis is defined as proliferation of myothelial and intralobular connective tissue (HAMPERL 1939; FOOTE and STEWART 1945; URBAN and ADAIR 1949; INGLEBY and GERSHON-COHEN 1960). This condition, also known as "myoid sclerosis," deforms and compresses the cysts of blunt duct adenosis. If these cysts contain psammomatous secretions, these secretory calcifications also become deformed (Fig. 7.10). Thus linear, comma-, v-, or wavy-shaped microcalcifications are formed. These can be confusingly similar to the pleomorphic microcalcifications observed in comedocarcinoma (see below; MACERLEAN and NATHAN 1972) (Fig. 7.11).

In cases of diffuse fibrosing adenosis, too, round/oval clusters can be identified according to the lobular distribution pattern (Fig. 7.12).

7.2.4 Fibroadenoma

Fibroadenoma develops from hyperplasia of the *intra*lobular connective tissue and cannot in its initial stage be histologically distinguished from fibrosing (sclerosing) adenosis. The processes described above, such as acinar cyst formation (i.e., adenosis) and hypertrophy of intralobular connective tissue (i.e., fibrosis, or rather the cyst deformation caused by this fibrosis), are also found in fibroadenoma. At the sites of excessive connective tissue proliferation the hypertrophic, elongated acini (canaliculi) are compressed so that fissures are formed. In cases where fibrotic nodules impinge on these crevices, pathologists refer to "*intracanalicular*" fibroadenoma. When several adjacent nodules are pushed into these fissures, *corkscrew-like* forms develop. The term *pericanalicular* fibroadenoma is used if the hypertrophic, elongated, and widened acini have not been pressed flat by the surrounding connective tissue because of its concentric or pericanalicular growth (Fig. 7.13). Both growth patterns of intralobular connective tissue occur simultaneously in the same fibroadenoma, so that pathologists almost always give the diagnosis peri- *and* intracanalicular fibroadenoma.

Calcifications in fibroadenoma comprise secretory calcifications occurring in preformed cavities. Previous assumptions that calcifications in fibroadenoma are due to necrobiosis (e.g., HOEFFKEN and LANYI 1973) are no longer valid since fibroadenograms have yielded information on the cavity structure of fibroadenomas (WAHLERS et al. 1977; SIGFUSSON et al. 1982). On the basis of these studies one can well imagine how calcifications develop in the elongated and more or less compressed and deformed acini (canaliculi) in fibroadenoma (Fig. 7.14). Monomorphous round calcifications as shown in Fig. 7.15 are rarely seen, and then exclusively in periductal fibroadenoma. They are larger than calcifications in microcystic adenosis, but their "septations" are an unmistakable reference to their original localization – within the lobule. The corkscrew-like calcifications are also characteristic of intracanalicular fibroadenoma (Fig. 7.16) and are not found in intraductal carcinomas. (They should not be confused with the vermiform, wavy microcalcifications presenting in carcinoma.)

As in all microcalcification clusters in the lobule, the cluster shape in fibroadenoma is typically round/oval in two views. Diagnosis is often facilitated by a sharply defined opaque mass with occasional "halo" effect. Problems in differential diagnosis occur only if the calcifications are very fine and/or the cluster is too small for its exact shape to be determined (Fig. 7.17). Figure 7.18 shows the progressive calcification of a fibroadenoma over a period of 7 years.

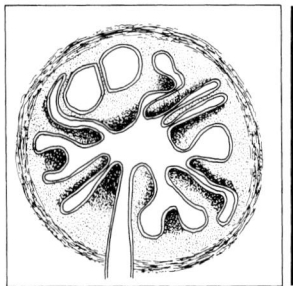

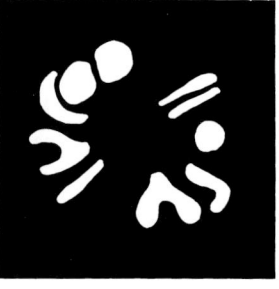

Fig. 7.10. a Schematic representation of the development of fibrosing (sclerosing) adenosis. Most of the acini have become deformed through proliferation of myothelial (*dark dotted*) and intralobular connective tissue. If these cavities contain calcium-containing secretions, the microcalcification pattern shown in **b** results

Differential Diagnosis of Microcalcifications

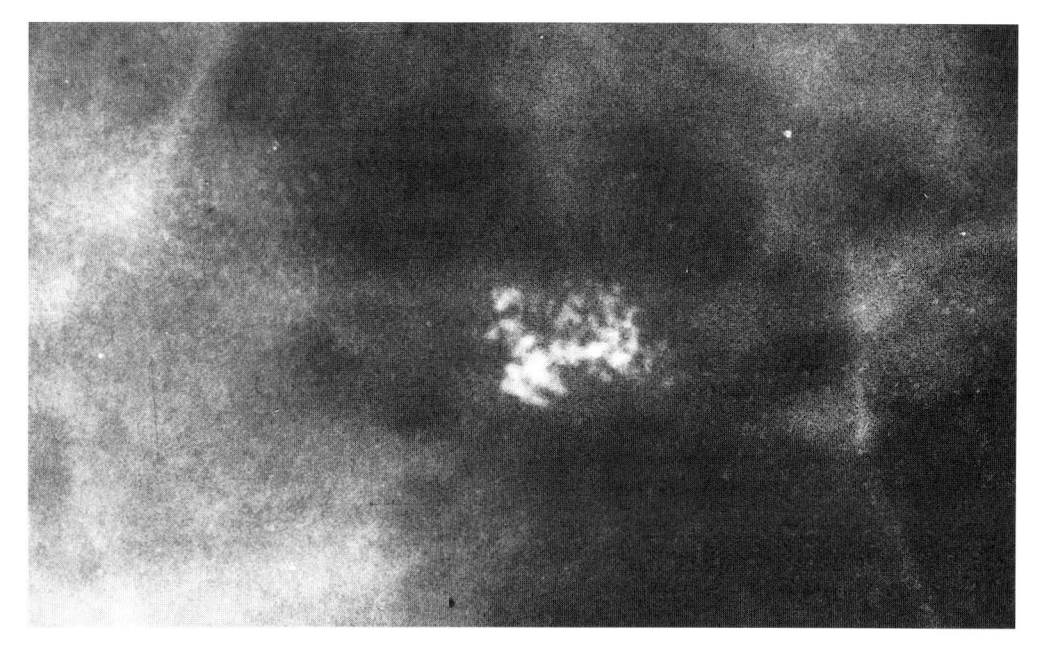

Fig. 7.11. Angled cluster of pleomorphic comma, linear, v-, and y-shaped microcalcifications, 6 mm in size. Histology: sclerosing adenosis

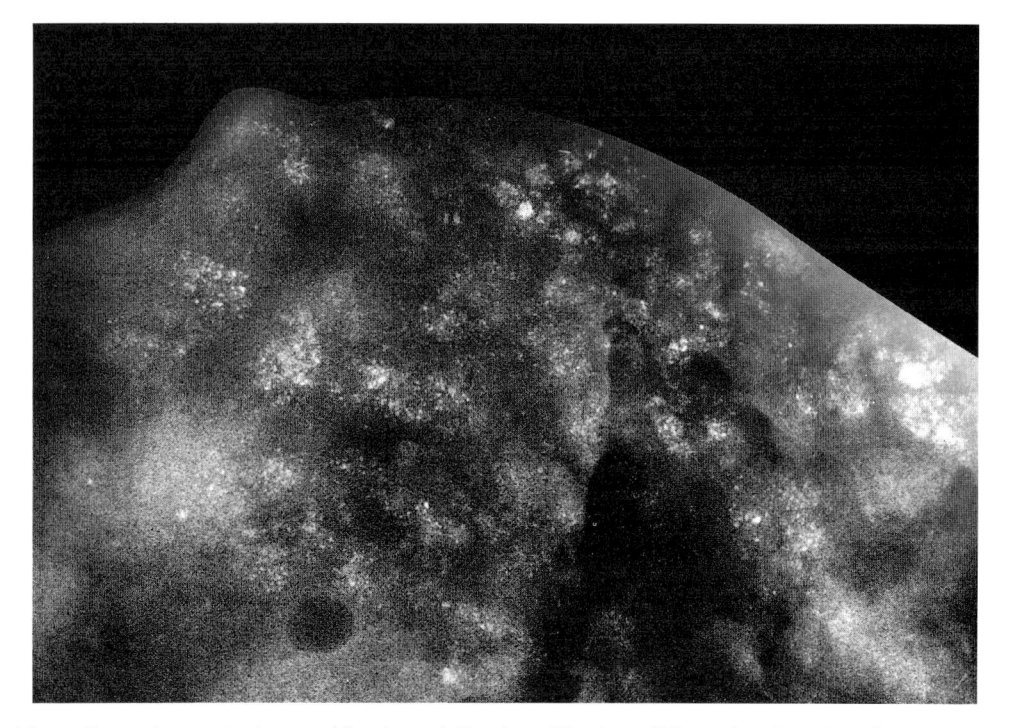

Fig. 7.12. Innumerable small, mostly round, pleomorphic microcalcifications. Histology: diffuse sclerosing adenosis

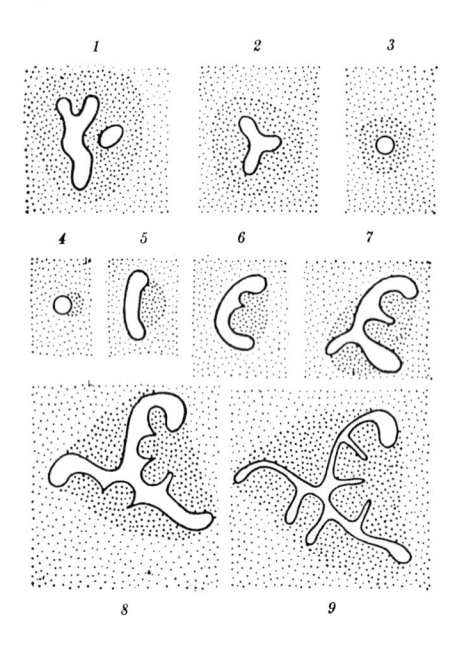

Fig. 7.13. Schematic representation of the development of pericanalicular (*1–3*) and intracanalicular (*4–9*) fibroadenoma (HAMPERL 1968). At the *center* of each drawing the proliferating acini are surrounded by the simultaneously proliferating connective tissue (*dark dotted*). Note the corkscrew-like configuration of the intracanalicular fibroadenoma (*6–9*)

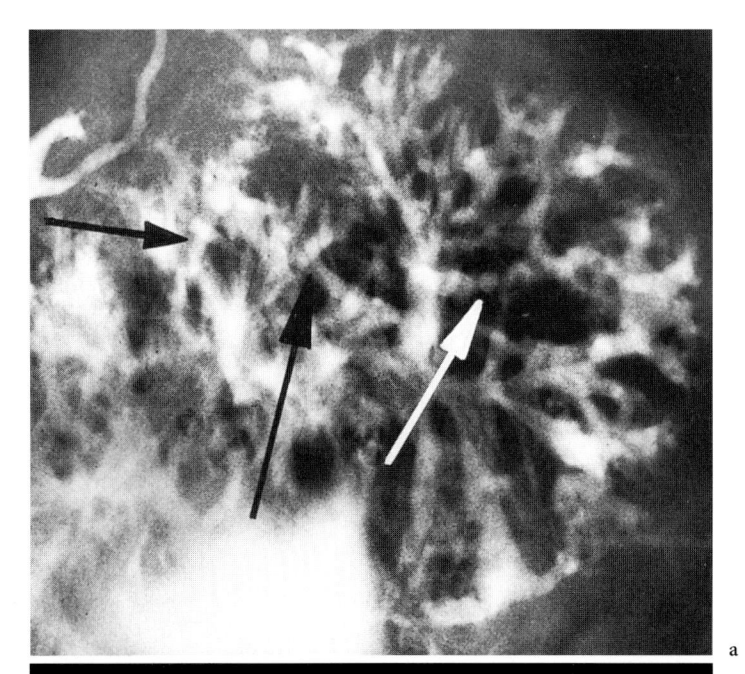

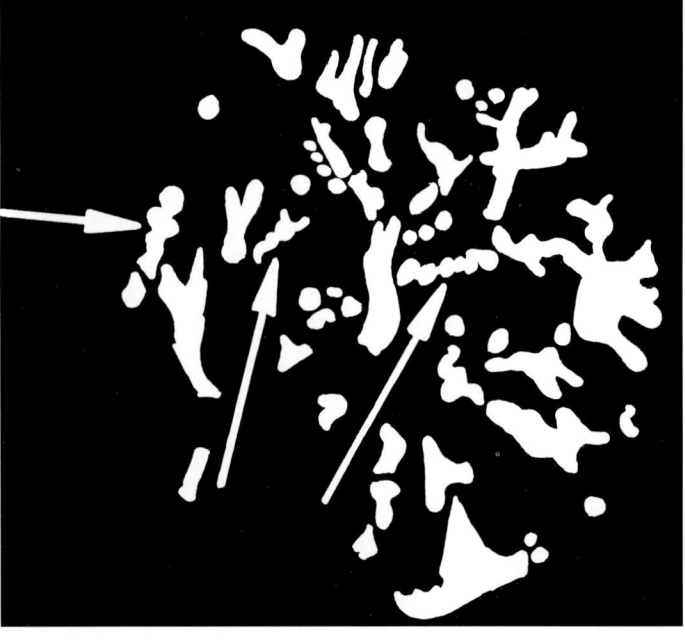

Fig. 7.14. a Magnified detail from a fibroadenogram (courtesy of Dr. R. Müller, Siegburg, FRG) which shows elongated, deformed acini (in this context: canaliculi). *Arrows* show the corkscrew-like "intracanalicular" indentations. **b** If microcalcifications were to develop in the cavities of **a**, one would see the typical microcalcification pattern of fibroadenoma. Possible corkscrew-like calcifications are marked with *arrows*

Fig. 7.15. Exclusively punctate microcalcifications in fibroadenoma with cystic cavities (histologically verified). The septa indicate the original intralobular localization of these microcalcifications. Faint oval opacity with halo effect (*arrow*)

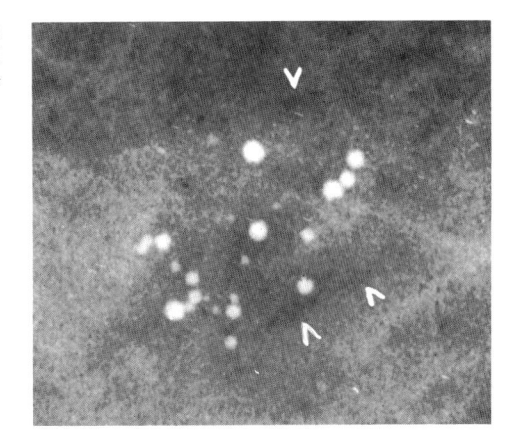

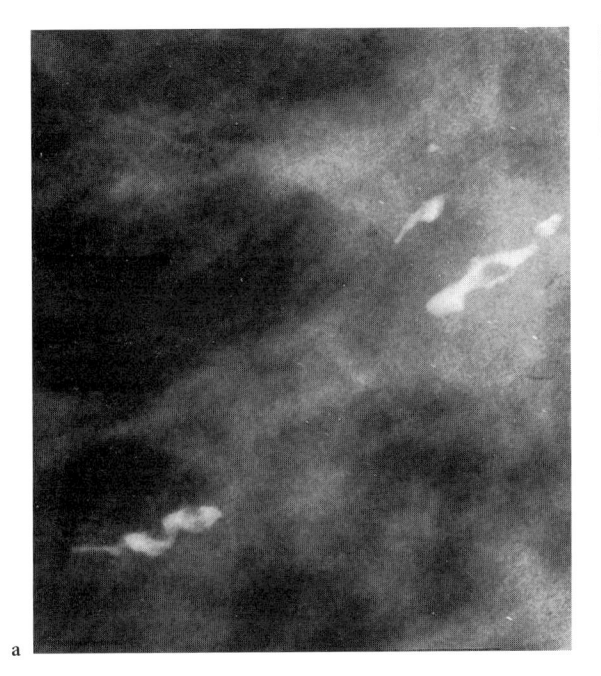

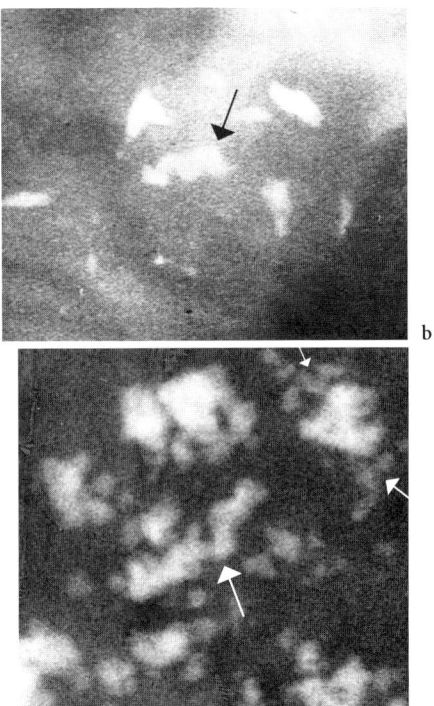

Fig. 7.16a–c. Selection of corkscrew-like microcalcifications in fibroadenoma. **a** Corkscrew-like microcalcifications which were the only feature of multiple fibroadenomas. **b** Corkscrew-like microcalcifications (*arrow*). **c** Detail: as well as the two smaller calcifications at the *upper right corner* (*arrows*), one can also see a large corkscrew-like microcalcification in the *center* (*arrow*)

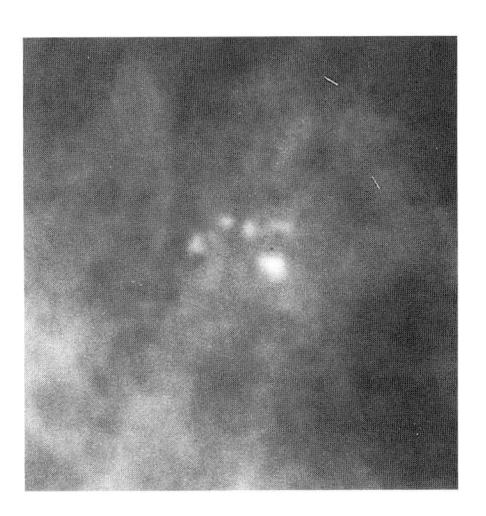

Fig. 7.17. Five-fine, tiny, somewhat pleomorphic microcalcifications. As the exact shape of the cluster, which was 4 mm in size, could not be determined (angled? oval?), a biopsy was performed. Histology: Fibroadenoma

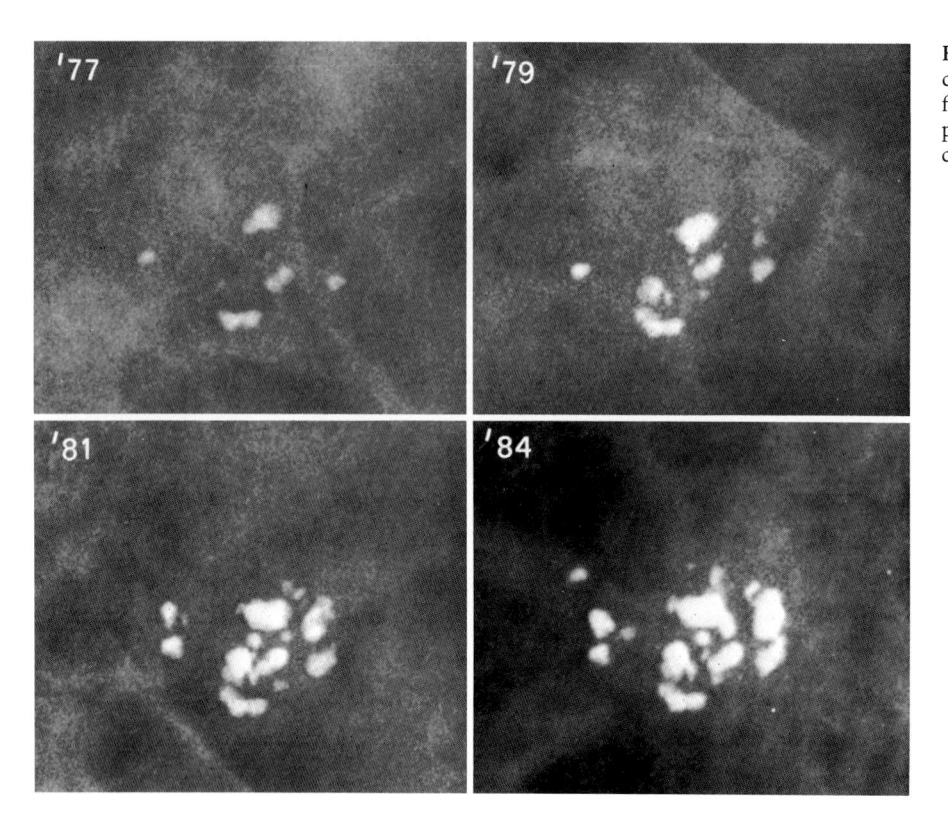

Fig. 7.18. Progressive calcification of a fibroadenoma over a period of 7 years. Oval cluster form

7.3 Microcalcifications of Ductal Origin

Ductal microcalcifications may originate in the following pathological processes:

1. Intraductal carcinoma (DCIS)
2. Secretory calcifications (e.g. comedo mastitis, benign duct ectasia)
3. Papillomatosis, papilloma

7.3.1 Intraductal Carcinoma (DCIS)

The various subtypes of intraductal carcinoma (DCIS) can also be interpreted as different stages of development.

In the initial stage of development the so-called *clinging* or *mural* carcinoma originates (AZZOPARDI 1979). At this stage there are at most only a few layers of malignant cells lining the lumer; in many cases there is only a single layer (Fig. 7.19a). Papillary projections evolve from the cells of the clinging carcinoma to give an overall "grass-like" appearance to the malignant milk duct epithelium (BÄSSLER 1978). Histologically this stage is described as *small papillary or micropapillary* carcinoma (Fig. 7.19b).

The "blades of grass" of the small papillary carcinoma become increasingly long; they double up and grow together to form an arch-like structure described by AZZOPARDI (1979) as a "Roman bridge" structure (Fig. 7.19c). The carcinomatous tissue extends more and more so that a sponge-like structure develops in the milk ducts. In histological sections of 5 μm thickness with the milk ducts usually in cross-section, pathologists refer to this as *sieve-like (cribriform) carcinoma* (Fig. 7.19c). The term "sponge-like" or "cavernous" carcinoma, however, would be more correct (cribriform, cavernous structures can also occur in benign papillomatosis or epitheliosis). When the cancerous tissue in the milk ducts becomes increasingly dense, the original grass-like appearance of papillary carcinoma gives way to the "scrub-" or "brush-like" structures of *solid* intraductal carcinoma (Fig. 7.19d).

Comedocarcinoma develops when the tissue of a solid carcinoma becomes necrotized at its center and the dead tissue is pressed out of the milk ducts as a comedo (BLOODGOOD 1934). More or less extensive tube-like cavities originate from the central necrosis.

The solid intraductal carcinoma tissue can eventually be completely destroyed, so that only one or two rows of malignant cells remain adhering to the duct wall and the lumen of the duct has once again become void. This condition is also defined as "clinging" carcinoma (AZZOPARDI 1979).

The pathological changes described above can occur simultaneously and in varying degrees in the milk ducts (Fig. 7.19e).

Calcifications rarely occur in clinging or small papillary carcinoma. If they do, they appear to be psammoma bodies microscopically (Fig. 7.20), as in blunt duct adenosis, fibrosing (sclerosing) adenosis, or milk of calcium cysts (LANYI 1986; HOLLAND et al. 1990; HOLLAND and HENDRIKS 1994).

Psammoma bodies are also found, sometimes en masse, in the cavities of sponge-like cavernous cribriform carcinoma (Fig. 7.21). A different type of calcification is found in comedocarcinoma, where the central and necrotic tissue has become calcified (Fig. 7.19e). Even complete calcification of necrotized comedocarcinoma is possible. Figure 7.22 summarizes the above-mentioned types of microcalcification as mirror images of the corresponding histology. All forms of calcifications described above can occur simultaneously since mixed histological subtypes of DCIS frequently coexist.

The analysis of 7028 individual microcalcifications in 121 intraductal carcinomas (Table 7.3) yielded the following results:

1. In small papillary/cribriform carcinoma, the punctate or granular shape was by far the most prevalent (73%).
2. In comedocarcinoma, 57% of microcalcifications were pleomorphic and only 43% were punctate/granular.
3. In combined forms ("mainly comedo, partly papillary," "comedo, papillary, cribriform," or "papillary, cribriform with comedo elements"), punctate microcalcifications presented in 55% and nonpunctate microcalcifications in 45% of the cases (LANYI 1983, 1986).

Similar results have been reported by STOMPER and CONNOLLY (1992), HOLLAND and HENDRIKS (1994), and CIATTO et al. (1994).

Table 7.3. Histologic diagnoses for 121 ductal carcinomas that were biopsied on the basis of microcalcifications alone, without a visible tumor shadow

Comedocarcinoma	60
Micropapillary/cribriform carcinoma	11
Mixed forms (comedo and cribriform)	40
Ductal carcinoma (further differentiation was not possible retrospectively)	10
	121

Complete monomorphism in the shape of the punctate microcalcifications was observed in only 4% of the cases, and almost exclusively in very small papillary/cribriform carcinomas (Fig. 7.23). Because the subgroups of DCIS virtually never occur in a pure form, punctate microcalcifications in papillary cribriform carcinomas are almost always accompanied by linear and branching calcifications characteristic of comedo elements. This minimal pleomorphism along with the cluster shape is almost invariably a sign of an intraductal localization, and therefore a malignant process (Figs. 7.24, 7.39).

The above-described microcalcifications exist as real particles which can be scraped from the carcinoma (Fig. 7.25) (LANYI 1983).

Intraductal localization, and with it the highly probable diagnosis of DCIS, results from a combination of the shape of individual microcalcifications and the shape of the cluster. The cluster shape of intraductal microcalcifications, whatever it may be, is determined by the form of the milk ducts (Fig. 7.26). The changes in the shape of the microcalcification clusters in different mammographic views represent an important differential diagnostic feature (Fig. 7.27).

Analysis of cluster shape in 153 groups of microcalcification in intraductal carcinoma (LANYI 1977, 1982) showed that in 88% of cases the angled shape prevailed (65% of these angled clusters were triangular or trapezoid in form). Five percent of the clusters were propeller or star shaped, 4% were linear, and 3% were not definable (Figs. 7.28–7.33). Sixty-five percent of the clusters were triangular or trapezoid in both views. In the remaining cases clusters occurred in combined forms (Figs. 7.34–7.36). The larger the clusters, the more likely they were to be triangular. The smaller the clusters, the more difficult it was to assess their form. A round/oval cluster shape is extremely seldom seen in DCIS [according to MITNICK et al. (1989) it occurs in only 3.7% of all carcinomas]. Such round/oval clusters were on average 0.7 mm in diameter.

The cluster shape is not always immediately obvious, but can be discerned by "joining the dots" along the outer border of the cluster, using a pencil with the aid of a magnifying glass. Irregularities in cluster shape, such as indentations or protuberances (Fig. 7.37), correspond to the anatomy of the milk ducts, as is known from galactography. Patches free from microcalcifications within a larger cluster are also a sign of an intraductal localization (Fig. 7.38).

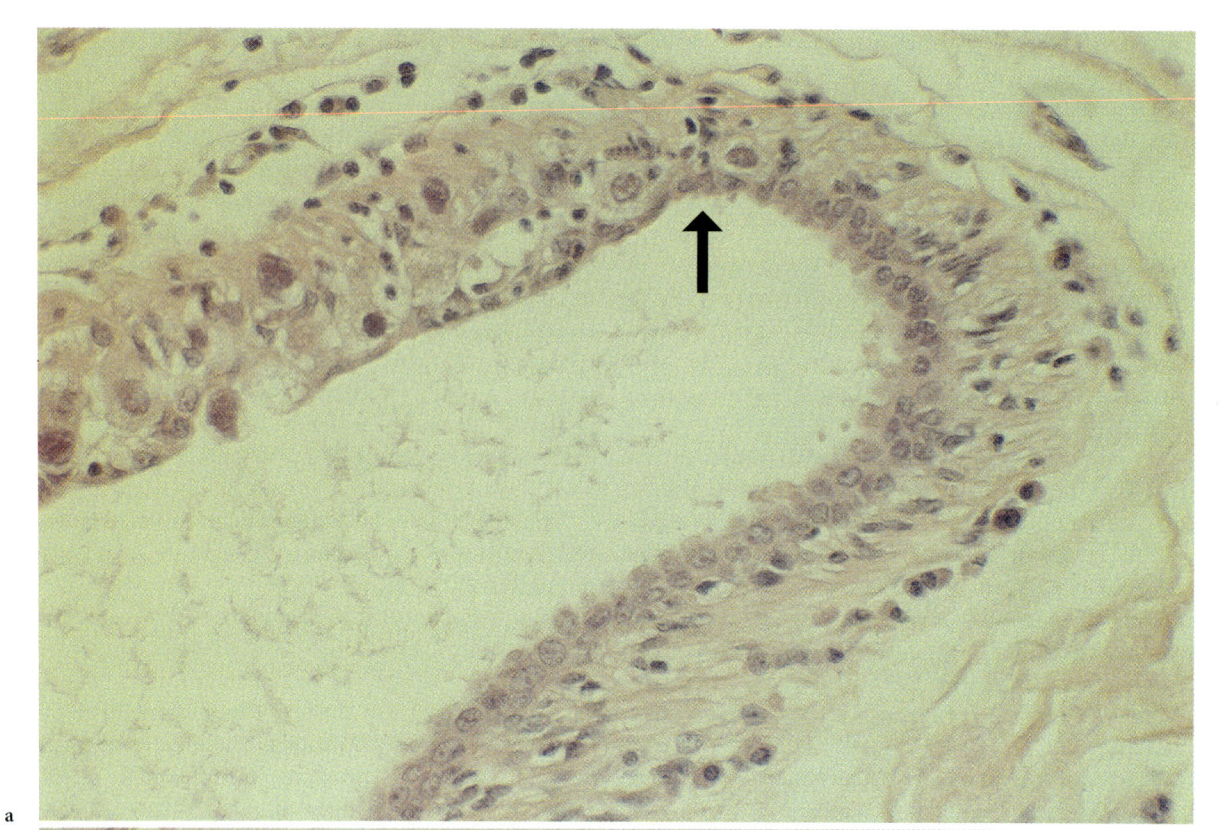

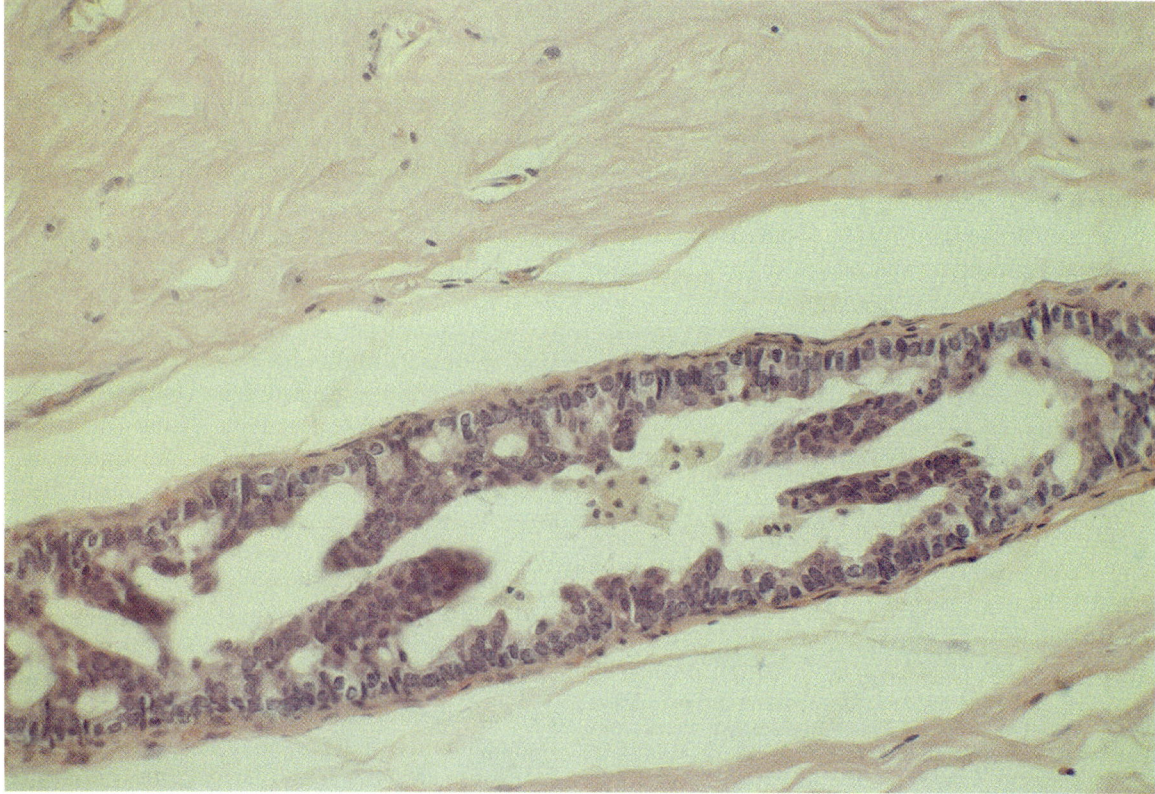

Fig. 7.19. a Cross-section of a milk duct: transition of normal epithelium to clinging carcinoma (*arrow*). **b** Longitudinal section of a milk duct with micropapillary carcinoma (courtesy of Prof. R. Stiens, Gummersbach, FRG). **c** Cross-section of several milk ducts. Cribriform carcinoma at the *center* with clinging and micropapillary elements and "Roman bridges" on the right (*arrows*) (courtesy of Prof. P. Citoler, Cologne, FRG). **d** Several milk ducts in cross-section filled with dense carcinomatous tissue. Central necrosis is seen in one of the ducts. **e** The oblique section of a milk duct shows all the various stages in the development of an intraductal carcinoma. *Left*: clinging carcinoma with Roman bridge; *right*: cribriform carcinoma and solid carcinoma centrally with necrosis and calcification (comedo) (courtesy of Prof. R. Stiens, Gummersbach, FRG)

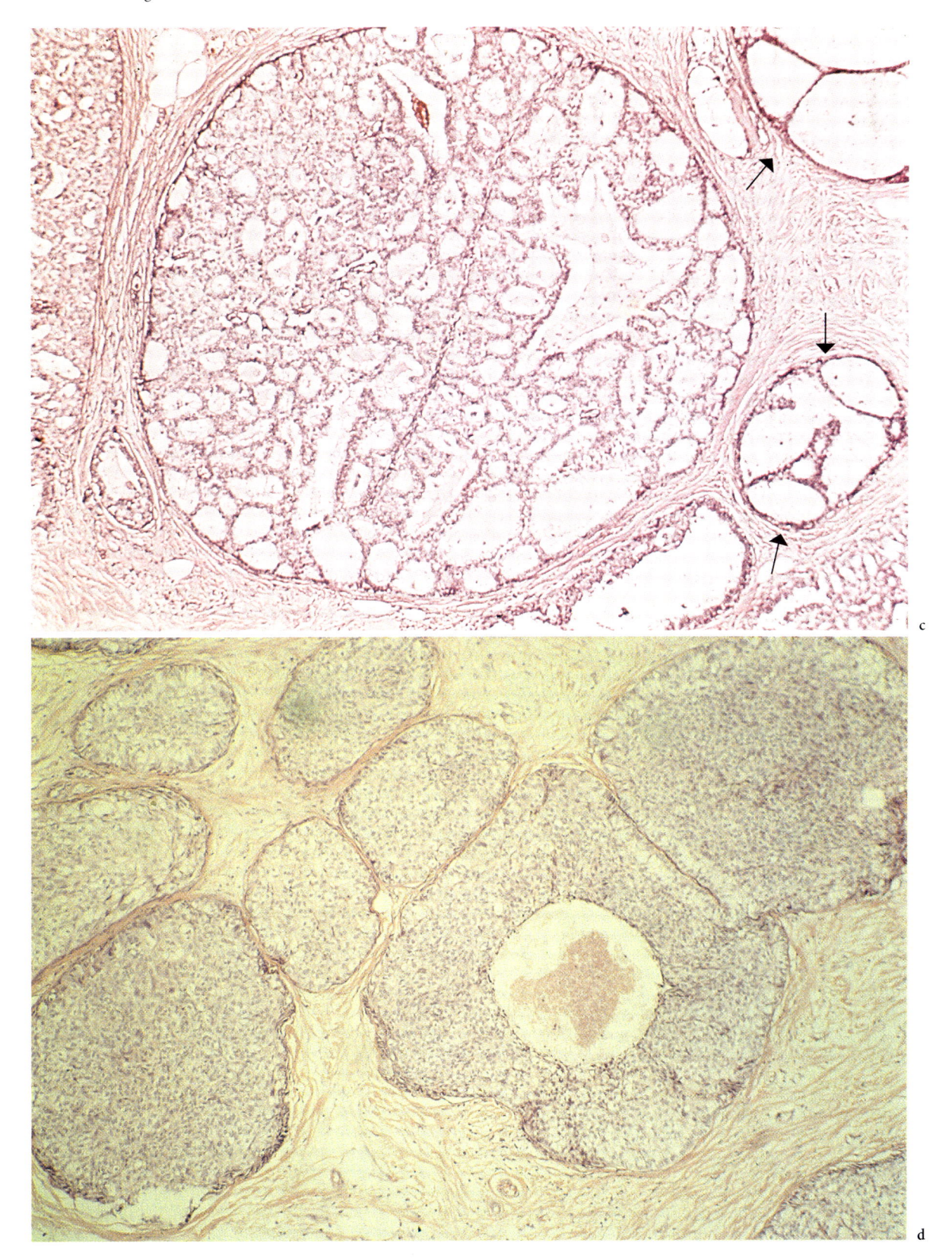

Differential Diagnosis of Microcalcifications

Fig. 7.19c,d

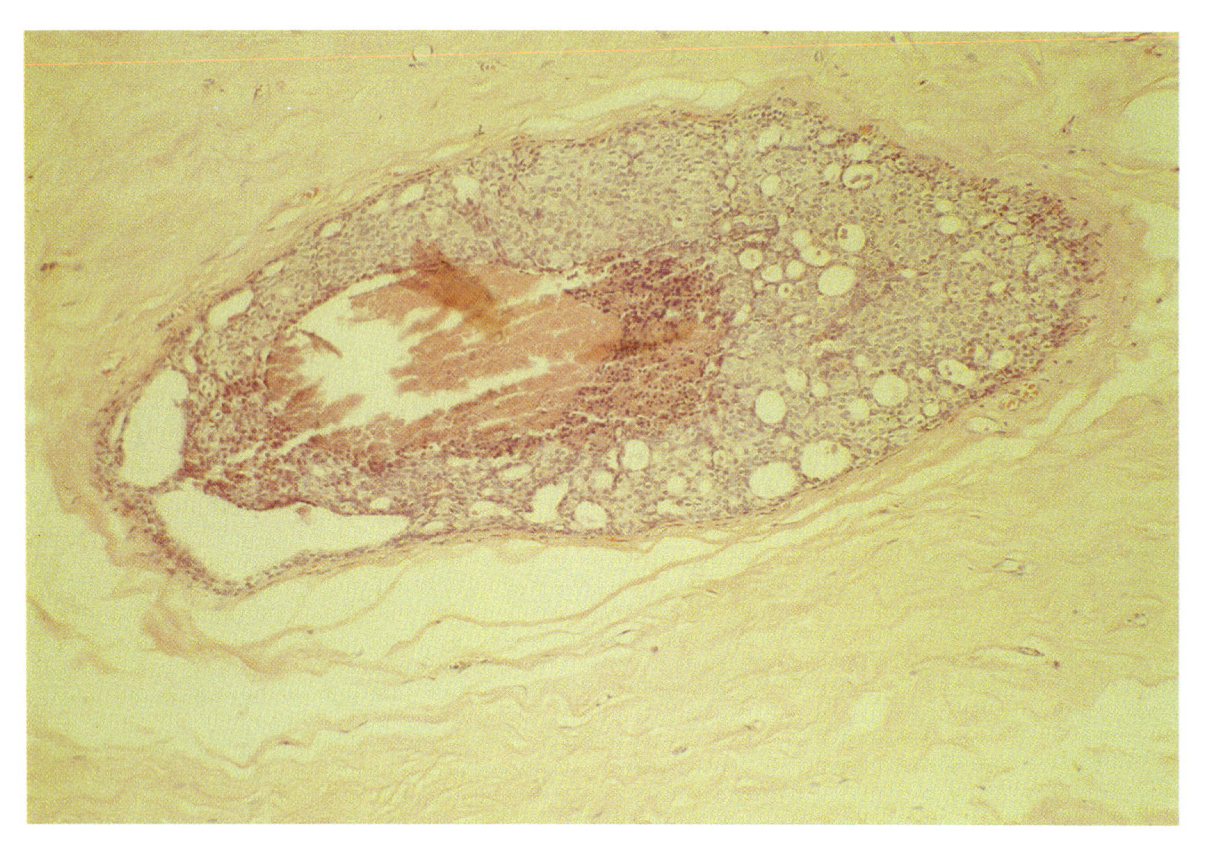

Fig. 7.19e

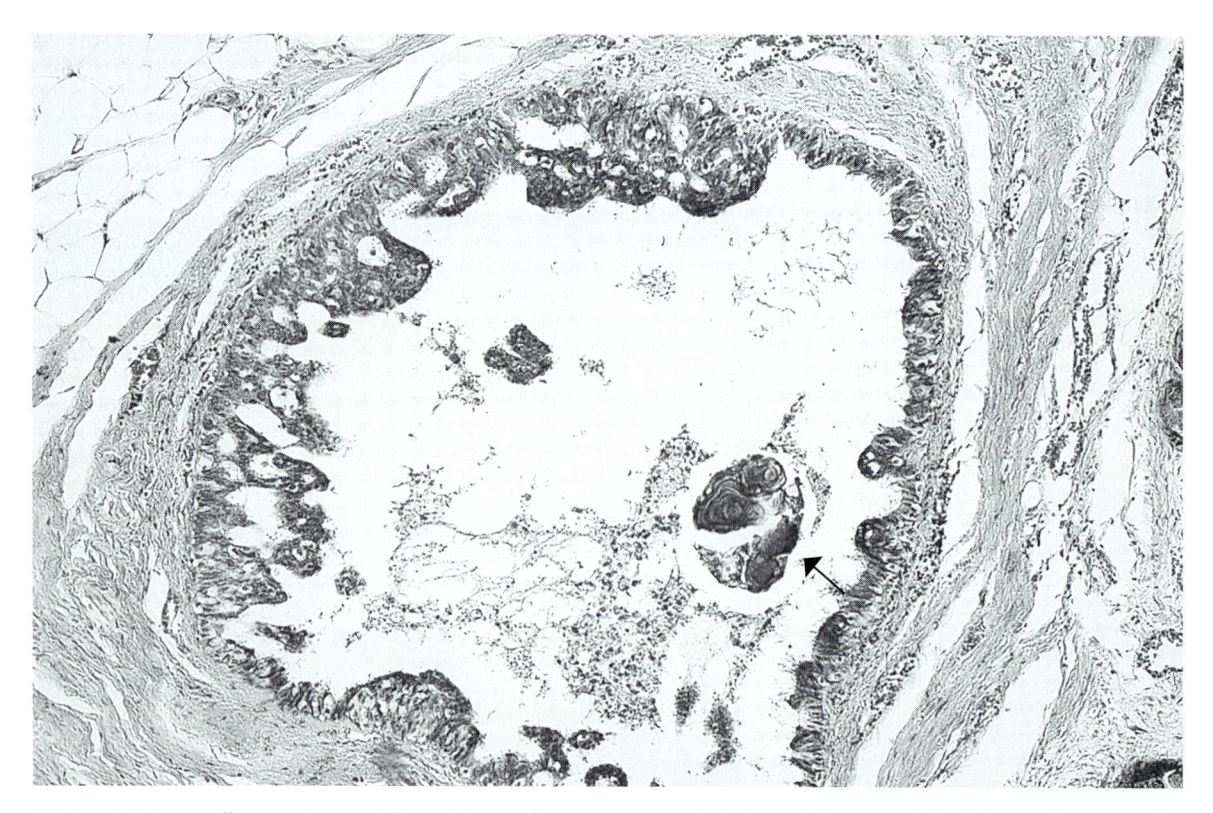

Fig. 7.20. Micropapillary carcinoma with secretions and one psammoma body (*arrow*) (courtesy of Prof. Caesar, Braunschweig, FRG)

This phenomenon is not observed in diffuse acinar calcifications.

The actual extent of DCIS can be far greater than that of the area of microcalcification; indeed, only a few microcalcifications may be seen in an extensive intraductal carcinoma (Fig. 7.39). Obviously, the tendency of the individual lesion to form microcalcifications is an important factor. Microcalcifications in the comedo type of carcinoma most clearly mirror the presence of intraductal growth of the carcinoma.

Increase over time in the number of microcalcifications was considered by MENGES et al. (1973, 1976) to be a useful differential diagnostic feature. However, in my own material, diagnosis was made on the basis of this feature in only 4% of all cases. A progressive increase in the number of microcalcifications is not characteristic of carcinoma, as this phenomenon can also be observed in secretory calcifications and in fibroadenoma (Fig. 7.18). PARKER et al. (1989) have reported on the disappearance of microcalcifications. An initial increase, then a decrease, followed by another increase or a change in the intensity of microcalcifications in an intraductal carcinoma is documented in Fig. 7.40.

After radiotherapy, microcalcifications may (a) remain unchanged, (b) become less discernible, or (c) disappear completely. The unchanged appearance of microcalcification after radiation therapy yields no evidence about tumor activity (LIBSHITZ et al. 1977).

Microcalcifications in male breast cancer have been extremely seldom observed (ROSEN and NADEL 1966; ROCEK et al. 1968; TABAR et al. 1972; PENTEK et al. 1975; BRYANT 1981). Radiomorphologically, there is no difference from microcalcifications found in intraductal carcinoma of the female breast.

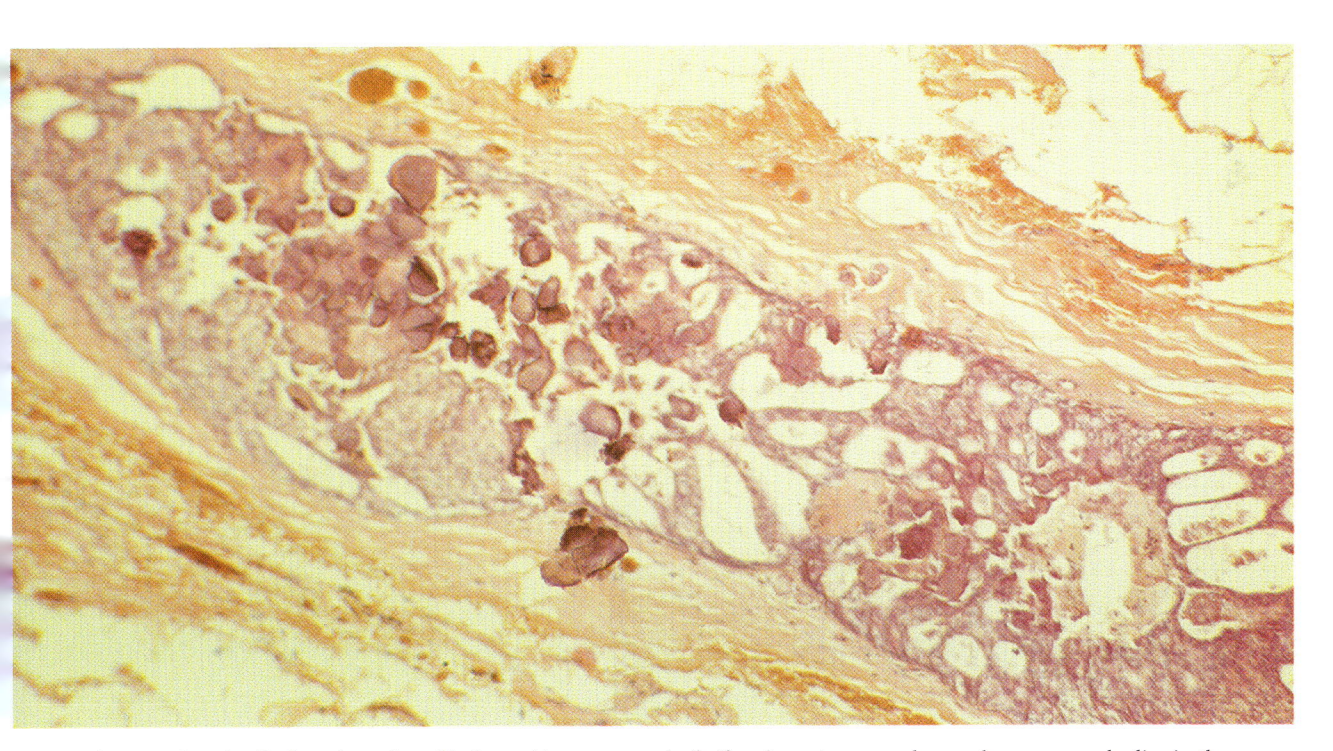

Fig. 7.21. Longitudinal section of a milk duct with cavernous (cribriform) carcinoma and several psammoma bodies in the cavities (courtesy of Prof. R. Stiens, Gummersbach, FRG)

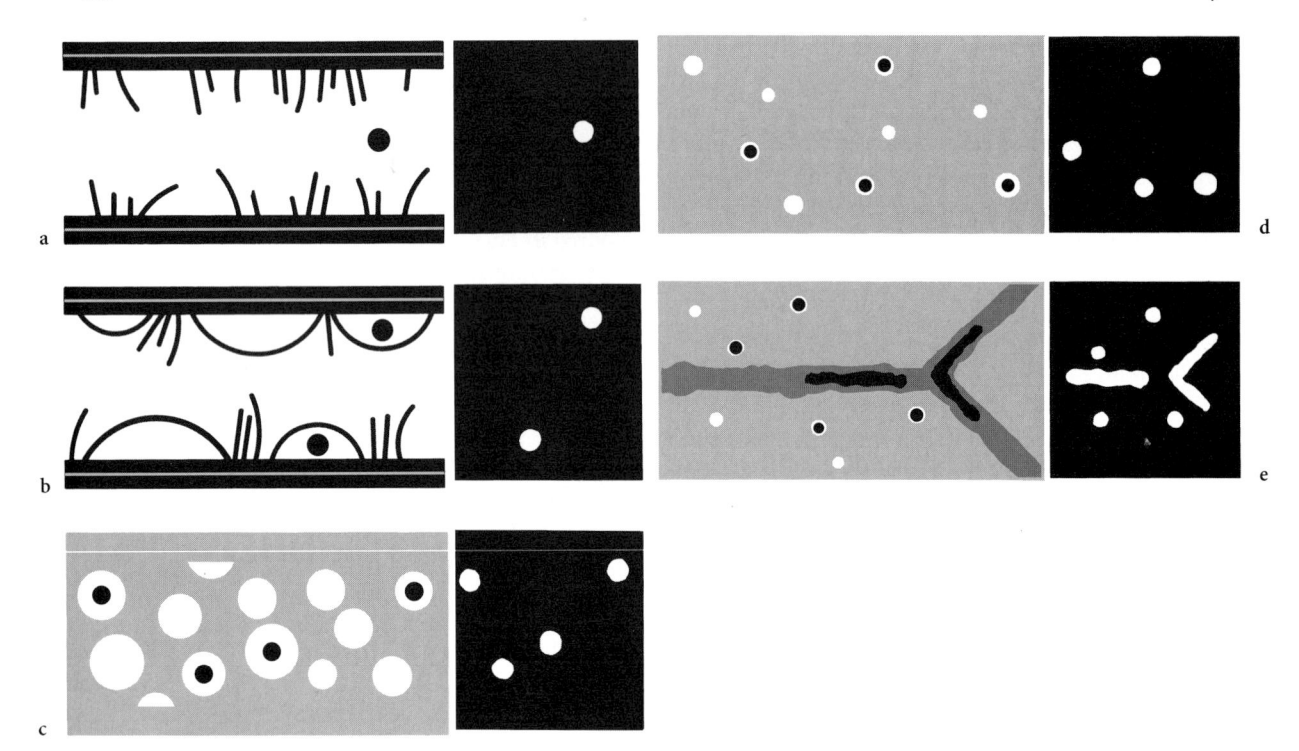

Fig. 7.22a–e. Schematic representation of forms of microcalcifications in intraductal carcinoma on mammogram (*right*), and corresponding histology (*left*). a Clinging and micropapillary carcinoma with isolated psammoma bodies. b Roman bridges with a few psammoma bodies. c Cavernous (cribriform) carcinoma with psammoma bodies. d Solid carcinoma with some remaining cavities and psammoma bodies. e Comedo carcinoma with central necrosis and psammoma bodies in the remaining cavities. On the mammogram, psammoma bodies appear punctate while centrally necrotic calcifications present as linear or branching calcifications

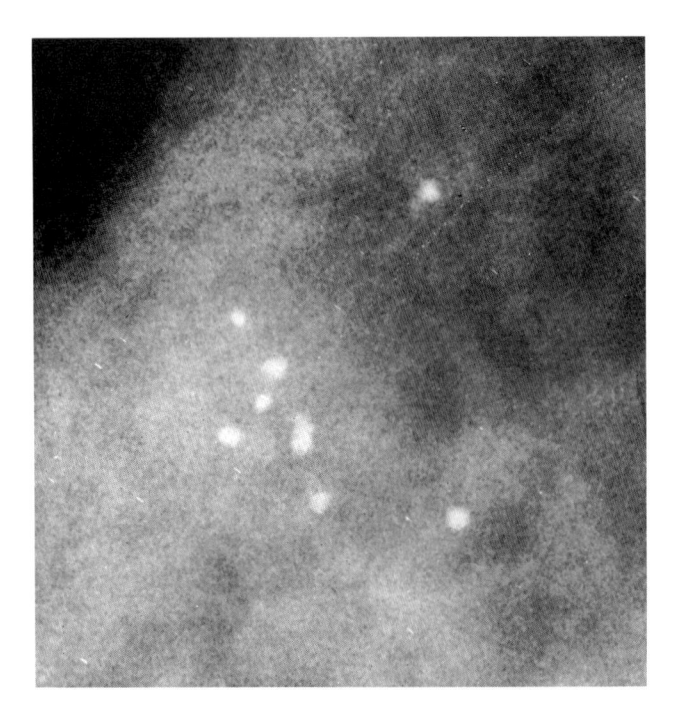

Fig. 7.23. Seven monomorphous punctate microcalcifications in a trapezoid cluster. Histology: micropapillary cribriform carcinoma

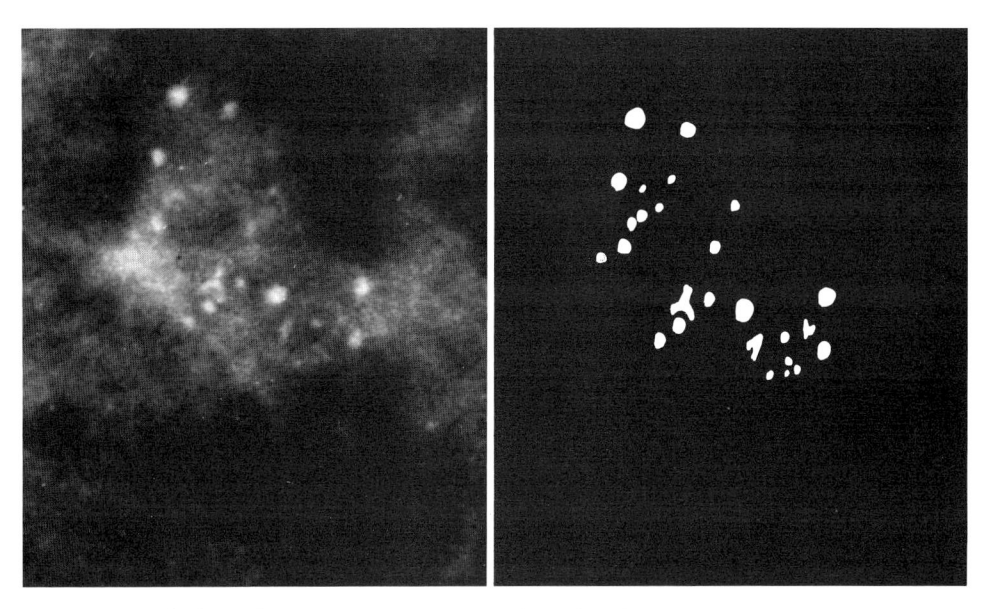

Differential Diagnosis of Microcalcifications

Fig. 7.24. Detail of a mammogram and schematic representation. As well as 22 punctate microcalcifications, three y- or v-shaped microcalcifications are also visible, leading to suspicion of intraductal carcinoma. Histology: micropapillary cribriform carcinoma with comedo elements

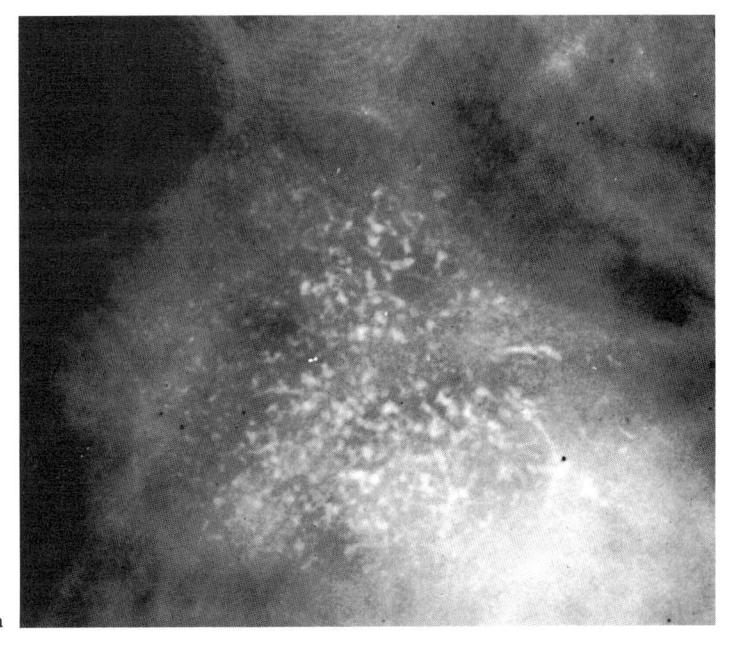

Fig. 7.25. a Detail of a mammogram: triangular cluster with mostly pleomorphic and isolated punctate microcalcifications. After histological verification (comedo carcinoma), the tissue was laminated and the microcalcifications extracted. These were then radiographed, and enlarged prints were produced. **b** Selection from more than 100 samples of extracted microcalcifications

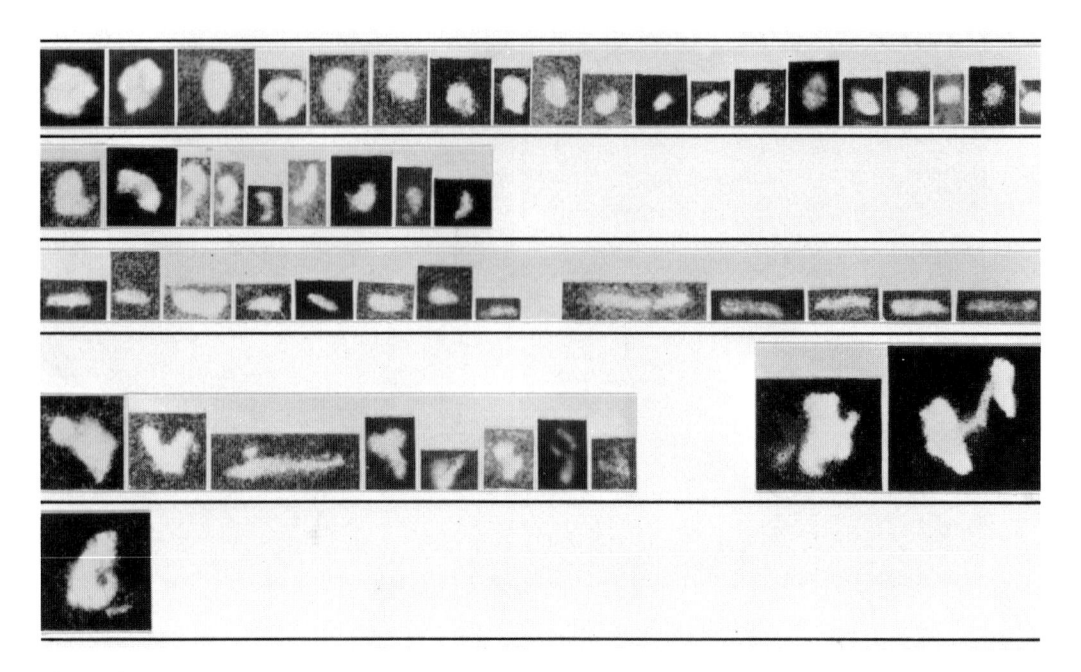

Fig. 7.25b

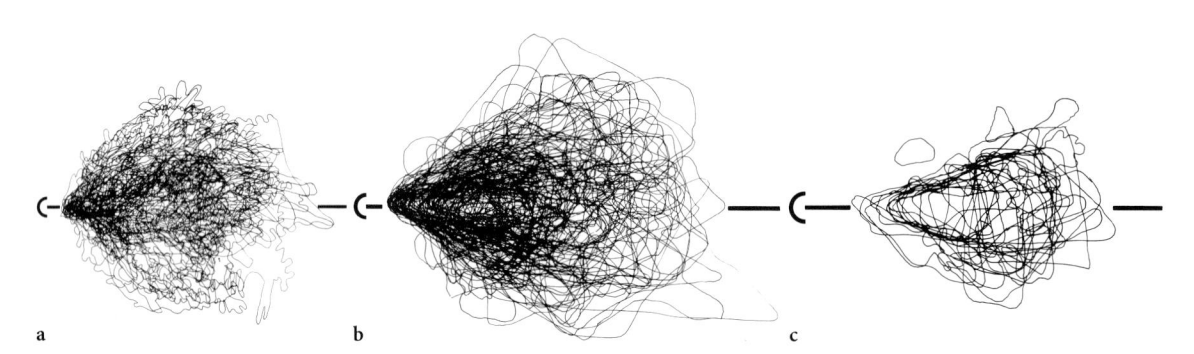

Fig. 7.26a–c. Using a magnifying glass, the contours of milk duct contents or intraductal microcalcifications of various origin were traced onto transparent foils. With the aid of an episcope they were projected to equal size, superimposed, and resketched. **a** Summation of 60 milk duct contours: triangular, wavy contours with dorsal indentations. **b** Summation of contours of 153 microcalcification clusters of malignant origin. The triangular shape is most predominant here, too. **c** Summation of contours of 29 benign intraductal microcalcification clusters (secretion calcification or intraductal epithelial proliferation). Again the most predominant form is the triangular

Differential Diagnosis of Microcalcifications 113

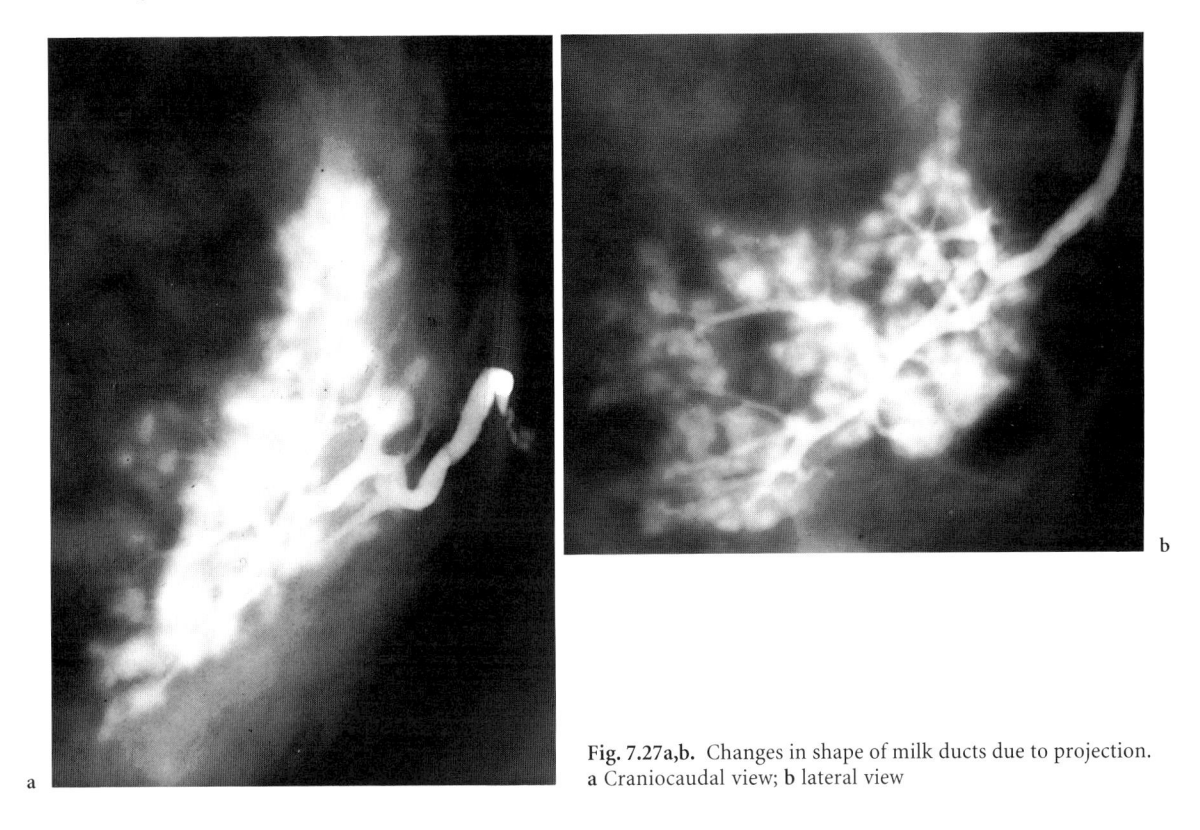

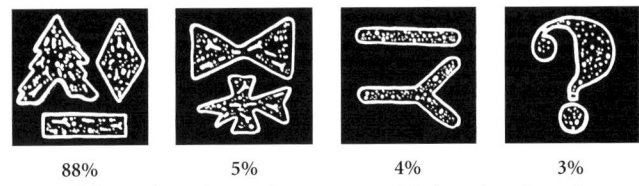

Fig. 7.27a,b. Changes in shape of milk ducts due to projection. **a** Craniocaudal view; **b** lateral view

88%   5%   4%   3%

Fig. 7.28. Frequency of the various cluster shapes among 153 intraductal carcinomas

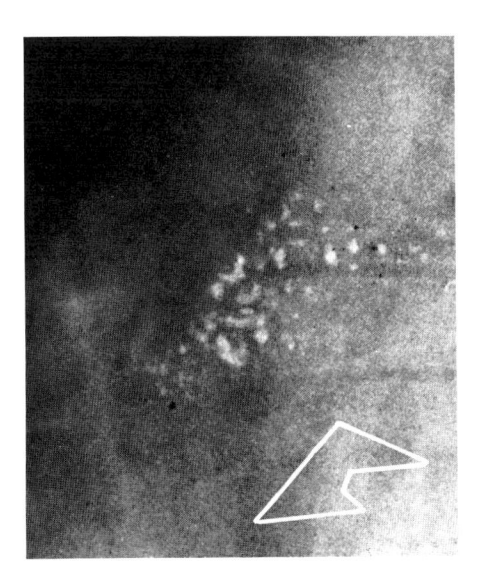

Fig. 7.29. Triangular cluster of mostly pleomorphic microcalcifications with dorsal indentation. Note the extremely straight lateral contour! Histology: comedocarcinoma

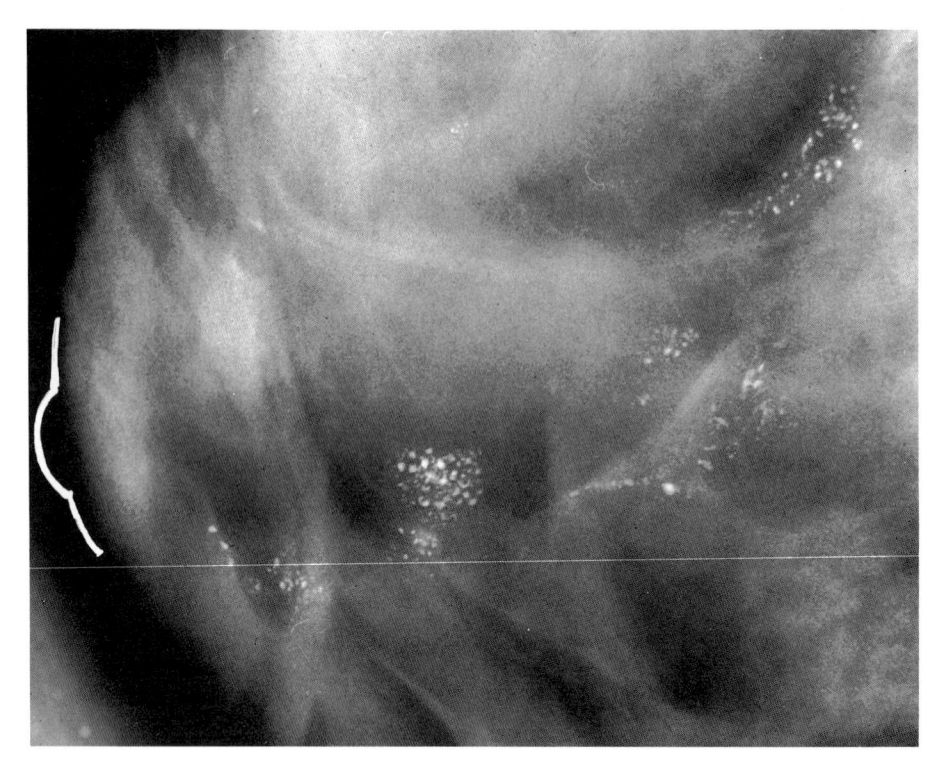

Fig. 7.30. Five triangular clusters with mostly pleomorphic and isolated punctate microcalcifications. Histology: carcinoma with cribriform and comedo elements

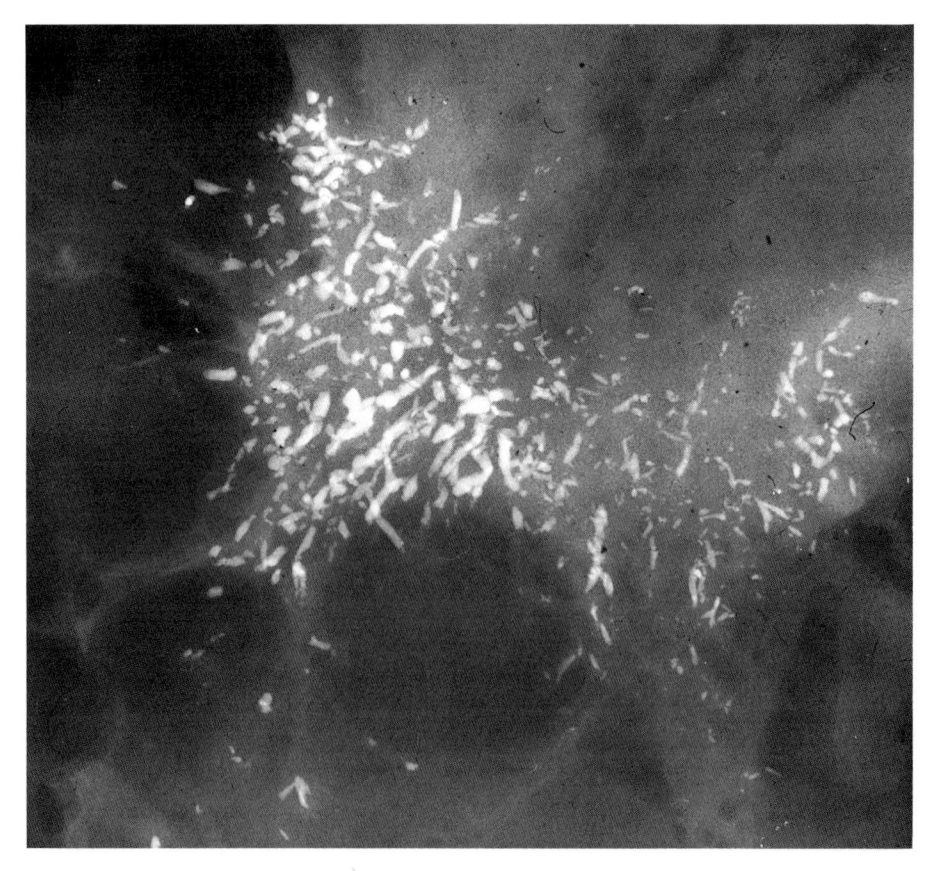

Fig. 7.31. Propeller-shaped cluster of mostly pleomorphic microcalcifications in a comedocarcinoma

Differential Diagnosis of Microcalcifications

Fig. 7.32. Star-shaped cluster with punctate and pleomorphic microcalcifications. Histology: predominantly comedocarcinoma

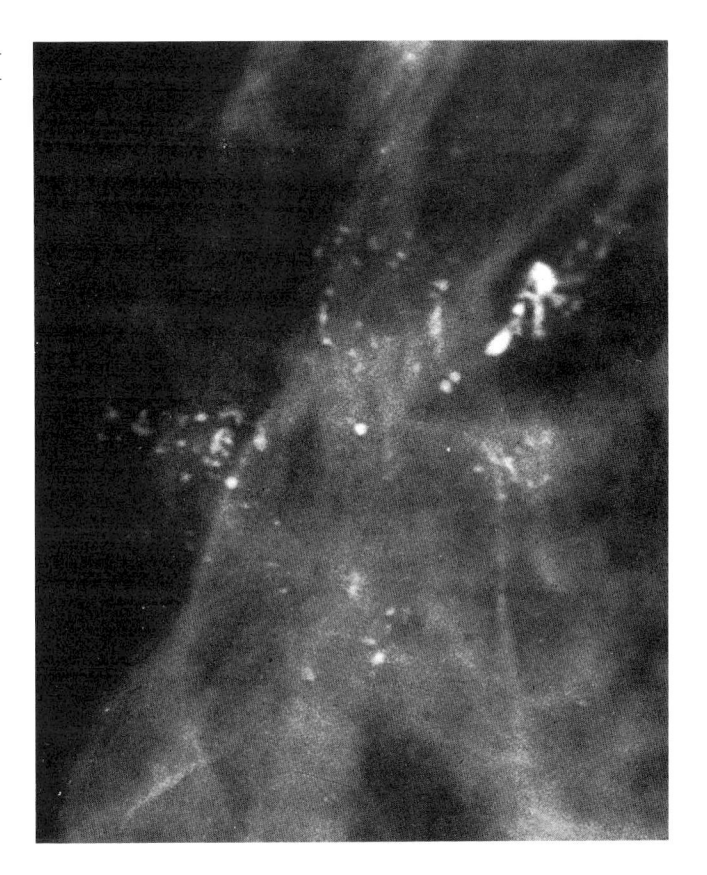

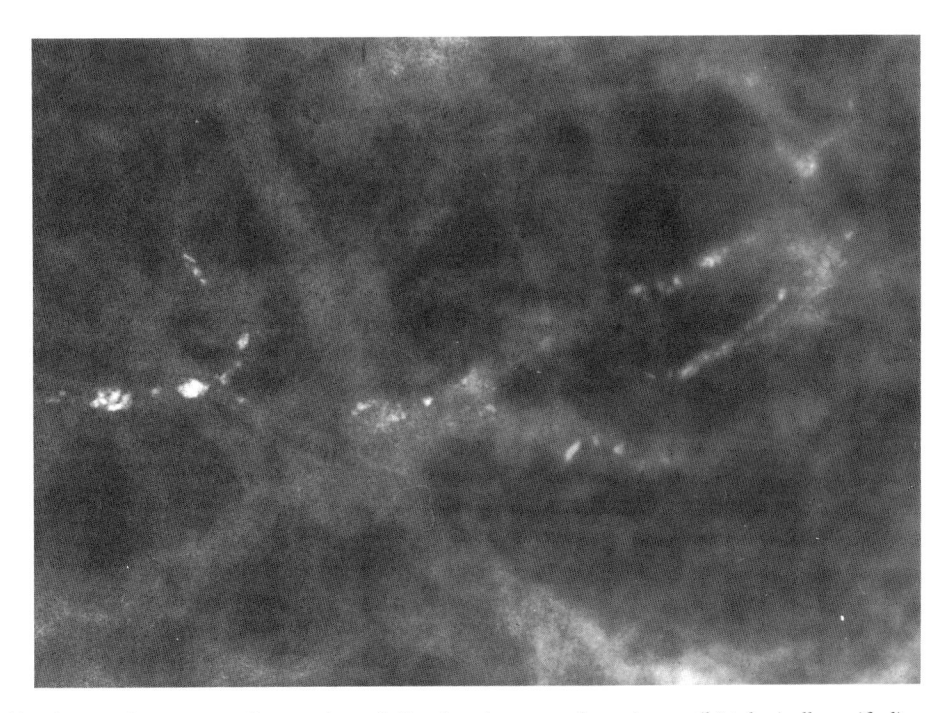

Fig. 7.33. Linear branch-like cluster of punctate or linear microcalcifications in a comedocarcinoma (histologically verified)

Fig. 7.34. Selection of different changes (due to projection) in cluster shape of microcalcifications in intraductal carcinoma. Each case is indicated by a letter

Fig. 7.35a,b. Changes in cluster shape in a comedocarcinoma associated with invasive ductal carcinoma. **a** Craniocaudal view; **b** lateral view

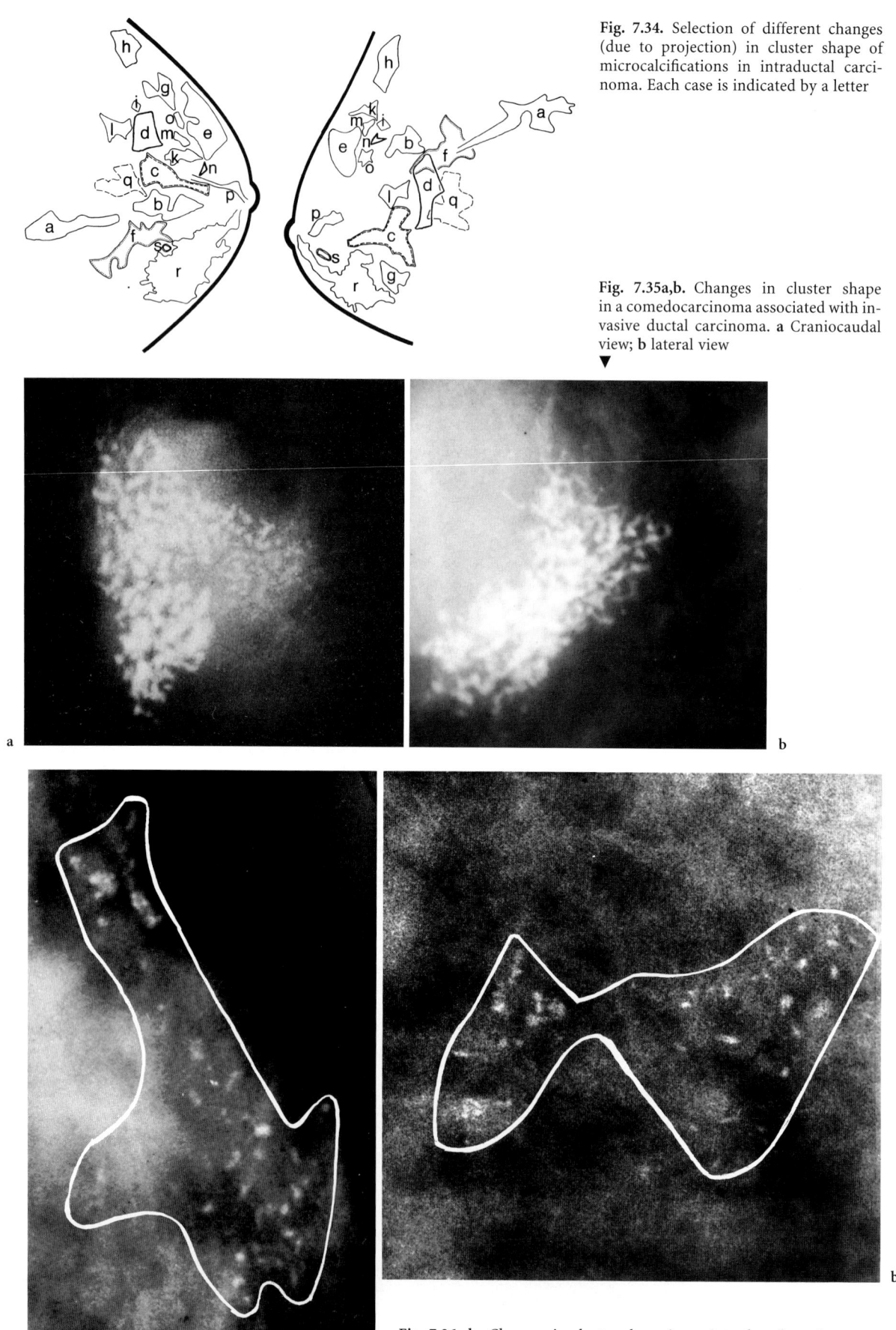

Fig. 7.36a,b. Changes in cluster shape in an intraductal carcinoma. **a** Lateral view; **b** craniocaudal view

Differential Diagnosis of Microcalcifications

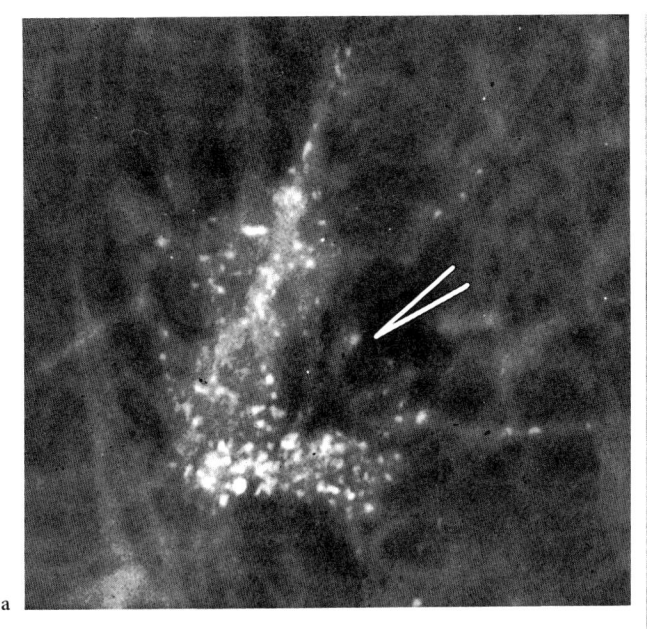

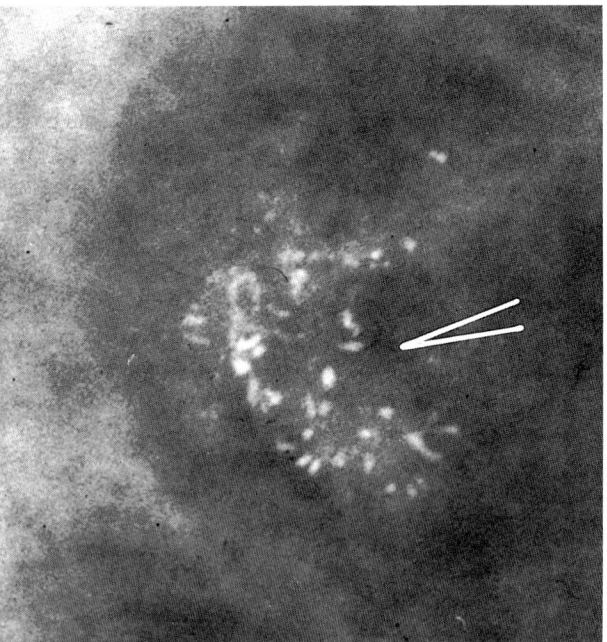

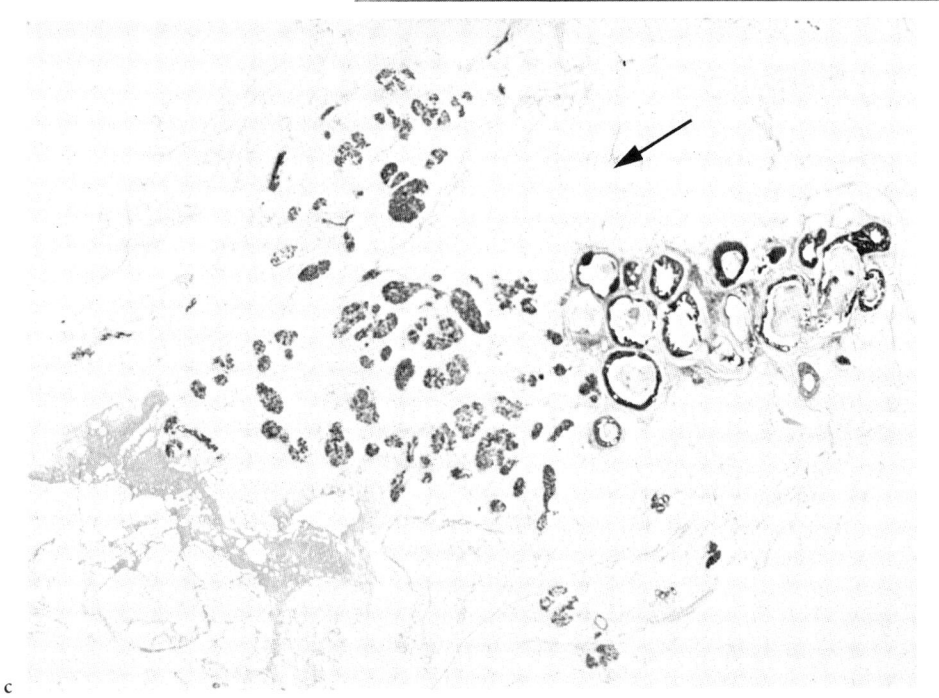

Fig. 7.37a,b. Two different cases of microcalcification clusters with varying degrees of punctate or pleomorphic microcalcification. Both clusters are triangular and both have dorsal indentation (swallowtail phenomenon). These changes correspond to intraductal carcinoma. **c** On the histological view of **b** both the triangular form and the dorsal indentation can be seen (courtesy of Prof. P. Citoler, Cologne, FRG)

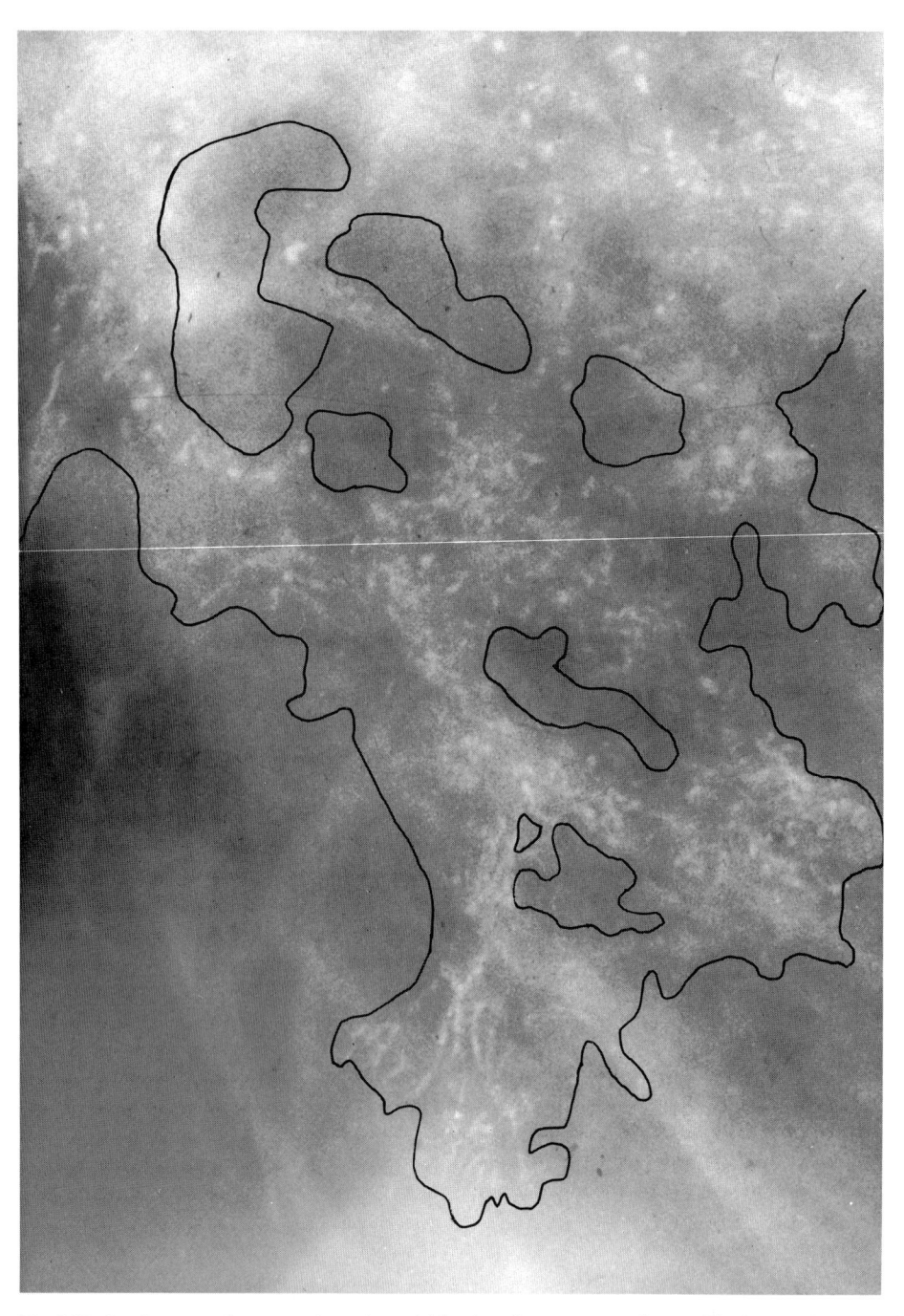

Fig. 7.38. Border area of an extensive microcalcification cluster in comedocarcinoma (×5). Predominantly pleomorphic microcalcifications. Small and large contour projections correspond to milk duct endings. Isolated patches free from microcalcifications correspond to interductal connective tissue or fat

Differential Diagnosis of Microcalcifications

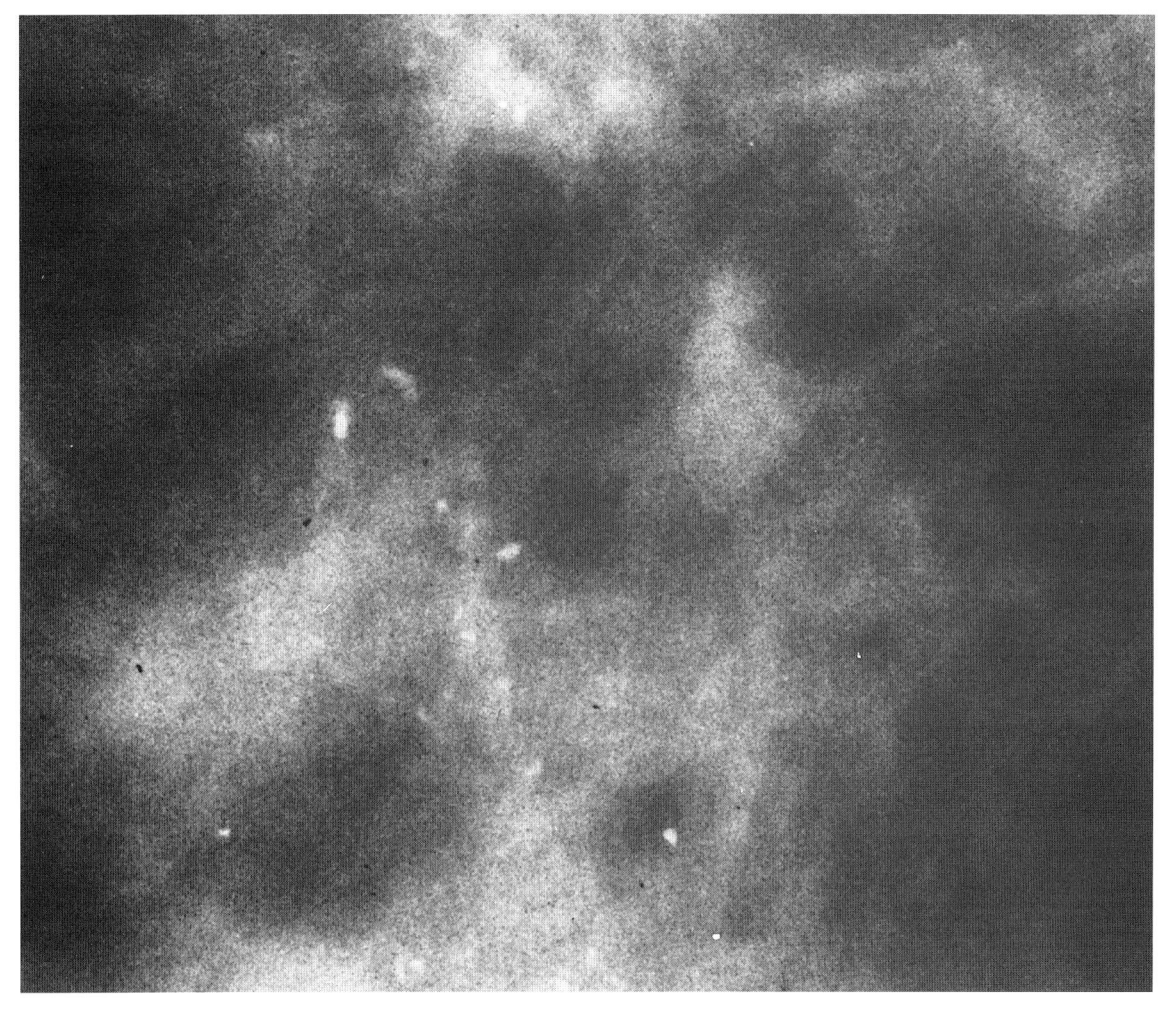

Fig. 7.39. Predominantly punctate and some tiny comma-shaped microcalcifications (minimal pleomorphism). The cluster shape cannot be clearly determined. Histology: extensive intraductal carcinoma with beginning invasion

7.3.2 Secretory Calcifications

Simultaneous occurrence of benign duct ectasia and secretion is known as *secretory disease* (Gershon-Cohen et al. 1956; Ingleby and Hermel 1956; Gershon-Cohen 1970). The retained secretion can become as thick as toothpaste, and clots of this can be squeezed onto the section surface, as is the case in comedocarcinoma. This so-called comedo mastitis cannot be distinguished macroscopically from comedocarcinoma (synonyms: obliterating mastitis, galactophoritis, whereby "-itis" implies a nonbacterial or so-called chemical mastitis).

It is usually easy to distinguish between the retained calcified secretions of benign duct ectasia and the microcalcifications seen in DCIS. If they are monomorphous, linear and facing towards the nipple "like a shoal of fish"(Willemin 1972), they are characteristic of calcified secretions (Fig. 7.41). They usually present bilaterally. Unresolvable problems can arise, however, if the microcalcifications are pleomorphic and the clusters circumscribed (Fig. 7.42) or if a necrotized intraductal comedocarcinoma and simultaneous a comedomastitis are completely calcified (Fig. 7.43).

7.3.3 Microcalcifications in Papillomatosis and Papilloma

Papillomatosis (syn.: ductal hyperplasia epitheliosis) may also be accompanied by microcalcifications. In this case one sees either dense calcified secretion (Fig. 7.44) or psammoma bodies if the papillomatosis is sponge-like with secondary lumens (Fig. 7.45).

Microcalcifications in sclerosing papilloma may be punctate, pleomorphic, or scaly. The cluster shape is generally round/oval, rather like a small fibroadenoma, though it can also be angular. In cases with spontaneous nipple discharge, galactography will indicate intraductal localization and a correct diagnosis becomes possible (Fig. 7.46).

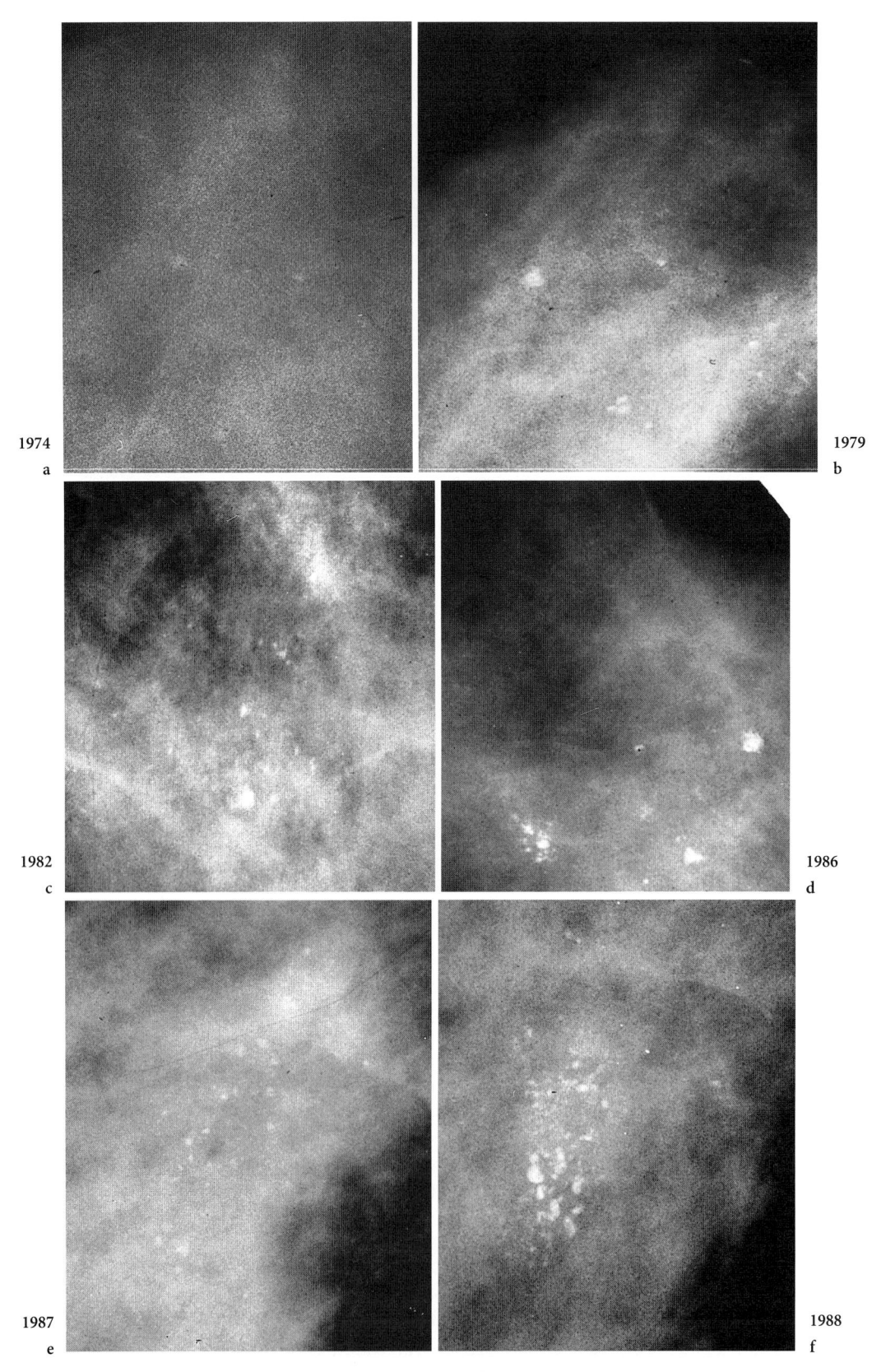

Fig. 7.40a–f. As the patient (a physician!) initially declined surgery, we had the opportunity to observe changes in the number and density of the microcalcifications in an intraductal carcinoma over a period of 14 years. When finally the histology was established, no invasion could be seen with light microscopy (consultation 1988)

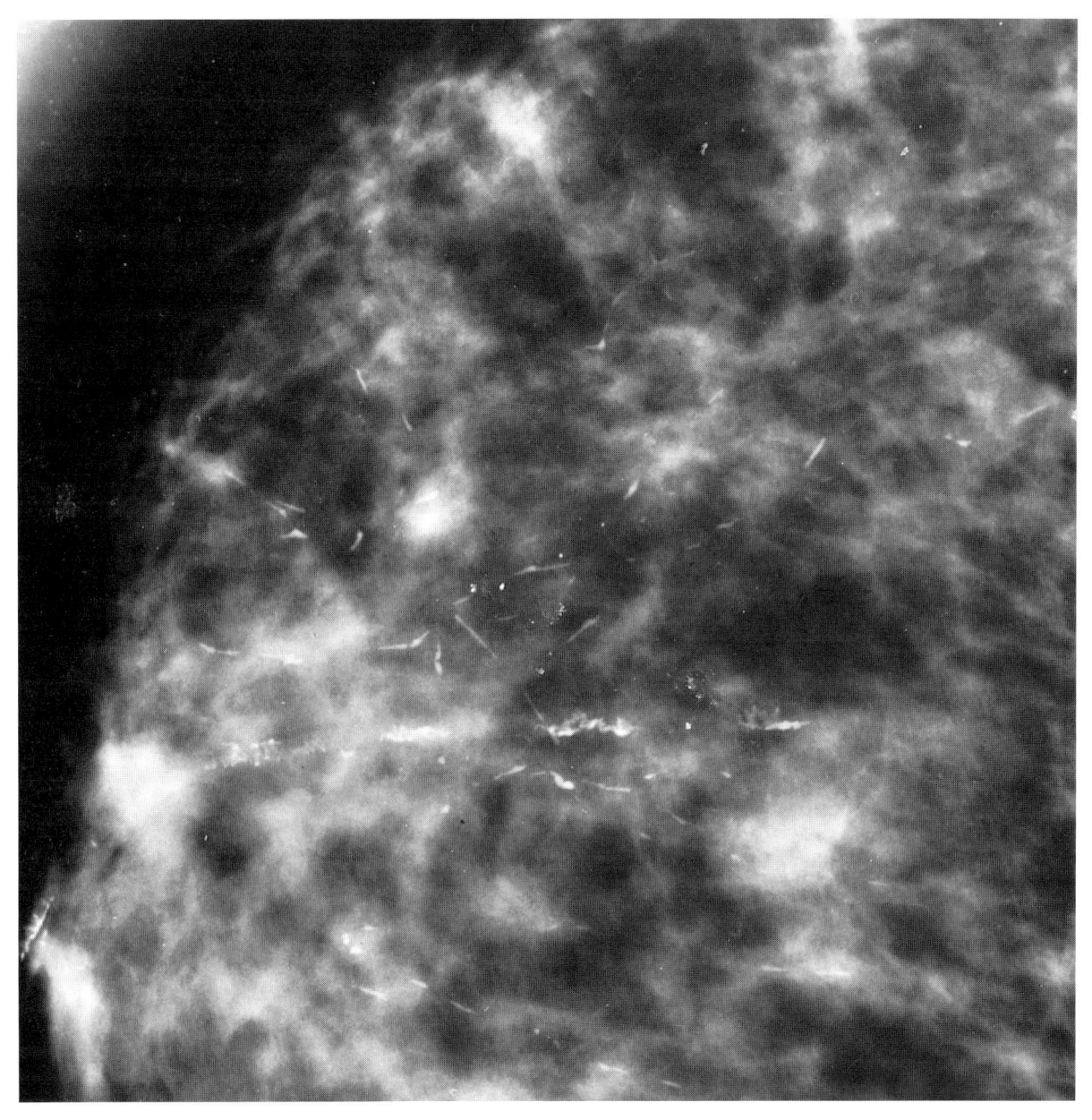

Fig. 7.41. Thin, monomorphous, linear microcalcifications facing towards the nipple; thickened, calcified secretion. Calcified artery found in the same case

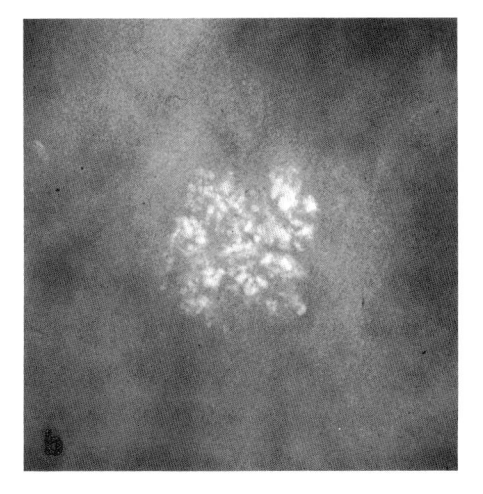

Fig. 7.42. Pleomorphic microcalcifications; the cluster is angular in both views. Histology: Chronic galactophoritis with intraductal calcification

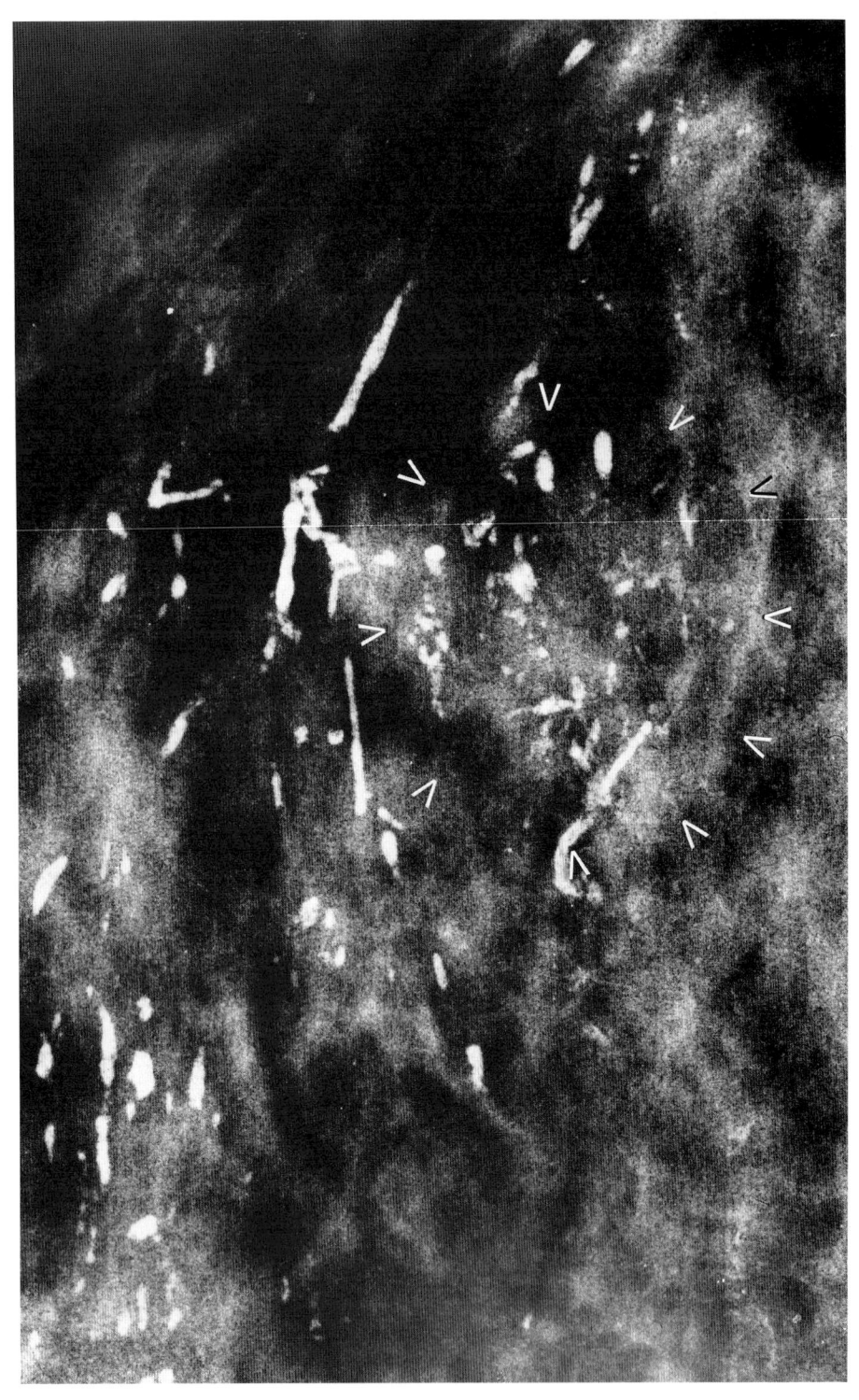

Fig. 7.43. Simultaneous manifestation of calcified secretions and microcalcifications in a comedocarcinoma. The calcified secretions are considerably longer and thicker, than the calcifications in the carcinoma (*arrows*) (Histology: Prof. P. Citoler, Cologne, FRG)

Fig. 7.44. Angular cluster of faint, pleomorphic microcalcifications in an area of multicentric papillomatosis with atypia

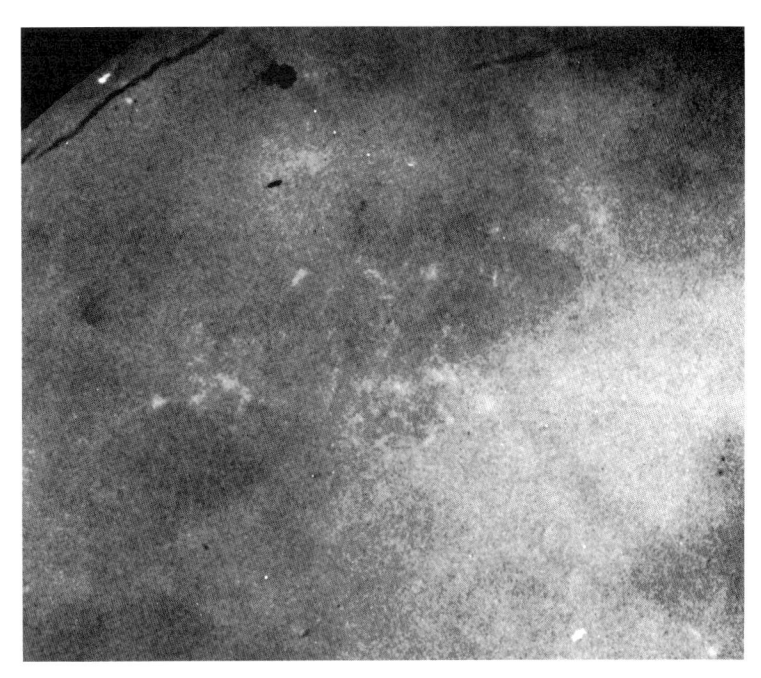

Fig. 7.45. Countless punctate microcalcifications in extensive papillomatosis
▼

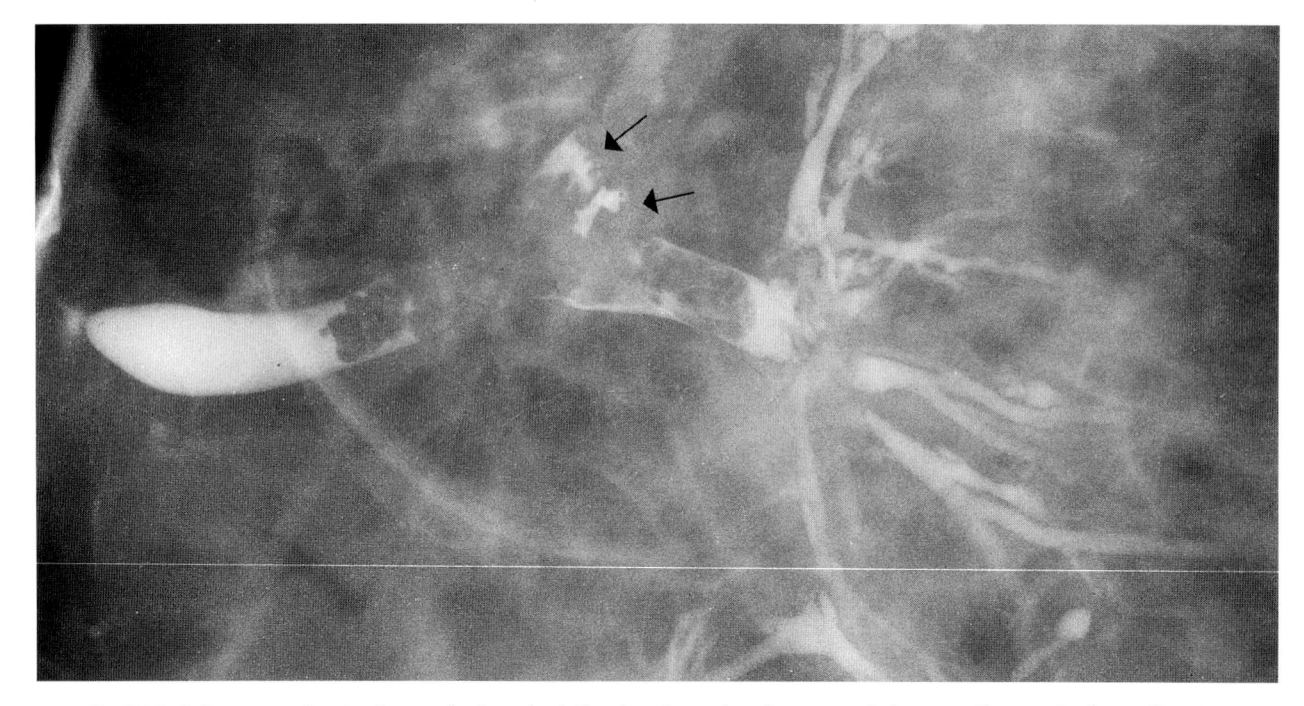

Fig. 7.46. Galactogram showing long scale-shaped calcifications (*arrow*) at the center of a large papilloma. Histology: Fibrosing, calcified papilloma

7.4 Simultaneous Occurrence of Acinar and Ductal Microcalcifications

In cases of intraductal carcinoma, ductal microcalcification can be accompanied by acinar calcifications, though this is extremely rare. The author has encountered only four such cases, one of which is shown in Fig. 7.47. As in these four cases the acinar microcalcifications were not histologically examined, it cannot be definitely ascertained whether this was a fortuitous coincidence of both forms of microcalcifications or a so-called lobular cancerization with acinar calcification. Cancerization of lobules means the retrograde spread of tumor from ducts or ductules into the lobules (Azzopardi 1979). Cytomorphologically, this is not LCIS but rather genuine ductal in situ carcinoma spreading back to the lobule. It may also be that the carcinomatous tissue in lobular cancerization becomes necrotic and calcified.

The author has only encountered two corresponding histological references in the literature: Fig. 10–11 in the book by Azzopardi (1979) and Fig. 11 in the publication of Kopans et al. (1990), the latter in connection with the apocrine nature of the carcinoma cells (the apocrine nature of these cells may be due to the hypersecretory activity of the cells). This assumption of Kopans et al. is in contrast to the experience of Gilles et al. (1994), who found intralobular microcalcifications in only one out of 17 apocrine carcinomas. These were located in benign microcysts (fortuitous simultaneous occurrence of microcalcifications). Whether the microcalcifications are due to lobular cancerization or a fortuitous simultaneous occurrence, the mammographer must not be tempted by the lobular appearance of some of the microcalcifications not to diagnose intraductal carcinoma.

In cases of *primary* and *secondary hyperparathyroidism*, calcifications seem to develop simultaneously within both the milk ducts and the lobules (Marinesen and Damian 1984). It is known that in this disease, soft tissue calcifications may occur in various organs (aorta, cornea, conjunctiva, joint capsules, skin, lung, heart). Sang y Han and Witten (1977) reported a case of secondary hyperparathyroidism with bilateral calcification of the glandular and ductal breast tissue. Interestingly in this case, regression of calcifications was observed after dialysis. The author observed two cases of secondary hyperparathyroidism due to renal insufficiency respectively bone metastases with extensive

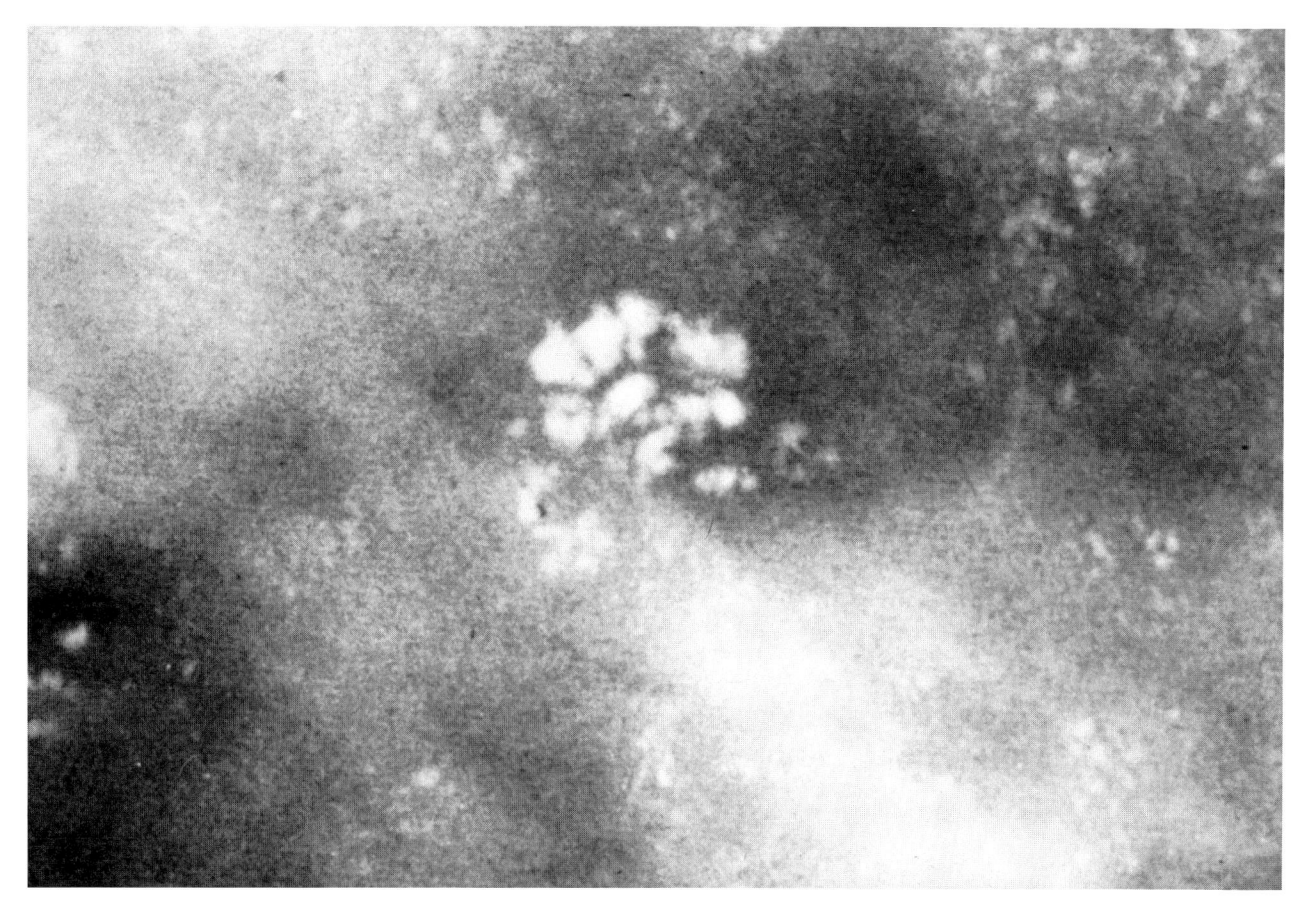

Differential Diagnosis of Microcalcifications

Fig. 7.47. Detail: *Centrally*: round, facetted cluster, of obviously lobular microcalcifications, surrounded by punctate and pleomorphic microcalcifications (see Fig. 7.3). Histology: intraductal carcinoma. Unfortunately the area with acinar microcalcifications was not analyzed

bilateral breast calcifications (Figs. 7.48, 7.49). EGAN (1988) also described a case of hypercalcemia with breast calcifications similar to that shown here. More or less extensive calcification of blood vessels, occasionally with small aneurysms, seems to be the rule. In EGAN's case the calcifications were shown histologically to be "stroma calcifications." Our cases were not histologically analyzed, but the acinar localization in the first case is undeniable (Fig. 7.48). The assumption that further calcifications are at least partially intraductal seems fairly certain. This is particularly true in Fig. 7.49.

7.5 Microcalcifications Outside of the Acini and Milk Ducts

Microcalcifications outside of the acini and milk ducts comprise calcified fat necrosis, arterial calcifications, calcifications in the axillary lymph nodes, calcified foreign bodies, and calcifications of the sebaceous glands.

7.5.1 Fat Necrosis

Fat necrosis always follows the same pattern of development independent of its cause. In the *posttraumatic* phase, the membranes of the fat cells are ruptured and neutral fat escapes. In the *resorptive* phase lipophagic cells absorb the neutral fat and vacuoles develop. In the phase of *repair* these cavities become encapsulated or scarred. Sometimes neutral fat remains in the cavities (so-called oil cyst). Calcified salt precipitations (saponified fat) may collect in the connective tissue capsule or in the scar tissue.

Calcified liponecrotic microcysts, first defined by LEBORGNE (1967), may occur in the following conditions:

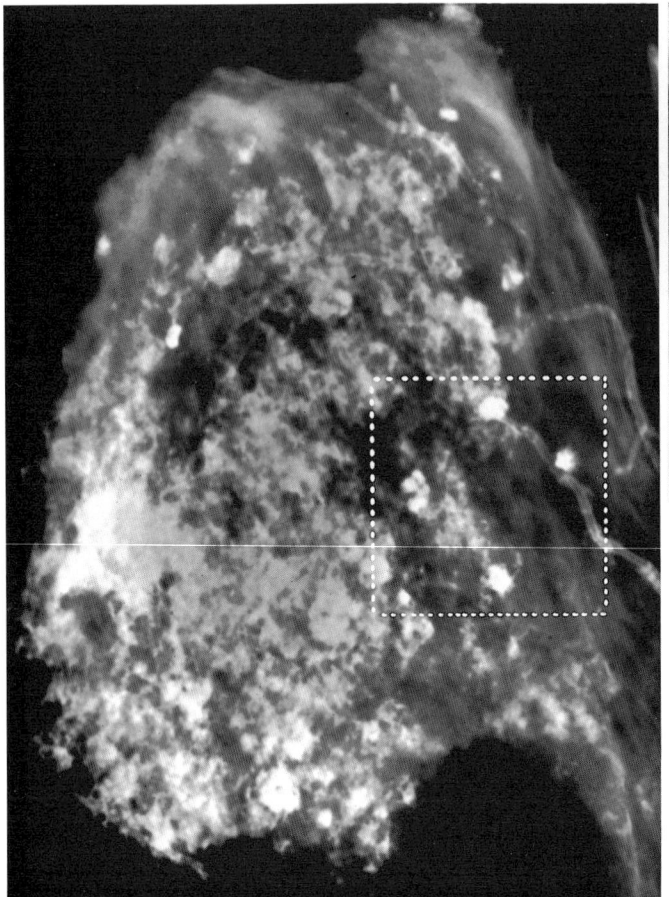

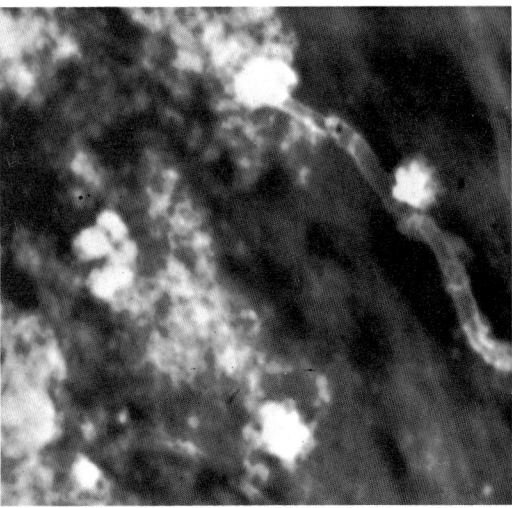

Fig. 7.48. a Mammogram (somewhat reduced in size); b detail. Microcalcifications, some of which are contained in lobular cysts (septa!) and some of which are definitely intraductal. Further microcalcifications cannot be definitely localized in the glandular acini or the ductal system. There is also calcification of arteries. Clinical diagnosis: renal insufficiency, hyperparathyreoidism

1. After iatrogenic or noniatrogenic trauma or, as described by BASSETT et al. (1982), after primary radiotherapy
2. After bacterial or abacterial inflammation (so-called plasma cell mastitis, burst cyst, nonpurulent panniculitis)

Liponecrotic microcysts are a common diagnosis. They usually occur as isolated findings, only rarely being multiple or disseminated (Fig. 7.50a). They are normally round, rarely oval, and are similar in size (2–3 mm in diameter). They characteristically present a central radiolucency with some scattered punctate or amorphic calcifications. Histologically these are calcifications of granulomatous tissue within fat vacuoles (Fig. 7.50b). Sometimes disappearance and reappearance of the same liponecrotic microcyst can be observed. Blister-like, sometimes oval calcifications can also be found in the vicinity of secretory calcifications. This is because the secretion escaping from the milk ducts induces a circumscribed abacterial inflammation with fat necrosis. LEBORGNE (1967) suspected some connection between liponecrotic cysts and carcinoma. This theory, however, has never been investigated. Amorphous, pleomorphic, and net-like conglomerations of calcifications, possibly in an angled configuration (Fig. 7.51), are rarely found in scar tissue. We agree with BASSETT et al. (1978) that the four cases observed by these authors presented some difficulty in the differentiation of truly benign calcifications from those of intraductal carcinoma.

7.5.2 Arterial Calcifications

Arterial calcifications can cause problems in differential diagnosis only if they are limited to a small stretch of one vessel, showing circumscribed calcification with a linear, punctate, or wavy configuration that may be mistaken for linear milk duct calcification. Attention to the parallelism of these linear cal-

Differential Diagnosis of Microcalcifications

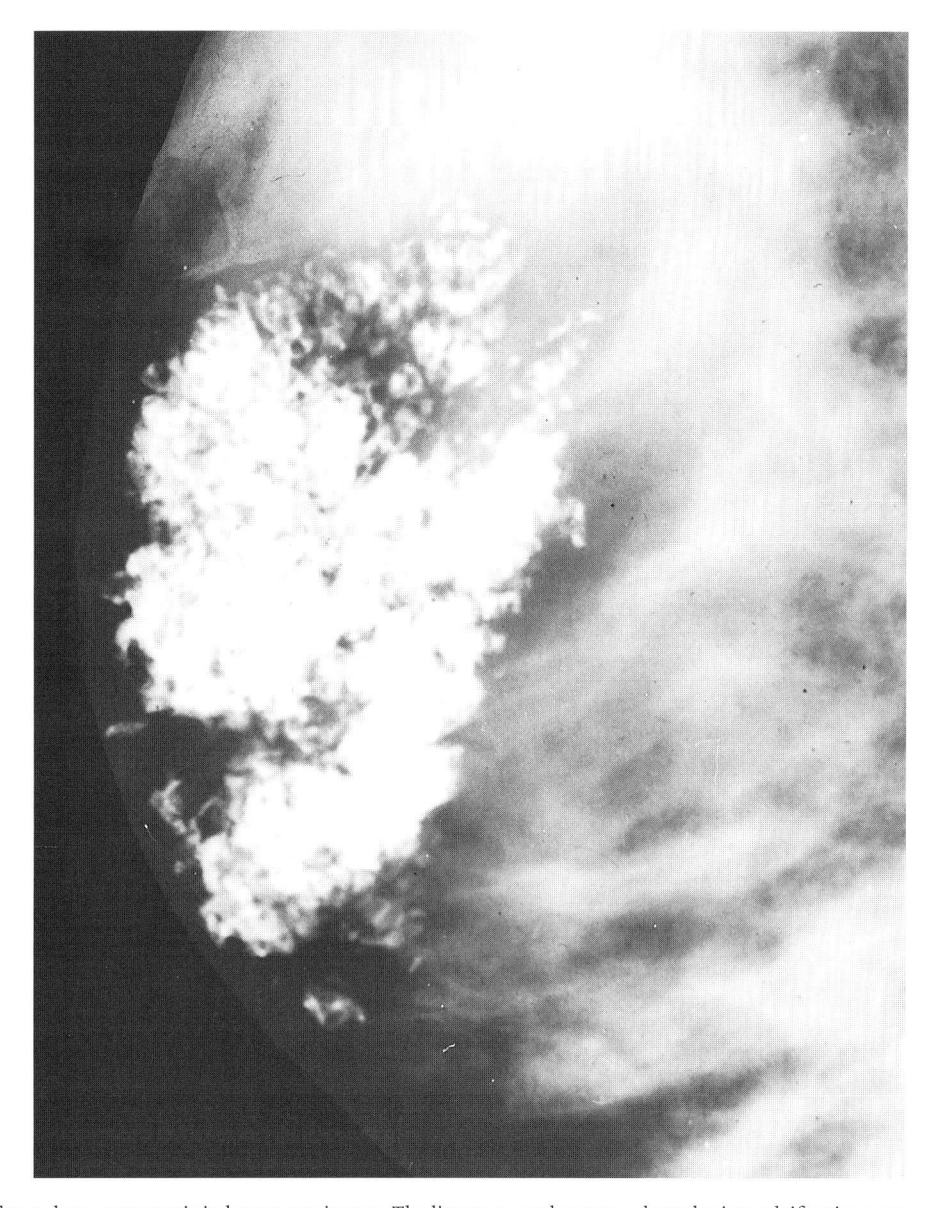

Fig. 7.49. Hypercalcemia due to bone metastasis in breast carcinoma. The linear, v-, and comma-shaped microcalcifications are localized intraductally. Arterial calcification

cifications (Fig. 7.52) will enable one to avoid misinterpretation.

Multiple calcified very small arteries, on the other hand, cause greater problems in differential diagnosis. These rather rare forms of calcification may occur in clusters or diffusely (Fig. 7.53). Besides short, bent, tube-like calcifications, those more characteristic of arteriosclerosis are also observed, so that, even without the corresponding case history, the incorrect diagnosis of calcified parasites can be avoided. If the polarity of the calcifications does not correspond to milk ducts (i.e., facing towards the nipple), intraductal calcifications can be excluded.

7.5.3 Calcifications in Axillary Lymph Nodes

Microcalcifications in axillary lymph node metastases are extremely rare (BJURSTAM 1978; HELVIE et al. 1988). One such case from the author's collection is shown in Fig. 7.54. Calcifications in benign inflammatory lymph node are usually larger. In the case illustrated in Fig. 7.55, the histological diagnosis was cat-scratch disease. Large calcifications also can be seen in tuberculous lymph nodes, or in axillary nodes ipsilateral to the arm used for BCG inoculation.

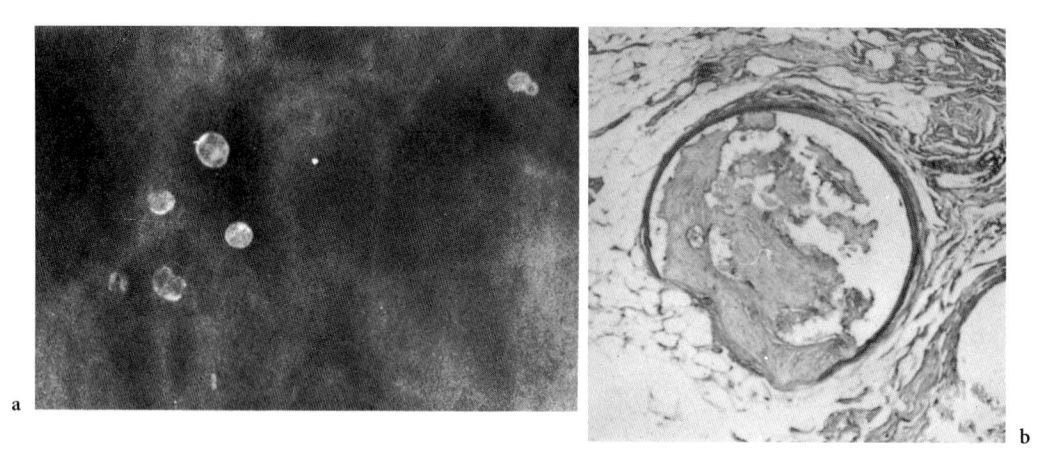

Fig. 7.50. a Ring-shaped calcifications of similar size, with amorphous calcium deposits at the center. Liponecrotic microcysts without any known trauma. **b** Histology of another case. Here the ring-shaped calcifications correspond to the calcified capsule, and the amorphous calcified center to intracystic granulation tissue

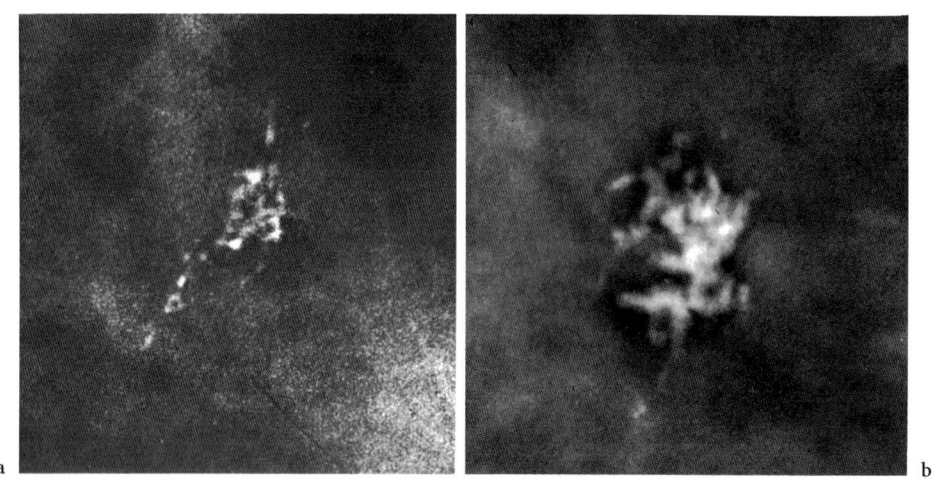

Fig. 7.51. Post biopsy: triangular configuration of punctate and pleomorphic microcalcifications in the area around the biopsy scar. Histology: nodular lipomatosis with large, scale-shaped calcifications

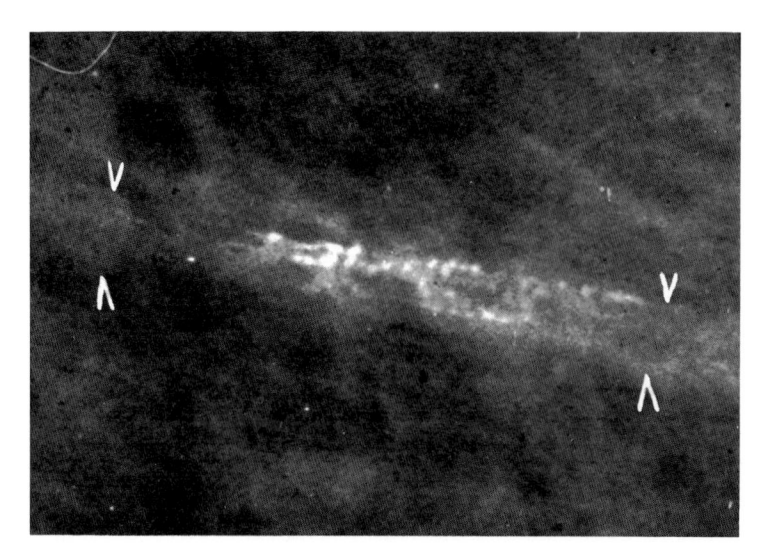

Fig. 7.52. Elongated cluster of predominantly punctate but occasionally linear microcalcifications which are arranged in two parallel lines. At the end of the cluster a strip of soft tissue opacity is visible (*arrow*). Partial calcification of an artery

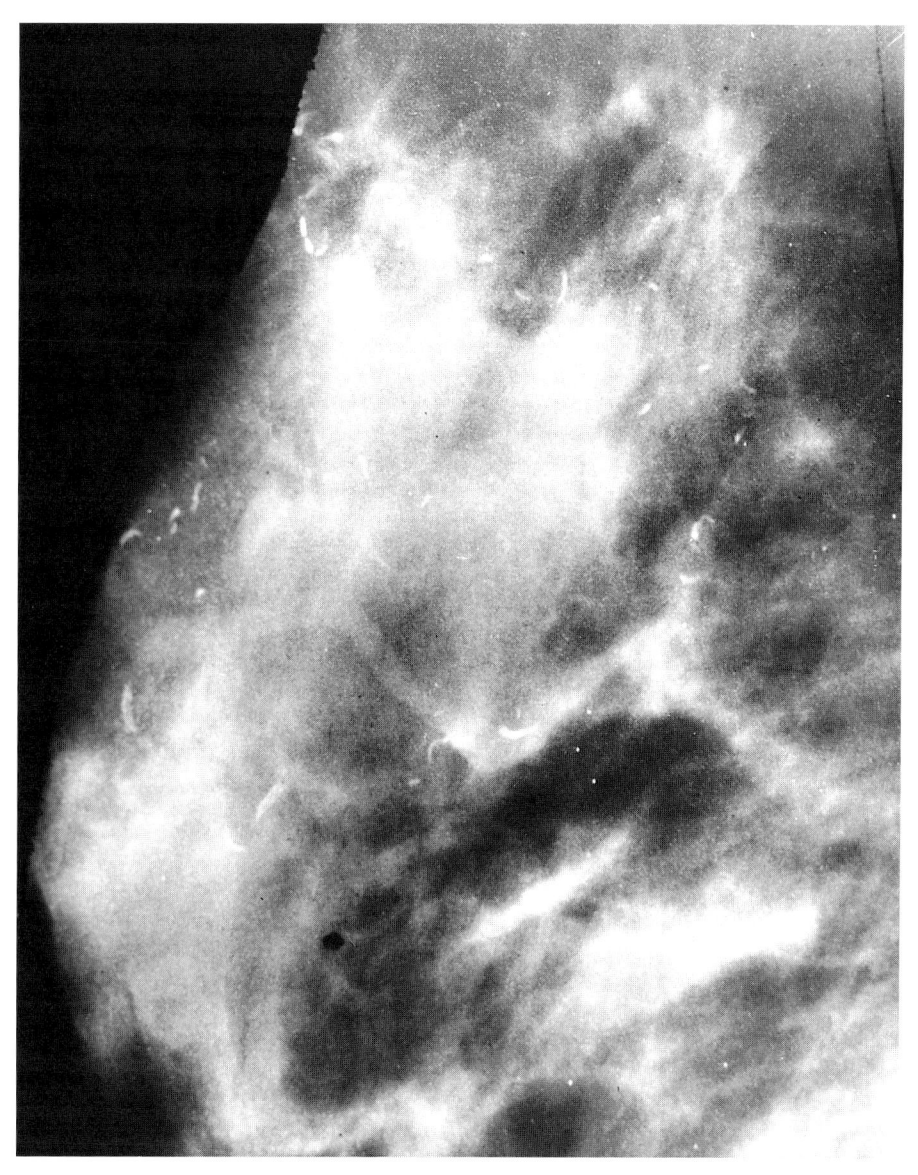

Fig. 7.53. Multiple calcified very small arteries

7.5.4 Calcified Foreign Bodies

Calcified foreign bodies, such as suture material (DAVIS et al. 1989; STACEY-CLEAR et al. 1992), or gold deposits in intramammary lymph nodes of patients suffering from rheumatoid arthritis who have undergone prolonged gold therapy (BRUWER et al. 1987), are rarely found.

Filariasis may be diffuse (Fig. 7.56) or clustered (BRITTON et al. 1992). This condition presents long, fine, snake-like, wavy calcifications. Neither their form nor their distribution is characteristic of milk duct calcifications. Calcified *Trichinella spiralis* within the pectoralis major muscle (trichinosis) may mimic breast calcifications on mammograms, as in one case reported by IKEDA and SICKLES (1988). EGAN (1988) shows one case of fine bullet fragments (from a gunshot wound) mimicking clustered microcalcifications.

After silicone injection for breast augmentation, calcifications may form at the rim of silicone granulomas scattered throughout the breasts (Fig. 7.57). The mammographic appearance is so characteristic that there is no problem in diagnosis, even if the patient does not admit to having had treatment, as was reported by INOUE et al. (1978). Breast calcifications can also form after paraffin injections (THIELS and DUMKE 1977; KOIDE and KATAYAMA 1979).

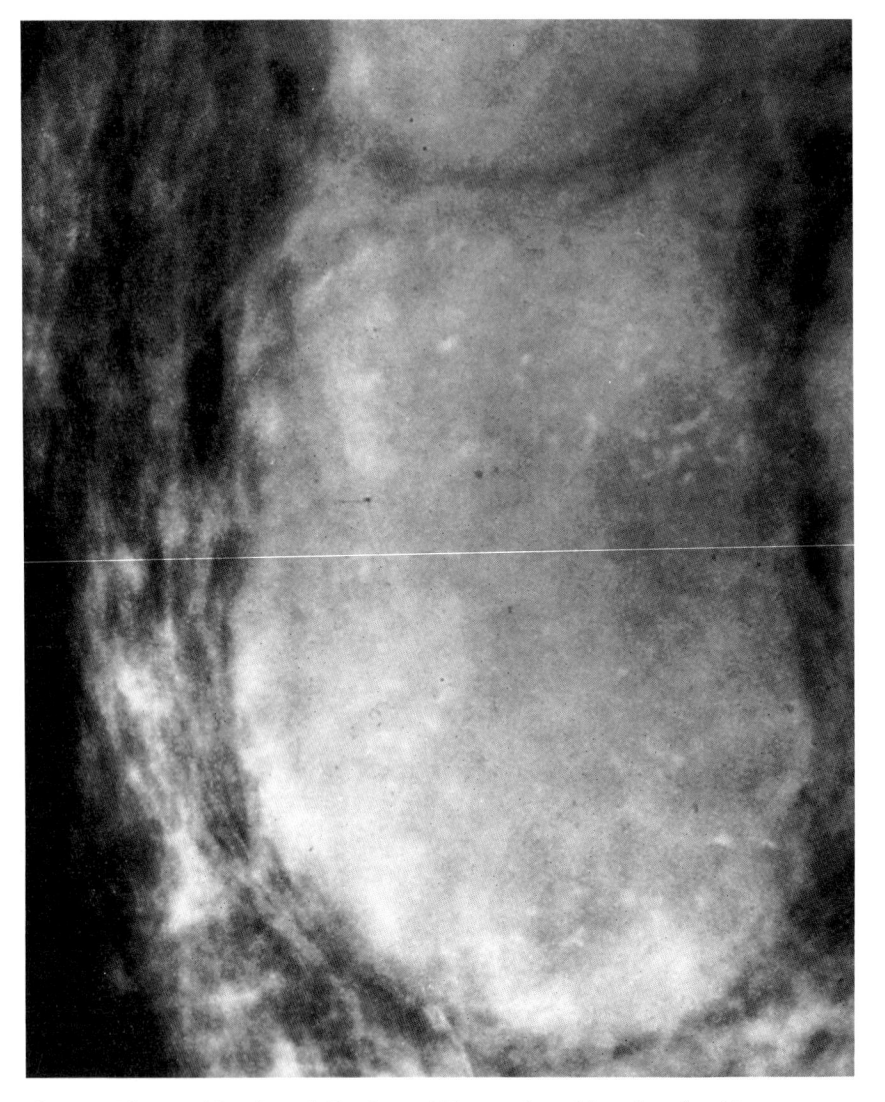

Fig. 7.54. Pleomorphic microcalcifications within an enlarged lymph node with metastases

7.5.5 Calcified Sebaceous Glands

Calcified sebaceous glands present in about 3% of all mammograms. Approximately half of these are clustered. They are in the order of 1–1.5 mm in size. Normally they are ring or dumbbell shaped with central radiolucency (Hoeffken and Lanyi 1973). Punctate or linear sebaceous calcifications are less common, but when they occur in close proximity to each other (i.e., clustered) they may cause problems in differential diagnosis unless their intracutaneous localization can be demonstrated. Only some clustered sebaceous gland microcalcifications can be reliably localized intracutaneously using standard mammograms. A tangential view (Fig. 7.58) usually solves the problem (Sickles 1986). An unchanging orientation of clustered skin calcifications when comparing current with previous mammograms is also said to indicate an intracutaneous site (Homer et al. 1994). If there is any further uncertainty, stereotaxic biopsy will correctly indicate intracutaneous localization (Linden and Sullivan 1989). In my own experience, however, this is not necessary.

Fig. 7.55. Scale-shaped lymph node calcifications in cat-scratch disease

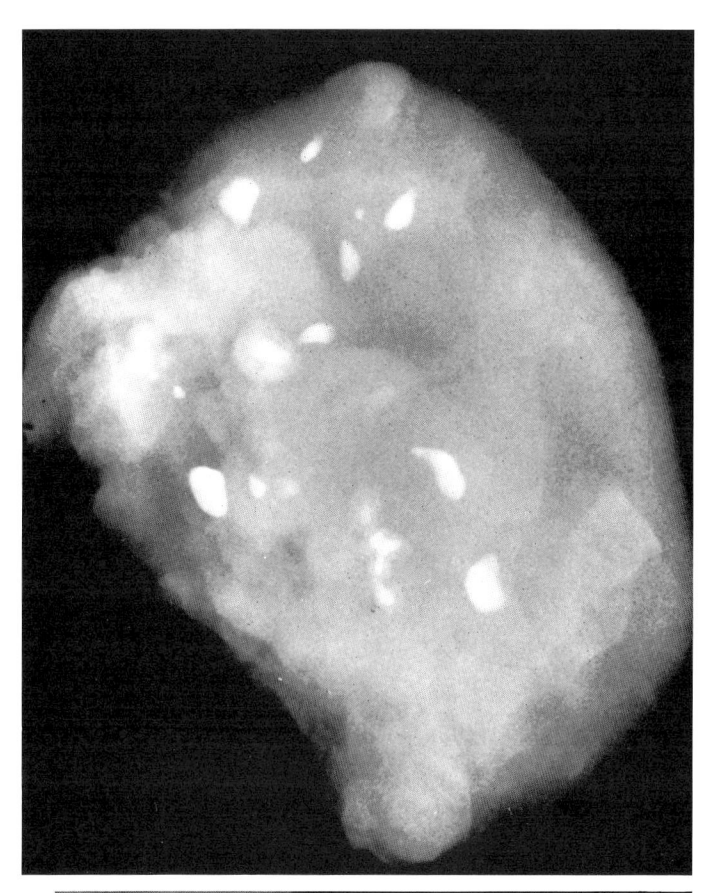

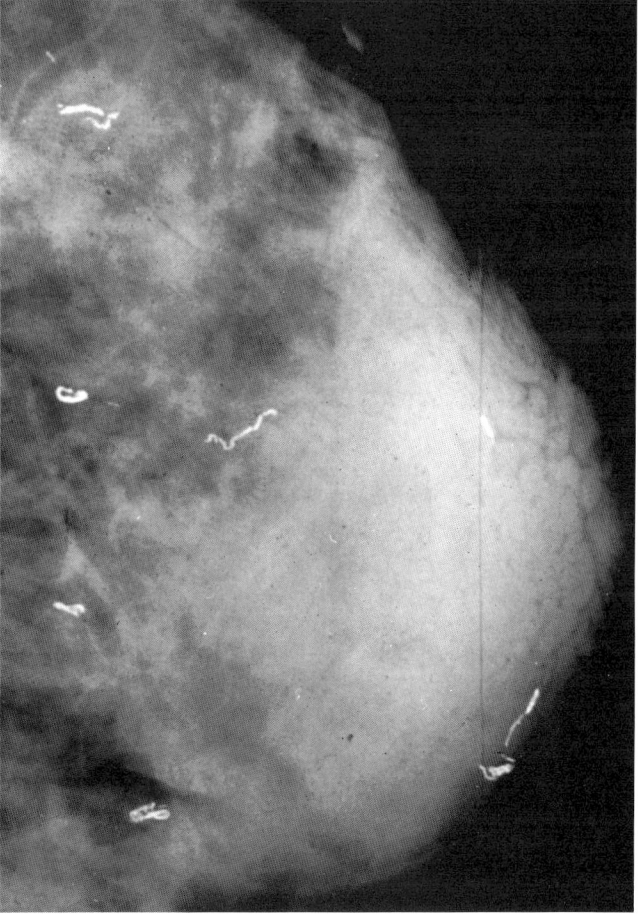

Fig. 7.56. Calcified filariae in a female African patient. Courtesy of Prof. Kiefer, Wiesbaden, Germany

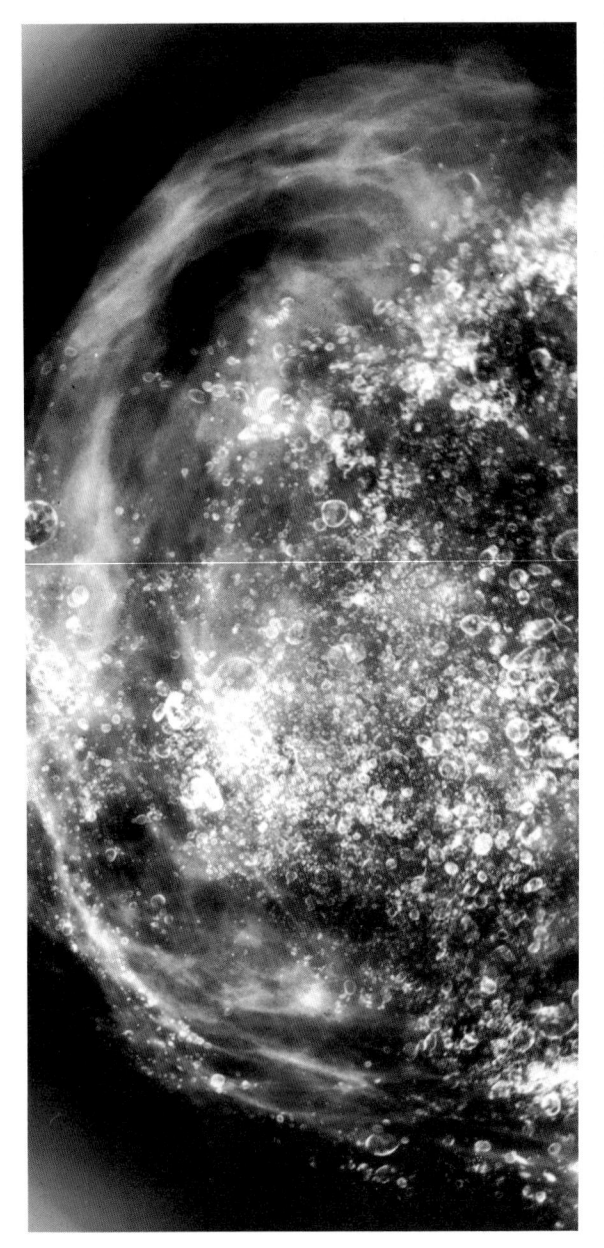

Fig. 7.57. Ring-like calcifications after silicone injection. Courtesy of Rado, MD, Bergheim, Germany

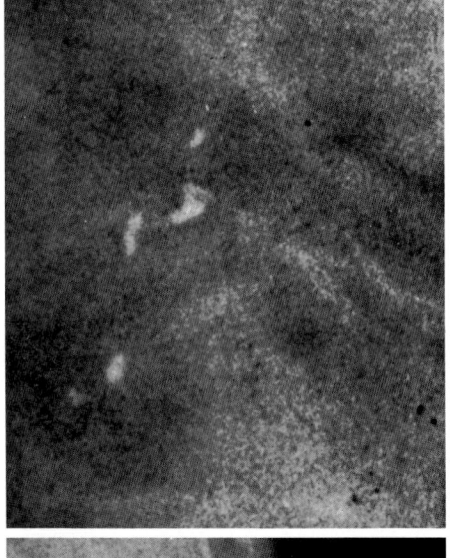

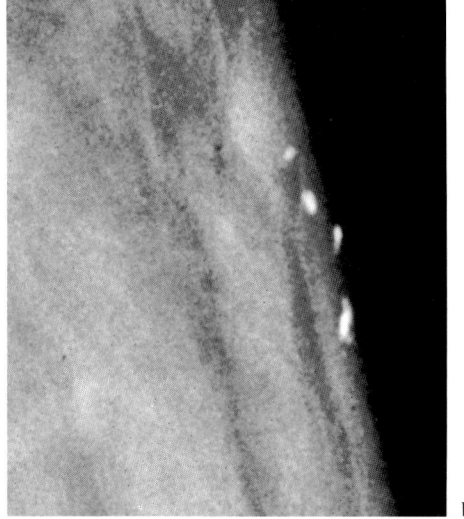

Fig. 7.58a,b. This patient had previously undergoe mastectomy of the other breast for carcinoma. In comparison with the preoperative mammogram an angled cluster of five punctate, linear, and comma-shaped microcalcifications has appeared. **a** As the microcalcifications seemed to be intramammary on both conventional views, intraductal calcifications were first suspected. **b** A tangential view solved the problem of differential diagnosis. The intracutaneous localization indicates benign sebaceous gland calcifications

7.6 Calcium-like Artifacts

Calcium-like artifacts may be due to (a) objects or foreign bodies in or on the skin or (b) defective film processing. Ointments containing zinc or powders (Fig. 7.59), or contrast medium which has been spilled onto the skin, may mimic microcalcifications. BROWN et al. (1981) reported that tattoo marks on the skin of the breast may appear as microcalcifications. Likewise, dust particles similar in absorption to calcium or metal chippings after repair of the tube lock can produce speckles on the mammogram similar to microcalcifications. During galactography contrast medium may escape from the nipple and spill onto the supporting tray and be rendered visible during a subsequent mammogram. Par-

Differential Diagnosis of Microcalcifications

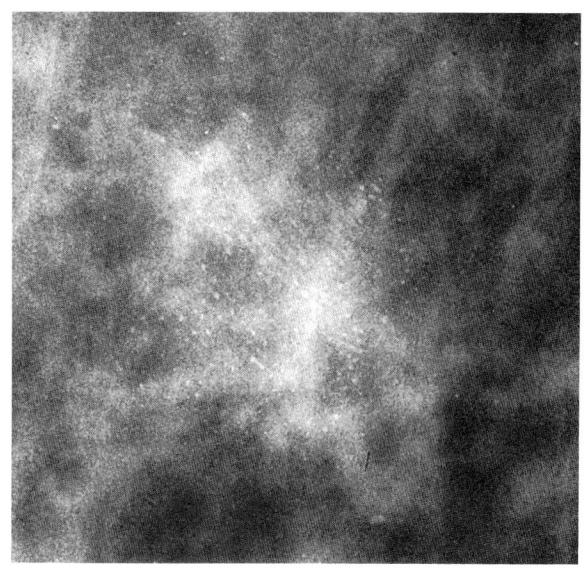

Fig. 7.59. Traces of powder (artifact)

Fig. 7.60. Fingerprint (artifact)

ticles of dirt on the cassette surface or the intensifying screen, or fingerprints on the film (Fig. 7.60), may also mimic intramammary microcalcifications. Dirty rollers in the film-developing machine can produce clusters of stains similar to microcalcifications. Such artifacts, whatever their cause, can rarely be localized to the breast on a second view. If there is any suspicion of artifacts, the mammogram must be repeated after thorough cleaning of the breast, the tube casing, the cassette, the screen, and the grid table.

7.7 Conclusion

It is strange that 45 years after LEBORGNE's discovery of microcalcifications, today there seems to be more uncertainty in their interpretation than in the early years after their detection. Insufficient training and lack of uniformity of diagnostic criteria have led to skepticism on the part of clinicians (HOMER 1984). As ABBES et al. (1988) stated, "The surgeon is often in a difficult position as the indication for biopsy has already been suggested." What, indeed, should the clinician think of a method with such equivocal diagnostic value? The search for ever smaller breast carcinomas and fear of litigation (because of delayed diagnosis of a small carcinoma) have led to a situation where smaller carcinomas are indeed detected but a higher percentage of biopsies are performed for benign lesions (SICKLES 1986). As pointed out by ABBES et al. (1988): "Abusive surgery in the name of cancer prophylaxis may result in excessive mutilation." Iatrogenic scars may cause problems in later differential diagnosis. Is it justified to expect three out of four symptom-free women to undergo unnecessary biopsies in order to find carcinomas in only one out of four of them? It is certainly justified to ask whether microcalcifications are a curse or a blessing for the women (LANYI 1985). Also in future screening projects the enormous expense and cost of unnecessary biopsies must be reduced. Radiologists have come to terms with this low yield of carcinomas with the analysis of microcalcifications, but the desire for a more reliable method of diagnosis has become stronger; thus LE TREUT et al. (1992) concluded, "The selection of the indications for a histological control on the basis of an accurate semiological study is ... essential."

Every physician has the right to indicate a follow-up examination and this is also true in the case of microcalcifications in mammography. SICKLES (1986) reexamined selected cases of "probably benign" microcalcifications (not characteristically benign but also not considered worthy of biopsy) at least twice in 6 to 12-month intervals. He reported that out of more than 1000 such cases, only three (still early-stage) carcinomas were detected in a period of at least 3 years. He proposed periodic follow-up as an alternative to biopsy for these cases of almost certainly benign microcalcifications.

Although obvious, it must be emphasized once again that top quality x-rays are an indispensable prerequisite for successful differential diagnosis of microcalcifications. Sharp magnification views are especially helpful in reducing the number of equivocal diagnoses (SICKLES 1980). It goes without saying that a magnifying lens should always be used.

Even the most meticulous radiologist will make false-positive diagnoses – usually in cases of small clusters of microcalcification in sclerosing adenosis or in fibroadenoma when the cluster form is difficult to evaluate or angled. As noted previously, my own success rate has never exceeded 70%. False-negative diagnoses also are repeatedly, though rarely, made in cases of small clustered microcalcifications. In these cases one should heed the advice of GERSHON-COHEN, which is, more or less, that if a radiologist fails to detect a clinically occult carcinoma in the breast in its early stage, he should be able to take comfort in the fact that, at the time of his diagnosis, there was no other method with which the lesion could have been discovered.

References

Abbes M, Vergnet F, Aubanel D (1988) Practical importance of breast microcalcifications: report on 112 cases. Eur J Surg Oncol 14:651–661

Azzopardi JG (1979) Problems in breast pathology. Saunders, Philadelphia

Basset LW, Gold RH, Cove HC (1978) Mammographic spectrum of traumatic fat necrosis: the fallibility of "pathognomic" signs of carcinoma. Am J Roentgenol 130:119

Basset LW, Gold RH, Mirra JM (1982) Nonneoplastic breast calcifications in lipid cysts: development after excision and primary irradiation AJR 138:335–338

Bässler R (1978) Pathologie der Brustdrüse (Spezielle pathologische Anatomie, vol 11). Springer, Berlin, Heidelberg, New York

Bauermeister DE, McClure H, Hall DA (1973) Specimen radiography – a mandatory adjunct to mammography. Am J Clin Pathol 59:782–789

Beute BJ, Kalisher L, Hutter RVP (1991) Lobular carcinoma in situ of the breast: clinical, pathologic and mammographic features. AJR 157:257–265

Bjurstam NG (1978) Radiography of the female breast and axilla. Acta Radiol Suppl 357

Bloodgood JC (1934) Comedocarcinoma (or comedoadenoma of the female breast). Am J Cancer 22:842

Britton CA, Sumkin J, Math M, Williams S (1992) Mammographic appearance of loiasis. AJR 159:51–52

Brown RC, Zuehlke RL, Ehrhardt JC, Jochimsen PR (1981) Tattoos simulating calcifications on xeroradiographs of the breast. Radiology 138:583

Bruwer A, Nelson GW, Spark RP (1987) Punctate intranodal gold deposits simulating microcalcifications on mammograms. Radiology 163:87–88

Bryant J (1981) Male breast cancer: a case of apocrine carcinoma with psammoma bodies. Hum Pathol 12:751

Ciatto S, Bianchi S, Vezzosi V (1994) Mammographic appearance of calcifications as a predictor of intraductal carcinoma histologic subtype. Eur Radiol 4:23–26

Citoler P (1978) Microcalcifications of the breast in early diagnosis of breast cancer. In: Grundmann E, Beck L (eds) Cancer campaign, vol 1. Gustav Fischer, Stuttgart, pp 113–118

Colbassini HJ, Feller WF, Cigtay OS, Chun B (1982) Mammographic and pathologic correlation of microcalcification in disease. Surg Gynecol Obstet 155:689–696

Davis SP, Stomper PC, Weidner N, Meyer JE (1989) Suture calcification mimicking recurrence in the irradiated breast: a potential pitfall in mammographic evaluation. Radiology 172:247–248

de Lafontan B, Daures JP, Salicru B et al. (1994) Isolated clustered microcalcifications: diagnostic value of mammography – series of 400 cases with surgical verification. Radiology 190:479–483

Egan RL (1964) Mammography. Thomas, Springfield, Illinois

Egan RL (1988) Breast imaging. Saunders, Philadelphia

Egan RL, McSweeney MB, Sewell CW (1980) Intramammary calcifications without an associated mass in benign and malignant diseases. Radiology 137:1–7

Foote FW, Stewart FW (1945) Comparative studies of cancerous versus non cancerous breasts. Am Surg 121:6

Galkin BM, Feig SA, Frasca P, Muir HD, Soriano RZ (1983) Photomicrographs of breast calcifications: correlation with histopathologic diagnosis. Radiographics 3:450–477

Gershon-Cohen J (1970) Atlas of mammography. Springer, Berlin, Heidelberg, New York

Gershon-Cohen J, Ingleby H, Hermel MB (1956) Calcification in secretory disease of the breast. AJR 76:132–135

Gershon-Cohen J, Yiu LS, Berger SM (1962) The diagnostic importance of calcareous patterns in roentgenography of breast cancer. Radiology 88:1117–1125

Gershon-Cohen J, Berger SM, Curcio BM (1966) Breast cancer with microcalcifications: diagnostic difficulties. Radiology 87:613–622

Gilles R, Lesnik A, Guinebrotjere JM, Tardivon A, Masselot J, Contosso C, Vanel D (1994) Apocrine carcinoma: clinical and mammographic features. Radiology 190: 495–497

Hamperl H (1939) Über die Myothelien (Myoepithelialen Elemente) der Brustdrüse. Virchows Arch (A) 305:171

Hamperl H (1968) Lehrbuch der allgemeinen Pathologie und pathologischen Anatomie Springer, Berlin, Heidelberg, New York

Hassler O (1969) Microradiographic investigations of calcifications of the female breast. Cancer 23:1103–1109

Helvie MA, Rebner M, Sickles EA, Oberman HA (1988) Calcifications in metastatic breast carcinoma in axillary lymph nodes. AJR 151:921–922

Helvie MA, Hessler C, Frank TS, Ikeda DM (1991) Atypical hyperplasia of the breast: mammographic appearance and histologic correlation. Radiology 179:759–764

Hoeffken WM, Lanyi M (1973) Mammography. Thieme, Stuttgart

Holland R, Hendriks JHCL (1994) Microcalcifications associated with ductal carcinoma in situ: mammographic-pathologic correlation. Semin Diagn Pathol 11:181–192

Holland R, Hendriks JHCL, Verteek ALM et al. (1990) Extent distribution and mammographic/histological correlations of breast ductal carcinoma in situ. Lancet 335:483–485

Homer MJ (1984) The mammography report. AJR 142:643–644

Homer MJ, Cooper AG, Pile-Spellman ER (1988) Milk of calcium in breast microcysts: manifestation as a solitary focal disease. AJR 150:789–790

Homer MJ, D'Orsi CJ, Sitzman SB (1994) Dermal calcifications in fixed orientation: the tattoo sign. Radiology 192:161–163

Hutter RVP, Snyder RE, Lucas JC, Foote FW, Farrow JH (1969) Clinical and pathologic correlation with mammographic findings in lobular carcinoma in situ. Cancer 23:826–839

Ikeda DM, Sickles EA (1988) Mammographic demonstration of pectoral muscle microcalcifications. AJR 151:475–476

Ingleby H, Gershon-Cohen J (1960) Comparative anatomy pathology and roentgenology of the breast. University of Pennsylvania Press, Philadelphia

Ingleby H, Hermel MB (1956) Calcification in secretory disease of the breast. Am J Roentgenol 76:132

Inoue Y, Ohya G, Maruyama M, Omoto R (1978) Die röntgenologischen Ver-änderungen nach Mammaplastik. Fortschr Roentgenstr 129:353

Kersschot E, Achten E, Hoste M et al. (1985) Microcalcifications: differential diagnostic limits. In: Colin C, Gordenne W (eds) Evaluation du risque de cancer mammaire, chimiotherapie premiere? Brussels, pp 69–79

Kindermann G, Rummel W, Bischoff J, Paterok E, Weishaar J, Willgeroth F, Ober KG (1979) Early detection of ductal breast cancer: the diagnostic procedure for grouped microcalcification. Tumori 65:547–553

Koide T, Katayama H (1979) Calcification in augmentation mammoplasty. Radiology 130:337

Kopans DB, Nguyen PI, Koerner FG et al. (1990) Mixed form, diffusely scattered calcifications in breast cancer with apocrine features. Radiology 177:807–811

Lanyi M (1977) Differentialdiagnose der Mikroverkalkungen. Die verkalkte mastopathische Mikrozyste. Radiologe 17:217–218

Lanyi M (1982) Formanalyse von 153 Mikroverkalkungen maligner Genese. Das "Dreieckprinzip". Fortschr Roentgenstr 136:77

Lanyi M (1983) Formanalyse von 5641 Mikroverkalkungen bei 100 Milchgangs-karzinomen: Die Polymorphie. Fortschr Roentgenstr 139:240

Lanyi M (1985) Microcalcifications in the breast – a blessing or a curse? A critical review. Diagn Imag Clin Med 54:126–145

Lanyi M (1986) Diagnosis and differential diagnosis of breast calcifications. Springer, Berlin, Heidelberg, New York

Lanyi M, Citoler P (1981) Differentialdiagnostik der Mikroverkalkungen: Die kleinzystische (blunt duct) Adenose. Fortschr Roentgenstr 134:225

Lanyi M, Neufang KFR (1984) Möglichkeiten und Grenzen der Differentialdiagnostik gruppierter intramammärer Mikroverkalkungen. Fortschr Roentgenstr 141:4

Leborgne R (1951) Diagnosis of tumors of the breast by simple roentgenography AJR 65:1–11

Leborgne R (1967) Esteatonecrosis quistica calcificata de la mama. Torax 16:172

Le Gal M, Durand JC, Laurent M, Pellier D (1976) Conduite a tenir devant une mammographie revelatrice de microcalcifications groupees, sans tumeur palpable. La Nouvelle Presse medicale 5:1623–1627

Le Gal M, Chavanne G, Pellier D (1984) Valeur diagnostique des microcalcifications groupees decouvertes par mammographies. (A propos de 227 cas avec verification histologique et sans tumeur du sein palpable). Bull Cancer (Paris) 71:57–64

Le Treut A, Barreau B, Kind M, Dilhuydy MH (1992) Les microcalcifications mammaires. J Radiol 73:527–541

Levitan H, Witten DM, Harrison EG (1964) Calcification in breast disease mammographic-pathologic correlation. AJR 92:29–39

Lewison EF (1964) Lobular carcinoma in situ of the breast. Mil Med 129:115

Libshitz HI, Montagne ED, Paulus DD (1977) Calcifications and the therapeutically irradiated breast. AJR 128:1021–1025

Linden SS, Sickles EA (1989) Sedimented calcium in benign breast cysts: the full spectrum of mammographic presentations. AJR 152:967–971

Linden SS, Sullivan DC (1989) Breast skin calcifications: localization with a stereotactic device. Radiology 171:570–571

MacErlean DP, Nathan BE (1972) Calcification in sclerosing adenosis simulating malignant breast calcification. Br J Radiol 45:944–945

Marinesen I, Damian A (1984) Primary hyperparathyreoidism associated with galactophorous ducts calcification. Endokrinologie 22:211

Martin JE, Moskowitz M, Milbrath JR (1979) Breast cancer missed by mammography. AJR 132:737–739

Menges V, Wellauer J, Engeler V, Stadelmann R (1973) Korrelation zahlenmäßig erfaßter Mikroverkalkungen auf dem Mammogramm und dadurch diagnos-tizierter Carcinome und Mastopathietypen. Radiologe 13:468–476

Menges V, Frank P, Prager P (1976) Zahlenmäßige Zunahme von Mikroverkalkungen, ein wichtiges röntgen-diagnostisches Kriterium für das okkulte Mammakarzinom. Fortschr Röntgenstr 124:372–378

Millis RR, Davies R, Stacey AJ (1976) The detection and significance of calcifications in the breast: a radiological and pathological study. Br J Radiol 49:12–26

Mirowitz SA, Kotner LM (1988) Metastatic breast cancer presenting as micro-calcifications in axillary lymph nodes. J Med Imaging 2:16–18

Mitnick JS, Roses DF, Harris MN, Feiner HD (1989) Circumscribed intra-ductal carcinoma of the breast. Radiology 170:423–425

Moskowitz M (1979) Screening is not diagnosis. Radiology 133:265–258

Muir BB, Lamb J, Anderson TJ, Kirkpatrick AE (1983) Microcalcification and its relationship to cancer of the breast: experience in a screening clinic. Clin Radiol 34:193–200

Murphy WA, De Schryver-Kecskemeti K (1978) Isolated clustered microcalcification in the breast: radiologic-pathologic correlation. Radiology 127:335–341

Parker MD, Clark RL, McLelland R, Daughtery K (1989) Disappearing breast calcifications. Radiology 172:677–680

Paterok EM, Rosenthal H, Richter S, Säbel M (1993) Occult calcified breast lesions. Eur Radiol 3:138–144

Péntek Z, Balogh J, Bakó B, Éliás S (1975) Mikrokalzifikation im männlichen Mammakarzinom. Fortschr Röntgenstr 123:90–91

Pope TL, Fechner RE, Wilhelm MC, Wanebo HJ, de Paredes WS (1988) Lobular carcinoma in situ of the breast: mammographic features. Radiology 168:63–66

Powell RW, McSweeney MB, Wilson CE (1983) X-ray calcifications as the only basis for breast biopsy. Ann Surg 197:555–559

Prorok JJ, Trostle DR, Scarlato M, Rachman R (1983) Excisional breast biopsy and roentgenographic examination for mammographically detected microcalcification. Am J Surg 145:684–686

Rebner M, Raju U (1994) Noninvasive breast cancer. Radiology 190:623–631

Rocek V, Sery Z, Sera D, Kamenicek O (1968) Verkalkungen beim männlichen Mammakarzinom. Fortschr Roentgenstr 109:679

Rogers JV, Powell RW (1972) Mammographic indications for biopsy of clinically normal breasts: correlation with pathologic findings in 72 cases. AJR 115:794–800

Roselli del Turco M, Ciatto S, Bravetti P, Pacini P (1986) The significance of mammographic calcifications in early breast cancer detection. Radiol Med (Torino) 72:7–12

Rosen IW, Nadel HI (1966) Roentgenographic demonstration of calcification in carcinoma of the male breast. Radiology 86:38

Rosen PP (1984) Lobular carcinoma in situ and intraductal carcinoma of the breast. In: McDivitt RW, Obermann HA, Ozello L, Kaufmann N (eds) The breast. International Academy of Pathology monograph. Williams and Wilkins, Baltimore

Rosen PP, Snyder RE, Robbins G (1974) Specimen radiography for nonpalpable breast lesions found by mammography: procedures and results. Cancer 34:2028–2033

Roses DF, Harris MN, Gorstein F, Gumport SL (1980) Biopsy for micro-calcification detected by mammography. Surgery 87:248–252

Sang Y Han, Witten DM (1977) Diffuse calcification of the breast in chronic renal failure. Am J Roentgenol 129:341–342

Schnitt SJ, Connolly JL, Tavassoli FA, Fechner RE, Kempson RL, Gelman R, Page DL (1992) Interobserver reproducibility in the diagnosis of ductal proliferative breast lesions using standardized criteria. Am J Surg Pathol 16:1133–1143

Schwartz GF, Feig SA, Rosenberg AL, Paterefsky AS, Schwartz AB (1984) Staging and treatment of clinically occult cancer. Cancer 53:1379

Sickles EA (1980) Further experience with microfocal spot magnification mammography in the assessment of clustered breast microcalcifications. Radiology 137:9–14

Sickles EA (1984) Mammographic features of "early" breast cancer. AJR 143:461–464

Sickles EA (1986) Breast calcifications: mammographic evaluation. Radiology 160:289–293

Sickles EA, Abele JS (1981) Milk of calcium within tiny benign breast cysts. Radiology 141:655–658

Sigfusson BF, Andersson I, Ljungberg O (1982) Percutaneous injection of contrast medium into breast lesions for radiographic exclusion of malignancy. Br J Radiol 55: 26–31

Sigfusson BF, Andersson I, Aspegren K, Janzon L, Linell F, Ljungberg O (1983) Clustered breast calcifications. Acta Radiol 24:273–281

Snyder RE (1966) Mammography and lobular carcinoma in situ. Surg Gynecol Obstet ••:255–260

Sonnenfeld MR, Frenna TH, Weidner N, Meyer JE (1991) Lobular carcinoma in situ: mammographic-pathologic correlation of results of needle-directed biopsy. Radiology 181:363–367

Stacey-Clear A, McCarthy KA, Hall DA et al. (1992) Calcified suture material in the breast after radiation therapy. Radiology 183:207–208

Stomper PC, Connolly JL (1992) Ductal carcinoma in situ of the breast: correlation between mammographic calcification and tumor subtype. AJR 159:483–485

Tabár L, Márton L, Kádas I (1972) Verkalkungen im männlichen Brustkrebs. Fortschr Roentgenstr 117:360–362

Thiels C, Dumke K (1977) Mammaverkalkung nach Paraffininjektion. Fortschr Roentgenstr 126:173

Tinnemans JGM, Wobbes T, Lubbers EJC, van der Sluis RF, de Boer HHM (1986) The significance of microcalcifications without palpable mass in the diagnosis of breast cancer. Surgery 99:652–657

Urban JA, Adair FE (1949) Sclerosing adenosis. Cancer 2: 625

Wahlers B, Plum R, Fischedick O (1977) Die perkutane Darstellung von Milchgängen in gutartigen Mammatumoren. Fortschr Roentgenstr 126:345–350

Willemin A (1972) Les images mammographiques. Karger, Basel

8 Imaging Evaluation of Spiculated Masses

D.D. Adler

CONTENTS

8.1 Introduction 137
8.2 Carcinoma 138
8.3 Postoperative Scar 140
8.4 Radial Scar 142
8.5 Conclusion 146
    References 146

8.1 Introduction

Accurate characterization of mammographic findings is essential in analysis of breast lesions. Standardized terminology is also critical and recent publication of the American College of Radiology's (ACR) Breast Imaging Reporting and Data System (BI-RADS) (1995) should result in more consistent reports and final assessment categories. The BI-RADS lexicon terminology will be used throughout this chapter.

Once a lesion has been identified, a tailored, diagnostic examination is usually indicated. This allows the radiologist to more carefully visualize and analyze the finding(s) in order that a differential diagnosis and recommendation be made. As applied to analysis of breast masses, shape and margins are the initial features that deserve attention, with the latter particularly important. The density of the mass relative to surrounding fibroglandular tissue, its location, and any associated findings may also be useful in further characterizing the mass.

The shape of a breast mass is best designated as either round, oval, lobulated, irregular, or architectural distortion. Having thus been identified, the margins of the mass must be carefully analyzed. Special views such as magnification images, often combined with spot compression, allow displacement of surrounding tissue and more detailed imaging of the borders of the mass. The margins should be described by one of the following terms: circumscribed, microlobulated, obscured, indistinct, or spiculated. Any of these descriptors can be combined with any of the shape descriptors. It is important to realize that a mass may have more than one type of margin (e.g., it may be partly circumscribed but partly obscured by overlying tissue, or circumscribed in part and spiculated along only a portion of the border). In such cases, the mass cannot be considered in the differential diagnosis for circumscribed margins as the spiculated or obscured component represents the "worse case."

Margins have been shown to be extremely important in assessing the likelihood of a benign or malignant mass. Macroscopic evaluation of breast cancers by Lane et al. (1961) showed that cancers with smooth edges have a better prognosis than those with irregular edges. Early work by Ingleby and Gershon-Cohen (1966) correlated the mammographic contour of over 250 breast cancers with histology and Apsimon et al. (1968) developed a classification system for gross tumor outline. Data show that if the margin is truly circumscribed, the risk of malignancy is on the order of 2% (Moskowitz 1983; Hall 1989) whereas a spiculated margin, particularly in the absence of prior biopsy is almost synonymous with carcinoma (Kopans 1989).

Prior to the development of standardized terminology, the term "stellate" was frequently used. The word "stellate" has been eliminated from the current ACR lexicon but prior publications utilizing "stellate" most often refer to the irregular mass with spiculated margins.

Gallager and Martin (1969) described three specific patterns of growth of breast cancer, correlating mastectomy specimens with mammographic appearances. The stellate tumor was considered the "classic" cancer characterized as irregular, star-shaped, with multiple slender, tapering, "tentaculate" projections." These tumors were found to have abundant fibrosis. A less common growth pattern

---

Dorit D. Adler, MD, Associate Professor of Radiology and Associate Director, Division of Breast Imaging, Department of Radiology, University of Michigan Hospitals, TC-2910P, 1500 E. Medical Center Drive, Ann Arbor, MI 48109-0326, USA

they described was designated "spiculate" and comprised a mass with short, fine "hairlike projections" extending from its periphery. These projections correlated with malignant cells extending between adipose cells. The BI-RADS definition of a spiculated margin is "the lesion ... characterized by lines radiating from the margins of a mass." Such characteristic "definitely malignant" masses have been shown to have the highest mammographic predictive value for cancer, ranging from 74% in the absence of clinical findings to 100% in the presence of a positive clinical examination (MOSKOWITZ 1983).

The importance of the mammographic finding of spicules is also being incorporated into new investigational computerized mammography methods. Programs for computer-aided diagnosis designed specifically to identify spicules have been described (KEGELMEYER et al. 1994). A computer vision method to detect spiculated lesions is employed and the radiologist is provided with the information from the computer analysis. Preliminary reports are promising, suggesting that sensitivity for detecting spiculated cancers may be improved with the aid of such computerized techniques.

The differential diagnosis of a mass with spiculated margins is relatively short. First and most significant is carcinoma. The onus rests upon the radiologist to explain why a mass with spiculated borders is *not* a malignancy. Other possible explanations might include the postoperative scar, radial scar, and sequelae of abscess, hematoma, fat necrosis, or any process resulting in marked fibrosis (SICKLES 1989).

8.2 Carcinoma

Some investigators have described the spiculated border as the only "truly diagnostic feature of malignancy" (KOPANS 1989). The significance of this radiographic sign was recognized early in the history of mammography. LEBORGNE (1951) noted that borders of malignant tumors were not only less likely to have the same "sharpness of outline" seen in many benign tumors, but were likely to have "ragged borders with numerous spicules of variable lengths, which radiate from the periphery into the surrounding mammary tissue. This spiculated border is characteristic of malignant tumors and discloses its eminently scirrhous nature." The thin strands may be only a few millimeters in length or extend over several centimeters.

The importance of breast spicules has been studied in detail, including attempts to obtain more accurate information on the extent of the carcinoma. VAN BOGAERT and HERMANS (1977) divided spicules into those without malignancy, those with malignancy along the entire length of the spicules, and a mixed type with malignancy only at the base of the spicule. Spiculated projections may represent areas of desmoplastic fibrosis without tumor that distort the surrounding tissue, or actual tumor infiltration extending into adjacent tissues. LINELL et al. (1980) viewed the tissue strands extending from the periphery of the tumor more as a result of retraction of structures towards the tumor. The fact that the spicules of breast cancers are sometimes difficult to identify in specimen radiography suggested to these investigators that the spicules were not stiff malignant outgrowths, but rather loose connective tissue bands that were cut off from the surrounding tissue at the time of surgery, thereby losing some of the spiculated appearance. It is the marked desmoplastic response elicited by some tumors that results in palpatory findings larger than mammographic and pathologic findings (LEBORGNE 1951).

Invasive duct carcinoma, also known as invasive duct carcinoma not otherwise specified (NOS), constitutes by far the largest group of breast cancers, accounting for 65%–80% of cases (ROSEN and OBERMAN 1993). The most common mammographic appearance of this neoplasm is that of a mass with spiculated margins (Fig. 8.1). The second most common type of invasive carcinoma, invasive lobular carcinoma, accounts for between 3% and 14% of invasive breast neoplasms (ROSEN and OBERMAN 1993). While this particular histologic tumor is known to elude early diagnosis both clinically and mammographically, a mass with spiculated margins has been identified in 26%–63% of invasive lobular cancers among recently reported mammographic series (HILLEREN et al. 1991; LE GAL et al. 1992; KRECKE and GISVOLD 1993; HELVIE et al. 1993) (Fig. 8.2). These cancers are known to result in higher rates of false-negative mammograms as a result of their tendency to be of relatively low density or isodense with surrounding tissue and their propensity not to disrupt local structures until late in their growth.

Due in part to their generally favorable prognosis, tubular carcinomas have received a great deal of attention despite their relative rarity. Tubular carcinomas have been reported to account for between 2% and 8% of invasive breast cancers (ROSEN and

Imaging Evaluation of Spiculated Masses

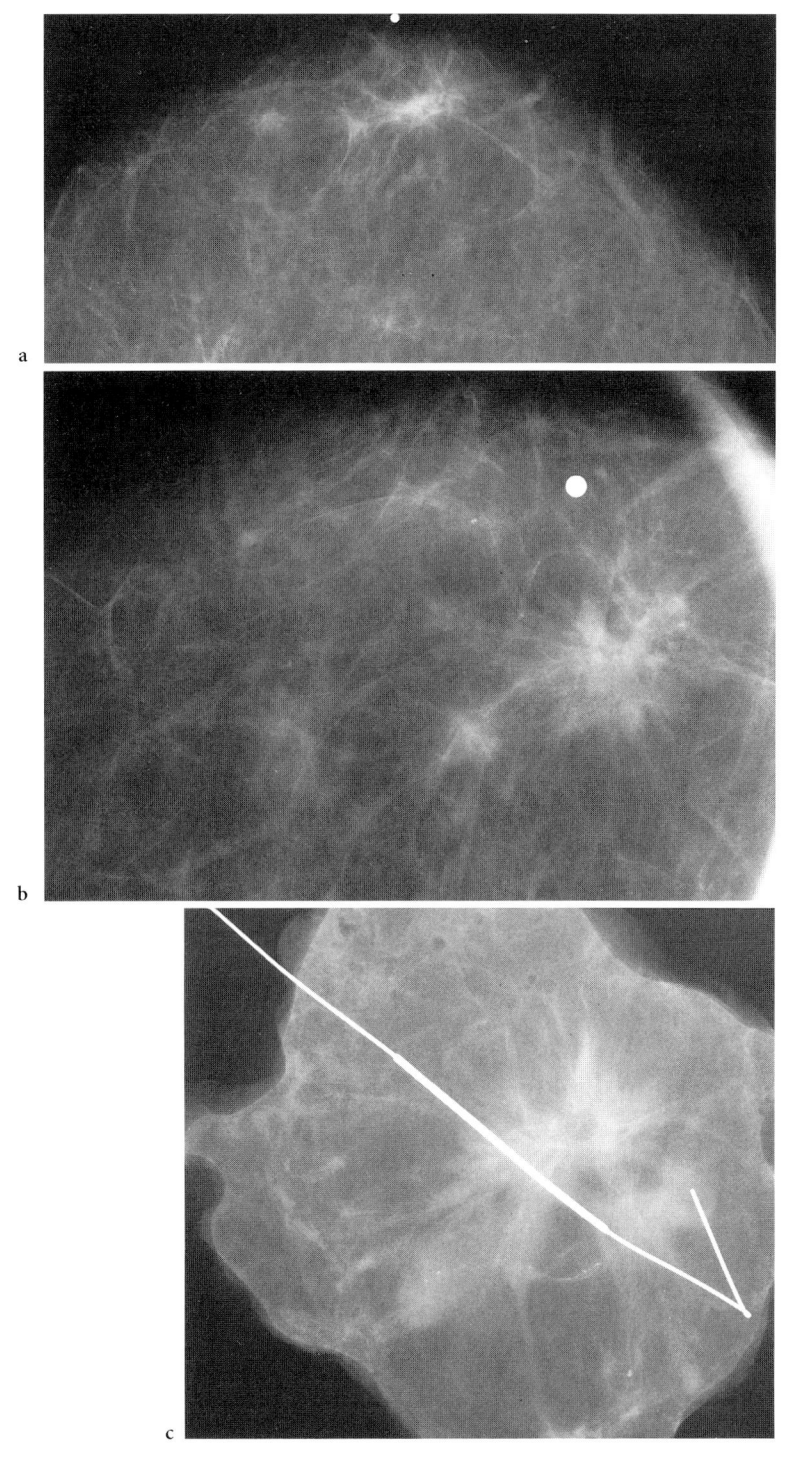

Fig. 8.1a–c. A 61-year-old woman presented for her annual mammogram. A left mastectomy had been performed 10 years earlier. Physical examination performed just prior to the mammogram revealed a vague thickening at the 12 o'clock position in the right breast, which was marked with a radiopaque BB. **a** The craniocaudal view shows an irregular mass in the region of the palpable thickening. **b** The spot magnification view better demonstrates the irregular mass with spiculated margins. Due to the vague palpatory finding, the lesion was localized under mammographic guidance. **c** Magnification view of the surgical specimen confirms excision of this 1.8-cm invasive ductal carcinoma

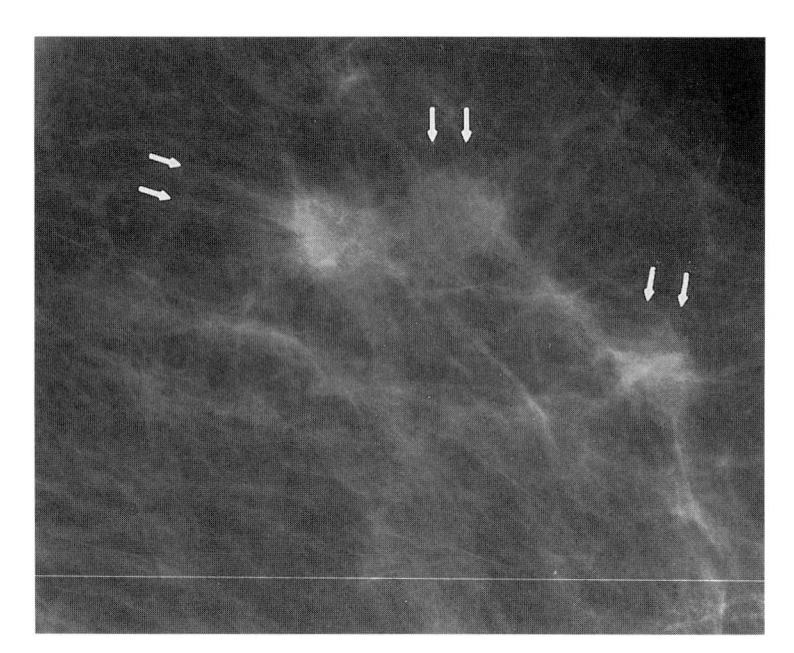

Fig. 8.2. Screening mammogram in a 64-year-old woman showing three contiguous masses with spiculated margins in the upper outer quadrant of the left breast. The fine spicules (*arrows*) are well seen on the magnification view. Histology revealed multifocal invasive lobular carcinoma

OBERMAN 1993), although LINELL et al. (1980) reported a frequency of 19% for tubular carcinomas. These investigators have long supported the theory that tubular carcinomas develop into larger and less differentiated tumors and that at the other end of the spectrum, many radial scars develop into tubular carcinomas. These theories have been widely debated, further explaining the disproportionate interest in this specific type of invasive tumor.

Histologically, the designation of tubular carcinoma has been used to describe a highly differentiated invasive cancer. Cells are arranged into neoplastic tubules which resemble normal breast ductules. The tubular growth pattern must comprise at least 75% of the tumor for inclusion in this category. The small randomly arranged tubules are usually lined by a single layer of uniform cells (ROSEN and OBERMAN 1993).

The earliest mammographic description of tubular carcinoma was published in 1978 by FEIG et al. Thirteen of 16 tubular cancers visualized mammographically appeared as "scirrhous masses," with none appearing as circumscribed masses or densities (Fig. 8.3). More recently, LEIBMAN et al. (1993) reported 11/13 tubular carcinomas appearing as small spiculated masses. Ninety-three percent of the tubular carcinomas seen on mammography described by ELSON et al. (1993) had spiculated margins. Pathologic correlation showed that the spicules represented both malignant cells and fibrous stroma. LEIBMAN et al. (1993) emphasized the relative smallness of these tumors compared with other invasive breast cancers and suggested that this feature could be used to differentiate tubular carcinoma from other forms of invasive breast cancer on mammography. Others have not found this feature to be specific enough to warrant such differentiation, although most agree that these tumors do generally have a more favorable prognosis with a relatively low propensity to metastasize compared to less well differentiated invasive adenocarcinomas. It is likely that tubular carcinomas represent a stage in the evolution of invasive ductal carcinoma characterized by a typical microscopic pattern, relatively small size, and relatively infrequent lymph node metastases (ROSEN and OBERMAN 1993). The tumor likely represents a slow-growing variant of invasive carcinoma and with increasing time, the growth pattern changes into that of the more typical invasive breast cancer (OBERMAN and FIDLER 1979).

8.3 Postoperative Scar

Following biopsy of a benign lesion, few or no changes are generally found at mammography. If surgical complications arise, if a large amount of tissue is removed, or if the breast is irradiated as part of treatment of breast cancer, sequelae of the biopsy may be radiographically apparent (KOPANS 1994).

The dense fibrous tissue that develops in a post-surgical scar often appears as an irregular mass with

Imaging Evaluation of Spiculated Masses

Fig. 8.3a,b. An asymptomatic 79-year-old woman found to have a 0.7-cm mass in the right upper outer quadrant on screening mammography. **a** The spiculated margin is well seen on the spot magnificatin view (*arrows*). **b** Specimen radiograph confirms excision of the mass. Pathologic diagnosis was a 0.6-cm tubular carcinoma

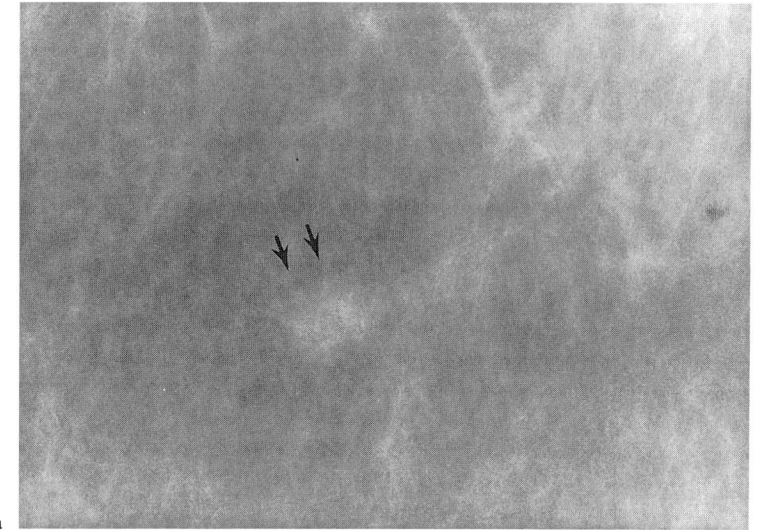

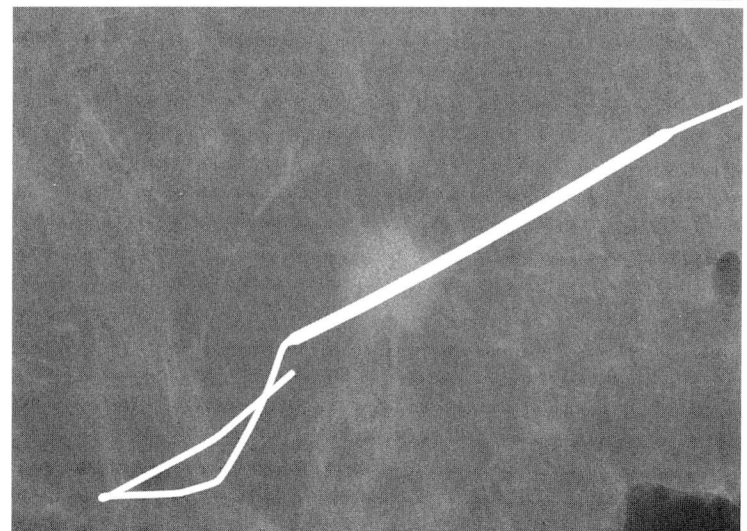

spiculated margins (SICKLES and HERZOG 1980) (Fig. 8.4). Retraction of surrounding tissue is not uncommon. Without the relevant clinical history, mammographic differentiation from carcinoma is essentially impossible. Herein lies the critical step of correlating radiographic findings with clinical examination and history.

It is important that the radiologist match the site of the patient's scar with the site of the radiographic finding, either by direct examination of the patient or using an accompanying diagram depicting all scars. Time of surgery is also significant inasmuch as history of a remote biopsy would not be consistent with either a new or enlarging mass, even if the latter is at the biopsy site. Rather, one would expect a stable or regressing lesion as scar retraction occurs. Progressive changes should raise concern for malignancy, with biopsy indicated.

In addition to correlating the site and time of the surgical procedure, another supportive radiographic feature of a postoperative scar is the variability of the appearance of the lesion at mammography (Fig. 8.5). This reflects the fact that the scar does not represent a true three-dimensional mass but rather, planar fibrous tissue which is likely to appear prominent in one projection and much less apparent in an orthogonal view.

A mass with spiculated margins considered to represent scarring at a recent biopsy site could be followed mammographically to confirm a stable or resolving lesion (SICKLES 1989). Should any question or inconsistency remain, biopsy should be suggested.

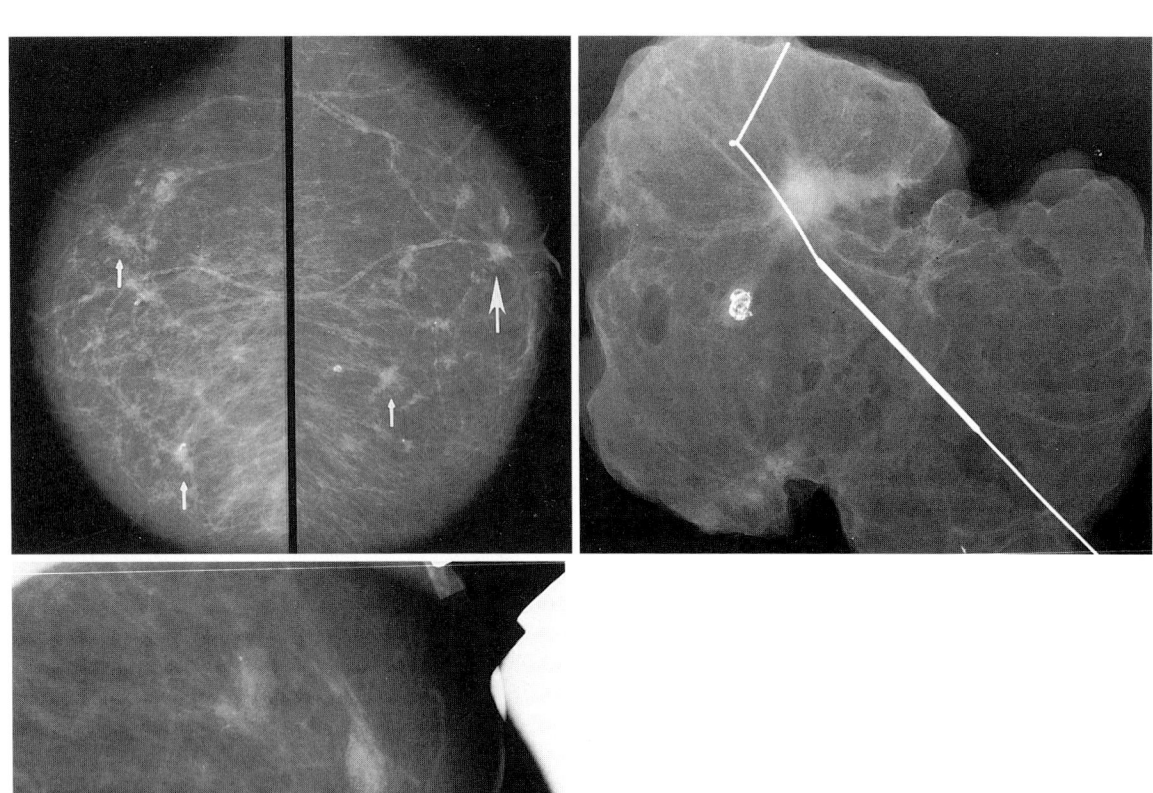

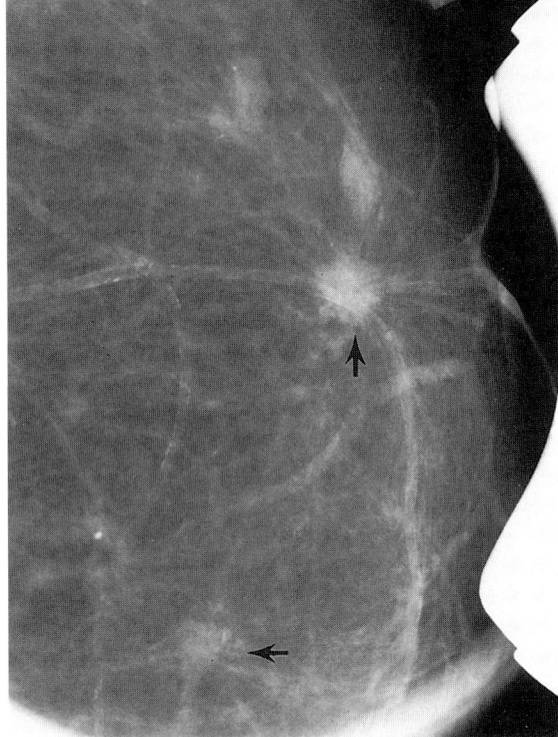

Fig. 8.4a–c. Bilateral mammography was performed in a 77-year-old woman after her physician palpated a breast mass superior to the left nipple in a region of scar tissue from an old surgical biopsy. **a** Bilateral lateromedial images show two small irregular masses with spiculated margins in each breast (*arrows*). The *large arrow* denotes the mass corresponding to the clinically palpable mass which is also causing nipple retraction. **b** The two masses in the left breast are seen on the lateral spot magnification view (*arrows*). **c** Magnification image of one of the left surgical specimens. Pathologic diagnosis was radial scar. The palpable left breast mass proved to be a dense scar with focal inflammation. Histologic examination of the two nonpalpable right breast masses revealed dense scar and fat necrosis although there had never been a previous biopsy of the right breast

Rarely, carcinomas may develop at the scar of a previous benign biopsy, further confusing the picture.

8.4 Radial Scar

Radial scars are benign lesions which, similar to tubular carcinomas, have been the subject of numerous publications in both the pathology and radiology literature despite their relative rarity (Fisher et al. 1979; Linell et al. 1980; Price et al. 1983; Wellings and Alpers 1984; Andersen and Gram 1984; Anderson and Battersby 1985; Nielsen et al. 1987; Mitnick et al. 1989; Adler et al. 1990; Orel et al. 1992; Ciatto et al. 1993). This likely is a result of the fact that at both radiographic and gross pathologic evaluation, these lesions can be confused with malignancy. In addition, there exists ongoing

Imaging Evaluation of Spiculated Masses 143

Fig. 8.5. a 52-year-old woman underwent lumpectomy and radiotherapy for treatment of her left breast cancer (*large arrows*). A small area of spiculation is consistent with the postoperative scar (*small arrow*) on the mammogram several years after treatment. **b** The scar is more apparent in the craniocaudal projection (*arrow*). **c** The postoperative distortion (*arrowheads*) and spicules (*arrows*) are well seen on the magnification view

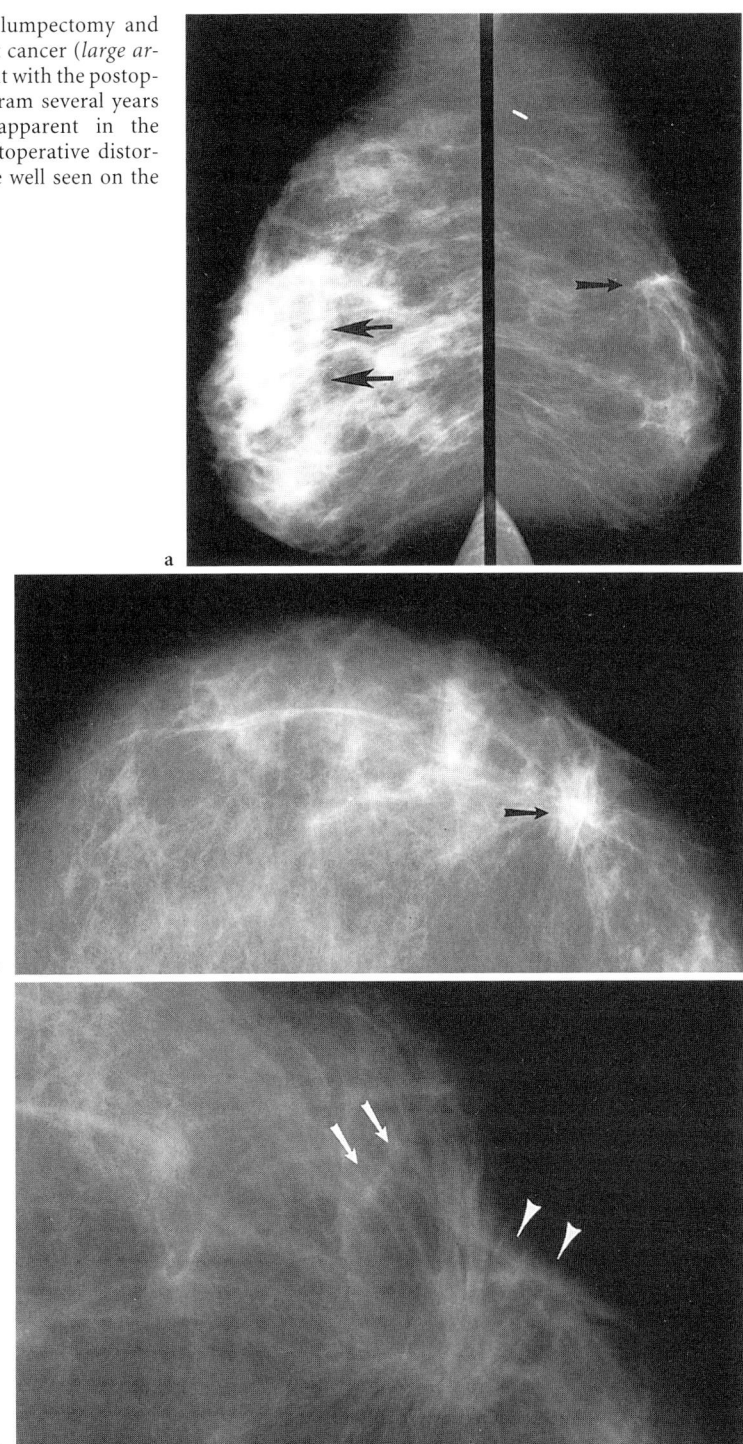

debate regarding the malignant potential of radial scars, particularly as the precursors of tubular carcinomas.

Many different terms have been applied to this entity, including radial sclerosing lesion, infiltrating epitheliosis, and indurative mastopathy (ROSEN and OBERMAN 1993). The commonly applied term of radial scar is potentially confusing in implying a postinflammatory etiology, which is not the case. All the terms, however, describe the radial appearance

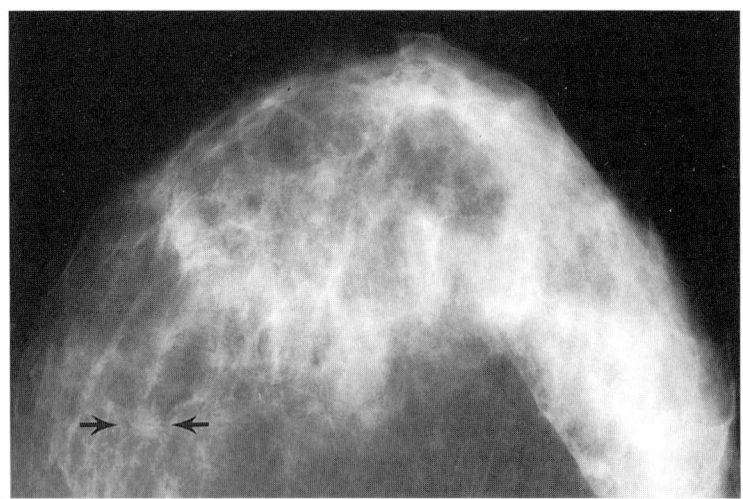

Fig. 8.6. a Left craniocaudal view in a 48-year-old asymptomatic woman demonstrates a 0.5-cm irregular mass with spiculated margins in the medial breast (*arrows*). **b** This is seen to better advantage on the spot magnification view (*arrows*). **c** The relatively lucent center of the mass seen on the magnified view of the surgical specimen is one of the signs described as suggestive of radial scar. Pathologic diagnosis was a 0.5-cm radial scar

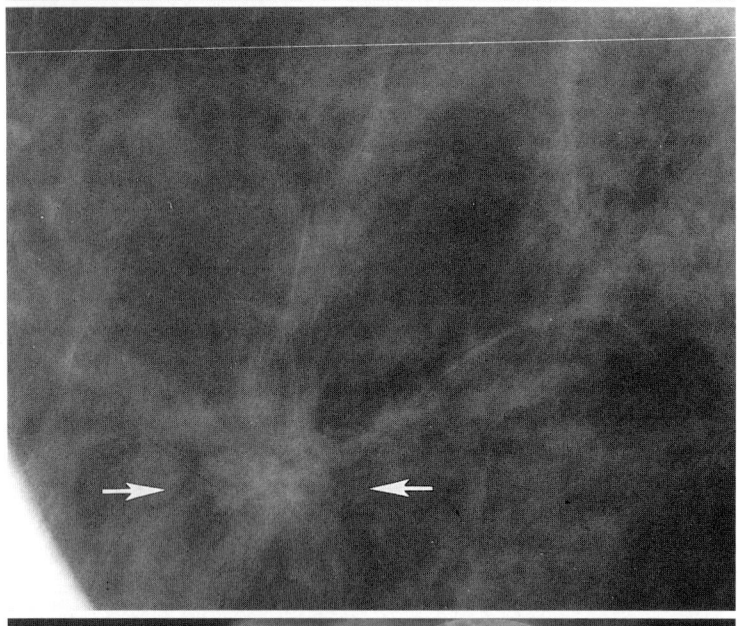

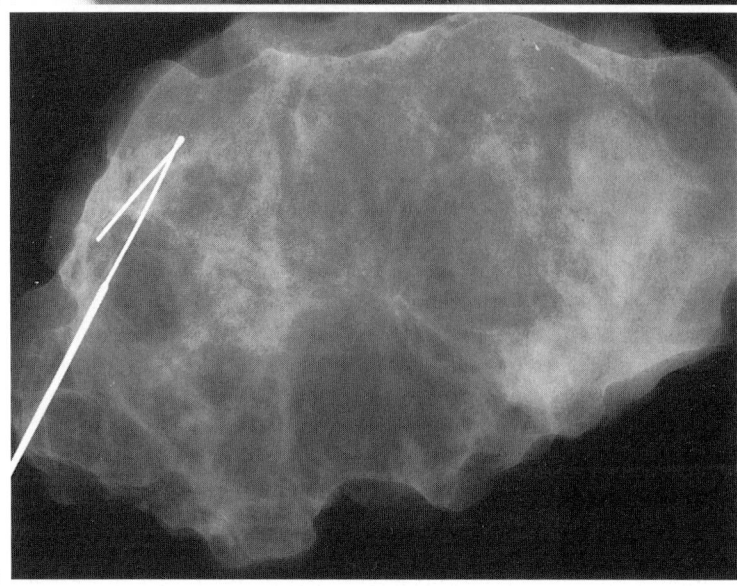

Imaging Evaluation of Spiculated Masses

Fig. 8.7. Right craniocaudal spot magnification view obtained in an asymptomatic 44-year-old woman reveals an irregular mass with spiculated margins (*arrows*). The mammographic appearance was considered highly suspicious for malignancy. Surgical excision showed a radial scar

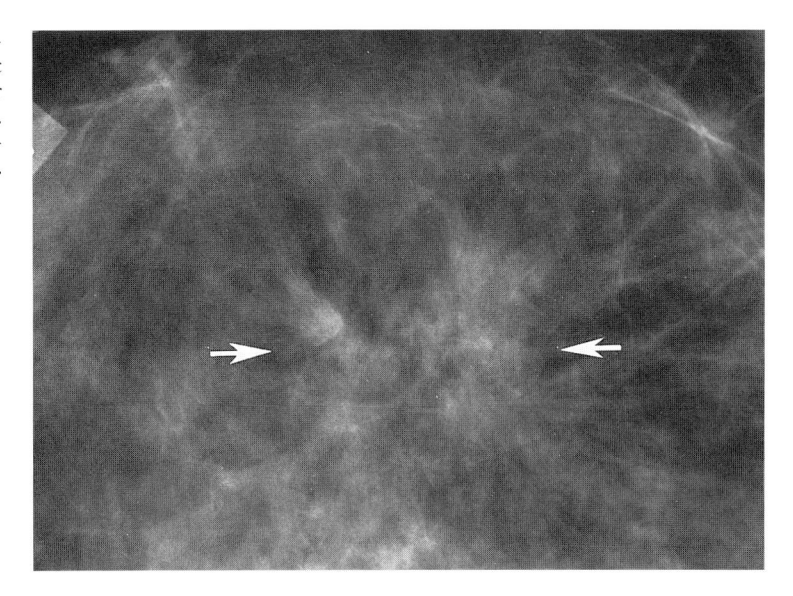

with a typical central region of hyalinizing fibrosis and elastosis containing entrapped ducts.

Most radial scars are detected microscopically and are not visualized mammographically. The lesion has been found at pathologic examination in nearly one-third of breasts examined in detailed autopsy studies (NEILSEN et al. 1985). They are commonly multiple and bilateral. Rarely are they clinically apparent.

The "typical" mammographic appearance of the radial scar was described by TABÁR and DEAN (1983) as being that of a lesion with a radiolucent center from which multiple long thin spicules radiate (Fig. 8.6); calcifications were considered unusual. While such an appearance may suggest the diagnosis of radial scar, numerous reports to date (MITNICK et al. 1989; ADLER et al. 1990; OREL et al. 1992; CIATTO et al. 1993) have demonstrated that this appearance is nonspecific, inasmuch as radial scars may have both a dense center and associated calcifications and conversely, carcinoma may mimic the "typical" radial scar. Current agreement is that in the absence of a postoperative scar, radiographic differentiation of carcinoma and radial scar is not possible and surgi-

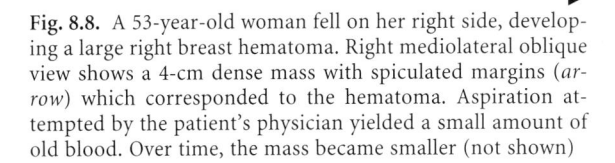

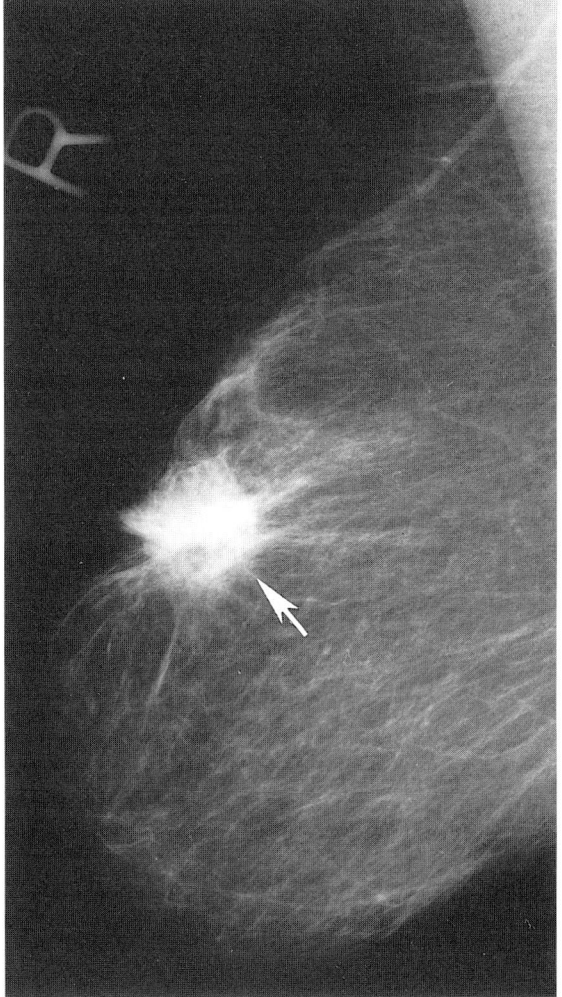

Fig. 8.8. A 53-year-old woman fell on her right side, developing a large right breast hematoma. Right mediolateral oblique view shows a 4-cm dense mass with spiculated margins (*arrow*) which corresponded to the hematoma. Aspiration attempted by the patient's physician yielded a small amount of old blood. Over time, the mass became smaller (not shown)

cal biopsy is needed in order to arrive at the correct diagnosis (Fig. 8.7). There are insufficient data to consider these lesions premalignant and excision is adequate treatment (ROSEN and OBERMAN 1993).

8.5 Conclusion

Stability of a radiographic finding is generally suggestive of a benign etiology, particularly with increasing time intervals. Data show, however, that lesions with spiculated margins should be considered malignant even if unchanged over time, unless a specific benign etiology can be attributed to the lesion (Fig. 8.8). MEYER and KOPANS (1981) reported five mammographically detected breast cancers, approximately 1 cm in size, that remained unchanged over intervals between 2 and 4.5 years. All proved to be invasive ductal carcinomas.

Radiographic visualization of a spiculated breast mass must raise prompt concern for breast cancer. As described, one may occasionally be able to explain such a finding secondary to benign changes. If not, however, biopsy is warranted.

References

Adler DD, Helvie MA, Oberman HA, Ikeda DM, Bhan AO (1990) Radial sclerosing lesion of the breast: mammographic features. Radiology 176:737-740
American College of Radiology (ACR) (1995) Breast imaging reporting and data system (BI-RADS™), 2nd edn. American College of Radiology, Reston, Va.
Andersen JA, Gram JB (1984) Radial scar in the female breast. Cancer 53:2557-2560
Anderson TJ, Battersby A (1985) Radial scars of benign and malignant breasts: comparative features and significance. J Pathol 147:23-32
Apsimon HT, Stewart HJ, Williams WJ (1968) Recording the gross outlines of breast tumours: a pathological assessment of the accuracy of radiographs of breast cancers. Br J Cancer 22:40-46
Ciatto S, Morrone D, Catarzi S, Del Turco MR, Bianchi S, Ambrogetti D, Cariddi A (1993) Radial scars of the breast: review of 38 consecutive mammographic diagnoses. Radiology 187:757-760
Elson BC, Helvie MA, Frank TS, Wilson TE, Adler DD (1993) Tubular carcinoma of the breast: mode of presentation, mammographic appearance, and frequency of nodal metastases. AJR 161:1173-1176
Feig SA, Shaber GS, Patchefsky AS, Schwartz GF, Edeiken J, Nerlinger R (1978) Tubular carcinoma of the breast: mammographic appearance and pathological correlation. Radiology 129:311-314
Fisher ER, Palekar AS, Kotwal N, Lipana N (1979) A nonencapsulated sclerosing lesion of the breast. Am J Clin Pathol 71:240-246
Gallager HS, Martin JE (1969) The study of mammary carcinoma by mammography and whole organ sectioning: early observations. Cancer 23:855-873
Hall FM (1989) Circumscribed intraductal carcinoma of the breast. Radiology 172:579
Helvie MA, Paramagul C, Oberman HA, Adler DD (1993) Invasive tubular carcinoma: imaging features and clinical detection. Invest Radiol 28:202-207
Hilleren DJ, Andersson IT, Lindholm K, Linnell F (1991) Invasive lobular carcinoma: mammographic findings in a 10-year experience. Radiology 178:149-154
Ingleby H, Gershon-Cohen J (1966) Comparative anatomy, pathology and roentgenology of the breast. University of Pennsylvania Press, Philadelphia, pp 309-376
Kegelmeyer WP, Pruneda JM, Bourland PD, Hillis A, Riggs MW, Nipper ML (1994) Computer-aided mammographic screening for spiculated lesions. Radiology 191:331-337
Kopans DB (1989) Breast imaging. Lippincott, Philadelpha
Kopans DB (1994) Conventional wisdom: observation, experience, anecdote, and science in breast imaging. AJR 162:299-303
Krecke KN, Gisvold JJ (1993) Invasive lobular carcinoma of the breast: mammographic findings and extent of disease at diagnosis in 184 patients. AJR 161:957-960
Lane N, Goksel H, Salerno RA, Haagensen CD (1961) Clinicopathologic analysis of the surgical curability of breast cancers: a minimum ten-year study of a personal series. Ann Surg 153:483-498
Le Gal M, Ollivier L, Asselain B, Meunier M, Laurent M, Vielh P, Neuenschwander S (1992) Mammographic features of 455 invasive lobular carcinomas. Radiology 185:705-708
Leborgne R (1951) Diagnosis of tumors of the breast by simple roentgenography: calcifications in carcinomas. AJR 65:1-11
Leibman AJ, Lewis M, Kruse B (1993) Tubular carcinoma of the breast: mammographic appearance. AJR 160:263-265
Linell F, Ljungberg O, Andersson I (1980) Breast carcinoma: aspects of early stages, progression and related problems. Acta Pathol Microbiol Immunol Scand 272 (Suppl):1-233
Meyer JE, Kopans DB (1981) Stability of a mammographic mass: a false sense of security. AJR 137:595-598
Mitnick JS, Vazquez MF, Harris MN, Rosen DF (1989) Differentiation of radial scar from scirrhous carcinoma of the breast: mammographic-pathologic correlation. Radiology 173:697-700
Moskowitz M (1983) The predictive value of certain mammographic signs in screening for breast cancer. Cancer 51:1007-1011
Nielsen M, Jensen J, Andersen JA (1985) An autopsy study of radial scar in the female breast. Histopathology 9:287-295
Nielsen M, Christensen L, Andersen J (1987) Radial scars in women with breast cancer. Cancer 59:1019-1025
Oberman HA, Fidler WJ (1979) Tubular carcinoma of the breast. Am J Surg Pathol 3:387-395
Orel SG, Evers K, Yeh I-T, Troupin RH (1992) Radial scar with microcalcifications: radiographic-pathologic correlation. Radiology 183:479-482
Price JL, Thomas BA, Gibbs NM (1983) The mammographic features of infiltrating epitheliosis. Clin Radiol 34:433-435

Rosen PP, Oberman HA (1993) Tumors of the mammary gland. Armed Forces Institute of Pathology, Bethesda, Maryland

Sickles EA (1989) Breast masses: mammographic evaluation. Radiology 173:297–303

Sickles EA, Herzog KA (1980) Intramammary scar tissue: a mimic of the mammographic appearance of carcinoma. AJR 135:349–352

Tabar L, Dean PB (1983) Teaching atlas of mammography. Thieme, Stuttgart

van Bogaert L-J, Hermans J (1977) Importance of spicules on clinical staging of carcinoma of the breast. Surg Gynecol Obstet 144:356–358

Wellings SR, Alpers CE (1984) Subgross pathologic features and incidence of radial scars in the breast. Hum Pathol 15:475–479

9 The Management of Nonpalpable Circumscribed Breast Masses

E.D. Pisano

CONTENTS

9.1 Introduction 149
9.2 Pathognomonically Benign Lesions 149
9.3 Other Definitively Benign Lesions
    That Require Additional Workup 150
9.4 Follow-up of Lesions Considered Probably Benign
    After Additional Workup 155
9.5 Other Factors That Influence the Need for Further
    Workup in the Setting of a Circumscribed Mass.... 163
9.6 Summary 165
    References 165

9.1 Introduction

Circumscribed breast masses are usually benign. The most important step in ensuring that a patient with a newly discovered, nonpalpable breast mass receives appropriate care is correct categorization of the mass. The proper workup and management of mammographically detected circumscribed breast masses will be described in this chapter.

Circumscribed masses can be divided into four broad categories: pathognomonically benign lesions on screening mammography, circumscribed masses that are shown to be definitively benign after further workup, circumscribed masses that are shown to be benign by virtue of stability at follow-up, and suspicious circumscribed masses. Other factors that might influence that need for further workup in such patients will also be discussed.

In general, almost all masses found on screening mammography require additional workup. Circumscribed lesions are found in as many as 8% of screening examinations (Stomper et al. 1991).

E. D. Pisano, MD, Associated Professor of Radiology and Chief of Breast Imaging, Department of Radiology, CB# 7510, Room 503, Old Infirmary Building, University of North Carolina at Chapel Hill, Chapel Hill, NC 27599-7510, USA

9.2 Pathognomonically Benign Lesions

There are a few types of mammographic lesions that are circumscribed and so typical that they are virtually pathognomonic to any experienced radiologist. This type of lesion requires no further workup once identified on a screening study. In fact, it is the radiologist's duty to avoid unnecessary tests for further evaluation of such lesions.

Typical intramammary nodes (Fig. 9.1) fall into this category. An intramammary node frequently has a circumscribed border and a central fatty hilus. Typically, nodes are less than 1 cm in size and lie in the upper outer quadrant of the breast, but they have been reported in all locations within the breast (Svane and Franzen 1993). When a node has such a pathognomonic benign appearance, no further workup is necessary and only routine screening is indicated.

Hamartomas (or adenofibrolipomas, or fibroadenolipomas, or lipofibroadenomas) may also have a characteristic appearance (Figs. 9.2, 9.3) (Helvie et al. 1989; Hessler et al. 1978). These lesions are composed pathologically of the types of cells that normally exist in the breast but they are arrayed in a disorganized pattern. These lesions often have well-defined borders and an outer capsule. The lesion itself contains a mixture of fat and fibroglandular density tissue. Sometimes the fat and fibroglandular density coexist in a whirling or nodular pattern. Such characteristic lesions do not require further evaluation. Again, only routine screening is indicated.

Lipomas also have a characteristic appearance with a well-defined capsule and absolutely no fibroglandular density tissue (Fig. 9.4). Oil cysts are characteristic when egg-shell calcification is seen surrounding a perfectly well-defined mass (Fig. 9.5) (Evers and Troupin 1991; Coren et al. 1974). Typical fibroadenomas (Fig. 9.6) with circumscribed borders and coarse, peripheral "popcorn" calcifications should also undergo only routine screening without additional views.

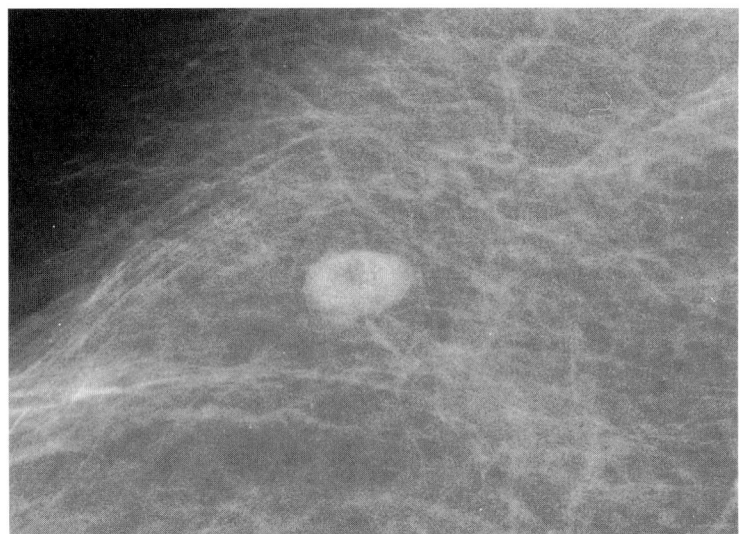

Fig. 9.1a,b. These two circumscribed masses, located in the upper outer quadrant of this 55-year-old patient's left breast, have all of the characteristics of typical intramammary lymph nodes. The larger one had been referred for percutaneous biopsy. This was deferred and subsequent 3-year follow-up of both masses has been unremarkable

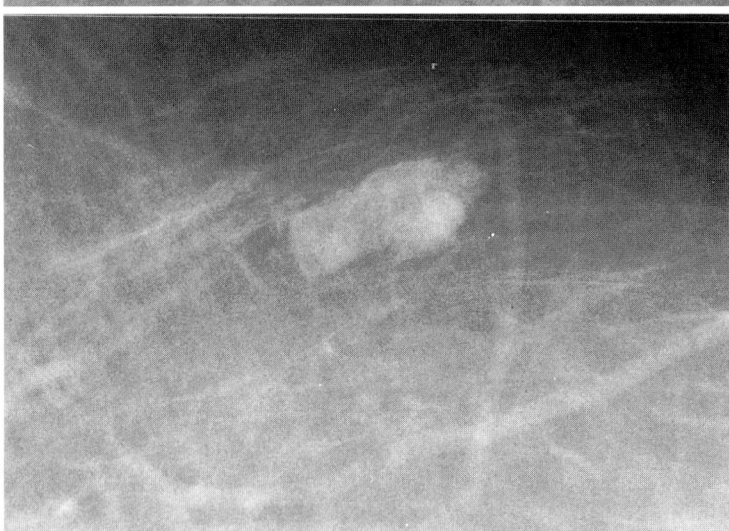

9.3 Other Definitively Benign Lesions That Require Additional Workup

If there is any doubt on screening regarding the presence of atypical features when the diagnosis of one of these pathognomonically benign lesions is suspected, it is, of course, best to obtain supplementary mammographic views (such as magnification mammography with or without spot compression). These additional views may serve to confirm a definitive benign diagnosis. Routine follow-up can be recommended after additional imaging is obtained, and the patient can be reassured that the area of concern on her screening examination appeared definitively benign after further work-up.

All other masses should be submitted to additional mammographic evaluation after they are found on screening (BERKOWITZ et al. 1989; SICKLES 1988; FEIG 1988). This usually involves the performance of spot compression magnification views, usually in two projections. This enables the radiologist to detect unsuspected irregularities, lack of definition in mass contour, internal calcifications, or associated architectural distortion (Figs. 9.7, 9.8).

The proper performance of magnification mammography requires meticulous attention to radiographic detail. Specifically, a 0.2 mm or smaller focal spot is required and patient motion must be kept to an absolute minimum. Furthermore, the lesion should be placed as near to the middle of the field of view as possible.

If calcifications are present, they should be carefully examined for number, shape, size, and density characteristics. Milk of calcium within microcysts

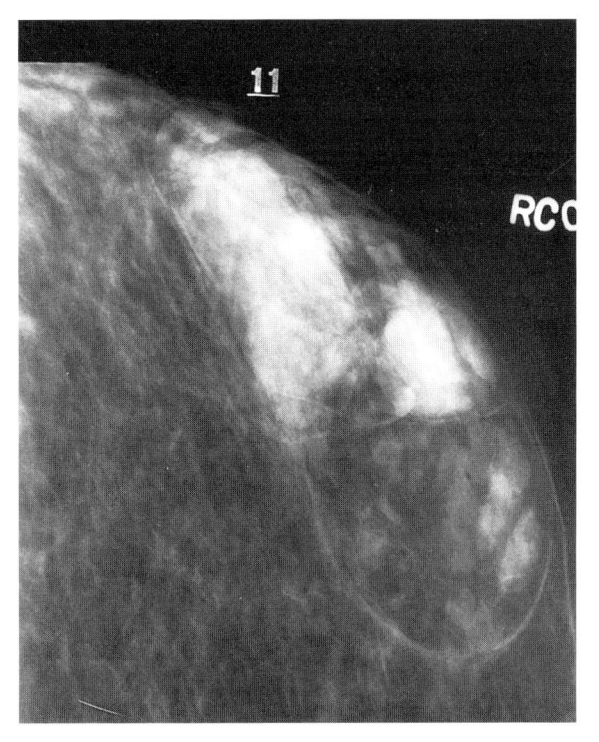

Fig. 9.2. Magnification view of this palpable lump in a 50-year-old patient reveals a mixed fat and fibroglandular density circumscribed mass with an obvious capsule. This is characteristic of a hamartoma

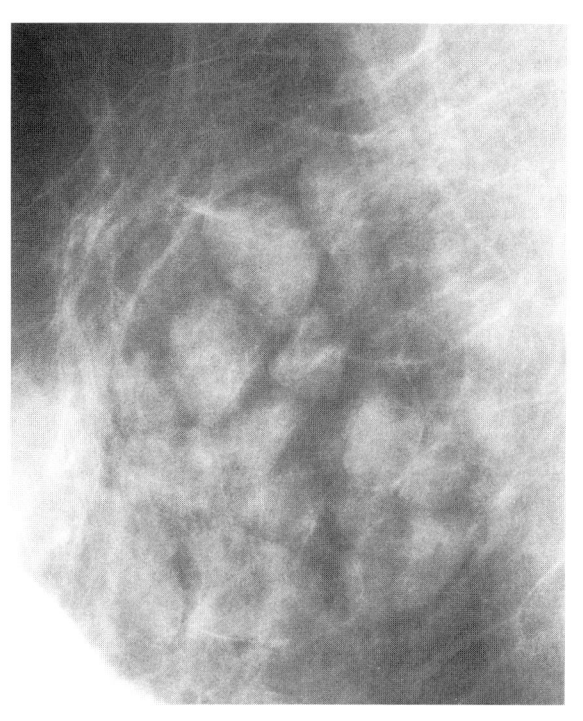

Fig. 9.3. This 35-year-old woman presented with a palpable mass that was soft and mobile, in a location that corresponded perfectly with this mixed fibroglandular tissue and fatty mass. This appearance is pathognomonic for a hamartoma and biopsy was deferred. This lesion has remained stable at physical examination and mammography during 4 years of follow-up

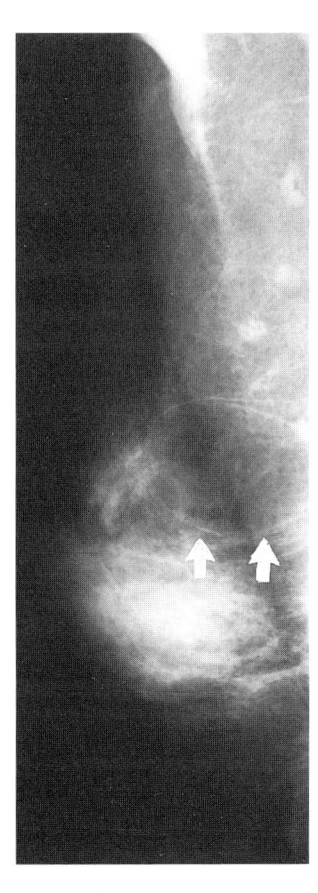

Fig. 9.4. Screening mammogram of this 58-year-old woman revealed a completely fatty circumscribed mass (*arrows*). This finding is pathognomonic for a lipoma and no further workup is indicated

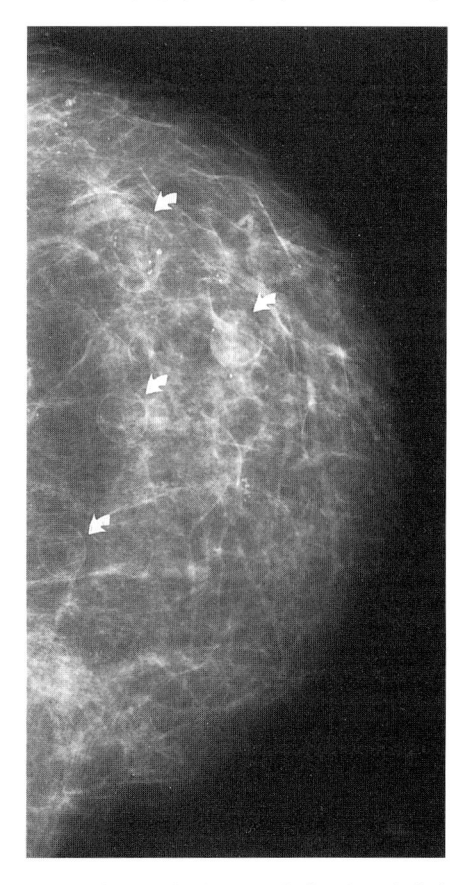

Fig. 9.5. This patient has multiple, round, faintly calcified masses throughout her breast, several of which are marked by *arrows*. These are characteristic lipid cysts, and no further workup is indicated

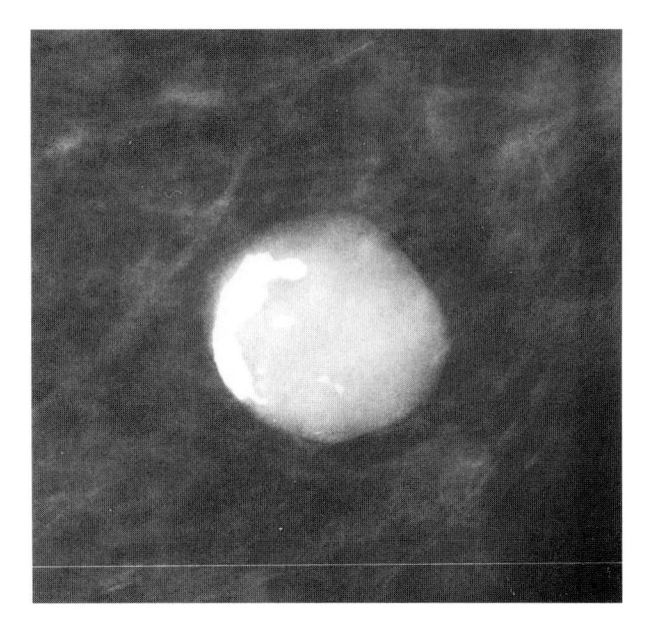

Fig. 9.6. This circumscribed mass with coarse calcifications is typical of a fibroadenoma

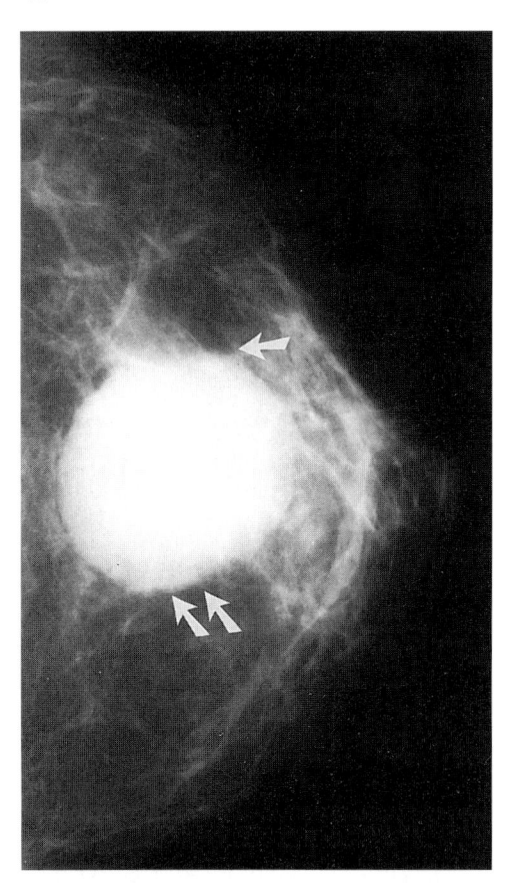

Fig. 9.8. This 63-year-old patient presented with a large palpable lump with predominantly circumscribed borders. Close inspection reveals some irregularity, however, (*arrows*). On biopsy this proved to be infiltrating ductal carcinoma. Despite the large size of the mass, the patient's lymph nodes were free of metastasis

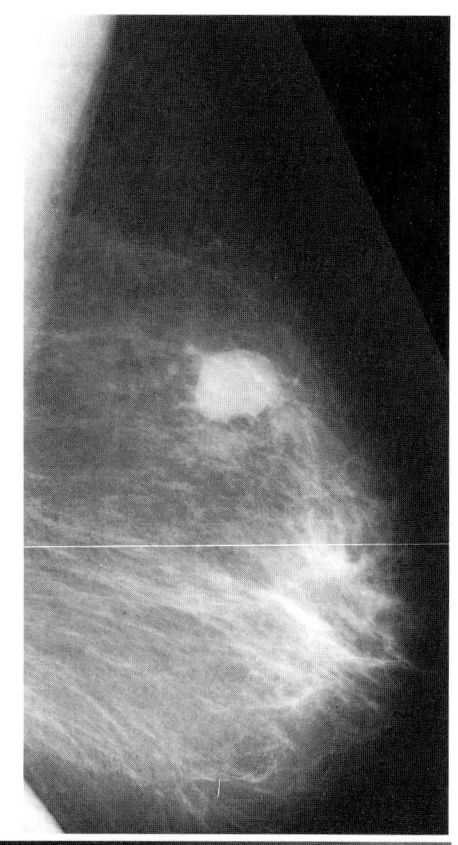

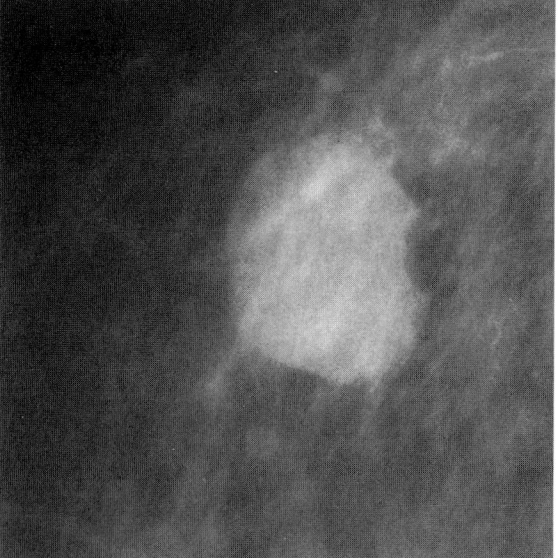

Fig. 9.7. a At first inspection, this mass appears relatively well circumscribed without associated features that are suspicious for malignancy. **b** Closer inspection reveals that the inferior border of the mass is somewhat irregular and indistinct. This prompted biopsy which revealed papillary carcinoma

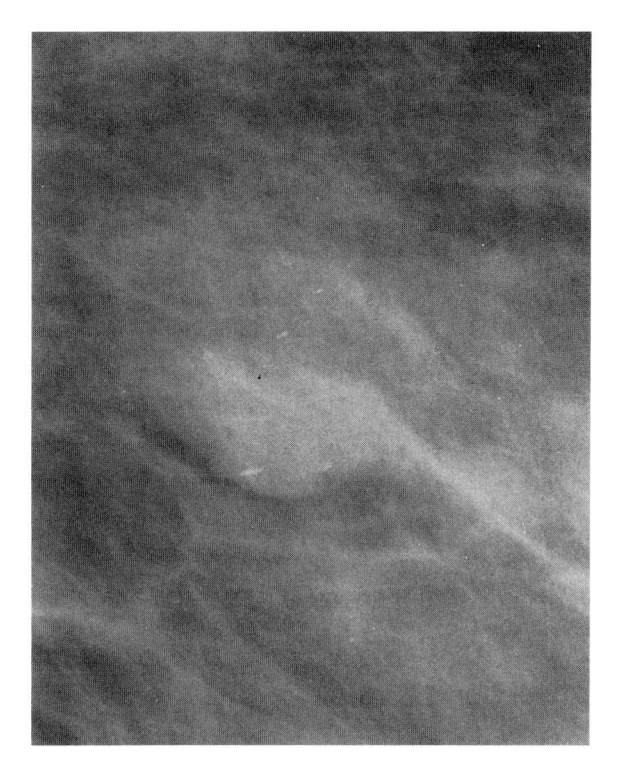

Fig. 9.9. Screening mammogram of this perimenopausal patient revealed a new moderately circumscribed mass. The true-lateral compression magnification view reveals calcifications that are characteristically benign, with the layering that is typical of milk of calcium in microcysts. Subsequent 2-year follow-up has revealed no mammographic or physical examination changes suggestive of malignancy

can be associated with circumscribed masses (Fig. 9.9). This can be diagnosed when the characteristic change in shape of the calcifications is noted between standard orthogonal views. On the craniocaudal view, such calcifications appear somewhat amorphous, like clouds or puddles. On the oblique view, the calcifications appear better defined and angular, even linear. On the standard or spot compression magnification view in the 90° lateral projection, the calcifications take on an absolutely diagnostic "teacup" appearance (horizontal superior margin, curvilinear inferior margin), with the calcifications settling into the dependent portions of the microcysts. Routine screening is all that is indicated in patients with this entity.

If a lesion still appears to be circumscribed with no suspicious features detected by additional views, ultrasonography should be performed to establish or exclude the diagnosis of simple cyst (FEIG 1989). A definitive cyst must be anechoic and demonstrate a smooth, sharp back wall with posterior enhancement and increased through-transmission of sound. It must also be round or oval and be readily compress-

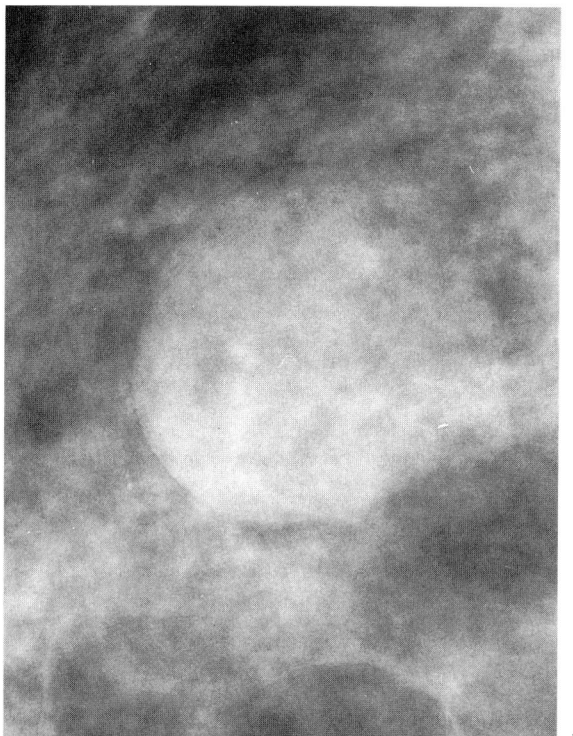

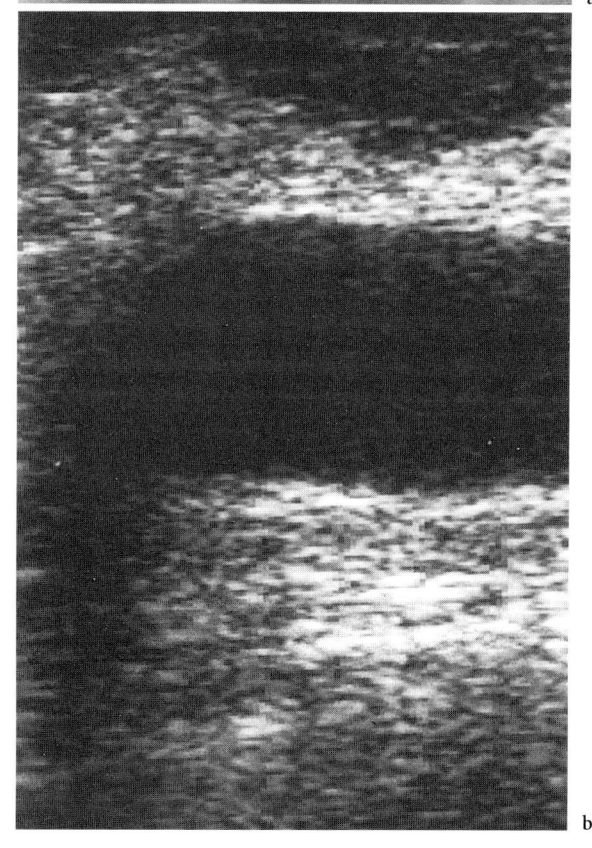

Fig. 9.10. a Screening mammogram of this 43-year-old patient revealed a large moderately circumscribed, partially obscured mass in the left breast. **b** Ultrasonography showed an anechoic mass with a sharp back wall and enhanced through-transmission. It readily changed shape with compression. Subsequent aspiration yielded characteristic clear yellow cyst fluid

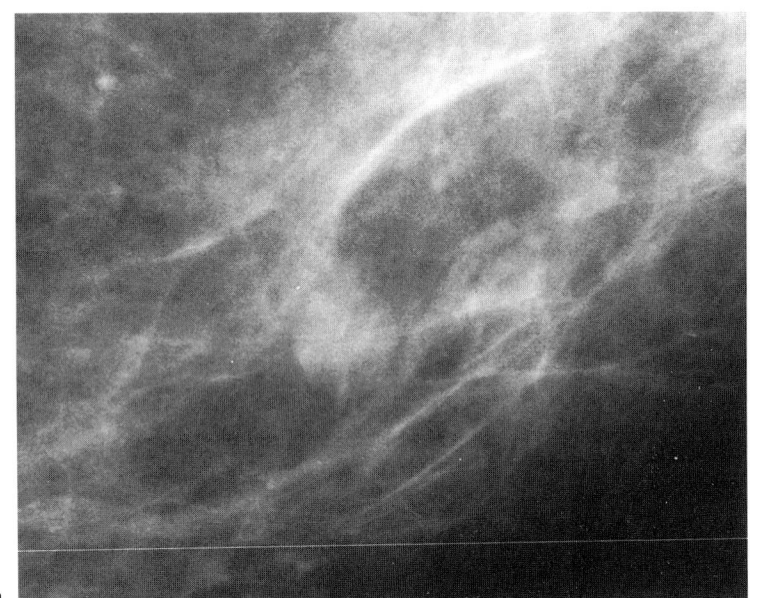

Fig. 9.11a,b. Close-up view (**a**) of the screening mammogram of this 70-year-old woman revealed a circumscribed mass that was indistinct on its superior border. When the patient returned for additional views to allow further evaluation of the mass, the ill-defined border was again seen on the spot compression view (**b**). Physical examination by the radiologist of the region of the abnormality revealed a skin lesion

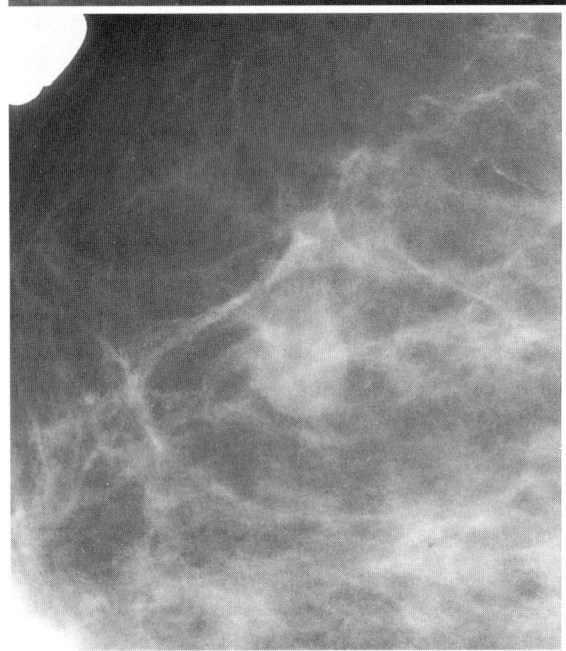

ible (Fig. 9.10). If any of these features is absent, a lesion cannot be diagnosed definitively as a simple cyst. It then would be considered as an atypical cyst (containing blood or other debris) or a solid mass. The advantage to the patient of definitively diagnosing a cyst is that she will not have to return for anything but routine screening mammography.

Another type of lesion that can be definitively worked up with additional views is a skin lesion. If a patient has a known mole or skin lesion in the same area as a mammographic abnormality, an additional mammogram should be obtained with a metallic marker placed over the cutaneous abnormality. Once a mammographic mass is shown to correspond to a skin lesion, it will be known to represent a skin lesion every time it is identified at future screening studies. Skin lesions tend to have circumscribed borders, since they are surrounded on almost all sides by air. The border that abuts the skin tends to be indistinct, just like a nipple shadow on a chest x-ray (Fig. 9.11).

Another type of circumscribed lesion that can be definitively proven benign after additional views is a galactocele (GOMEZ et al. 1986). This kind of mass occurs only in patients who are or recently have been

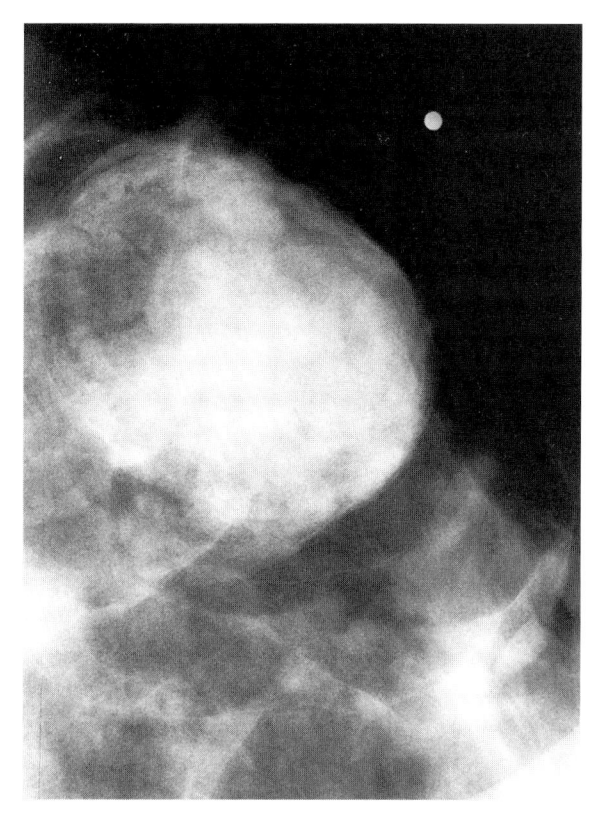

The Management of Nonpalpable Circumscribed Breast Masses 155

Fig. 9.12. Note the mixture of fat and fibroglandular density tissue seen on this spot compression magnification view of a moderately circumscribed palpable lump in a 33-year-old lactating patient. Subsequent aspiration proved the lesion to be a galactocele

lactating. If such a patient undergoes mammography, a galactocele often appears as a mixed fat and fibroglandular density mass. If the diagnosis is in doubt from the standard views, that is, if the lesion appears to contain only fibroglandular density tissue, a cross-table lateral view might be helpful for further evaluation. That view might show a characteristic fluid-fluid level, the fatty parts of the milk layering above the proteinaceous parts (SICKLES and VOGELAAR 1981). This finding is absolutely characteristic, and when it is present, no further workup of the mass is necessary and the radiologist can assure the patient that her mammographic abnormality requires no further evaluation (Fig. 9.12).

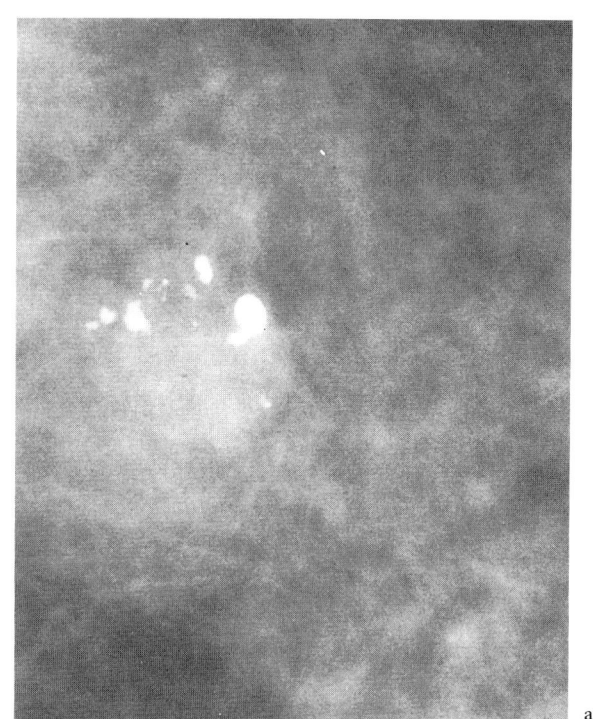

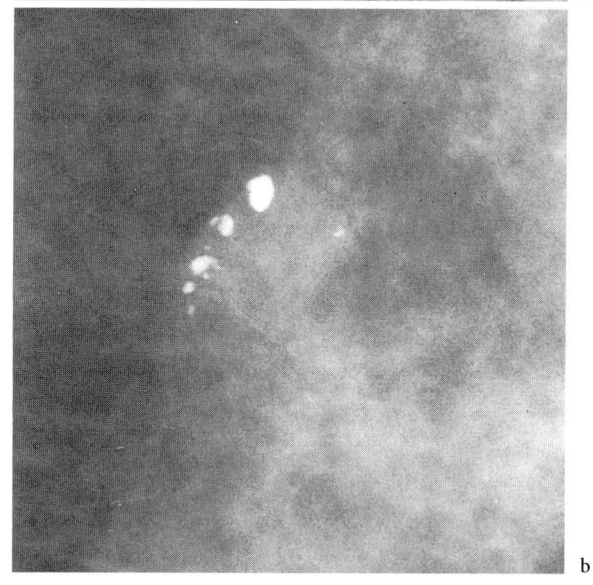

Fig. 9.13a,b. This partially circumscribed, mostly obscured mass with predominantly coarse peripheral calcifications has been managed with mammographic surveillance only and has remained stable for 5 years. It almost certainly represents a fibroadenoma

9.4 Follow-up of Lesions Considered Probably Benign after Additional Workup

What should the radiologist recommend for the circumscribed mass that is not definitely cystic, and is not pathognomonically benign?

There is a growing body of literature that supports short-term follow-up of such lesions, regardless of the lesion's size or patient's age. Specifically, SICKLES (1994) has recently reported the results of a prospective study of 1403 such patients in which 6-month follow-up, followed by 12–18 month, 24–30 month,

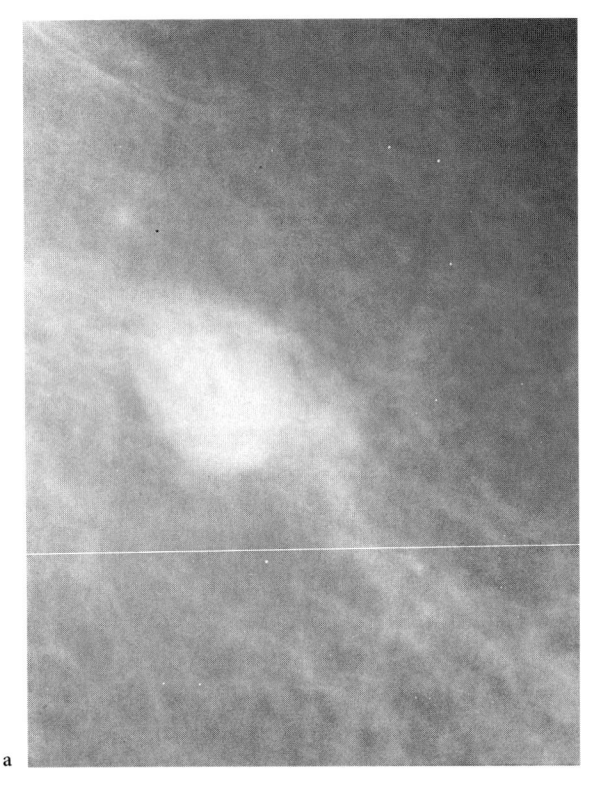

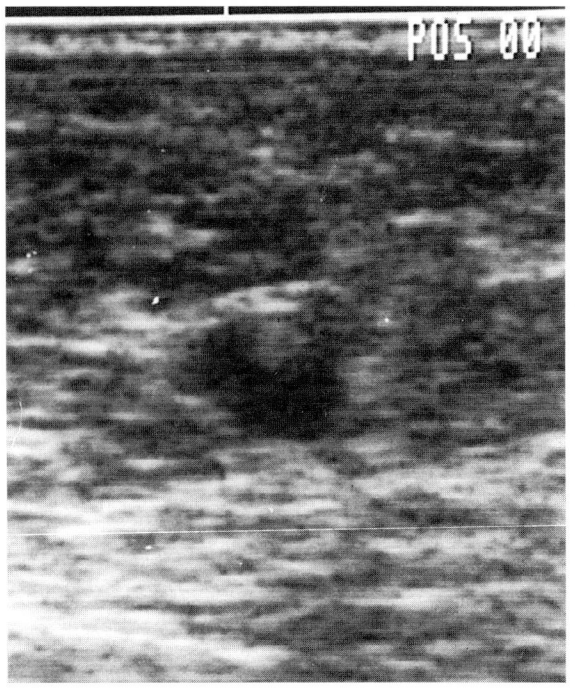

Fig. 9.14a,b. Mammograms of this 60-year-old patient revealed this circumscribed mass in the axillary portion of her breast (**a**). It appeared to have grown a few millimeters since the prior examination 3 years earlier. **b** Ultrasonography revealed a heterogeneous round mass. Biopsy was performed which revealed fibrocystic change

and 36–42 month mammography, was performed. Of the 1403 women for whom follow-up had been recommended, 958 (68.3%) completed the follow-up regimen out to 36–42 months. The remainder were contacted by phone to assess their breast health status. Only 19 patients (1.4%) of this large cohort proved ultimately to have cancer in the lesion being followed, with the follow-up interval being at least 36 months at the time of the report. Of these 19 patients, only one patient had (one) positive lymph node at surgery and that patient had no evidence of distant disease at 127 months of follow-up. Of the 19 patients

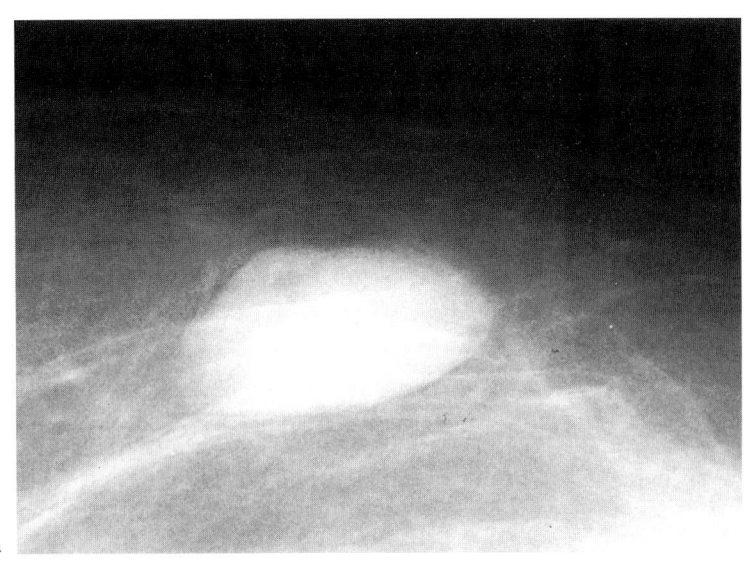

Fig. 9.15a–c. Initial screening mammogram of this 74-year-old patient showed a mass with circumscribed borders on the mediolateral oblique view (**a**) and partially indistinct borders on the craniocaudal view (**b**). Spot compression magnification views (**c**) were blurred because of patient motion but raised concern that the lesion was indistinct. Open biopsy revealed focal fibrosis

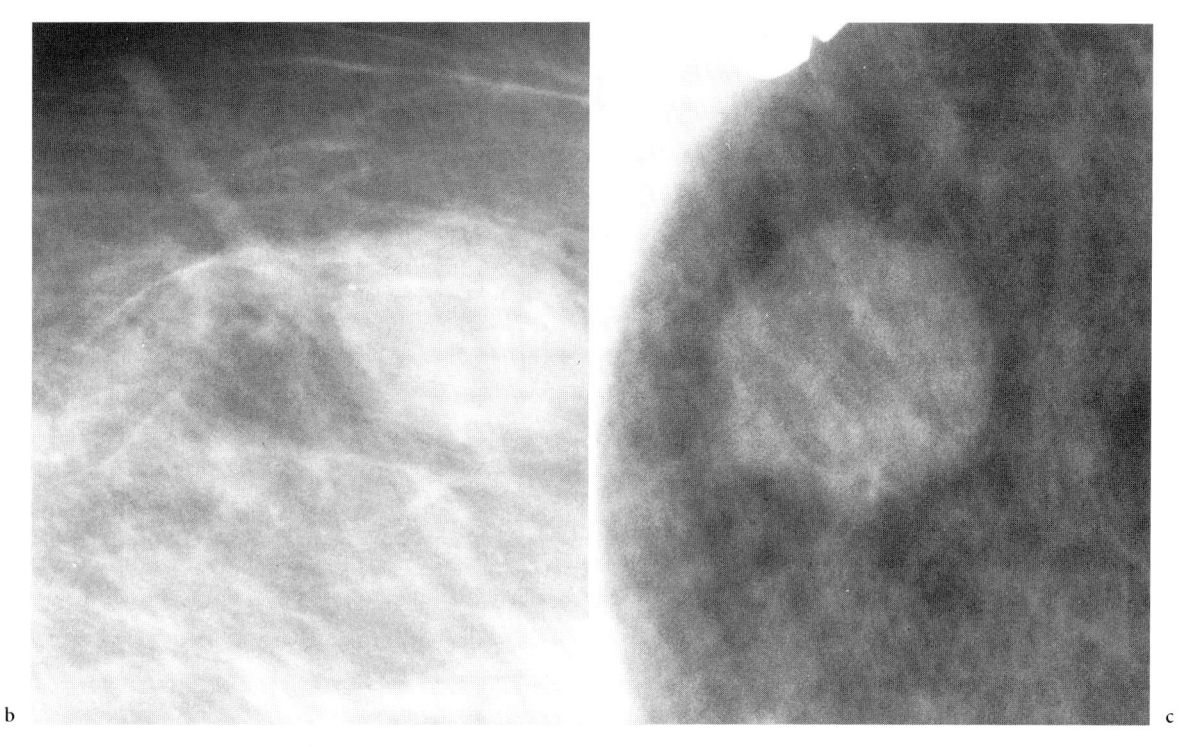

The Management of Nonpalpable Circumscribed Breast Masses 157

Fig. 9.15b,c.

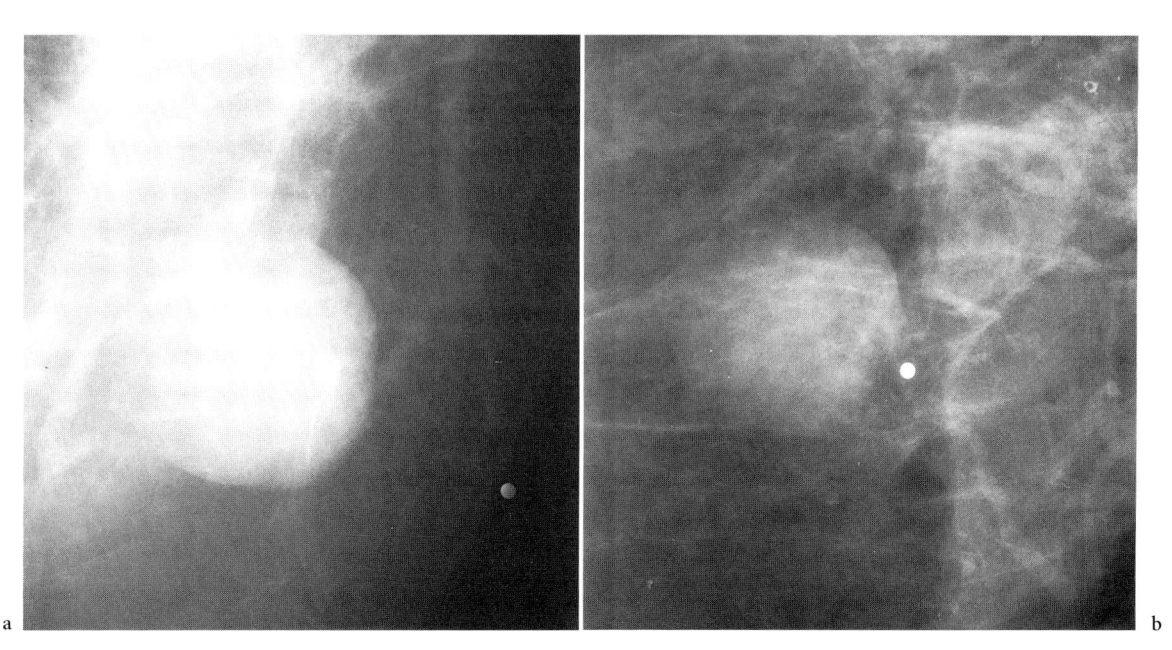

Fig. 9.16a–c. This 61-year-old patient reported a palpable lump that had been unchanged for more than 30 years in her left breast. It has been sampled percutaneously many years previously, yielding benign results. a,b Mammography revealed a predominantly circumscribed mass with some obscured and minimally indistinct borders on magnification views. c Ultrasonography revealed a circumscribed hypoechoic mass with enhanced through-transmission, findings suggestive of the diagnosis of fibroadenoma. Because of clinical concern, open biopsy was performed which revealed a fibroadenoma

Fig. 9.16c.

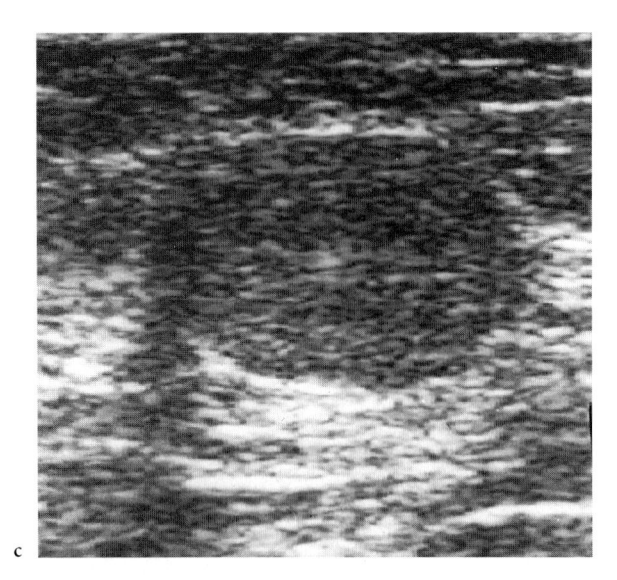

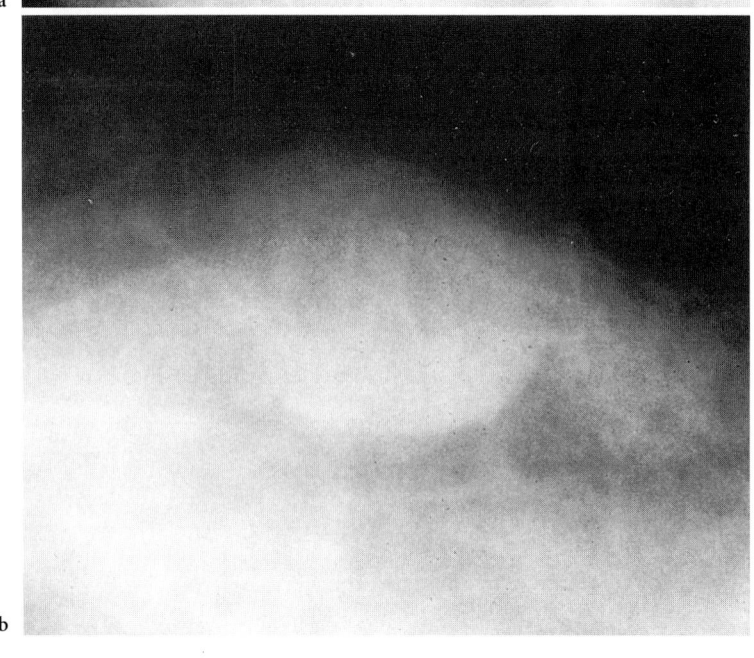

Fig. 9.17a,b. This circumscribed mass has somewhat obscured borders on these standard mediolateral oblique (**a**) and craniocaudal (**b**) views. The patient desired biopsy, which revealed sclerosing adenosis

Fig. 9.18. a Initial screening mammogram revealing a typical lipid cyst (of fat necrosis), "many years" after a breast biopsy. **b** Subsequent mammogram 4 years later showing an associated developing density with architectural distortion. Biopsy of this region revealed only a lipid cyst with surrounding inflammation and fibrosis

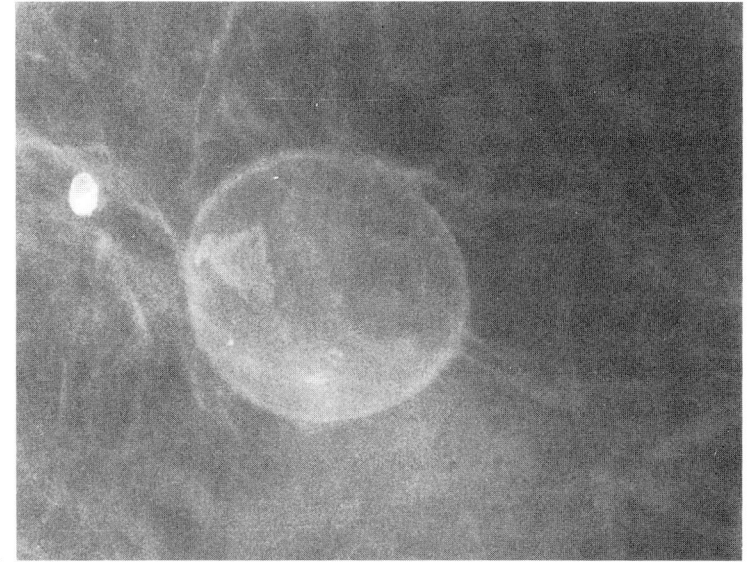

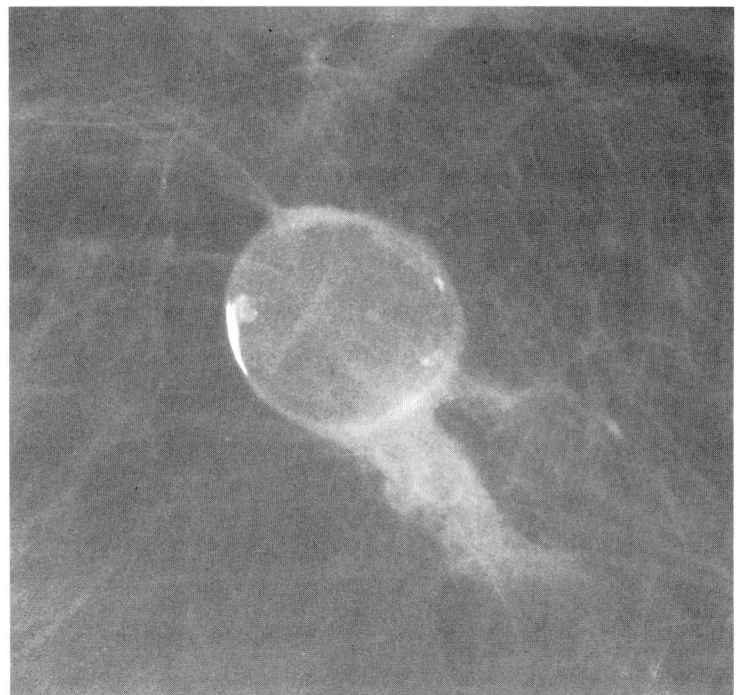

who proved to have cancer, 18 were diagnosed when they were still stage 1. The only other patient who was diagnosed at stage II had a 24-mm tumor. Seventeen out of the 19 cancer patients were ultimately diagnosed as having cancer by virtue of a mammographic change while only two of the lesions were diagnosed because they became palpable (SICKLES 1991, 1994). These data, and the results of other large series, (VARAS et al. 1992; DYESS et al. 1992) support the utility of a conservative approach to the management of these kinds of lesions.

Sickles' data show very little difference in the positive predictive value for these types of lesions even when patient age or lesion size is considered. Even for lesions between 10 and 15 mm in size, the likelihood of malignancy in a circumscribed lesion was only 1.6%, and for patients over age 50 with a circumscribed lesion, the likelihood of malignancy was only 1.7% (SICKLES 1991, 1994).

Familiarity with such results gives radiologists strong justification for follow-up of such lesions, should they need to defend their opinion in the rare case that does prove malignant (Figs. 9.13–9.15) (BRENNER and SICKLES 1989).

The types of benign solid lesions that may appear as circumscribed masses on mammography include fibroadenomas, sclerosing adenosis, focal fibrosis, fat necrosis, plasma cell mastitis, intraductal papillomas, and giant fibroadenoma (cystosarcoma phylloides) (Figs. 9.16–9.21), as well as variants of the previously described characteristically benign masses (FEIG 1992; COLE-BEUGLET 1983; GERSHON-COHEN and MOORE 1960). Hematomas may also present as well-circumscribed masses (Fig. 9.22); this diagnosis is usually obvious from the clinical setting.

It is again important to emphasize that follow-up is appropriate only for lesions for which complete mammographic work-up has been performed and that still prove to be circumscribed, *without other features suspicious for malignancy*. Suspicious features include spiculation or indistinctness of the lesion border (Fig. 9.23), suspicious calcifications, and architectural distortion (Fig. 9.18). In addition, if a lesion changes on mammography or becomes pal-

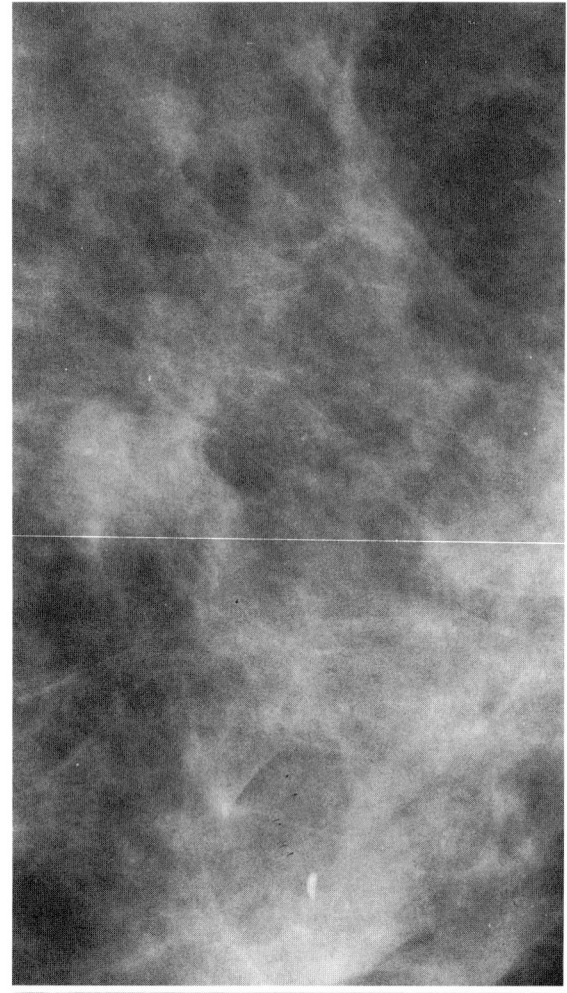

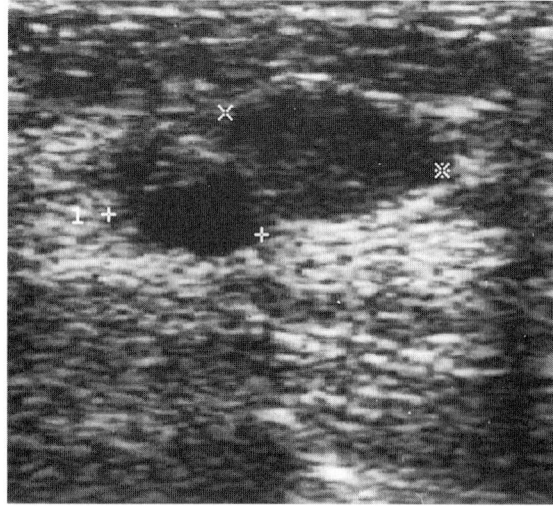

Fig. 9.19. a This new subareolar mass found on screening mammography in a 42-year-old patient appears indistinct and obscured on the spot compression magnification view, and was totally obscured on the opposite view. **b** Ultrasonography revealed a mixed cystic and solid lesion. Fine-needle aspiration was interpreted as showing clusters of papillary cells, but a papillary neoplasm could not be exluded. Subsequent open surgical biopsy proved the lesion to be a sclerosing papilloma

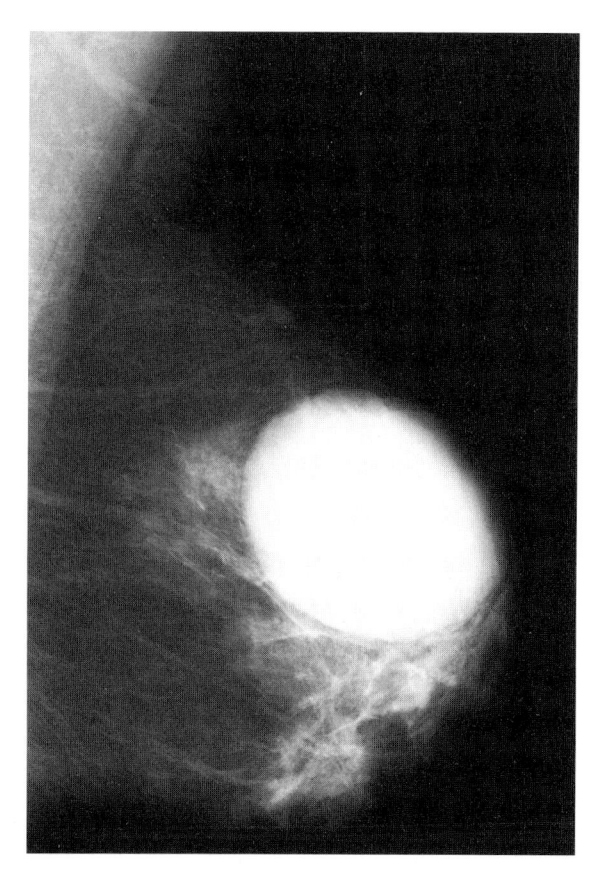

Fig. 9.20. This patient noticed a palpable lump in her breast. All of its borders appear circumscribed, with no evidence of irregularity. Surgical excision demonstrated a giant fibroadenoma (phylloides tumor) with some focal atypia

The Management of Nonpalpable Circumscribed Breast Masses 161

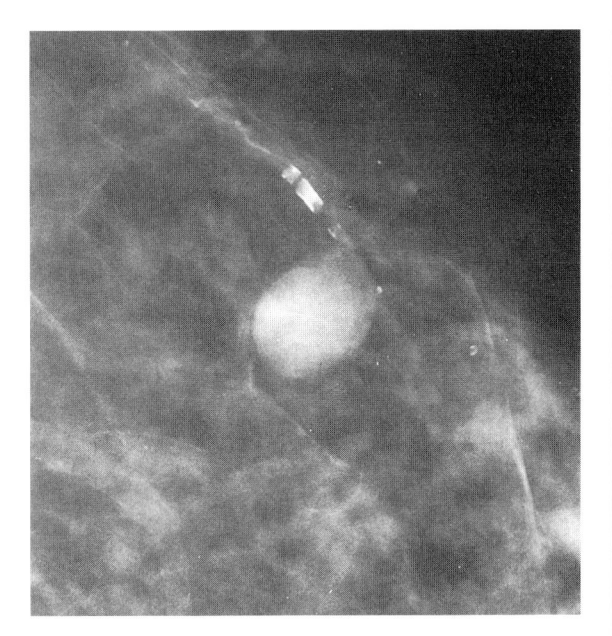

Fig. 9.21. This small perfectly circumscribed mass was readily palpable and therefore it was biopsied despite its benign mammographic appearance. It proved to be a papilloma

pable during the follow-up interval (Figs. 9.14, 9.15), it falls into the more suspicious category and biopsy should then be performed. Even for those types of lesions, according to Sickles' data, only 15 out of 131 proved to be malignant, for a positive predictive value of approximately 11% (SICKLES 1994).

The types of primary breast cancer that most frequently are circumscribed at mammography are mucinous (or colloid) carcinoma and medullary carcinoma (Fig. 9.24) (MEYER et al. 1989) but invasive ductal and lobular carcinomas also can have circumscribed borders (IKEDA and ANDERSSON 1989; HELVIE et al. 1993; MITNICK 1989). In fact, MOSKOWITZ reported that 17% of all nonpalpable cancers found as masses were smooth and circumscribed (MOSKOWITZ 1983).

Metastases to the breast also tend to be circumscribed, and can be solitary or multiple (Fig. 9.25) (CHAIGNAUD et al. 1994; AMICHETTI et al. 1990; BOHMAN et al. 1982; PAULUS and LIBSHITZ 1982). Non-Hodgkin's lymphoma of the breast also most frequently presents as a circumscribed mass (PAULUS 1990). In addition, recurrent breast cancer

Fig. 9.22. a Mammogram obtained 6 months after an open surgical biopsy (for suspicious calcifications that proved to be benign), revealing a large circumscribed mass at the biopsy site. This was presumed to represent a postoperative hematoma. b Subsequent follow-up mammogram 8 months later revealing partial resolution of the mass

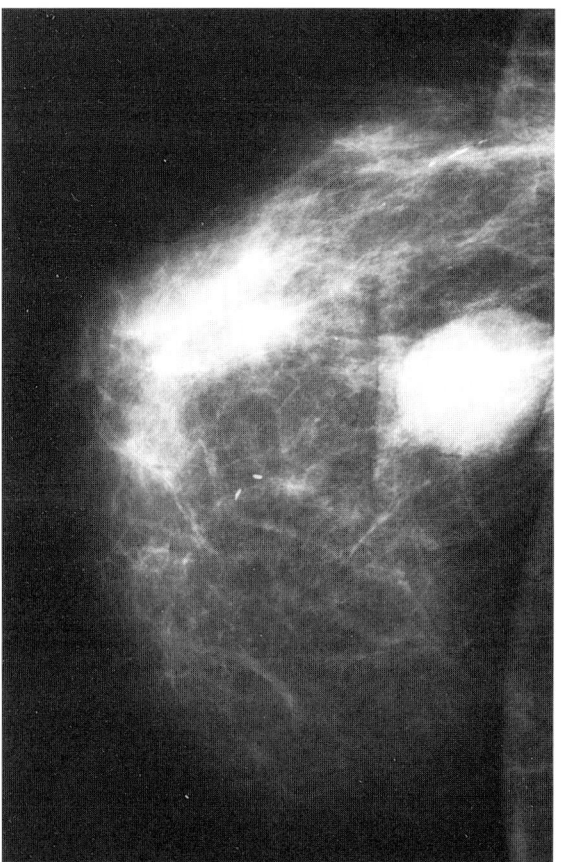

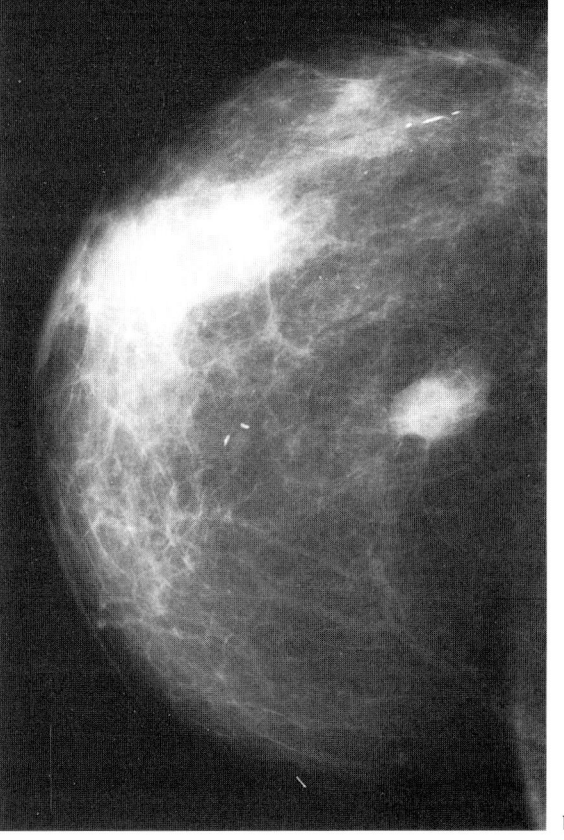

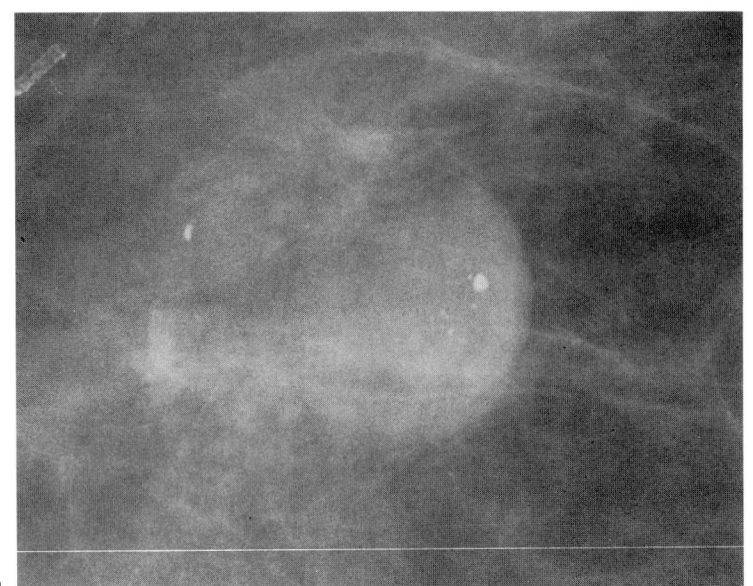

Fig. 9.23. a This 68-year-old patient developed a 1-cm moderately circumscribed mass with associated calcifications. The calcifications are very similar in size and shape to two coarse large calcifications. This characterization suggests that the calcifications are benign. **b** Ultrasonography revealed the mass to be round and hypoechoic (*not* anechoic), with some increased through-transmission and back-wall enhancement. Thus, the mass is not a simple cyst. Because of questions about the lesion border characteristics and the sonographic findings, a needle was placed into the mass. A few milliliters of greenish-black fluid were drained from the lesion. Subsequent mammograms showed no residual evidence of the mass

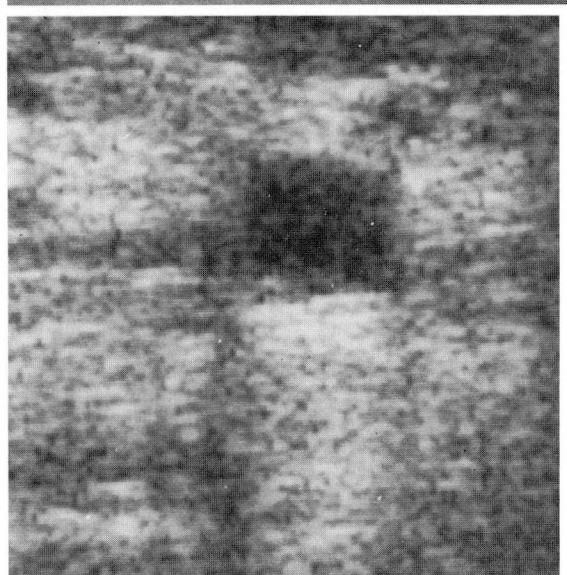

most frequently presents as a circumscribed mass (Fig. 9.26) (RISSANEN et al. 1993).

What type of biopsy should be performed for circumscribed lesions that change on physical examination or mammography during the follow-up period? Either percutaneous or open surgical biopsy is acceptable, as long as a definitive diagnosis is achieved. Percutaneous biopsy can be performed with sonographic or stereotactic guidance. If sonographic guidance is used, care should be taken to assure that the lesion biopsied definitely corresponds to the mammographic abnormality. This can usually be accomplished by placing a metallic marker on the sonographically visible lesion and obtaining a mammogram to confirm that the marker lies over the mammographically apparent mass. A postdrainage mammogram also can be obtained to confirm that a mammographically apparent lesion disappears after a cyst has been drained.

If percutaneous biopsy is used, the results obtained must be correlated carefully with the mammographic appearance of the lesion (JACKSON and REYNOLDS 1991). The types of diagnoses that can be considered definitively benign in the setting of a circumscribed mass that has grown slightly on mammography during the follow-up period include fibroadenoma, lymph node, hamartoma, fat necrosis, papilloma, and nonproliferative fibrocystic change without atypia. This type of lesion could

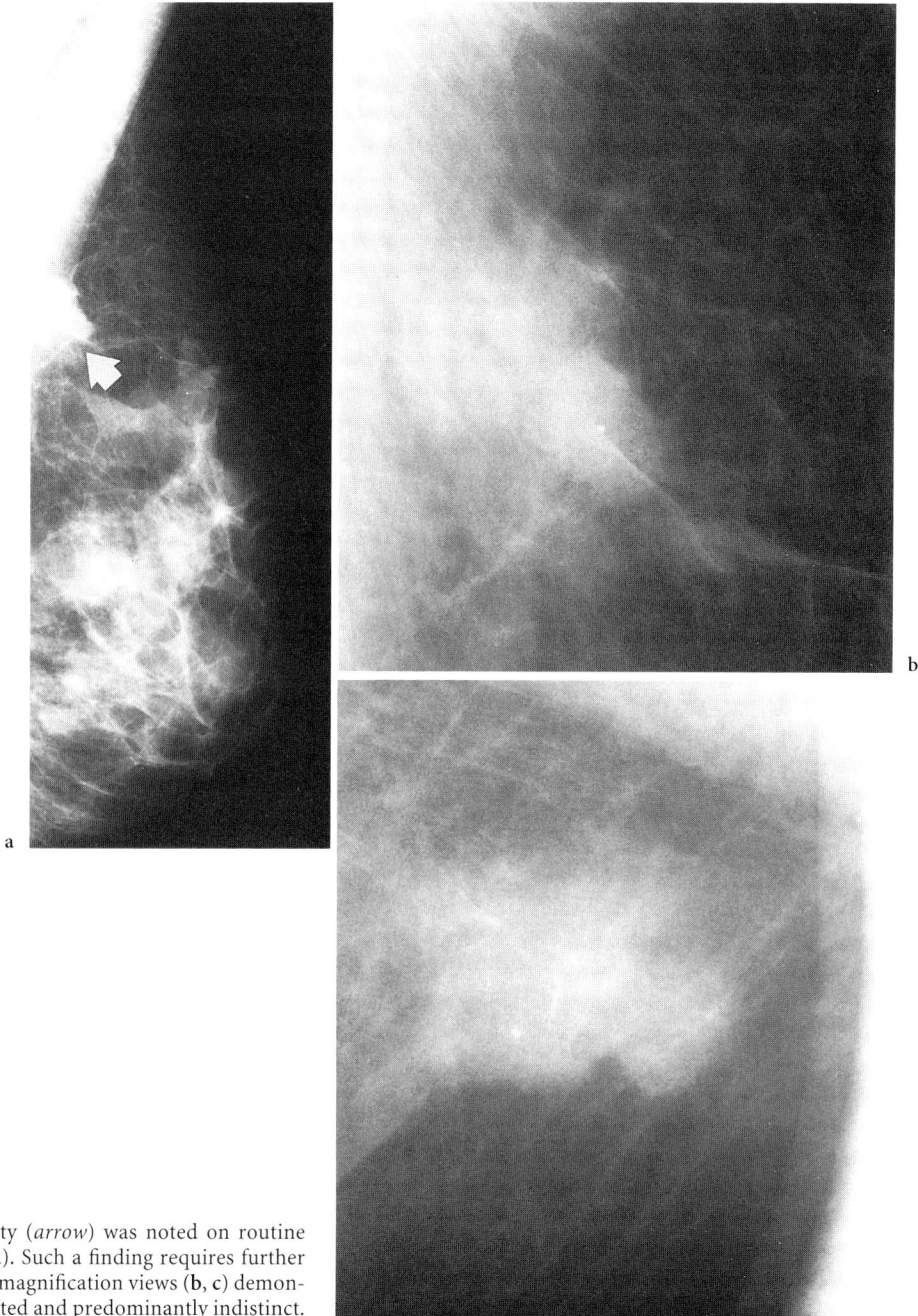

The Management of Nonpalpable Circumscribed Breast Masses 163

Fig. 9.24a–c. This neodensity (*arrow*) was noted on routine screening mammography (**a**). Such a finding requires further work-up. Spot compression magnification views (**b**, **c**) demonstrate that the mass is lobulated and predominantly indistinct. Biopsy showed it to be a mucinous carcinoma

probably be safely followed at 6-, 12-, 24-, and 36-month intervals.

There is no benign diagnosis that should be believed without complete surgical excision in the setting of a primarily circumscribed mass that has acquired suspicious mammographic features such as spiculation, architectural distortion, or pleomorphic calcifications.

9.5 Other Factors That Influence the Need for Further Workup in the Setting of a Circumscribed Mass

Ideally, to keep screening costs low and to avoid unnecessary morbidity, almost all circumscribed masses should be managed without open surgical biopsy. However, there are a few circumstances,

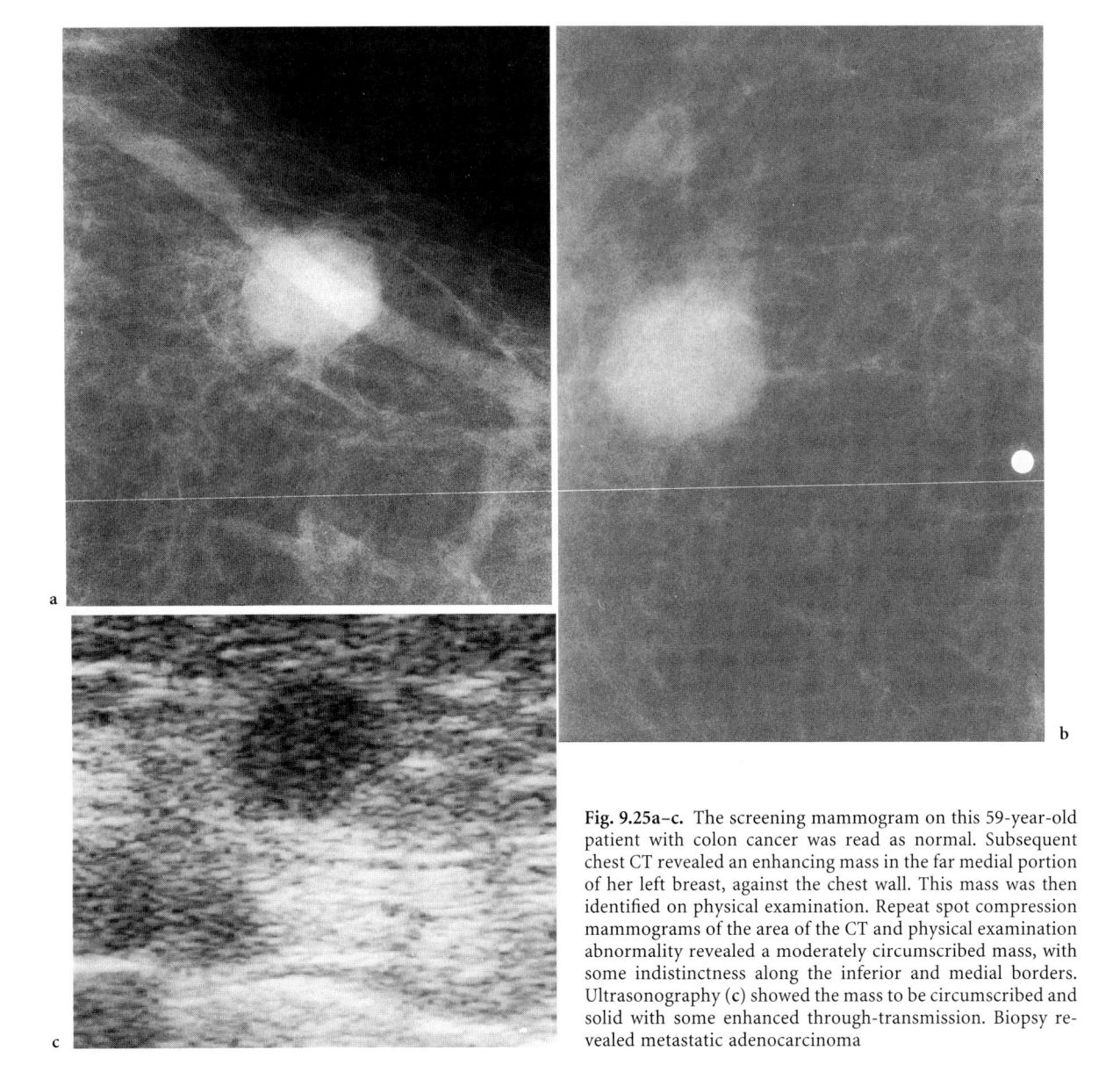

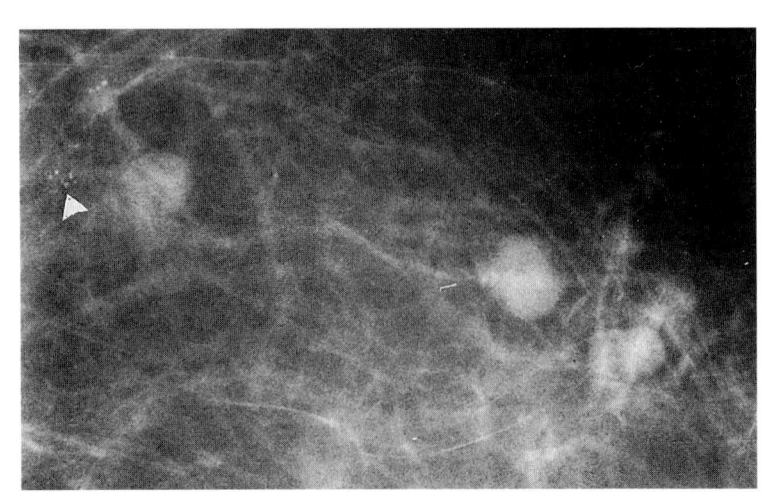

Fig. 9.25a–c. The screening mammogram on this 59-year-old patient with colon cancer was read as normal. Subsequent chest CT revealed an enhancing mass in the far medial portion of her left breast, against the chest wall. This mass was then identified on physical examination. Repeat spot compression mammograms of the area of the CT and physical examination abnormality revealed a moderately circumscribed mass, with some indistinctness along the inferior and medial borders. Ultrasonography (**c**) showed the mass to be circumscribed and solid with some enhanced through-transmission. Biopsy revealed metastatic adenocarcinoma

Fig. 9.26. This woman had undergone lumpectomy and radiation therapy for an infiltrating ductal carcinoma in 1986. Four years later, routine follow-up revealed three small moderately circumscribed masses in the region of her prior tumor. These and the associated pleomorphic calcifications (*arrowhead*) proved to be recurrent tumor on biopsy

other than those already discussed, in which biopsy will be necessary.

The patient may not be comfortable with the uncertainty, however, slight, of follow-up for a mammographic abnormality. Some patients are extremely cancer-phobic and anxious. If attempts are made to educate such patients about the reasonableness of follow-up and the patient still desires histologic confirmation of the benign nature of her lesion, biopsy is probably the best course of action.

Furthermore, there are some women who are at such high risk for breast cancer that the threshold for biopsy might reasonably be set lower. These include patients with a prior personal history of ductal or lobular carcinoma, lobular neoplasia, or atypical ductal hyperplasia. A circumscribed lesion occurring in a premenopausal patient with a mother and/or sister with premenopausal breast cancer might also justify a more aggressive management strategy, that is, biopsy. There is no literature that specifically addresses the risk of carcinoma in a circumscribed lesion in this subset of patients. It is possible that percutaneous biopsy might suffice in confirming a benign diagnosis of what is admittedly a probably benign lesion, even in such circumstances.

9.6 Summary

Circumscribed lesions of the breast are almost always benign. Definitively benign diagnoses can be made for some lesions, either directly from screening mammography examinations or after complete breast imaging evaluation. Most of the remaining lesions are properly managed by periodic mammographic follow-up. However, if change occurs during the surveillance period, either at mammography or at clinical examination, biopsy is then justified.

References

Amichetti M, Perani B, Boi S (1990) Metastases to the breast from extramammary malignancies. Oncology 47:257–260
Berkowitz JE, Gatewood OMB, Gayler BW (1989) Equivocal mammographic findings: evaluation with spot compression. Radiology 171:369–371
Bohman LG, Bassett LW, Gold RH (1982) Breast metastases from extramammary malignancies. Radiology 144:309–312
Brenner RJ, Sickles EA (1989) Acceptability of periodic follow-up as an alternative to biopsy for mammographically detected lesions interpreted as probably benign. Radiology 171:645–646
Chaignaud B, Hall TJ, Powers C, Subramony C, Scott-Conner CEH (1994) Diagnosis and natural history of extramammary tumors metastatic to the breast. J Am Coll Surg 179:49–53
Cole-Beuglet C, Soriano RZ, Kurtz AB (1983) Fibroadenoma of the breast: sonomammography correlated with pathology in 122 patients. AJR 140:369–375
Coren GS, Libshitz HI, Patchefsky AS (1974) Fat necrosis of the breast: mammographic and thermographic findings. Br J Radiol 47:758–762
Dyess DL, Lorino CO, Grieco A, Ferrara JJ (1992) Selective nonoperative management of solid breast masses. Am Surg 58:437–440
Evers K, Troupin RH (1991) Lipid cyst: classic and atypical appearances. AJR 157:271–274
Feig SA (1988) The importance of supplementary mammographic views to diagnostic accuracy. AJR 151:40–41
Feig SA (1989) The role of ultrasound in a breast imaging center. Semin Ultrasound CT MR 10:90–105
Feig SA (1992) Breast masses. Mammographic and sonographic evaluation. Radiol Clin North Am 30:67–92
Gershon-Cohen J, Moore L (1960) Roentgenography of giant fibroadenoma of the breast (cystosarcoma phylloides). Radiology 74:619–625
Gomez A, Mata JM, Donoso L, Rams A (1986) Galactocele: three distinctive radiographic appearances. Radiology 158:43–44
Helvie MA, Adler DD, Rebner M, Oberman HA (1989) Breast hamartomas: variable mammographic appearances. Radiology 170:417–421
Helvie MA, Paramagul C, Oberman HA, Adler DD (1993) Invasive lobular carcinoma. Imaging features and clinical detection. Invest Radiol 28:202–207
Hessler C, Schnyder P, Ozzello L (1978) Hamartoma of the breast: diagnostic observation in 16 cases. Radiology 126:95–98
Ikeda DM, Andersson I (1989) Ductal carcinoma in situ: atypical mammographic appearances. Radiology 172:661–666
Jackson VP, Reynolds HE (1991) Stereotactic needle-core biopsy and fine-needle aspiration cytologic evaluation of nonpalpable breast lesions. Radiology 181:633–634
Meyer JE, Amin E, Lindfors KK (1989) Medullary carcinoma of the breast: mammographic and ultrasound appearance. Radiology 170:79–82
Mitnick JS, Roses DF, Harris MN, Feiner HD (1989) Circumscribed intraductal carcinoma of the breast. Radiology 170:423–425
Moskowitz M (1983) The predictive value of certain mammographic signs in screening for breast cancer. Cancer 51:1007–1011
Paulus DD (1990) Lymphoma of the breast. Radiol Clin North Am 28:833–840
Paulus DD, Libshitz HI (1982) Metastasis to the breast. Radiol Clin North Am 20:561–568
Rissanen RJ, Makarainen HP, Mattila SI, Lindholm EL, Heikkinen MI, Kiviniemi HO (1993) Breast cancer recurrence after mastectomy: diagnosis with mammography and US. Radiology 188:463–467
Sickles EA (1988) Practical solutions to common mammographic problems: tailoring the examination. AJR 151:31–39
Sickles EA (1991) Periodic mammographic follow-up of probably benign lesions: results of 3184 consecutive cases. Radiology 179:463–468
Sickles EA (1994) Nonpalpable, circumscribed, noncalcified solid breast masses: likelihood of malignancy based on lesion size and age of patient. Radiology 192:439–442

Sickles EA, Vogelaar PW (1981) Fluid level within a galactocele: diagnosis aided by lateral projection mammogram with horizontal beam. Breast 7:32–33

Stomper PC, Leibowich S, Meyer JE (1991) The prevalence and distribution of well-circumscribed nodules on screening mammography: analysis of 1500 mammograms. Breast Dis 4:197–203

Svane G, Franzen S (1993) Radiologic appearance of nonpalpable intramammary lymph nodes. Acta Radiol 34:577–580

Varas X, Leborgne F, Leborgne JH (1992) Nonpalpable, probably benign lesions: role of follow-up mammography. Radiology 184:409–414

10 Management of Lesions Appearing Probably Benign at Mammography

E.A. Sickles

CONTENTS

10.1 Introduction.................................. 167
10.2 Mammographic Features of Probably Benign Lesions....................................... 168
10.3 Clinical Results of Periodic Mammographic Surveillance.................................. 168
10.4 Unresolved Issues............................ 169
10.5 Summary..................................... 171
    References.................................... 171

10.1 Introduction

Using mammography, radiologists often identify nonpalpable lesions that are interpreted as having a very low probability of malignancy. This chapter covers the several approaches, especially periodic mammographic surveillance, to subsequent management of these lesions. Follow-up mammography examinations usually are recommended as an alternative to open surgical biopsy or percutaneous imaging-guided tissue diagnosis (via aspiration cytology or core biopsy), in order to avert the morbidity and substantial cost of these more invasive procedures (Homer 1981; Moskowitz 1983; Homer 1987; Wolfe et al. 1987; Hall et al. 1988; Moskowitz 1988; Moskowitz 1989; Brenner and Sickles 1989; Hall 1990; Adler and Helvie 1990; Helvie et al. 1991; Sickles 1991a; Varas et al. 1992; Sickles and Parker 1993).

There is very strong evidence supporting management with periodic mammographic follow-up, coming from two studies of prospectively identified, consecutive cases, each derived from a series of more than 20000 mammography examinations (Sickles 1991a; Varas et al. 1992). These studies, from the University of California at San Francisco (UCSF) and the Hospital Pereira Rossell in Montevideo, Uruguay, as well as other smaller and less well controlled investigations (Wolfe et al. 1987; Hall et al. 1988; Helvie et al. 1991; de Waal 1991), show that the frequency of cancer among probably benign lesions ranges from 0.5% to 1.7%. Management by periodic mammographic surveillance is justified by demonstration (a) that probably benign lesions indeed have an extremely low likelihood of malignancy, (b) that careful mammographic surveillance almost always will identify by interval change those few lesions that actually are malignant, and (c) that cancers will be identified during follow-up while the tumors still have a favorable prognosis (Hall et al. 1988; Sickles 1991a; Varas et al. 1992).

The radiologist is well advised to describe these lesions as being "probably benign" rather than "minimally suspicious" or any other terminology implying suspicion of malignancy (Sickles 1991a; Sickles 1991b). The term "probably benign" conveys with much greater conviction the overwhelming likelihood that these lesions truly are benign and that management by observation is a reasonable, safe alternative to immediate tissue diagnosis.

One must distinguish from probably benign lesions those mammographic findings which are so clearly benign that periodic follow-up is not required and for which subsequent imaging should be limited to routine screening mammography. Such characteristically benign lesions include simple cysts diagnosed by aspiration or ultrasonography (Sickles et al. 1984), sedimented calcium within tiny benign cysts (Linden and Sickles 1989), dermal calcifications even if clustered (Kopans et al. 1983; Homer et al. 1994), arterial calcification (Sickles and Galvin 1985; Moshyedi et al. 1995), most calcified fibroadenomas, dystrophic and/or sutural postsurgical calcification, intraductal and/or periductal calcifications of benign duct ectasia (secretory calcifications), discrete masses that are entirely or partially fatty in content, and masses that demonstrate the size, shape, and location typical of

E.A. Sickles, MD, Professor, Department of Radiology, University of California School of Medicine, San Francisco, and Chief, Breast Imaging Section, Department of Radiology, University of California Medical Center, Box 0628, San Francisco, CA 94143-0628, USA

intramammary lymph nodes (SICKLES 1986; SICKLES 1989a).

10.2 Mammographic Features of Probably Benign Lesions

Mammographic findings interpreted as being probably benign with recommendation for periodic surveillance consist of two major categories, localized and generalized. Localized findings are characterized by a focal distribution, occurring in one segment of one breast. This includes: (a) a cluster of tiny calcifications when fine-detail images demonstrate that all of the particles are round or oval in shape; (b) a noncalcified solid nonpalpable mass with round, oval, or lobular contour and circumscribed margins where not obscured by adjacent fibroglandular tissue; (c) a nonpalpable focal asymmetric density, defined as a discrete opacity readily visible on two orthogonal projection mammograms, with concave-outward margins and/or interspersed with fat; and (d) several miscellaneous focal findings, including a single dilated duct (if not associated with spontaneous nipple discharge) and a subtle area of architectural distortion without central increased opacity (when occurring at a known biopsy site).

The second major category of probably benign findings is characterized by a generalized distribution, involving multiple similar lesions (usually three or more lesions, either tiny calcifications or masses) randomly distributed in both breasts. The most important radiological feature prompting "probably benign" interpretation for generalized-distribution findings is the similarity of all the component parts of such scattered lesions. A distinction sometimes is made between two subtypes of widely distributed tiny calcifications: multiple discrete clusters of round or oval-shaped calcifications, and numerous bilateral scattered and randomly clustered calcifications.

10.3 Clinical Results of Periodic Mammographic Surveillance

Likelihoods of malignancy have been demonstrated for the various mammographic findings that prompt a probably benign diagnosis. Table 10.1 lists the presenting findings of the 26 cancers that were identified during the course of mammographic surveillance in the UCSF and Montevideo studies (SICKLES 1991a; VARAS et al. 1992). The majority of these cancers presented as solitary noncalcified circumscribed

Table 10.1. Specific mammographic findings of 3719 probably benign lesions and of the 26 breast cancers detected among them

Finding	Cases ($n = 3719$)	Cancers ($n = 26$)[a]
Localized microcalcifications	1338	5 (0.4)
Solid circumscribed mass	878	16 (1.8)
Focal asymmetric density	502	3 (0.6)
Generalized microcalcifications	619	1 (0.2)
Multiple solid circumscribed masses	329	1 (0.3)
Miscellaneous	53	0 (0)

[a] Numbers in parentheses are percentages

solid nodules, with a positive predictive value of 1.8%. The other probably benign findings each had a positive predictive value of less than 1%. The positive predictive value for all probably benign lesions combined was 0.7%.

The rendering of a probably benign interpretation usually requires additional imaging to supplement that provided by conventional two-view-per-breast screening mammography. Ultrasonography should be done for the nonpalpable, circumscribed, noncalcified mass to establish or exclude the diagnosis of simple cyst (SICKLES et al. 1984; JOKICH et al. 1992). Solid masses, densities, and lesions involving microcalcifications should undergo fine-detail imaging, especially spot-compression magnification mammography, to more clearly portray the shapes and marginal characteristics of these lesions, and also to serve as a source for comparison in case additional fine-detail images are obtained subsequently during mammographic surveillance (SICKLES 1979; SICKLES 1987; SICKLES 1989b; SICKLES 1995a). It is my standard practice not to make probably benign interpretations directly from screening examinations; rather, additional imaging is performed first.

There is no universally accepted protocol of periodic mammographic surveillance for probably benign lesions. However, both patients and their responsible physicians should be fully informed about the rationale for and timing of recommended follow-up mammography, and specifically of its use as an alternative to open surgical biopsy or percutaneous imaging-guided tissue sampling. It also should be understood in advance that any interval change in a probably benign mammographic finding which raises even a slight suspicion of malignancy would result in the recommendation for prompt tissue diagnosis. The most widely used surveillance protocol calls for repeat mammography of the ipsilateral breast in 6 months, involving orthogonal projection radiographs using whatever technique most effectively portrayed the lesion on initial workup. Subsequently, bilateral mammography is obtained 6 months later, followed by one or two additional bilateral annual examinations. Thus, mammographic surveillance involves three or four follow-up examinations spanning a 2- or 3-year period, although this actually represents only one (unilateral) examination more than what ordinarily is recommended as routine annual screening in the United States (SICKLES 1995b).

When such a surveillance protocol is competently and confidently presented to patients and referring physicians, there will be overwhelming initial acceptance. At UCSF, fewer than 2.5% of women with probably benign lesions choose to have immediate tissue diagnosis instead of periodic mammographic follow-up (SICKLES 1991a; SICKLES 1994b). However, compliance with the full extent of the surveillance protocol is far less complete. In the UCSF series, although almost all patients underwent at least one follow-up examination, only 45% had all four recommended examinations (SICKLES 1991a).

The findings of the large-scale prospective UCSF and Montevideo studies demonstrate that mammographic surveillance of probably benign lesions will correctly identify almost all of the lesions that actually are malignant, usually while the tumors remain nonpalpable and curable (SICKLES 1991a; VARAS et al. 1992). Indeed, 24 of the 26 cancers in these studies were biopsied because surveillance mammography showed interval progression of lesions prior to the development of palpable findings. Furthermore, prognostic factors were very favorable for the 26 malignancies detected during follow-up. All but one of the cancers was either ductal carcinoma in situ or a T1 invasive carcinoma (2 cm or less in greatest dimension). Axillary lymph node metastasis was found in only 15% (4/26) of the cancers. Finally, all of the 17 UCSF cancer patients have been free of recurrent tumor after a median follow-up period of more than 8 years; in the Montevideo series, which has an average follow-up of 23 months, only one of the nine cancer patients has shown evidence of recurrence, in this case involving distant metastasis from a T1N0 cancer. These several indicators of good prognosis are similar to those reported for large-scale *screening* programs using modern mammography (SICKLES 1992; THURFJELL and LINDGREN 1994; WARREN BURHENNE et al. 1995). Therefore, there does not appear to be clinically measurable harm to patients due to periodic mammographic follow-up of those few probably benign lesions that actually are malignant, even though the cancers in these women are diagnosed and treated months to years after initial detection.

The UCSF and Montevideo studies also show that by managing probably benign lesions with mammographic surveillance, the biopsy yield of cancer would increase from the current United States average of 15%–30% up to approximately 40%, without a substantial reduction in the detection of small cancers (SICKLES 1991a; VARAS et al. 1992). During the periods of case accrual in both studies, the biopsy yield of cancer for nonpalpable lesions read as suspicious for malignancy ranged from 38% to 47%. These results were obtained during periods in which only 0.5%–1.7% of probably benign interpretations eventually proved to represent malignant lesions.

Conservative management of probably benign lesions has several other important advantages. Substituting mammographic surveillance for open surgical biopsy will substantially reduce morbidity and monetary costs, thereby benefitting both patients and third-party payers. In the United States and in most other countries, there also will be similar benefits, primarily involving cost reduction, when periodic mammographic follow-up is used rather than percutaneous imaging-guided tissue sampling procedures such as fine-needle aspiration and core biopsy (SICKLES and PARKER 1993; SULLIVAN 1994; SICKLES 1995b). However, it is likely that the most significant effect of adopting surveillance instead of tissue diagnosis for probably benign lesions is that by increasing the cost-effectiveness of breast imaging, this will help to remove a major remaining barrier to the utilization of screening mammography (EDDY et al. 1988).

10.4 Unresolved Issues

Despite the building consensus that probably benign lesions should be followed with periodic mammographic surveillance, several issues remain unresolved concerning diagnosis and management. First, in an effort to further reduce costs, some radiologists prefer to eliminate the full problem-solving imaging workup that traditionally is completed before making a probably benign diagnosis (HALL 1995). Rather, in selected cases, these radiologists recommend periodic follow-up solely on the basis of findings identified at screening mammography. In my opinion, this approach is unwise (SICKLES 1995a). The one-time use of breast ultrasonography or spot-compression magnification mammography permits many benign lesions to be classified definitively as benign (cysts, summation shadows, most intramammary lymph nodes), at a cost similar to that of the 6-month follow-up imaging that instead would have been performed later. The problem-solving imaging workup also will occasionally help the radiologist to correctly identify a circumscribed cancer as being suspect for malignancy, thereby resulting in more prompt tissue diagnosis and treatment. Finally, an initial set of fine-detail mammograms (supplementing conventional images) provides the baseline from which stability is best assessed during subsequent mammographic surveillance. Notwithstanding these arguments, because there are no controlled clinical studies comparing the efficacy of recommending mammographic follow-up on the basis of screening versus full problem-solving examination, it is likely that debate on this subject will continue.

Another unresolved issue concerning probably benign lesions is whether to use patient age and lesion size (for probably benign solitary masses) as additional criteria in choosing between the management alternatives of mammographic surveillance and immediate tissue diagnosis. An attitudinal survey of the Fellows of the Society of Breast Imaging indicates that although 92% of expert radiologists accept periodic mammograpic follow-up as proper management of such lesions, more than 80% utilize a size threshold (ranging from 0.5 cm to 2.0 cm) above which they recommend biopsy despite the presence of otherwise probably benign mammographic features (HALL 1993). Although the great majority of respondents reported recommending biopsy of larger masses and masses in older women, based on empirical observations that lesions in these subgroups carry a higher likelihood of malignancy, a few other respondents recommended the opposite strategy (biopsy of smaller masses and masses in younger women), based on the supposition that this approach is likely to identify those masses which are malignant while more of the tumors remain curable.

A recent update of results from the UCSF study of probably benign lesions provides the only objective evidence on the validity of using age and size thresholds to decide between management with mammographic surveillance and immediate biopsy (SICKLES 1994a). These data confirmed prior observations that the likelihood of malignancy was slightly increased for older women and for larger masses, but the differences among age and size subgroups were found to be very small and did not approach statistical significance. Most important, neither age nor size criteria defined subgroups of masses that had sufficiently high probability of malignancy to support management with immediate biopsy. Indeed, in the subgroup for which masses were most likely to be malignant, involving women aged 50 and older, there were 60 benign masses for each cancer. Results also indicated that neither age nor size criteria defined subgroups for which management with immediate biopsy could be justified in order to permit diagnosis while more cancers remain curable; the vast majority of cancers in all subgroups were stage 0 or stage 1 tumors despite diagnosis many months after initial detection. Therefore, overall results of the updated UCSF study suggest that probably benign masses should undergo periodic mammographic surveillance regardless of patient age or lesion size.

The last major unresolved issue involving mammographic follow-up of probably benign lesions concerns the specific details of the surveillance protocol. A survey of expert American radiologists, conducted in 1980, indicated a wide diversity of opinion about the proper timing, frequency, and duration of follow-up examinations (HOMER 1981). Furthermore, the subsequently published clinical studies, although instrumental in establishing the validity of management by follow-up, have not been particularly helpful in defining the optimal surveillance protocol. None of the studies compare the efficacy of different protocols, each of the studies utilizes a somewhat different approach to follow-up, and the largest series of cases involves only 15 cancers detected by mammography during the course of surveillance.

However, the similarity of results observed in the various studies not only suggests that any of the specific follow-up protocols in these studies is likely to produce satisfactory clinical outcomes, but also encourages those seeking consensus to identify the common elements inherent in all the published protocols. Based on these common elements, the first follow-up examination should be done 4–6 months after initial evaluation of a probably benign lesion. Most radiologists recommend this early recall examination, despite the very low frequency at which cancer is identified (2/15 cancers and 2/3184 cases in the UCSF series), in order to identify the even fewer *rapidly growing* cancers while still early-stage tumors. If the early recall examination shows mammographic stability, thereby greatly reducing the likelihood of a fast-growing malignancy, further follow-up usually proceeds at longer intervals. In the United States, where routine annual screening is recommended, it is easy to understand why these subsequent examinations involve both breasts, begin 1 year after initial evaluation, and are done at yearly intervals. Indeed, the great majority of probably benign lesions later found to be breast cancer are first identified at either the 1-year or 2-year follow-up examinations (SICKLES 1991a). Also unresolved is the total duration of surveillance. Most radiologists continue follow-up for a 2-year period, but some prefer longer duration protocols of 3 or more years, despite the extremely low frequency at which cancer is found on later examinations (only 1/15 cancers and 1/3184 cases in the UCSF series). The rationale behind prolonged surveillance, which is most prevalent in the United States, is that it involves examination no more often than should be done anyway for routine screening purposes.

10.5 Summary

Large-scale, independently conducted studies involving prospectively identified, consecutive cases establish the validity of managing probably benign breast lesions with periodic mammographic surveillance rather than prompt biopsy. Indeed, this approach to standard mammographic interpretation is now very widely accepted; the American College of Radiology even includes "probably benign – short interval follow-up suggested" as one of the five allowable final assessment categories in the Breast Imaging Reporting and Data System (BIRADS), which it encourages all radiologists to utilize (American College of Radiology 1993).

As yet unresolved issues concerning probably benign lesions include whether initial full-problem solving imaging should be required in all cases, whether to use patient age and lesion size (for solitary masses) as additional criteria in choosing between the alternatives of mammographic follow-up and immediate tissue diagnosis, and the specific timing, frequency, and duration of follow-up examinations that constitute the surveillance protocol. However, there is general consensus that probably benign interpretations should involve: (a) cases restricted to nonpalpable lesions; (b) use of the specific interpretive criteria described in the published reports; and (c) preinterpretation comparison with prior mammograms, if available, in order to identify new or progressing lesions so that they will undergo prompt biopsy (it makes little sense to recommend periodic follow-up for a lesion that has already demonstrated interval progression, when the very demonstration of interval progression during surveillance is what prompts biopsy instead of continued follow-up).

References

Adler DD, Helvie MA (1990) The "probably benign" breast lesion: work-up and management. In: Sickles EA, Kopans DB (eds) ACR categorical course syllabus on breast imaging. American College of Radiology, Reston VA, pp 57–61

American College of Radiology (1993) Breast imaging reporting and data system. American College of Radiology, Reston VA

Brenner RJ, Sickles EA (1989) Acceptability of periodic follow-up as an alternative to biopsy for mammographically detected lesions interpreted as probably benign. Radiology 171:645–646

de Waal JC (1991) Periodic mammographic follow-up of probably benign lesions. Letter to the editor. Radiology 181:608

Eddy DM, Hasselblad V, McGivney W, Hendee W (1988) The value of mammography screening in women under age 50 years. JAMA 259:1512–1519

Hall FM (1990) Mammographic second opinions prior to biopsy of nonpalpable breast lesions. Arch Surg 125:298–299

Hall FM (1993) Statistics, opinions, and controversies among expert mammographers. Breast Dis 6:173–175

Hall FM (1995) Probably benign breast nodules: follow-up of selected cases without initial full problem-solving imaging. Editorial. Radiology 194:305

Hall FM, Storella JM, Silverstone DZ, Wyshak G (1988) Nonpalpable breast lesions: recommendations for biopsy based on suspicion of carcinoma at mammography. Radiology 167:353–358

Helvie MA, Pennes DR, Rebner M, Adler DD (1991) Mammographic follow-up of low suspicion lesions: compliance rate and diagnostic yield. Radiology 178:155–158

Homer MJ (1981) Nonpalpable mammographic abnormalities: timing the follow-up studies. Am J Roentgenol 136:923–926

Homer MJ (1987) Imaging features and management of characteristically benign and probably benign breast lesions. Radiol Clin North Am 25:939–951

Homer MJ, D'Orsi CJ, Sitzman SB (1994) Dermal calcifications in fixed orientation: the tattoo sign. Radiology 192:161–163

Jokich PM, Monticciolo DL, Adler YT (1992) Breast ultrasonography. Radiol Clin North Am 30:993–1009

Kopans DB, Meyer JE, Homer MJ, Grabbe J (1983) Dermal deposits mistaken for breast calcifications. Am J Roentgenol 149:592–594

Linden SS, Sickles EA (1989) Sedimented calcium in benign breast cysts: the full spectrum of mammographic presentations. Am J Roentgenol 152:967–971

Moshyedi AC, Puthawala AH, Kurland RJ, O'Leary DH (1995) Breast arterial calcification: association with coronary artery disease. Work in progress. Radiology 194:181–183

Moskowitz M (1983) The predictive value of certain mammographic signs in screening for breast cancer. Cancer 51:1007–1011

Moskowitz M (1988) Follow-up of benign mammographic lesions. JAMA 260:3669

Moskowitz M (1989) Impact of a priori medical decisions on screening for breast cancer. Radiology 171:605–608

Sickles EA (1979) Microfocal spot magnification mammography using xeroradiographic and screen-film recording systems. Radiology 131:599–607

Sickles EA (1986) Breast calcifications: mammographic evaluation. State of the art. Radiology 160:289–293

Sickles EA (1987) Magnification mammography. In: Bassett LW, Gold RH (eds) Breast cancer detection: mammography and other methods in breast imaging, 2nd edn. Grune & Stratton, Orlando, Fl., pp 111–117

Sickles EA (1989a) Breast masses: mammographic evaluation. State of the art. Radiology 173:297–303

Sickles EA (1989b) Combining spot-compression and other special views to maximize mammographic information. Letter to the editor. Radiology 173:571

Sickles EA (1991a) Periodic mammographic follow-up of probably benign lesions: results in 3184 consecutive cases. Radiology 179:463–468

Sickles EA (1991b) Periodic mammographic follow-up of probably benign lesions. Reply to letter to the editor. Radiology 181:905

Sickles EA (1992) Quality assurance. How to audit your own mammography practice. Radiol Clin North Am 30:265–275

Sickles EA (1994a) Nonpalpable, circumscribed, noncalcified solid breast masses: likelihood of malignancy based on lesion size and age of patient. Radiology 192:439–442

Sickles EA (1994b) Management of probably benign lesions of the breast. Reply to letter to the editor. Radiology 193:582–583

Sickles EA (1995a) Probably benign breast nodules: follow-up of all cases requires initial full problem-solving imaging. Editorial. Radiology 194:305–306

Sickles EA (1995b) Management of probably benign breast lesions. Reply to letter to the editor. Radiology 194:912

Sickles EA, Galvin HB (1985) Breast arterial calcification in association with diabetes mellitus: too weak a correlation to have clinical utility. Radiology 155:577–579

Sickles EA, Parker SH (1993) Appropriate role of core breast biopsy in the management of probably benign lesions. Radiology 188:315

Sickles EA, Filly RA, Callen PW (1984) Benign breast lesions: ultrasound detection and diagnosis. Radiology 151:467–470

Sullivan DC (1994) Needle core biopsy of mammographic lesions. Am J Roentgenol 162:601–608

Thurfjell EL, Lindgren JAA (1994) Population-based mammography screening in Swedish clinical practice: prevalence and incidence screening in Uppsala County. Radiology 193:351–357

Varas X, Leborgne F, Leborgne JH (1992) Nonpalpable probably benign lesions: role of follow-up mammography. Radiology 184:409–414

Warren Burhenne LJ, Burhenne HJ, Kan L (1995) Quality-oriented mass mammography screening. Radiology 194:185–188

Wolfe JN, Buck KA, Salane M, Parekh NJ (1987) Xeroradiography of the breast: overview of 21 057 consecutive cases. Radiology 165:305–311

11 Radiation Risk of Mammography

S.A. Feig and R.E. Hendrick

CONTENTS

11.1 Introduction................................. 173
11.2 Risk Assessment 173
11.3 Dose-Response Models...................... 174
11.4 Latent Period and Duration.................. 175
11.5 Age at Exposure 175
11.6 Additive and Relative Risk Models 176
11.7 Radiation Dose 177
11.8 Quantifying Risks and Benefits 177
   References................................. 179

11.1 Introduction

No woman has ever been shown to have developed breast cancer as a result of mammography, not even from multiple studies received over many years with doses higher than the current average dose to the glandular tissues of the breast of approximately 2.5 mGy (250 mrad) (McLelland et al. 1991). However, the possibility of such risk has been raised because of excess breast cancers observed among populations exposed to much higher doses of 1–20 Gy (100–2000 rad). These mainly include Japanese A-bomb survivors (Kato and Schull 1982; McGregor et al. 1977; Preston et al. 1987; Preston and Pierce 1988; Shimizu et al. 1988, 1989; Tokunaga et al. 1979, 1984, 1987), North American tuberculosis sanatoria patients from Massachusetts (Boice et al. 1979; Hrubec et al. 1989) and Canada who underwent multiple chest fluoroscopies (Howe et al. 1982; Howe 1984; Miller et al. 1989), women from New York State (Mettler et al. 1969; Shore et al. 1977, 1986) and Sweden (Baral et al. 1977; Mattson et al. 1993) treated with radiation therapy

---

S.A. Feig, MD, Professor of Radiology, Jefferson Medical College, Director, Breast Imaging, Department of Radiology, Thomas Jefferson University Hospital, 1100 Walnut Street, Philadelphia, PA 19107, USA
R.E. Hendrick, PhD, Associate Professor and Chief, Division of Radiological Sciences, Department of Radiology, C278, University of Colorado, Health Sciences Center, 4200 E. Ninth Avenue, Denver, CO 80262, USA

for benign breast conditions such as postpartum mastitis, infants treated in New York State for thymic enlargement with radiation therapy (Hildreth et al. 1989), and women who had been treated in California with radiation therapy for Hodgkin's disease (Hancock et al. 1993). This chapter will estimate the hypothetical risk from mammography based on the latest radiation risk estimates provided by the National Academy of Sciences–National Research Council Committee on the Biological Effects of Ionizing Radiation (BEIR V Committee 1990) and compare such risk to the projected benefits from screening.

11.2 Risk Assessment

The need for a new report on radiation risk by the BEIR V Committee was based on a revision of A-bomb dosimetry, longer term follow-up of the Japanese survivors, and availability of newer computational techniques and models for risk estimates. Due to the lower estimates for both exposure dose and neutron component with the new DS86 A-bomb dosimetry, estimates for Kerma (kinetic energy released in matter) and absorbed breast doses are less. Since the number of breast cancers in the exposed population per year is fixed while estimates of absorbed breast dose are lower, the breast cancer risk estimates in the BEIR V report (BEIR V Committee 1990) are higher than those in the previous 1985 NIH report (National Institutes of Health 1985).

The BEIR V estimates for excess breast cancer mortality were based on data from the Canadian fluoroscopy study (Miller et al. 1989) and the Radiation Effects Research Foundation (RERF) Life Span Study (LSS) of A-bomb survivors (Shimizu et al. 1989). Estimates for excess breast cancer incidence were based on a subset of women from the Japanese A-bomb survivor LSS incidence series for whom revised dose estimates were available (Tokunaga et al. 1987), the New York acute postpartum mastitis study (Shore et al. 1986), and data on women in the Massachusetts tuberculosis fluoroscopy cohort (HRUBEC et al. 1989) (Table 11.1).

Each of these populations has both strengths and limitations with respect to radiation risk estimates for the small, fractionated doses from multiple annual mammographic exposures to American women. The Japanese A-bomb survivor cohort represents a large study population exposed to a wide range of doses yet it is non-Caucasian and received its entire dose in a single exposure. The Massachusetts fluoroscopy cohort was a U.S. population receiving highly fractionated exposures but the number of women involved was statistically small and the presence of tuberculosis could have affected cancer risk estimates. The Canadian fluoroscopy patients were a large population of North American women receiving fractionated exposures but they also had tuberculosis. The risk estimate for the Nova Scotia component of the Canadian fluoroscopy patients was found to be six times higher than that for women in the other provinces, possibly since the Nova Scotia patients were fluoroscoped while they faced the x-ray tube while elsewhere the patients were usually fluoroscoped from the back. Dose estimates for the Rochester, New York women receiving radiation therapy for postpartum mastitis were highly accurate, but their risk estimate was higher than that for the other groups, probably due to the hormonal and hyperplastic effects of pregnancy and the presence of inflammatory breast disease. Moreover, this cohort was relatively small.

Estimating the risk of breast cancer from radiation is complex. Different estimates for radiation risk for breast cancer have been made by various committees over the past 15 years, most notably, by the National Cancer Institute (NCI) Ad Hoc Working Group on the risks associated with mammography in mass screening for the detection of breast cancer (UPTON et al. 1977), by the Committee on the Biological Effects of Ionizing Radiation (BEIR III) of the National Academy of Sciences (BEIR III 1980), and by the National Institutes of Health (NIH) Ad Hoc Committee to Develop Radioepidemiological Tables (National Institutes of Health 1985). Each committee, including the BEIR V group in 1990, has had to base their estimate not only on the best data available at that time, but also on a selection of other options such as dose-response models, latent period, age at exposure, and additive and relative risk models.

The risk estimate will depend on both dose and selection of a dose-response relation (linear, quadratic, or linear-quadratic). Risk will also vary according to age at time of exposure. It may be predicted either as a number of excess cases or deaths (additive risk) or as a percent increase in the natural breast cancer incidence or death rate (relative risk). Risk will also depend on time; after exposure there will be a risk-free latent period followed by a period of risk of a given duration. Moreover, risk could be either constant or variable during this latter period.

11.3 Dose-Response Models

Although studies of populations exposed to high doses provide proof of carcinogenic risk to the breast at these levels of radiation, these same studies contain no direct evidence of risk from doses in the mammographic range. Because radiation-induced and spontaneously occurring breast cancers cannot be distinguished histologically (TOKUOKA et al. 1984; DVORETSKY et al. 1980), the presence of radiation-induced breast cancers can only be inferred in a statistical sense. This type of demonstration of risk

Table 11.1. Characteristics of study populations used for BEIR V breast cancer risk estimates

Study population	Reference	Endpoint	Cases	Person-years
A-bomb survivors	TOKUNAGA et al. (1987)	Incidence	376	940 300
	SHIMIZU et al. (1989)	Mortality	153	1 163 200
Canadian fluoroscopy patients (non-Nova Scotia)	MILLER et al. (1989)	Mortality	402	721 000
Massachusetts fluoroscopy	HRUBEC et al. (1989)	Incidence	74	30 932
New York radiotherapy	SHORE et al. (1986)	Incidence	115	45 000

becomes harder and harder to obtain as lower and lower doses are considered. If excess risk is proportional to dose, the number of women needed to test an excess is inversely proportional to the square of the dose. For example, if 1000 exposed and 1000 control women are needed to test risk at 1 Gy, then two groups of 100 000 women each are necessary at 0.1 Gy and two groups of 10 000 000 women each are necessary at 1 cGy (LAND 1980).

If there is any risk to the breast from low doses, the magnitude of this risk could be estimated by means of dose-response curves which describe three possible relationships between radiation dose and radiogenic cancer incidence (Fig. 11.1). In the linear dose-response model, incidence is directly proportional to dose: if the dose is diminished by a factor of 10, the excess cancer incidence will also be reduced by the same factor. With the quadratic dose-response relationship, the effect is proportional to the dose squared: if the dose is reduced by a factor of 10, the number of excess cancers would be reduced by a factor of 100. The linear-quadratic dose-response relationship predicts a risk intermediate between the risks expected from pure linear and pure quadratic models. It is generally agreed that the linear dose-response model represents the upper limits of risk and that the quadratic model defines the lower limits of risk.

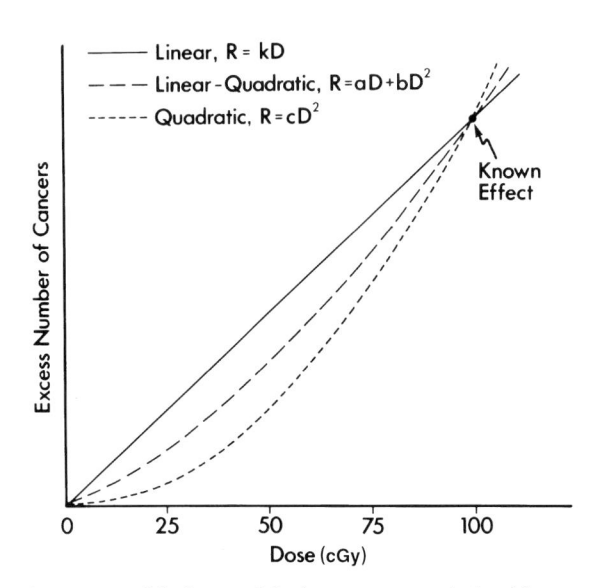

Fig. 11.1. Models for possible dose-response relationships at low doses. Most estimates for the hypothetical breast cancer risk from mammography have employed a linear dose-response model with the understanding that this projection represents the upper limits of such risk

Most data on radiation-induced breast cancer in humans do not clearly favor any one of the three different risk models for doses below 1 Gy (100 rads) (FEIG and EHRLICH 1990). All of these studies contain a paucity of data on doses below 0.5 Gy (50 rads) and none provides any direct information concerning risks from doses less than 0.1 Gy (10 rads). Even the best indirect evidence provided by the Japanese data has a limited ability to discriminate among the three models. Although most, but not all, experiments on a wide variety of radiation-induced animal tumors exhibit a quadratic dose-response relationship at these doses (BEIR III 1980), it might be argued that a similar relationship may not necessarily hold for radiation response in humans. For these reasons, risk estimates for radiation-induced breast cancer provided by the BEIR V Committee employed a linear dose-response relationship.

11.4 Latent Period and Duration

The latent period refers to the minimal length of time between exposure and earliest demonstration of excess cancer in the population. Because radiogenic breast cancers do not occur earlier than the spontaneous variety, the latent period may depend on age at exposure. The BEIR V report assumed a latent period of about 10 years after exposure before the risk of breast cancer induction due to radiation is nonnegligible. It also assumed that the period of excess risk may persist for the patient's lifetime since all populations have continued to exhibit excess breast cancer risk on the longest follow-up studies, 30–45 years after exposure (HRUBEC et al. 1989; MILLER et al. 1989; SHIMIZU et al. 1989; SHORE et al. 1986; TOKUNAGA et al. 1987).

11.5 Age at Exposure

All but one of the population studies demonstrate a strong dependence of risk on the age of the women at the time of exposure, with exposure at younger ages causing higher risks (BARAL et al. 1977; BOICE et al. 1979; HANCOCK et al. 1993; HOWE 1984; HOWE et al. 1982; MATTSON et al. 1993; PRESTON et al. 1987; SHIMIZU et al. 1989; TOKUNAGA et al. 1987). New York women treated with radiotherapy for postpartum mastitis (SHORE et al. 1986) constitute the only group which has not shown any relationship of risk to age at exposure. However, their breasts were in a proliferative state with elevated hormonal stimulation associated with parturition and lactation. The BEIR V report concluded that "there is little evidence of any increased risk to women exposed after age 40."

11.6 Additive and Relative Risk Models

Additive and relative risk models represent two different methods of estimating excess risk (stated as either excess breast cancer incidence or mortality) following radiation. Additive (absolute) risk estimates are given as the number of excess cancers/million women/year/cGy (rad). Relative risk estimates are given as the percent increase in the natural breast cancer incidence/year/cGy (rad). With both models, risk estimates are higher for exposure at younger ages. With the additive risk model, the risk projection remains constant each year after the latent period (Fig. 11.2). With the relative risk model, the absolute risk projection increases with age after exposure since relative risk represents a fixed percentage of the natural (spontaneous) breast cancer incidence, which also increases with age (Fig. 11.3).

Early studies were unable to determine which of these models was more appropriate, but later analyses of Japanese A-bomb survivors (KATO and SCHULL 1982; PRESTON et al. 1987; SHIMIZU et al. 1988), Canadian fluoroscopy patients (HOWE 1984), and New York radiotherapy patients (SHORE et al. 1986) strongly favored a constant relative risk model. Analyses such as the NIH-85 Report observed that for the same age-at-exposure cohort, excess breast cancer incidence increased each year in proportion to the natural breast cancer incidence and did not

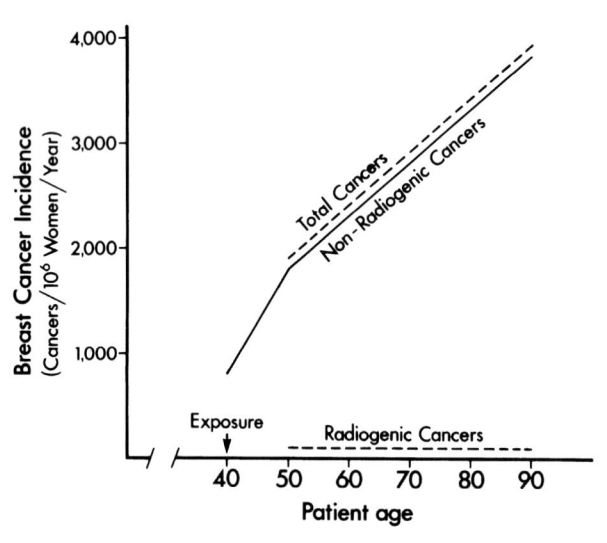

Fig. 11.2. Constant additive risk model

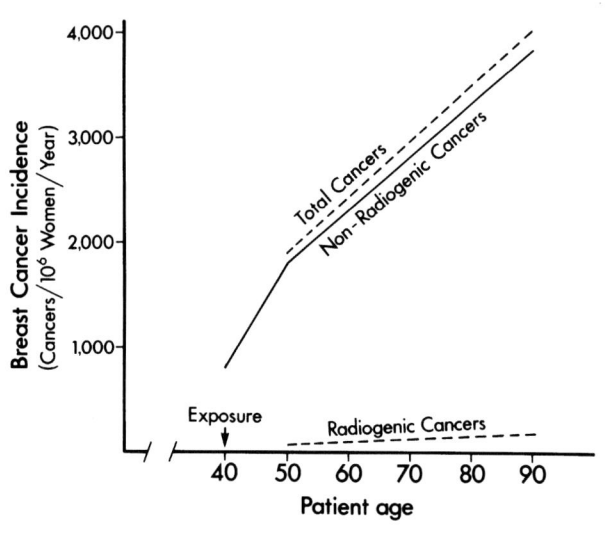

Fig. 11.3. Constant relative risk model

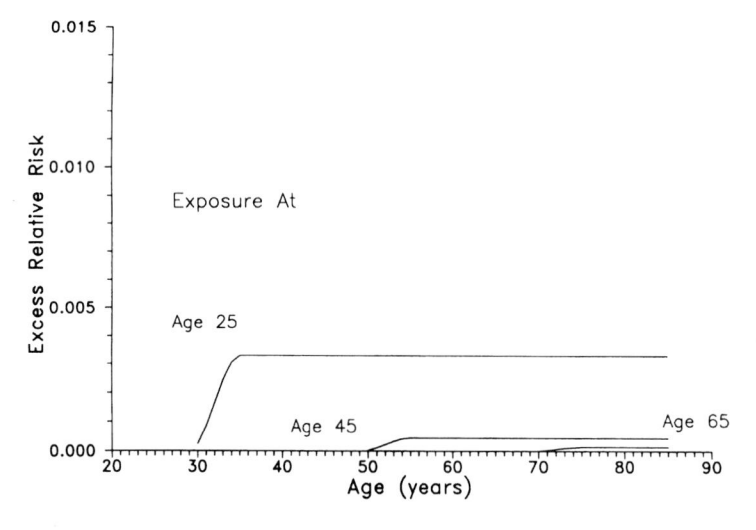

Fig. 11.4. Relative risk estimates for excess breast cancer incidence for absorbed dose of 1 cGy (1 rad) according to age at exposure. Based on data from National Institute of Health Ad Hoc Committee to Develop Radioepidemiological Tables (NIH-85)

Fig. 11.5. Relative risk estimates for excess breast cancer incidence for absorbed glandular dose of 1 cGy (1 rad) according to age at exposure. Based on data from National Academy of Sciences, National Research Council Committee on the Biological Effects of Ionizing Radiation (BEIR V)

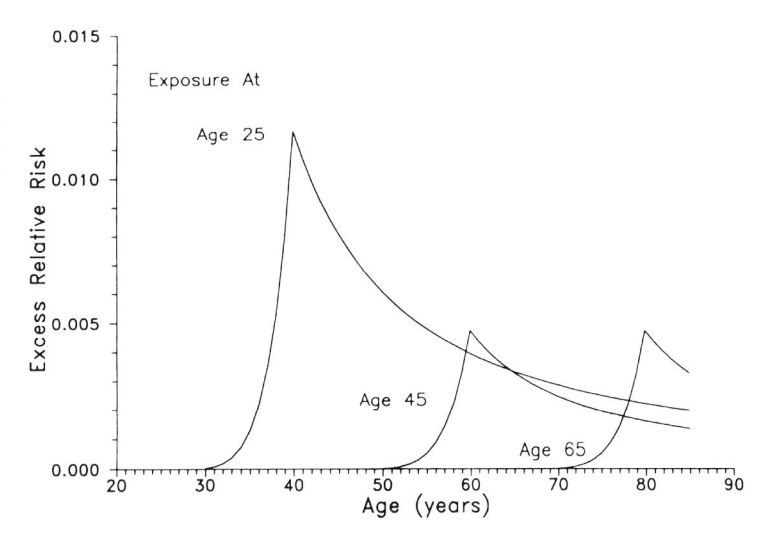

conform to a pattern of constant excess incidence over time.

Although the BEIR V report is similar to the NIH-85 report in favoring a relative rather than an additive risk model, BEIR V represents a departure from previous reports in employing a time-dependent rather than a time-independent (constant) relative risk model. In such a time-dependent model, relative risk varies over time during the follow-up period, reaching a peak at 15–20 years after exposure and then declining (Figs. 11.4, 11.5).

11.7 Radiation Dose

The mean glandular dose for a breast of average size and composition using Min-R Screen/Min-R M Film would be 2.3 mGy (0.23 rad) for a two-view per breast grid study (Haus 1987), similar to the average 2.5 mGy (0.25 rad) dose for film-screen studies in the ACR Mammography Accreditation Program (McLelland et al. 1991). This dose can be reduced by about 30% by means of 3-min extended processing (Kimme-Smith et al. 1989; Tabar and Haus 1989) or 40% by using Min-R Medium Screens with Min-R M Film (Tabar and Haus 1989). In this paper, risk estimates will assume a 2.5 mGy (0.25 rad) mean breast dose. Assumption of other dose values would affect risk proportionately.

11.8 Quantifying Risks and Benefits

The final steps in obtaining estimates for radiation risk should be selection of either an additive or a relative risk model and selection of excess incidence and/or mortality as the measured endpoint.

Using incidence data, the BEIR V Committee found that the excess relative risk for A-bomb survivors was 50% greater than that in the Massachusetts fluoroscopy and New York radiotherapy series but that the difference was not statistically significant ($P = 0.4$). The additive excess incidence rate per unit dose in the Japanese A-bomb population was 50% lower than in the two U.S. cohorts. The difference was statistically significant ($P = 0.01$). Based on these data, the BEIR V Committee decided to use a relative risk model to estimate excess incidence using pooled data from the three incidence series.

Using mortality data, estimated relative risk for A-bomb survivors was two to three times higher than that for Canadian provinces other than Nova Scotia and about half that for Nova Scotia women. These differences were not statistically significant ($P = 0.12$ and $P = 0.2$ respectively). Additive risk estimates were found to fit the mortality data equally well.

Based on these results, the BEIR V Committee decided to use a time-dependent relative risk model for both breast cancer incidence and mortality. These models can then be used to obtain numerical estimates for the risk from mammography, which can then be compared to the expected benefit from screening.

For women exposed at age 45 to 1 cGy (1 rad), excess breast cancer incidence would show a nonnegligible increase by 10 years post-exposure. There would be a peak 0.5% increase in the breast cancer incidence by age 60 (15 years post-exposure) which would drop to a 0.2% increase by age 70 (25 years post-exposure) (Fig. 11.5). Assuming a mean breast dose of 2.5 mGy (0.25 rad) from a two-view per breast mammography examination taken with a grid, the incidence at age 60 would be increased only 0.125% and would drop to a 0.05% increase by age 70.

The BEIR V report also includes lifetime risk estimates for mortality from radiogenic breast cancer. It obtains these by multiplying the time-dependent relative risk estimates for mortality (Fig. 11.6) to survival probabilities for an unexposed population and then sums the results for each year. For example, the report estimates 20 excess breast cancer deaths resulting from exposure of each of 100 000 women to 10 rem at age 45. Using a 2.5 mGy (0.25 rad) mean glandular dose from mammography, it can be seen that mammographic examination of one million women at age 45 could result in five excess breast cancer deaths during their lifetime. This lifetime risk of death (five in one million) would be about the same as traveling 5000 miles by plane (round trip New York City to Los Angeles), 450 miles by car (round trip New York City to Boston), smoking three cigarettes, or simply being alive for 15 min at age 60 (National Safety Council 1988; POCHIN 1978).

A more clinically meaningful perspective on risk can be obtained by comparing the number of deaths potentially caused by radiation with the number of breast cancer deaths averted through screening. Data from the Cancer Statistics Review (1973–1988) indicate that among one million U.S. women age 45, approximately 1500 breast cancers should surface clinically during a year and that in the absence of screening a long-term 50% breast cancer mortality can eventually be expected, resulting in 750 deaths from breast cancer (National Cancer Institute 1991). Assuming that a single mammographic screening of these women would reduce that number of deaths by either 20%, 40%, or 60%, this would mean that either 150, 300, or 450 breast cancer deaths would be averted, clearly a favorable result compared with a theoretical risk of five deaths from screening mammography. Screening at older ages would result in greater benefits since the natural incidence of breast cancer increases with age.

Table 11.2. Breast cancer risk from 2.5 mGy (0.25 rad) at age 45 years, assuming subsequent periodic screening

Mortality reduction due to subsequent screening	Lifetime risk: excess deaths/million women
0%	5.0
20%	4.0
40%	3.0
60%	2.0

Risk estimate based on BEIR V Report (1990)

Table 11.3. Breast cancer deaths averted per death caused by a single screening at age 45 years, with a dose of 2.5 mGy (0.25 rad) from a two-view per breast mammogram

	Mortality reduction		
	20%	40%	60%
Assuming no further screening	30	60	90
Assuming subsequent screening	37.5	100	225

Risk estimate based on BEIR V Report, National Research Council (1990)

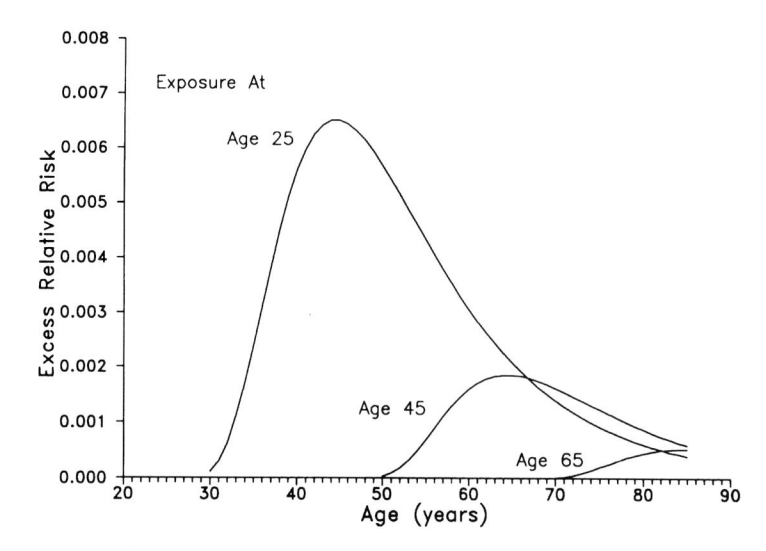

Fig. 11.6. Relative risk estimates for excess breast cancer mortality for an absorbed glandular dose of 1 cGy (1 rad) as a function of age for exposure at various ages. Based on the BEIR V Report

Continued annual screening would reduce the number of potential breast cancer deaths from the initial screening since subsequent screening would detect a proportion of radiogenic cancers at a curable stage (Table 11.2). Benefit/risk ratios for deaths averted/deaths caused by mammographic screening under several possible levels of benefit are shown in Table 11.3. Therefore, the risk from mammography appears to be small compared with the range of mortality reduction achievable through screening.

References

Baral E, Larrson LE, Mattson B (1977) Breast cancer following irradiation of the breast. Cancer 40:2905–2910

BEIR III Committee on the Biological Effects of Ionizing Radiation (1980) The effects on populations of exposure to low levels of ionizing radiation. National Academy of Sciences, Washington DC

BEIR V Committee on the Biological Effects of Ionizing Radiation (1990) Health effects of exposure to low levels of ionizing radiation. National Academy Press, Washington DC

Boice JD, Land CE, Shore RE, Norman JE, Tokunaga M (1979) Risk of breast cancer following low-dose radiation exposure. Radiology 131:589–597

Dvoretsky PM, Woodard E, Bonfiglio TA, Hempelmann LH, Morse IP (1980) The pathology of breast cancer in women irradiated for acute postpartum mastitis. Cancer 46:2257–2262

Feig SA, Ehrlich SM (1990) Estimation of radiation risk from screening mammography: recent trends and comparison with expected benefits. Radiology 174:638–647

Hancock SL, Tucker MA, Hoppe RT (1993) Breast cancer after treatment of Hodgkin's disease. J Natl Cancer Inst 85:25–31

Haus AG (1987) Recent advances in screen-film mammography. Radiol Clin North Am 25:913–928

Hildreth NG, Shore RE, Dvoretsky PM (1989) The risk of breast cancer after irradiation of the thymus in infancy. N Engl J Med 321:1281–1284

Howe GR (1984) Epidemiology of radiogenic breast cancer. In: Boice JD, Fraumeni JF (eds) Radiation carcinogenesis: epidemiology and biological significance. Raven Press, New York, p 119

Howe GR, Miller AB, Sherman GJ (1982) Breast cancer mortality following fluoroscopic irradiation in a cohort of tuberculosis patients. Cancer Detect Prev 5:175–178

Hrubec Z, Boice JD, Monson RR, Rosenstein R (1989) Breast cancer after multiple chest fluoroscopies: second follow-up of Massachusetts women with tuberculosis. Cancer Res 49:229–234

Kato H, Schull WJ (1982) Studies of the mortality of A-bomb survivors. 7. Mortality, 1950–1978. I. Cancer mortality. Radiat Res 90:395–432

Kimme-Smith C, Rothschild PA, Bassett LW, Gold RH, Moler C (1989) Mammographic film processor temperature, development time, and chemistry: effect on dose, contrast, and noise. AJR 152:35–40

Land CE (1980) Estimating cancer risk from low doses of ionizing radiation. Science 290: 1197–1203

Mattson A, Bengt-Inge R, Hall P, Wilking N, Rutqvist LE (1993) Radiation-induced breast cancer: long-term follow-up of radiation therapy for benign breast disease. J Natl Cancer Inst 85:1679–1685

McGregor DH, Land CE, Choi K, Tokuoka S, Liu PI, Wakabayashi T, Beebe GW (1977) Breast cancer incidence among atomic bomb survivors, Hiroshima and Nagasaki, 1950–1969. J Natl Cancer Inst 59:799–811

McLelland R, Hendrick RE, Wilcox P, Zinninger MD (1991) The American College of Radiology mammography accreditation program. Am J Roentgenol 157:473–479

Mettler FA, Hempelmann LH, Dutton AM, Pifer JW, Toyooka ET, Ames WR (1969) Breast neoplasms in women treated with x-rays for acute post-partum mastitis. A pilot study. J Natl Cancer Inst 43:803–811

Miller AB, Howe GR, Sherman GJ, et al. (1989) Mortality from breast cancer after irradiation during fluoroscopic examinations in patients being treated for tuberculosis. N Engl J Med 321:1285–1289

National Cancer Institute, Division of Cancer Prevention and Control (1991) Annual Cancer Statistics Review, Including Cancer Trends 1955–1990. NIH Publication No. 91, National Institutes of Health, National Cancer Institute, Bethesda MD

National Institutes of Health Ad Hoc Working Group to Develop Radioepidemiological Tables (1985) Report of the National Institutes of Health Ad Hoc Working Group to Develop Radioepidemiological Tables. NIH Publication No. 85-2748, National Institutes of Health, National Cancer Institute, Bethesda MD

National Safety Council (1988) Transportation accident passenger death rates 1987. NSC Washington DC

Pochin EE (1978) Why be quantitative about radiation risks? Lecture no. 2 in: The Lauriston S Taylor Lecture Series in Radiation Protection and Measurements. National Council on Radiation Protection and Measurements, Washington DC

Preston DL, Pierce DA (1988) The effect of changes in dosimetry on cancer mortality risk estimates in atomic bomb survivors. Radiat Res 114:437–466

Preston DL, Kato H, Kopecky KJ, Fujita S (1987) Studies of the mortality of A-bomb survivors: cancer mortality, 1950–1982. Radiat Res 111:151–178

Shimizu Y, Kato H, Schull WJ (1988) Life span study report 11. II. Cancer mortality in the years 1950–1985 based on the recently revised doses (DS86). RERF TR/5-88. Radiation Effects Research Foundation, Hiroshima, Japan

Shimizu Y, Kato H, Schull WJ, Preston DL, Fujita S, Pierce DA (1989) Studies of the mortality of A-bomb survivors. 9. Mortality, 1950–1985. I. Comparison or risk coefficients for site-specific cancer mortality based on DS86 and T65 DR shielded kerma and organ doses. Radiat Res 118:502–524

Shore RE, Hempelmann L, Kowaluk E, Mansur PS, Pasternack BS, Albert RE, Haughie GE (1977) Breast neoplasms in women treated with x-rays for acute postpartum mastitis. J Natl Cancer Inst 59:813–822

Shore RE, Hildreth N, Woodard ED, Dvoretsky P, Hempelmann L, Pasternack B (1986) Breast cancer among women given x-ray therapy for acute postpartum mastitis. J Natl Cancer Inst 77:689–696

Tabar L, Haus AG (1989) Processing of mammographic films: technical and clinical considerations. Radiology 173:65–69

Tokunaga M, Norman JE, Asano M (1979) Malignant breast tumors among atomic bomb survivors. Hiroshima and Nagasaki, 1950–1974. J Natl Cancer Inst 62:1347–1359

Tokunaga M, Land CE, Yamamoto T, et al. (1984) Breast cancer among atomic bomb survivors. In: Boice JD, Fraumeni JF (eds) Radiation carcinogenesis: epidemiology and biological significance. Raven Press, New York, p 45

Tokunaga M, Land CE, Yamamoto T, et al. (1987) Incidence of female breast cancer among atomic bomb survivors,

Hiroshima and Nagasaki, 1950–1980. Radiat Res 112:243–272

Tokuoka S, Asano M, Tsutomu Y, et al. (1984) Histologic review of breast cancer cases in survivors of atomic bombs in Hiroshima and Nagasaki, Japan. Cancer 54:849–854

Upton AC, Beebe GW, Brown JM, Quimby EH, Shellabarger C (1977) Report of the NCI Ad Hoc Working Group on the risks associated with mammography in the mass screening for the detection of breast cancer. J Natl Cancer Inst 59:481–493

12 Echomammography: Technique and Results

J. TEUBNER

CONTENTS

12.1	Introduction	181
12.2	Basic Technical Principles	182
12.3	Scanning Techniques	183
12.4	Real-Time Examination Technique	184
12.5	Sonographic Visualization of Breast Tumors	185
12.5.1	Echogenicity of the Lesion	185
12.5.2	Macroscopic Growth Pattern of the Tumorous Mass	186
12.5.3	Background Pattern of the Host Tissue	186
12.6	Sonographic Diagnostic Criteria	187
12.7	Normal Anatomy	189
12.8	Fibrocystic Disease (Mastopathy)	191
12.8.1	Circumscribed Mastopathic Changes	192
12.8.2	Intra- and Periductal Mastopathic Changes	194
12.8.3	Diffuse Mastopathic Changes	196
12.9	Cysts	196
12.10	Benign Solid Lesions	199
12.10.1	Fibroadenomas	199
12.10.2	Hamartomas	200
12.10.3	Adenomas	200
12.10.4	Lipomas	201
12.10.5	Abscesses	201
12.10.6	Chronic or Interstitial Mastitis	201
12.10.7	Scars	203
12.10.8	Fat Necrosis	203
12.10.9	Oil Cysts	203
12.10.10	Lesions Following Breast Augmentation Mammoplasty	203
12.11	Malignant Diseases	204
12.11.1	Intraductal Carcinoma	204
12.11.2	Invasive Ductal Carcinoma	207
12.11.3	Spiculated Carcinoma	209
12.11.4	Circumscribed Carcinoma	210
12.11.5	Diffusely Infiltrating Carcinoma	211
12.11.6	Inflammatory Carcinoma	212
12.12	Diagnostic Value of Ultrasonography in Breast Cancer Diagnosis	212
	References	217

12.1 Introduction

The first studies on ultrasound examination of the breast were performed in the early 1950s (HOWRY et al. 1954; WILD and REID 1952, 1954), but it was 20 years later, after the introduction of gray-scale imaging, that diagnostic sonographic visualization of complex breast structures became possible (JELLINS et al. 1971; KOSSOFF 1972). At that time, however, the resolution necessary for early breast cancer detection could not be achieved.

Up to the end of the 1970s automatic immersion scanners or compound scanners with hand-held probes with or without water bags were exclusively used. With these static methods, diagnostic criteria were established that are still valid today (COLE-BEUGLET and BEIQUE 1975; COLE-BEUGLET et al. 1980; DALE et al. 1975; GROS et al. 1977; KASUMI et al. 1982; KOBAYASHI 1979; KOSSOFF et al. 1976; TEIXIDOR and KAZAM 1977).

In the early 1980s, high-resolution 5- to 10-MHz real-time scanners were introduced (FLEISCHER et al. 1983; FRIEDRICH 1980; LEES 1981; TEUBNER et al. 1981; WEISS et al. 1978). The main advantages of these systems are that they enable *dynamic* breast imaging (TEUBNER et al. 1982, 1985a; VILARO et al. 1989). These advantages are due to the improved three-dimensional visualization and assessment of breast lesions with "real-time" examination of the tissue, evaluation of the tissue elasticity and observation of changes in tissue absorption with varying compression (TEUBNER et al. 1985b; UENO et al. 1988; SALVADOR et al. 1994; WALZ et al. 1994), direct correlation of physical and ultrasonic findings, and unrestricted choice of any scanning plane. Initially, however, this dynamic examination procedure was regarded critically because of its perceived disadvantages in not being transferable from expert to novice users, the difficulty of systematic documentation, the poor reproducibility of findings (limited field of view/free choice of scanning planes), and the limited resolution in the near field (EGAN and EGAN 1984; FLEISCHER et al. 1985).

Extensive clinical application of breast ultrasonography was initially impeded because of a considerable overlap in the diagnostic criteria of benign and malignant lesions. Therefore, its main indication was often only seen in the differentiation between

---

J. TEUBNER, MD, MSc, Department of Radiology, Faculty of Clinical Medicine Mannheim, University of Heidelberg, Theodor Kutzer Ufer, 68167 Mannheim, Germany

cystic and solid lesions (Bassett et al. 1987; Cole-Beuglet et al. 1983b; Dempsey 1988; Feig 1989; Kopans et al. 1982). Other publications stated that all solid-appearing lesions are potentially malignant, regardless of their sonographic characteristics; thus biopsy was recommended in order to be on the safe side (Cole-Beuglet et al. 1983a–c; Jackson et al. 1986; Heywang et al. 1984). Similar considerations led to its rejection as a screening method [in particular, it proved difficult to differentiate small lesions (Hirst 1994; Pamilo et al. 1991)] and in early cancer detection (Sickles et al. 1983; Teubner 1985c). On the other hand, many positive reports existed on the differential diagnosis of larger solid breast lesions (Fornage et al. 1989; Harper et al. 1983; Kobayashi 1979; Leucht et al. 1988; Majewski et al. 1986; Smallwood et al. 1986; Teubner et al. 1985a; Ueno et al. 1985, 1988). The merits of breast ultrasonography as a diagnostic tool were increasingly recognized and then proven with the introduction of high-resolution real-time ultrasonography (Maslak 1985). Today breast ultrasonography is seen as the most important adjunct examination to mammography for appropriately selected patients (Stavros et al. 1995; Gordon 1995; Jackson 1995). State-of-the-art hand-held high-frequency linear-array probes allow imaging of small nonpalpable carcinomas less than 1 cm in diameter, which can be further differentiated through ultrasound-guided fine-needle aspiration biopsy (Fornage et al. 1990). However, breast ultrasound examination still has no proven role in screening asymptomatic women for nonpalpable carcinoma.

The supplementary role of breast ultrasonography to mammography is due to the physical differences in image generation. The acousto-mechanical properties of the various breast tissue components are independent of their x-ray absorption properties, which leads to differing sonographic and mammographic tissue contrasts; thereby ultrasonography can improve considerably the visualization of tumors in radio-dense breasts. Additionally, as a cross-sectional imaging technique, breast ultrasonography enables tissue visualization free from overprojection, thus rendering possible detailed contour analysis of lesions, exact determination of tumor size, and assessment of internal tissue compositions as well as improved assessment of lesions located in the breast periphery or close to the chest wall.

The role of breast ultrasonography is also important in the detection and staging of lymph node metastases. Thus, ultrasonography opens up new possibilities in the diagnosis of equivocal mammographic findings, in the early diagnosis of carcinoma, and in the follow-up of tumor patients, as will be addressed later.

12.2 Basic Technical Principles

Ultrasonic image generation is based on the pulse-echo process, i.e., the generation of high-frequency sound impulses alternating with the electronic registration of sound waves which are reflected from tissue interfaces. In breast ultrasonography frequencies between 5 and 10 MHz are applied.

The resolution property of the transducer differs laterally and axially to the direction of sound propagation and depends on the transmission frequency, the pulse length, the beam focusing, and the tissue depth visualized. In linear-array scanners the lateral resolution (parallel to the scanning plane) is electronically controlled through varying selectable focal zones, whereas the in-plane focal zone (along the short axis) is fixed and determined by the width of the probe surface and a mechanically applied lens. By shifting the in-plane focal zone through appropriate stand-off devices (gel-pad, etc.) towards the superficial tissue layers, visualization of lesions located beneath the skin can be strongly enhanced, resulting in improved differentiation of small cystic versus solid tissue components and better contour analysis by reduction of slice thickness artifacts.

Mechanical sector scanners generally have an incorporated water path and a single-element or annular-array transducer which has identical lateral and in-plane resolution properties. Their contrast resolution is often better than that of linear-array scanners although the considerably slower image generation may affect the examination procedure. The trapezoid scan form with oblique incidences of sound waves on the lateral edges may produce additional shadowing artifacts.

Contrast resolution plays a decisive role in tissue discrimination. It is determined by the three-dimensional beam profile which is made up of the central beam and the "side lobes." The smaller the side lobes, the less sound energy is received from the off-axis area, i.e., the area adjacent to the actual tissue structure, thus enhancing the tissue contrast. The beam profile of the probe is manufacturer-dependent and determines whether the equipment yields "good" or "poor" tissue discrimination.

The axial resolution largely depends on the pulse length and varies only slightly from system to system. It therefore plays only a subordinate role in the overall resolution.

A higher transmission frequency improves the resolution by better beam focusing. However, sound absorption by the tissue increases, thus reducing the maximum penetration depth. For this reason frequencies of ≥10 MHz can only be used for detailed analysis in close-up views or with small breasts.

12.3 Scanning Techniques

The technical development of breast ultrasonography is characterized by diverging methodological approaches. Over recent decades almost all sonographic imaging procedures have been tested and new examination modalities are still being developed. This is because the breast is to be considered a sonographically difficult organ for the following reasons:

- Inhomogeneous tissue composition (fat, glandular, and connective tissue) with marked variation in the individual echo pattern and sound course with consequent multiple refraction artifacts along border areas, hindering the detection of small breast lesions
- Pliability of the breast and superficial location of tissue layers, causing difficulties in sound coupling and near-field focusing
- Overlap of diagnostic criteria of benign and malignant lesions, demanding an exquisite echographic image quality
- Volume rendering of the breast and its documentation (problems of reproducibility and follow-up)

Additionally the technical development has been influenced by two different clinical goals:

a) *Replacement* of other imaging procedures such as mammography as an independent examination procedure
b) Provision of a *complementary* examination technique for palpable or equivocal mammographic findings

ad a): For the total volume-rendering examination of the breast, automated dedicated breast scanners were developed (water path and immersion scanners).

With water bag scanners, the examination was carried out with the water bag positioned on the breast with the patient in a supine position. A single-element tranducer was mechanically moved in the water bag on an arc-like or linear scan (JELLINS et al. 1971). With this equipment, static cross-sectional images of the whole breast were documented in millimeter increments. In particular Japanese authors performed studies with this type of equipment in the mid-1970s (KOBAYASHI 1977). The biplane scanner was a further development of this scanning technique (KELLY-FRY et al. 1987; JACKSON et al. 1986). All water path scanners combined the advantages of an almost completely automated imaging process and a better correlation of palpatory and sonographic findings compared with immersion scanners, as well as allowing easier choice of the scan plane and direction with respect to the individual breast.

With immersion scanners the patient was placed prone over a water tank with her breasts immersed freely. Transducers with long focal lengths were used individually in a linear or sector scan, or in combination, as a compound scan which could be programmed for various slice distances and scan directions.

Despite the pioneering scientific work of Australian (KOSSOFF et al. 1976; JELLINS et al. 1982) and American authors (COLE-BEUGLET et al. 1980, 1983a), these systems had no lasting influence. This is due to various clinical disadvantages compared to other automated hand-held systems: poor sound transmission in uncompressed immersed breast tissue, time-of-flight artifacts frustrating expected compound capabilities, lack of correlation with palpatory findings, lack of feasibility of dynamic compression tests, long examination times (VAN KAICK et al. 1980; TEUBNER et al. 1982), and failure of the method to fulfill its expected role in breast screening (KOPANS 1984; SICKLES et al. 1983).

ad b): Prior to real-time scanners, hand-held slow compound scanners were state of the art. In general small-area (6 mmø) short-focused mechanical 5-MHz probes were used in direct skin contact (TEIXIDOR and KAZAM 1977; GROS et al. 1977; VAN KAICK et al. 1980). This equipment was suitable for the sonographic evaluation of localized palpatory or mammographic findings. However, slow image generation, inconvenient handling requiring considerable skill, and shortcomings in the examination of the whole breast proved disadvantageous.

All other hand-held scanning techniques are based on real-time technology and are preferred because they are cheaper, faster, and more applicable for interventional guidance. Initially only mechanical sector scanners with moderate resolution were available (DALE and GROS 1977; FRIEDRICH and KROLL 1981). In general, sector-scanning probes are less advisable for breast ultrasonography because of their oblique angle of sound incidence on the curved breast contour and on intramammary anatomical structures. A sector angle of ±20° with an integrated water path is just about acceptable. Mechanical or electronic scanners with larger sector angles (>60°) and without a water path are unsuitable because of the poor image quality in the near-field range and lateral image distortion.

State-of-the-art high-resolution real-time scanners are equipped with electronically focused linear-array probes of 5- to 10-MHz sound frequencies. For total breast examinations, probes with a scanning width of 4.5–6.5 cm are recommended. Smaller (<3.5 cm), high-frequency (10- to 13-MHz) transducers are only suitable for detailed evaluation of superficially located lesions or for ultrasound-guided biopsy. Nowadays, with miniaturized individual crystals and a large number of channels, scan line densities of 3–10 lines per millimeter can be achieved. When the individual crystal elements are coupled to individual electronic delay circuits, a self-focusing concave wave-front can be generated, mimicking a mechanical acoustical lens. A decisive advantage of this technology is that the focal zone can be freely defined for the various tissue depths. This principle is applied in both transmission (variable fixed focus) and receiver mode (dynamic focusing).

Directly below the surface of the transducer (in the so-called beam-forming zone) the resolution is not particularly good. Therefore, in order to better visualize superficial tissue structures near to the skin, a water path should be used. This results in better focus adaptation as well as producing a kind of self-demarcation of palpable lesions in the image through a wavy skin contour caused by protrusion or dimpling effects from the underlying lesions (FRIEDRICH 1987).

12.4 Real-Time Examination Technique

In order to reduce the required imaging depth, for better beam penetration (due to tissue compression), and for the reproducible depiction of pathological findings, the breast should be flattened and compressed during ultrasonography, thus immobilizing the breast against shifting displacements. This can be achieved by placing the patient in a supine position (flattening the breast by its own weight), elevating the arm (breast fixation by stretching of the skin and the pectoralis muscle), and using a pillow for shoulder support in patients with larger breasts (moderate oblique positioning for additional breast stabilization).

The transducer is held in direct skin contact. A water path or gel pad should be used for examination of lesions just below the skin surface. Generally the first two focal zones are selected (ventral parenchymal border at a depth of 5–10 mm, pectoralis muscle at a depth of 30–45 mm).

The examination starts with standardized gain settings. Usually the time-gain control (TGC) requires only moderate individual adjustments (lower absorption in fatty breasts, higher absorption in some cases of mastopathy). The optimum main gain settings should be adjusted according to the echogenicity of fatty tissue. The latter should not appear too dark in order to be able to distinguish between hypoechoic carcinoma and cysts.

The transducer is systematically moved over the skin, performing parasagittal scanning planes with continuous transversal increments (from lateral to medial and back again) and preventing scanning gaps by overlapping all imaged tissue windows. In order to avoid absorption and scattering artifacts, uniformly controlled tissue compression by the transducer and perpendicular insonation (perceived by a strong reflectivity of the fascia pectoralis) is necessary.

The elasticity, mobility, and delineation of a lesion with regard to the neighboring tissue can be evaluated through palpation of the mass during the sonographic examination. All palpable tissue thickenings or sonographically defined masses can thus be dynamically examined by applying various degrees of compression and varying the beam incidence and scanning planes ("sonopalpation").

The diagnostic criteria are already established during the real-time examination as some of the dynamic features such as elasticity, fixation, and disruption of architecture cannot be observed retrospectively on the static image. These criteria always refer to the three-dimensional image impression of the entire examined tissue volume. Every significant finding should be photographically documented in at least two scan planes (radial and antiradial) with the transducer orientation and position of the suspicious area indicated on the pictogram. Any visible changes of the contour or absorption characteristics of a lesion by compresion vs. decompression should be documented. Particular tissue characteristics, such as an "echogenic border sign", which may be only obvious during the dynamic examination process should be marked on the images additionally.

Additional diagnostic evaluation of unclear lesions can be achieved using small-area high-resolution (10- to 13-MHz) probes for better visualization of focal intraductal tumor extensions or a multifocal growth pattern. These small probes are not suitable for systematic examination of the breast as scanning gaps may occur and some subtle architectural distortions (especially in cases of echogenic scirrhous carcinoma) can only be recognized when the retractive pattern facing towards the lesion can be traced over a longer stretch of tissue.

12.5 Sonographic Visualization of Breast Tumors

Apart from tumor size and the resolution characteristics of the ultrasound equipment, the detection of any benign or malignant lesion is mainly influenced by three parameters:

1. The echogenicity of the lesion
2. The macroscopic growth pattern of the tumorous mass
3. The background pattern of the host tissue

12.5.1 Echogenicity of the Lesion

The echogenicity of any biological tissue is determined by the reflectivity, size, distance, and three-dimensional alignment of acoustic scattering centers (THIJSSEN and OOSTERVELD 1990), whereby the reflectivity of an interface increases with the differential impedance of the adjacent tissue components. The acoustic impedance ($Z = \rho \times c$) is mainly influenced by the velocity of ultrasound (c), since there are only slight differences between the specific densities (ρ) of different soft tissues within the breast. For the various tissue components the acoustic impedance gradually increases as follows (tissue components are shown in ascending order; "artificial" components are in parentheses): (air), (silicone), fatty tissue, cystic fluid, epithelial structures, fibrous tissue, hyalinosis, (calcifications).

Tissue structures consisting of *only one* of the aforementioned components induce a low echo response: for example, pure fatty tissue of the subcutaneous layer, pure epithelial proliferations in medullary carcinomas, debris in necrotizing tumors, or the pure fibrohyalinosis in the center of ductal invasive carcinomas typically appear hypoechoic. This may also explain the diffuse hypoechoic appearance of developing juvenile breast tissue (dense corpus fibrosum containing only subtle fat inclusions and few epithelial structures) and some kinds of mastopathy (in cases of either predominantly fibrous or adenoid tissue).

On the other hand, any intermingling of these components results in heterogeneous bioacoustic tissue compositions, leading to an increase in global echogenicity. The strongest effects are caused by slight interpositions of one of the extrema as either fat inclusions or strands of collagen (FIELDS and DUNN 1973; TEUBNER et al. 1983). This explains the high reflectivity of the infiltrating tumor periphery ("halo sign") as well as the existence of primary echogenic carcinomas (i.e., intraductal, diffusely infiltrating lobular, or highly differentiated tubular carcinomas).

Prerequisites for sonographic tumor demonstration are (1) the disruption of the preexistent glandular matrix and (2) replacement by another tissue with different acoustic echogenicity. From this point of view, therefore, sonography cannot distinguish a lactiferous duct coated by normal glandular epithelium from a duct that harbors an intraductal carcinoma: insofar as there is no extensive invasion or massive enlargement of the ducts (in cases of advanced ductal carcinoma in situ), the matrix of the mammary gland is being preserved so that no alteration in echo pattern can be expected in intraductal carcinomas as compared with the surrounding unaffected glandular tissue. Even small microcalcifications (smaller than the wavelength, i.e., $\ll 300\,\mu m$) are usually not detectable in these tumor types, since the echo pattern of the glandular tissue contains almost the same preexistent "speckle" sizes and echointensity. Only microcalcifications in the center of hypoechoic tumors present with easily recognizable high-density echoes (KASUMI 1988). Macrocalcifications (bigger than the beam width) as well as close conglomerates of clustered microcalcifications will additionally cast shadow zones (FILIPCZYNSKI and LYPACEWICZ 1984), making their perception easier.

The recognition of absorption or enhancement effects produced by tissue lesions is important for sonographic differential diagnosis. Shadowing and dorsal enhancement are caused by different absorption, reflection, and scattering effects of the lesion as compared with the neighboring tissue. Hereby, attenuation is predominantly due to increased absorption of energy which is frequently the result of increased fibrous content of a localized tissue area (KOBAYASHI 1979). Echogenicity and absorption should be regarded as independent entities in B-mode interpretation (KOSSOFF 1988).

12.5.2 Macroscopic Growth Pattern of the Tumorous Mass

As mentioned above, noninvasive and minimally invasive intraductal carcinomas are representatives of *non-tumor-forming types* (sonographically invisible), since the echogenicity of the affected glandular segments will not be changed. In some cases, radial scanning is helpful when enlarged and deformed ducts can be revealed (TEBOUL 1991; KAMIO et al. 1992). A second type of sonographically occult (non-tumor-forming) cancer is diffusely infiltrating carcinoma.

Because of the existence of echogenic carcinomas, malignancy cannot be excluded solely by ultrasonography. Therefore any patient with a clinically or mammographically suspicious lesion but "normal" sonographic findings must have a tissue diagnosis.

Most invasive carcinomas, if visible sonographically, appear as hypoechoic *tumor-forming types* with good contrast from echogenic glandular tissue. The roughness of the contour is largely determined by the growth pattern. Even within a hypoechoic background of involutional fatty breasts, invasive carcinomas are detectable when disruption of the remaining fibroglandular ligaments or an "echogenic border" of the infiltrative zone is recognizable (TEUBNER 1985) (see Fig. 12.31a). Problems arise, however, in smooth-marginated lesions (mucoid carcinoma, medullary carcinoma, fibroadenoma), which may remain hidden in fatty breast tissue since they may have a comparatively similar appearance to intramammary fat lobules. Beside static contour features the results of dynamic tests (elasticity, movability) and other secondary signs discernible during real-time evaluation (architectual distortion) provide additional information for differential diagnosis.

12.5.3 Background Pattern of the Host Tissue

The mammary gland is characterized by a combination of epithelial structures (ducts, lobules), loose intralobular connective tissue surrounding the lobules, and fatty inclusions which are embedded in dense interlobular connective tissue of the supporting glandular body. This complex matrix is generally responsible for a marked and homogeneous echogenicity of the glandular tissue, providing high contrast against the usually hypoechoic-appearing carcinomas.

Larger interspersed fat inclusions, circumscribed fibrotic areas, or focal zones of adenosis appear hypoechoic (TEUBNER et al. 1983) and may be responsible for inhomogeneous echo patterns. Similar inhomogeneities also can be produced by absorption artifacts at fat-fibrous interfaces, which generally exist at the surface of the mammary gland (line shadows at Cooper's ligaments and Duret's crest), in the retromammillary space (nipple shadowing), or at inner fat islands (lateral shadowing), or may originate from focal fat inclusions in mastopathic tissue (diffuse tissue absorptions). These absorption artifacts are more or less predominant depending on the tissue compression and the angle of incidence of insonation, both of which can be influenced by the examiner. Therefore the best sound transmission will be achieved by moderate tissue compression resulting in alignment of tissue interfaces so as to be perpendicular to the ultrasonic beam.

All inhomogeneities and inconstant background patterns reduce efficiency in the recognition of pathologies. Examination-dependent artifacts are disadvantageous special effects in breast ultrasonography that are not observed in other organs with a homogeneous texture (liver, thyroid, testicle, etc.), and thus make breast ultrasonography more difficult.

Other difficulties arise from macroscopic focal fat lobules: In these cases smooth-margined lesions (fibroadenoma, mucous carcinoma, etc.) can be hidden by the overlying intramammary fat lobules (TEUBNER et al. 1985a), which in turn can lead to false-positive diagnoses by mimicking smooth-marginated tumors. Real-time analysis of tissue elasticity is an important tool for differential diagnosis in these cases.

Apart from these individual inhomogeneities, three other age-dependent low-echo background patterns sometimes render the recognition of pathological findings difficult:

1. The juvenile breast (predominant connective tissue/few epithelial structures)
2. The hormonally stimulated breast in pregnant or nursing patients (hypertrophic glandular tissue)
3. The postmenopausal involutional breast (replacement of glandular tissue by fat)

In these cases the background appears hypoechoic since *one* tissue component almost completely replaces all others (i.e., fibrosis vs adenosis vs fat).

12.6 Sonographic Diagnostic Criteria

The sonographic evaluation of a mass lesion is divided into three steps:

1. *Global characterization of the surrounding breast tissue.* The echographic contrast between a mass and the surrounding tissue is very important for clear demarcation between the lesion and unaffected tissue. First, a general description of the echographic structure and of the host tissue is given (echogenicity, homogeneity, degree of fat interposition, involution) in order to assess the detectability of a lesion relative to its surroundings.

2. *Analysis of the region of interest (ROI).* Sonographically defined lesions can be characterized by the following evaluative criteria. The precise topographic localization of a mass relative to the surrounding anatomical structures, its size (diameter in the radial, antiradial, and ventroposterior directions, including a possible echogenic border), and its dynamic parameters (fixation in tissue) must be determined during the real-time examination, as retrospectively some of these features may be misinterpreted or cannot be documented on the static sonographic image. A *hyperechoic* carcinoma, for example, can be recognized during real-time examination by the interruption of adjacent tissue structures and its relative inelasticity, whereas the same tumor can be misinterpreted as a *hypoechoic* mass retrospectively in cases of dorsal shadowing simulating an irregularly defined hypoechoic lesion (see Fig. 12.34). This explains why carcinomas were almost exclusively observed to be hypoechoic in the past using static ultrasound examination techniques, whereas with dynamic real-time scanning more than 8% of carcinomas are seen to be "predominantly hyperechoic" (this term is applicable to tumors consisting to more than 70% of hyperechoic tissue, and thus being for more echogenic than fat tissue and comparable in echogenicity to glandular tissue) (TEUBNER 1993). If there is no well-defined lesion during ultrasound examination, at a site of

Table 12.1. Sonographic differential diagnosis of solid breast masses: the listed diagnostic criteria are individually of variable and limited predictive value, but in sum suggest the differentiation of benign from malignant masses (however, not with accuracy as great as tissue diagnosis)

Diagnostic criterion	Sonographic classification		
	Benign	Equivocal	Malignant
Shape	Round/oval	Lobulated	Irregular/jagged/diffusely infiltrative
Geometry	Flat (length/width <<1)	–	High (length/width >1)
Contour	Sharp (encapsuled)	Smooth	Unsharp/diffuse
Tumor front	Capsule: strong anterior/posterior echoes	–	"Echogenic border": ill-defined hyperreflective tumor periphery
Internal echo strength	Strong as glandular tissue or intermediate (> fatty tissue) (requirement: tissue elasticity!)	Weak (≤ fatty tissue) or nearly anechoic	a) Heterogeneous mixed echogenicity (side by side areas of different echo strength: low to strong echoes) b) Hyperreflective nonelastic lesions
Internal echo distribution	Uniform	–	Heterogeneous/coarse
Absorption	Strong posterior echo enhancement	Intermediate	Shadowing (only if not calcified)
Refraction	Strong bilateral shadowing	No lateral shadowing	–
Elasticity	Highly elastic (>20% compressible) Surface easily deformable	Nonelastic	–
Movability	Surrounding tissue gliding over the surface of the lesion	Lesion fixed on surrounding glandular tissue	Lesion fixed on skin or underlying pectoral fascia
Relation to palpation	Exact correspondence of visualized tumor size and palpatory finding	Little discrepancy between sonographic tumor size and size of palpatory finding	Distinct difference between size as assessed by palpation and hypoechoic center of the lesion
Relationship to surroundings	Deformed or displaced by surrounding tissues (like fatty lobules)	Displacement of protrusion into surrounding tissues	Disruption of tissue architecture/ infiltration into preexisting structures

mammographic or palpable abnormality, subtle changes in the echo pattern, loss of tissue elasticity, or thickening of breast parenchyma should be searched for.

3. *Differential diagnosis*. In the diagnostic evaluation of "defined" breast lesions, one must first differentiate between *cystic* and *solid* lesions. Criteria for cystic lesions are an anechoic center, a capsule-like border, dorsal echo enhancement, bilateral shadowing, and pliability of the lesion.

The next diagnostic step deals with the attempt to discriminate between benign and malignant solid lesions, applying the criteria listed in Table 12.1. If there is no clearly defined mass and the tissue can be clearly analyzed, the ROI can be classified as sonographically "normal", always recognizing that some cancers are sonographically invisible. It will be defined as "benign" if there is any echomorphological but nonmalignant correlation established between the clinical findings or an equivocal mammogram. Such correlations are for example sideasymmetry or a thin subcutaneous layer of fat with a prominent ventral parenchymal border (see Fig. 12.4).

Tissue areas are classified as "nondiagnostic" when the tissue cannot be analyzed sufficiently (due to technical difficulties or diffuse absorption artifacts in the ROI), making the exclusion of a tumorous mass impossible.

Sonographic evaluative criteria can be divided into four groups:

1. Morphological features (contour)
   a) Shape and sharpness of the outline of the mass
   b) Orientation of the mass (depth/width ratio)

Table 12.2. Diagnostic value of different diagnostic criteria: results of a prospective blinded study (TEUBNER 1993)

Sonographic criteria	Histology malignant ($n = 89$)	Histology benign ($n = 105$)	PV+[a]	Clinical decision[b]
Shape				
Round/oval	25% (22/89)	67% (70/105)	24% (22/92)	Benign
Lobulated	16% (14/89)	19% (20/105)	41% (14/34)	Equivocal
Irregular	60% (53/89)	14% (15/105)	78% (53/68)	Malignant
Contour				
Smooth	20% (18/89)	76% (80/105)	18% (18/98)	Benign
Jagged/diffuse	80% (71/89)	24% (25/205)	74% (71/96)	Malignant
Tumor front				
Strong anterior/posterior echoes	4% (4/89)	40% (42/105)	9% (4/46)	Benign
No reactive alterations	25% (22/89)	52% (55/105)	29% (22/77)	
Echogenic border	71% (63/89)	8% (8/105)	89% (63/71)	Malignant
Internal echoes (strength)				
Intermediate (> fatty tissue)	12% (11/89)	43% (45/105)	20% (11/56)	Benign
Strong (≈ glandular tissue)	5% (4/89)	9% (9/105)	31% (4/13)	Equivocal
Weak (≤ fatty tissue)	29% (26/89)	28% (30/105)	46% (26/56)	
Nearly anechoic/absent	31% (28/89)	18% (19/105)	60% (28/47)	
Mixed echogenicity (absent/strong)	23% (20/89)	2% (2/105)	91% (20/22)	Malignant
Internal echoes (distribution)				
Uniform	20% (18/89)	67% (70/105)	20% (18/88)	Benign
Absent echoes	7% (6/89)	7% (7/105)	46% (6/13)	Equivocal
Nonuniform	73% (65/89)	26% (28/105)	70% (65/93)	Malignant
Posterior echoes (accentuation/attenuation)				
Enhanced	12% (11/89)	27% (28/105)	28% (11/39)	Benign
Intermediate	42% (37/89)	57% (60/105)	38% (37/97)	Equivocal
Attenuated	46% (41/89)	16% (17/105)	71% (41/58)	Malignant
Bilateral shadowing				
Marked	11% (10/89)	15% (16/105)	38% (10/26)	Equivocal
Weak/unilateral	19% (17/89)	31% (32/105)	35% (17/49)	
Absent	70% (62/89)	54% (57/105)	52% (62/119)	
Elasticity				
Deformable	1% (1/89)	26% (27/105)	4% (1/28)	Benign
Not deformable	99% (88/89)	74% (78/105)	53% (88/166)	Equivocal

[a] PV+ (positive predictive value) is the likelihood that a lesion yielding a positive test in a specific criterion is actually malignant
[b] CD = benign if PV+ ≤ 30%; CD = equivocal if 30% < PV+ < 70%; CD = malignant if PV+ ≤ 70%

2. Combined acoustic/morphologic properties (texture, sound transmission)
   a) Echogenicity of the tumor
   b) Echo texture (homogeneous/inhomogeneous)
   c) Heterogeneity of the echo pattern within a mass (second-order statistics: patchwork of areas of varying echogenicity)
   d) Echogenicity of the margin of the lesion ("echogenic border")
   e) Echogenicity of the area behind a lesion influenced by absorption and refraction effects
3. Dynamic criteria
   a) Mobility and compressibility of a mass during real-time examination
   b) Compression effect (changes in the sonographic properties of a mass under varying degrees of compression, i.e., internal echo pattern and absorption)
4. Secondary phenomena
   a) Difference in size between the hypoechoic tumor center and the palpable lesion (desmoplastic reactive changes of surrounding tissue, "pseudolipoma" induced by retraction phenomena in scirrhous carcinoma)
   b) Relationship to adjacent tissue structures (displacement vs infitting into or disrupt of the existing tissue architecture)

The predictive value of each criterion was analyzed on the basis of 89 malignant and 105 benign biopsies in a consecutive series of 194 sonographically visualized lesions (TEUBNER et al. 1994) (Table 12.2).

12.7 Normal Anatomy

In breast ultrasonography one can differentiate the following tissue layers: skin and nipple, subcutaneous fat and preglandular fat layer (separated by the superficial fascia), glandular tissue, prepectoral fatty tissue, breast muscle, contours of the ribs, and the intercostal muscle layer.

Border echoes can be observed on all perpendicularly insonated interfaces between fatty and connective tissue. Therefore the skin (double contour with water path), the septa dividing the fat lobules,

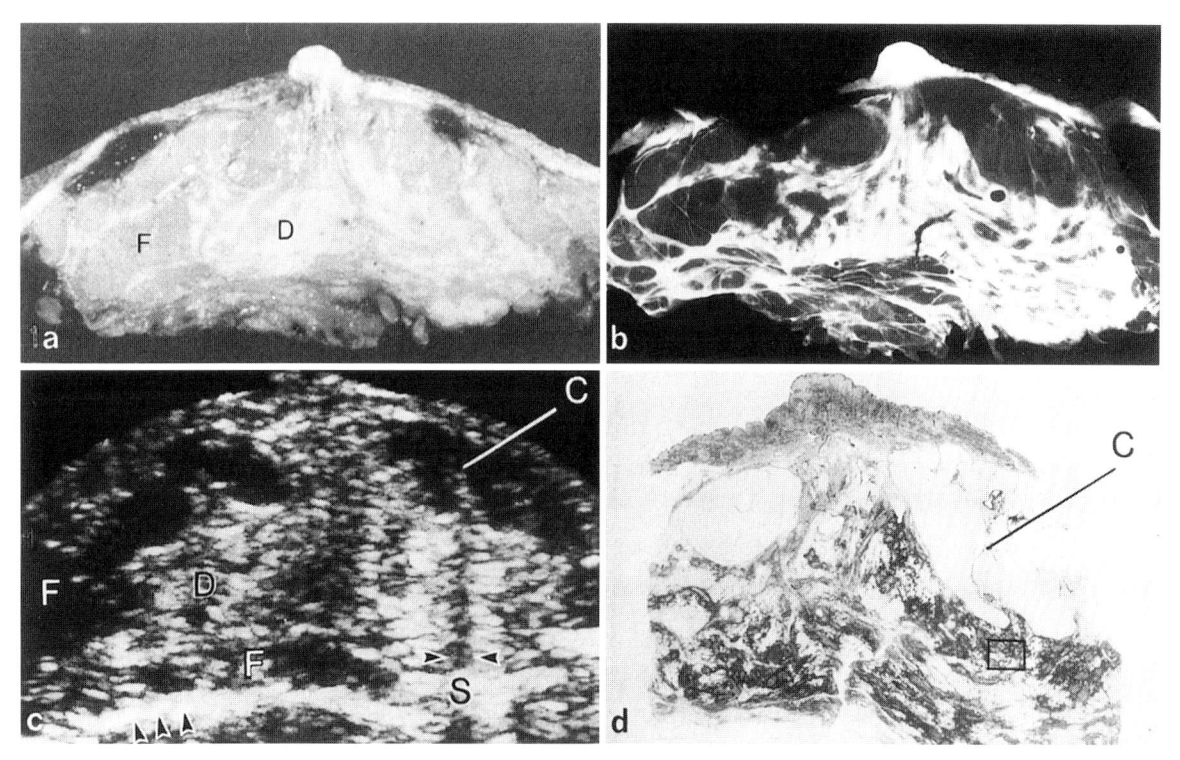

Fig. 12.1a–d. Correlative morphological study of a normal breast specimen. a Anatomical gross slice through the nipple with bright dense glandular tissue (D) surrounded by yellow fatty tissue (F). b Specimen radiograph of the same 3-mm-thick breast section demonstrating high absorption in the dense glandular tissue (*bright*) and low absorption in the fatty tissue (*dark*). c Sonogram of the entire breast showing echodense glandular tissue (D), less echogenic fatty tissue (F), and shadow zones(s) behind the mamilla and at a Cooper's ligament (C) Pectoral fascia marked by arrowheads. d Inhomogeneous tissue composition of glandular tissue with dense interlobular connective tissue (*dark*), loose intralobular connective tissue (*gray*), and translucent fatty tissue

Type I

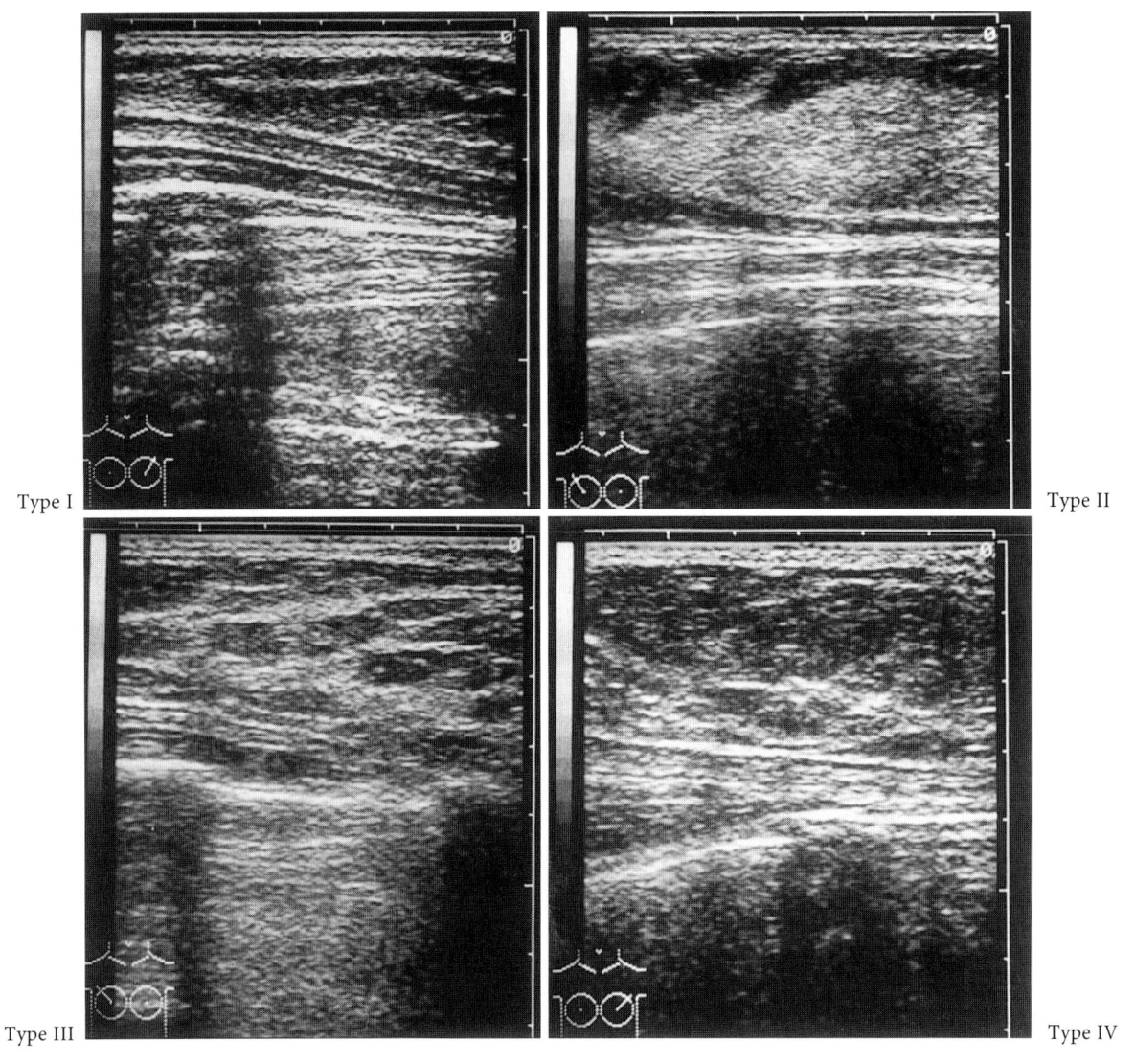

Type II

Type III

Type IV

Fig. 12.2. Age-related echo pattern of a normal breast. *Type I*: Hypoechoic glandular tissue in a young patient (17 years). Same echogenicity of the gland as compared with surrounding fatty tissue. A bright reflection is seen at the ventral border of the gland (fat-to-connective tissue interface). *Type II*: Homogeneous highly reflective glandular tissue in a 30-year-old woman. *Type III*: Dispersed glandular tissue with some interspersed flat, oval fatty islets (38 years). *Type IV*: Fatty involutional breast (hypoechoic) with rare highly reflective strands of remaining glandular tissue in a 62-year-old patient

Cooper's ligaments, the surface of the mammary gland, the pectoral fascia, the periosteum of the ribs, and the pleura generate intense reflections.

The echogenicity of the various tissue layers depends on the tissue composition and can vary greatly from patient to patient. The skin is 1–2 mm in thickness and is of moderate echogenicity, whereas the areola and nipple are usually areas with sparse echoes. In the area behind the nipple there may be so-called nipple shadowing from the fibrotic milk duct structures which are perpendicular to the skin. The perimammary fatty tissue yields only low echoes, in strong contrast to the normally intensely reflective glandular tissue. There may be some marring refraction shadowing along the serrated ventral border of the parenchymal fascia, the so-called Duret's crest. These anatomical features are illustrated in Fig. 12.1.

The retroglandular border forms a smooth line which runs parallel to the underlying muscle. Due to tissue compression in the supine position, the separating prepectoral fat layer is only some millimeters thick during breast ultrasonography. In contrast, on mammography the lateral compression causes more fatty tissue to be pressed into the retromammary space in order to obtain a better view of the retroglandular border close to the chest wall. The topographic relation of a mass to the pectoralis muscle (movability) can be established through dynamic tests, thus yielding additional diagnostic information to that provided by mammography and better assessment or exclusion of chest wall infiltrations.

Muscle tissue is usually of moderate echogenicity and presents a lamella-like structure running parallel to the muscle fibers. The calcified parts of the ribs show strong shadowing whereas the sternal cartilaginous segments appear as well-defined oval areas of weak echogenicity in the sagittal plane. Since the latter are sonolucent, evaluation of the underlying parasternal lymphatic drainage area is not affected.

The evaluation of the various breast parenchymal patterns is very important for the detectability of breast lesions: The appearance of the fibroglandular layer can vary greatly with the patient's age and individual constitution. The glandular tissue may be homogeneously hypoechoic in juvenile breasts, in adenoid hyperplasia occurring during pregnancy, and in the atrophied fatty glandular tissue of the older patient, or may present with an inhomogeneous echo pattern, interspersed with fat inclusion or circumscribed fibrotic or adenoid areas. The menstrual cycle has no effect on the interpretation of the sonogram, so there are no problems in appointment planning for breast ultrasonography.

There are four age-related echographic types of breast parenchyma (Figs. 12.2, 12.3):

Type I: Compact hypoechoic glandular tissue (Fig. 12.2a). The glandular tissue is of similar echogenicity to the subcutaneous fat, which forms a thin layer separating the skin and the superficial margin of the glandular tissue. Distinction between these structures is therefore often only possible during the dynamic scanning process and with perpendicular sound incidence on the superficial fascia of the gland (highly echogenic line). This type is predominantly found in younger women under 30 years old, and depending on the age of the patient it is observed in 20%–50% of cases. It also may be present during pregnancy and periods of lactation.

Type II: Compact hyperechoic glandular tissue (Fig. 12.2b). The hyperreflective glandular tissue can be clearly distinguished from the surrounding hypoechoic fatty tissue. The thickness of this layer of fat varies with the age and constitution of patients. The subcutaneous layer is more developed than

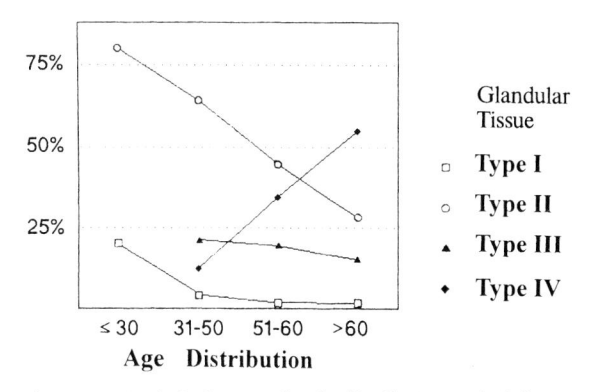

Fig. 12.3. Statistical age-related distribution of different sonographic glandular patterns (TEUBNER 1993)

the prepectoral layer. This type is mostly observed in middle-aged women but can also be seen in the menopausal breast in 36% of cases. Usually (77%) the glandular tissue is of inhomogeneously interspersed structure. Occasionally (4%) the retroareolar tissue is interspersed with areas of tube-like structures ("sponge type" with a mottled pattern).

Type III: Glandular tissue interspersed with inclusions of fat lobules (Fig. 12.2c). This type of glandular tissue is interspersed with clearly defined, oval-shaped inclusions of fatty tissue. On static scans these inclusions may be misdiagnosed as pathological structures. Viewing these structures under compression in the dynamic scan, their elasticity and continuity with each other can be identified and differentiation from other solid lesions is usually quite clear-cut. This category is observed in about 20% of patients over the age of 40 years, whereby the amount of adipose inclusions increases with the patient's age.

Type IV: Involuted adipose breast (Fig. 12.2d). The glandular tissue of the involuted breast of older patients has become atrophic and is replaced by hypoechoic adipose tissue. The adipose tissue is interlaced with hyperechoic trabeculae consisting of connective tissue fibers and residual parenchyma. Occasionally a hyperechoic compact area of glandular tissue presents in the retroareolar region. This type of breast structure can be seen in more than 55% of patients over the age of 60.

12.8 Fibrocystic Change (Mastopathy)

Mastopathy is a collective term for a manifold group of diffuse or focal proliferative and regressive changes in the breast. As these changes often occur in asymptomatic women, they are not considered as a real disease entity in their uncomplicated histological form. Rather they represent a physiological condition depending on hormonal influences. Mastopathy is usually first noticed by the examining physician and not by the patient. The *clinical* findings may involve diffuse areas of induration or defined nodularity which may be accompanied by premenstrual tenderness. Occasionally nipple discharge may be the only clinical symptom of this stage.

As patients with fibrocystic changes usually have radiodense glandular tissue (P2/DY) in which tumors can be difficult to detect or to exclude, mammography may not depict palpable lesions with sufficient clarity. Dense areas with or without microcalcifications may also present on mammography without any clinical findings. Thus, the mammographic and/or clinical appearance may suggest the need for biopsy.

Because of its very different principle of image generation, ultrasonography can yield valuable information in the cases, if there are focal or diffuse differences in the acoustic properties of the affected tissue components. On the other hand, ultrasonography offers little additional diagnostic information when microcalcifications are seen on the mammogram in the absence of a palpable lesion. This is because no clear sonographic finding can be correlated with the pattern of microcalcifications, whether benign or malignant (TEUBNER et al. 1990). In these cases the further diagnostic workup depends on the result of spot-compression magnification mammography of the microcalcifications (TEUBNER et al. 1987). Because of its histological variation, the clinical, mammographic, and sonographic appearance of fibrocystic change is heterogeneous. In most cases ultrasonography is unable to demonstrate the changes in tissue structure (TEUBNER et al. 1985a), but if macroscopic anatomical changes are involved, focal, peri- or intraductal, or diffuse sonographic patterns can be recognized, as discussed in the following sections.

12.8.1 Circumscribed Mastopathic Changes

In cases of uncomplicated mastopathy, glandular thickening accompanied by a reduction in the thickness of the subcutaneous fat layer is observed (Fig. 12.4). In such cases a palpable nodule can quite easily be correlated sonographically with the locally increased amount of parenchyma: under a thin layer of subcutaneous fat the breast parenchyma can be palpated as a firm mass, whereas surrounded by a normal subcutaneous fat layer the breast parenchyma appears obviously to be of normal elasticity. As long as the mammogram is inconspicuous and the lesion appears to be pliable or compressible under "sonopalpation", it is probably benign and further surveillance by ultrasonography and mammography should be carried out.

In mastopathic nodules with microcystic or fibrotic changes the sonographic parenchymal pattern is quite inhomogeneous. Using very high-resolution probes (>10 MHz) the microcystic changes can be identified and differentiated from purely solid (generally fibrotic) lesions (Fig. 12.5). Evaluation of the elasticity of the tissue is also very important in these cases. The more pronounced these architectural changes are, the greater the probability of proliferating fibrocystic disease, in which cell atypia cannot be excluded using imaging modalities. Sampling by core biopsy or open biopsy should be preferred to simple follow-up in these patients. Macrocystic mastopathy with larger cysts, on the other hand, rarely causes problems of differential diagnosis.

Circumscribed fibrotic areas may present as well-defined areas of lower echogenicity (Fig. 12.6) and may be misdiagnosed at ultrasonography as tumor masses if the "lesion" is not clearly margined. In some cases there may be dorsal shadowing which disappears under tissue compression, if the lesion remains elastic.

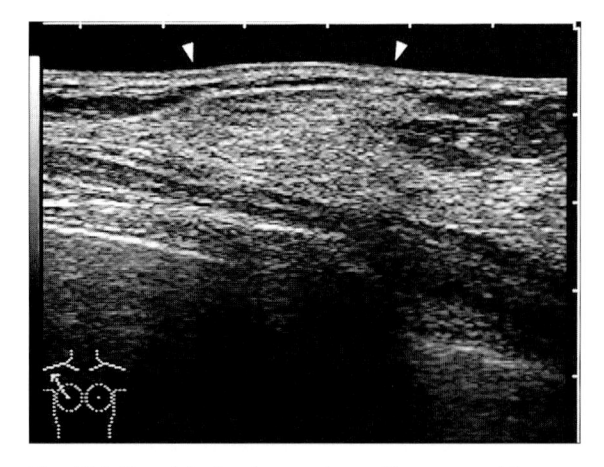

Fig. 12.4. Pseudolesion in a patient with mastopathic complaints. Focal thickening of glandular tissue (*arrowheads*) and reduction of the subcutaneous fat layer resulted in a circumscribed, firm palpatory finding

Echomammography: Technique and Results 193

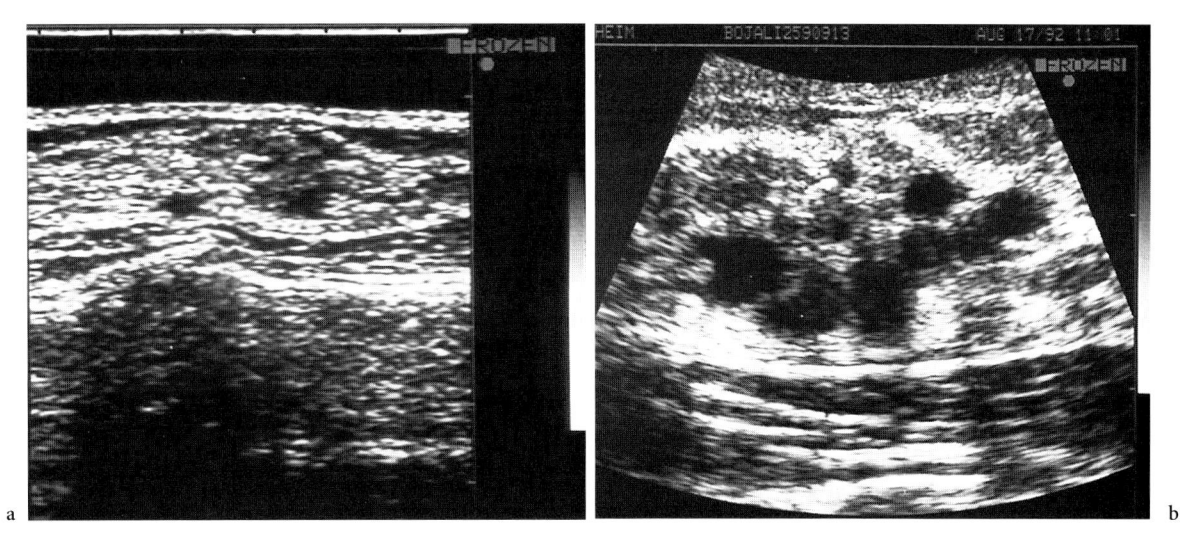

Fig. 12.5a,b. Circumscribed fibrocystic lesion. **a** Examination with a medium-resolution transducer (5-MHz linear array) demonstrates an ill-defined, suspicious appearing 1.5-cm-diameter lesion. **b** Further evaluation with a high-resolution probe (13-MHz annular array) reveals multiple grape-like microcysts (maximum diameter: 1–3 mm)

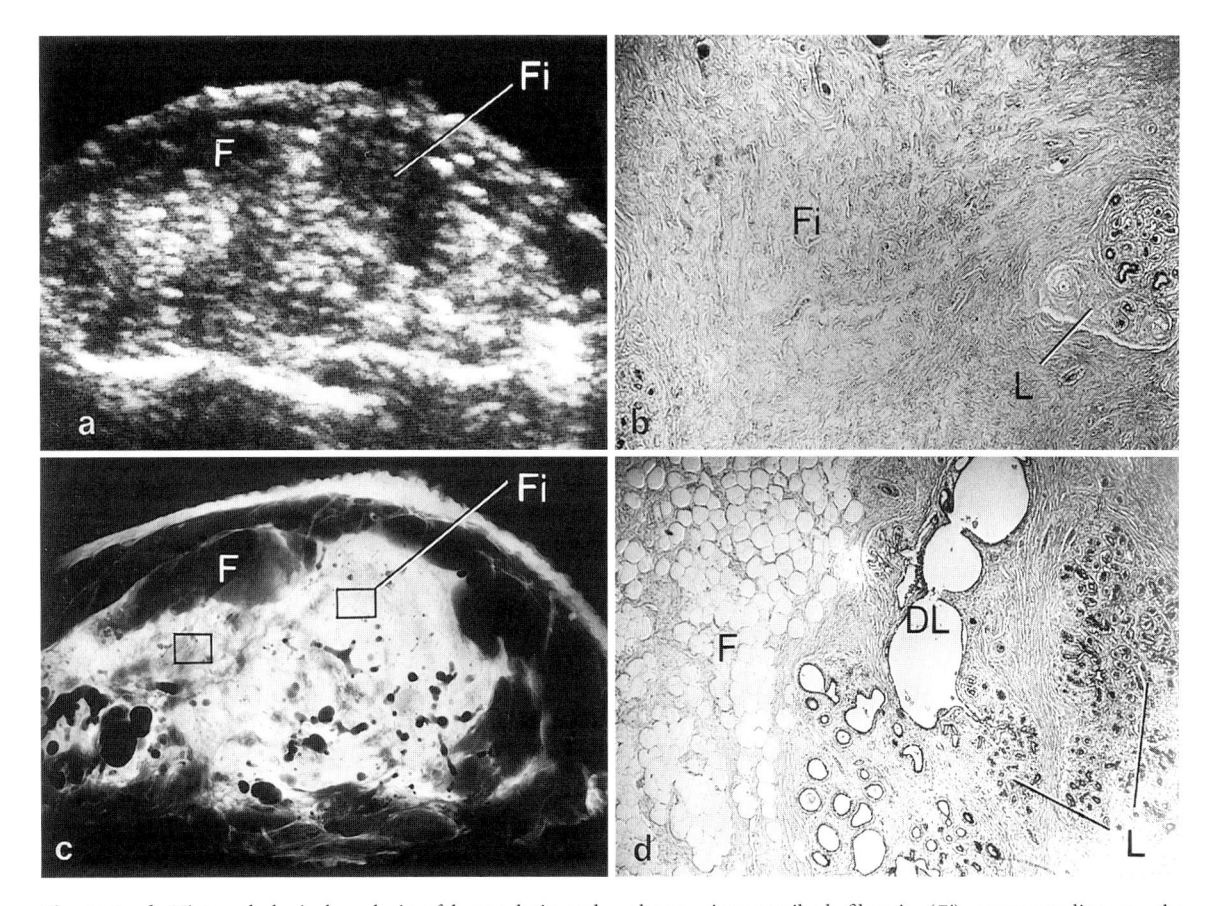

Fig. 12.6a–d. Histopathological analysis of hypoechoic and echogenic tissue areas in fibrocystic disease. **a** Well-defined hypoechoic "lesion" (*Fi*) with a similar echotexture to fatty tissue (*F*). **b** Medium-power magnification of the hypoechoic area, revealing homogeneous fibrosis (subtle acoustic interfaces). **c** Specimen radiograph of the same gross section also shows circumscribed fibrosis (*Fi*) corresponding to the hypoechoic area on the sonogram. **d** Microscopic view of a representative echodense tissue area reveals an inhomogeneous tissue composition (multiple acoustic interfaces) consisting of cystically altered glandular lobules (*L*), dilated ducts (*DL*), and interspersed fatty tissue

It is well known that the echogenicity of parenchymal abdominal organs increases with the amount of connective tissue (fibrosis). Paradoxically, in the mammary gland the opposite is the case, as the transition from the normally inhomogeneous tissue composition of breast parenchyma (microsopic patchwork of adenoid, fatty, and fibrous components) to predominance of fibrosis (one tissue component) results in an acoustic homogenization of the tissue. In the following example, comparison of a sonographic section and the corresponding specimen radiograph of the gross slice in Fig. 12.6 shows a superficial zone of low echogenicity at the anterior border of the parenchyma which could be mistaken for fatty tissue. In fact this hypoechoic region corresponds to homogeneously radiodense tissue with no fat inclusions! Histological analysis of this area explains this discrepancy: the glandular lobules are pushed apart by a large amount of homogeneous interlobular fibrosis (Fig. 12.6b). Thus, the echogenicity of this relatively homogeneous area is reduced. Histological sections of echodense areas, on the other hand, demonstrate a very different fine-tissue structure (Fig. 12.6c). Acinar lumens are widened almost to resemble cysts, the lobules are located more closely together, and the interlobular connective tissue is interspersed with tiny fatty islets and interlaced with dilated ductules. Enhanced echogenicity is due to the numerous microscopic interfaces of different acoustic impedance.

Similarly, areas of circumscribed adenosis are hypoechoic. However, unlike areas of dense fibrosis in mastopathy, adenosis shows discrete posterior echo enhancement and tissues remain easily compressible.

Radial scars and *complex sclerosing lesions* are characterized by a stellate zone of fibrosis and elastosis. Histologically these benign tumor-like lesions present a glandular pattern mimicking infiltrating processes scattered throughout the fibroelastic tissue (THONO et al. 1994). It is difficult to distinguish these so-called intramammary scars from tubular carcinoma, which in turn may actually develop from radial scars, so in fact these changes may be considered as potentially precancerous lesions. On the mammogram they appear similar to scirrhous carcinoma lacking, however, the central nidus of fibrosis (TABAR and DEAN 1985). During breast ultrasonography, too, these lesions cannot be distinguished from malignant masses. Depending on their tissue environment, there are both hyper- and hypoechoic variants, the latter usually presenting with high absorption (Fig. 12.7). Hence ultrasonography makes no contribution in the differential diagnosis of these lesions.

12.8.2 Intra- and Periductal Mastopathic Changes

Lactiferous duct structures with lumina of more than 1 mm in diameter can be visualized using high-resolution (>10 MHz) scanners. Hence the somewhat wider lactiferous sinus in the retroareolar region are often visible in asymptomatic patients. The transition from the normal width of the ducts to "ductectasia" has not been clearly defined [the author personally applies the term ductectasia to ducts >3 mm in diameter (Fig. 12.8)]. As dilated ducts are clinically irrelevant insofar as they present no intraductal proliferation, it does not appear very important to classify them exactly. Uncompli-

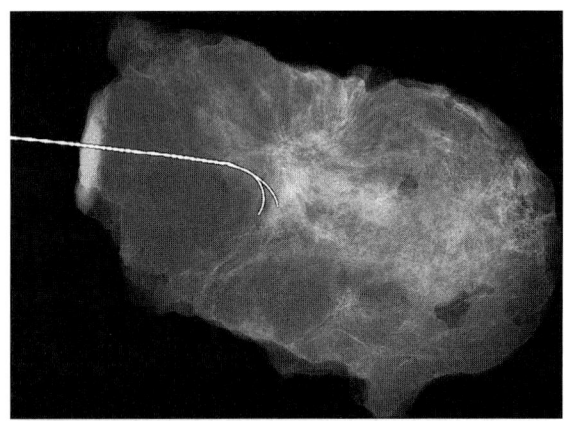

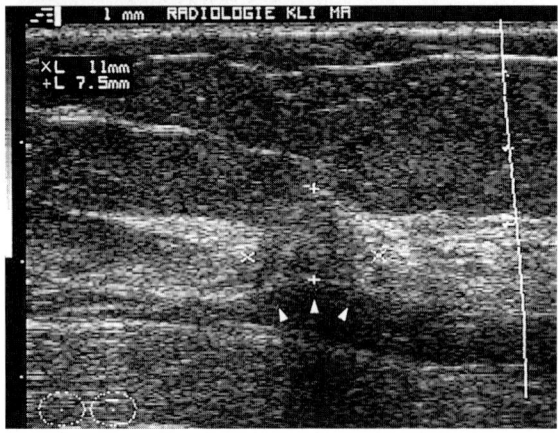

Fig. 12.7a,b. Radial scar. **a** Specimen radiograph demonstrating a typical stellate lesion without central density. **b** Ultrasonography demonstrates a focal gathering of glandular structures (*arrows*) with subtle loss of echogenicity. Insignificant dorsal shadowing is present. On palpation the area of the stellate lesion was less elastic than the surrounding fibroglandular tissue

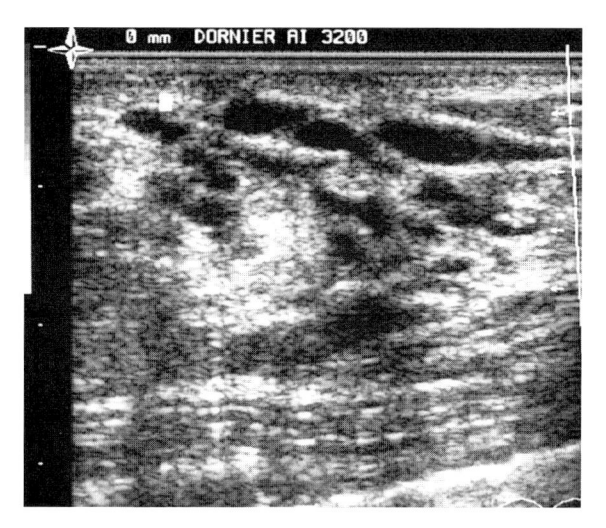

Fig. 12.8. Dilated ducts behind the areola (lumen width 1–3 mm) clearly visible with high-resolution 7.5-MHz linear array transducer. No pathological finding

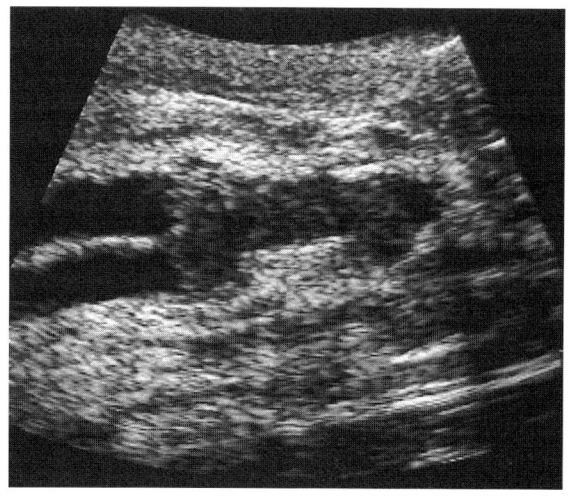

Fig. 12.9. Patient with bloody nipple discharge. Galactography failed because of inverted nipple. High-resolution 13-MHz ultrasonography revealed a dilated duct segment (lumen 3 mm) with a solid intraductal tubular mass (3 × 15 mm). Histology: benign intraductal papilloma

cated dilated ducts are depicted during ultrasonography as straight hypo- or anechoic tubular structures with smooth walls. Serpiginous ductal structures with irregular outlines (see Fig. 12.26), absent hyperechoic wall echoes, and hypoechoic content, especially in the surroundings of carcinomas, may indicate diffuse (malignant or benign) intraductal proliferation.

The detection of *intraductal papillomas* depends greatly on the width of the lumen and the echogenicity of the ductal content. Within dilated anechoic ducts, benign epithelial proliferations may present as hyperechoic polypoid irregular ductal protuberances (Fig. 12.9). Using ultrasonography, morphological discrimination between intraductal papilloma and intraductal carcinoma, particularly in its early stage, is not possible. Along with galactography, however, ultrasonography is helpful in the guidance of the preoperative dye marking of these lesions.

Periductal fibrosis typically presents as sponge-like interspersing of hypo- and hyperechoic structures, within single segments or the whole parenchyma. Tubular hypoechoic structures, at times interlacing and measuring about 3 mm in diameter, extend radially from the nipple towards the periphery. Using radial scanning orientations, the ductal course can be recognized easily whereas antiradial scans demonstrate a mottled pattern (Fig. 12.10). Because of the close relation to the ductal structures, this phenomenon is often mistaken for ductectasia. As these changes also occur in

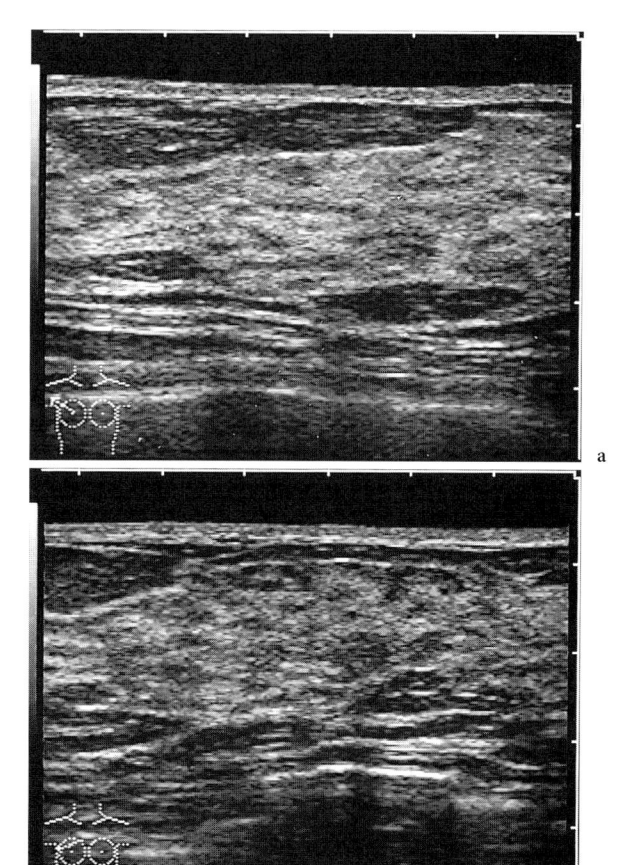

Fig. 12.10a,b. Periductal fibrosis. a Ductal pattern on the radial scanning orientation. b Mottled pattern on the antiradial scan direction

tissue so that delineation of the glandular tissue is often rendered possible only by the hyperechoic anterior fascia of the parenchyma. This is often accompanied by a reduced elasticity of the tissue and an increase in sound absorption. Intense shadowing may be present in patients with chronic nephropathy, tertiary hyperparathyroidism, or insulin-dependent diabetes mellitus. This can lead to both sonographic and mammographic misinterpretation and is often mistaken for diffuse infiltrating carcinomas (Fig. 12.11).

12.9 Cysts

All additional diagnostic information provided by ultrasonography, as compared with mammography, greatly depends on the type of lesion. Simple cysts are the easiest to diagnose reliably. These are round, oval, or lobulated anechoic lesions with smooth wall contours, usually bilateral refraction shadows due to their capsule-like borders, and dorsal echo enhancement. Simple cysts as small as 2 mm in diameter can be reliably detected using high-resolution systems (Fig. 12.12). Sometimes septations are observed which, however, can be distinguished from intercystic vegetations by dynamic scanning.

The most important differential diagnostic criteria between cysts and solid lesions are the anechoic center and the capsule-like borders of cysts. As 30% of carcinomas also display only weak echoes

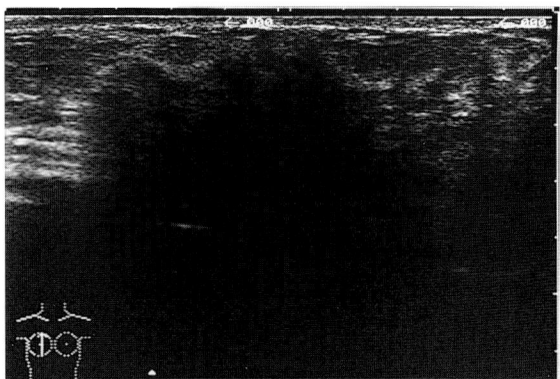

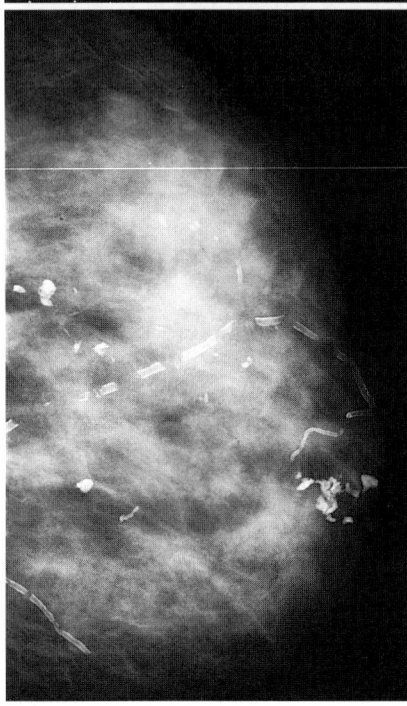

Fig. 12.11a,b. Diabetic fibrous disease. The patient presented with hard lumpy induration of two-thirds of the breast. She had a 15-year history of insulin-dependent diabetic mellitus and chronic nephropathy with tertiary hyperparathyroidism. **a** Ultrasonography showed a nonelastic highly absorptive gland retaining the normal crest-shaped surface. Ultrasonography-guided core cut biopsy revealed diffuse hyalinosis. **b** Corresponding mammogram with dense fibrotic tissue and multiple calcified arteries

asymptomatic patients, their importance is not well defined.

12.8.3 Diffuse Mastopathic Changes

Other diffuse hypoechoic structural changes are the result of fibrosis of breast tissue. The echogenicity of these areas may sometimes resemble that of fatty

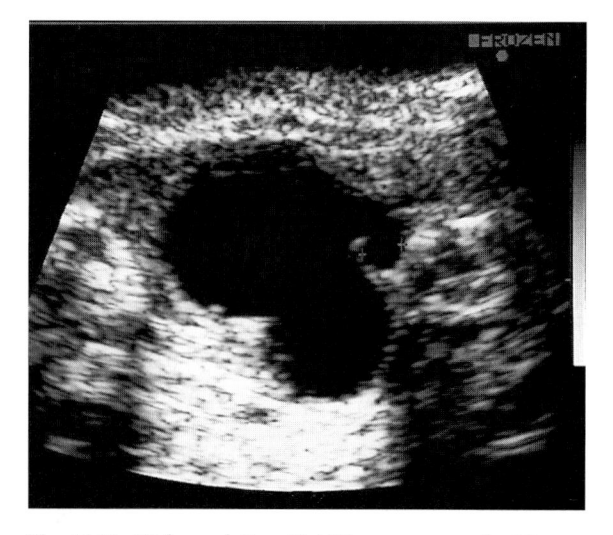

Fig. 12.12. High-resolution 13-MHz sonogram of a 10-mm-diameter cyst. The lobulated contour was caused by incomplete septation. A small 1.2-mm-diameter "knapsack" cyst is clearly delineated

Echomammography: Technique and Results

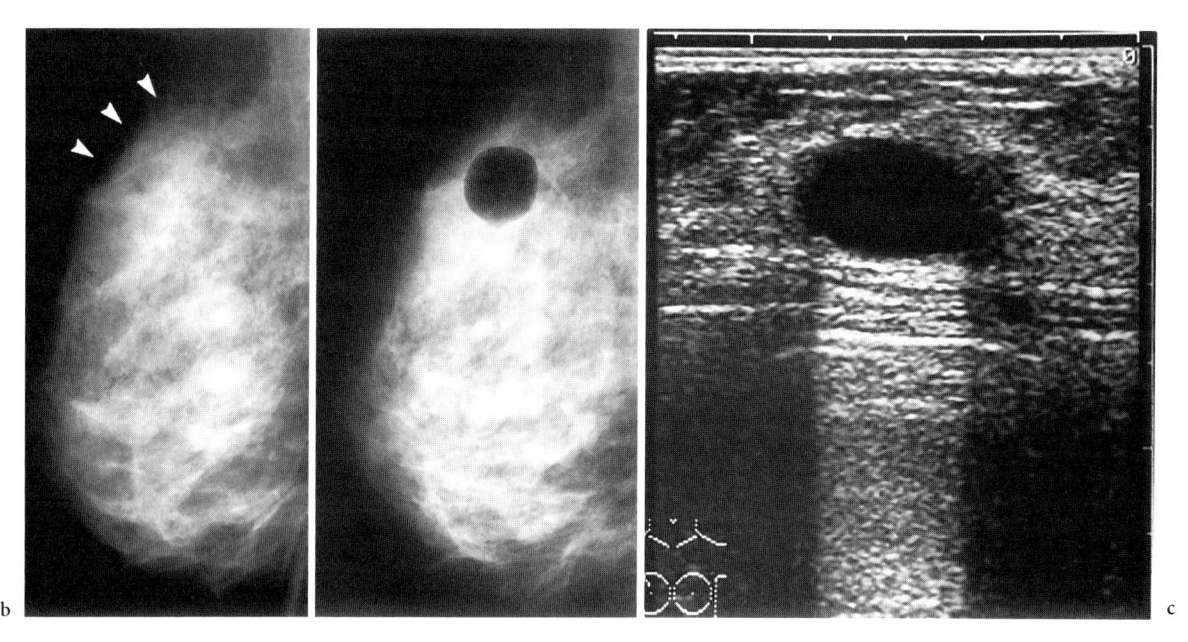

Fig. 12.13a–c. Patient with clinically suspicious firm mass of the outer upper quadrant. **a** No correlate of palpatory finding (*arrowheads*) in a mammographically dense, nondiagnostic breast. **c** Ultrasonography revealed a simple cyst. **b** Pneumocystography confirmed smooth cystic walls. Conclusion: ultrasonography avoided unnecessary biopsy

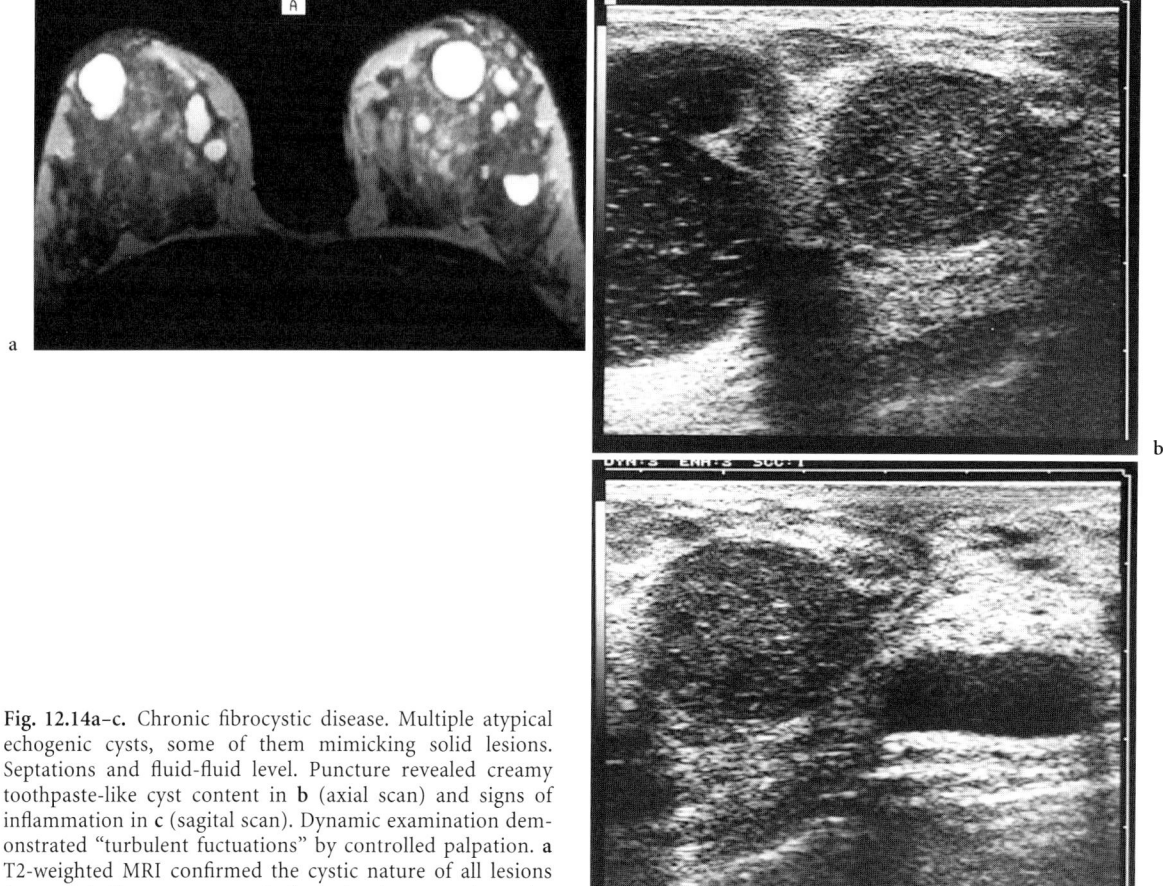

Fig. 12.14a–c. Chronic fibrocystic disease. Multiple atypical echogenic cysts, some of them mimicking solid lesions. Septations and fluid-fluid level. Puncture revealed creamy toothpaste-like cyst content in **b** (axial scan) and signs of inflammation in **c** (sagital scan). Dynamic examination demonstrated "turbulent fuctuations" by controlled palpation. **a** T2-weighted MRI confirmed the cystic nature of all lesions (comment: there was no pathological enhancement on dynamic postcontrast T1 evaluation)

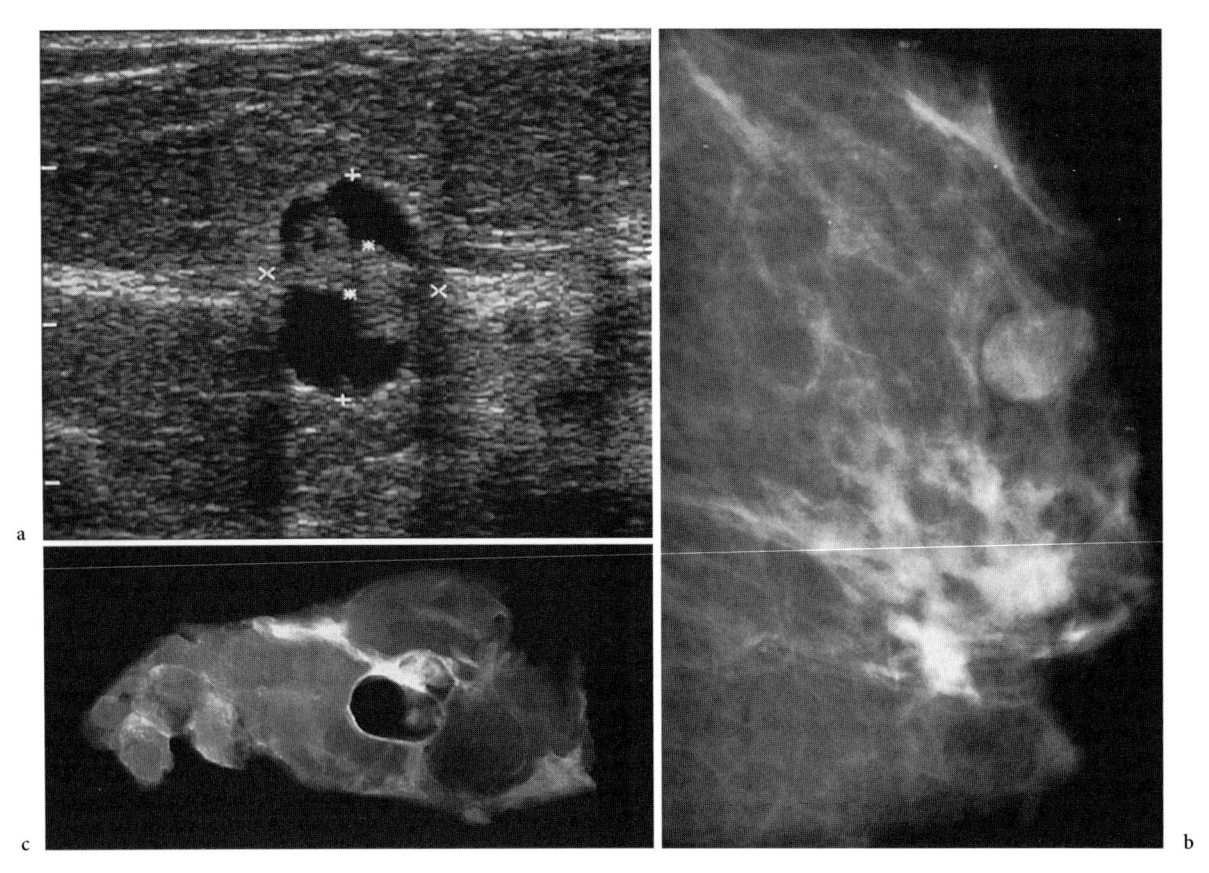

Fig. 12.15a–c. Intracystic papilloma (3×11 mm): correlation of sonogram (a) mammogram (b) and specimen radiograph (c)

centrally, this distinction can only be reliable when optimal gain settings and state-of-the art equipment are used.

The diagnosis of cysts is of great importance in the evaluation of palpable lesions in mammographically dense (non-diagnostic) breasts. Before the advent of sonography, these lesions were fine-needle aspirated and in cases of unsuccessful fluid aspiration, they were biopsied by surgery. This is no longer necessary as an exact cyst aspiration can be performed under ultrasonographic guidance (Fig. 12.13).

About half of all cysts are compressible. Demonstration of compressibility can be of some diagnostic value if the center of a cyst does not appear anechoic [e.g., due to thickened intercystic fluid or inflamed cysts with a high cell or protein content (Fig. 12.14)] or if the borders are not entirely sharp.

If intracystic lesions are detected by ultrasonography, aspiration should not be performed since the pneumocystogram will not yield further information in these cases (Fig. 12.15). Even cytolology cannot reliably differentiate between a benign papilloma and an intracystic papillary carcinoma. The sonographic differential diagnostic criteria are equally unreliable (Kasumi and Sakuma 1994). Therefore, the next step should always be surgical biopsy. Bigger intracystic papillomas as well as papillary carcinoma can fill the cyst lumen completely and display the characteristics of any other benign-appearing solid lesion.

12.10 Benign Solid Lesions

12.10.1 Fibroadenomas

Fibroadenomas are the most common benign tumors and are often found in younger women. They usually are solitary lesions usually measuring about 1–2 cm and seldom more than 4 cm in diameter. Multiple fibroadenomas or fibroadenomatosis is observed in less than 10% of cases. In more than 70% of all cases fibroadenomas present with typical "benign" criteria such as (Fig. 12.16) (FORNAGE et al. 1989; TEUBNER et al. 1985a):

- Round, oval, sometimes lobulated contour
- Sharp borders with strong capsule echoes
- Homogeneous hypoechoic internal pattern
- Bilateral refractive shadowing
- Posterior enhancement
- Horizontal orientation (D/W ratio <0.7)
- >20% compressibility

Sonographic delineation of fibroadenomas is easy in radiodense breasts of younger women, but detection may be difficult in fatty breasts of older women as fat tissue has an almost equal echogenicity to fibroadenoma (Fig. 12.17). More information can be gained from the dynamic scan. Fibroadenomas are less pliable than fat inclusions (fat lobules), whose continuity with other fat lobules can easily be recognized during real-time examination.

With advancing age fibroadenomas develop hyaline degeneration sometimes accompanied by calcium deposits, losing their typically "benign" characteristics. Larger sclerotic fibroadenomas may have irregular walls and inhomogeneous internal echoes (Fig. 12.18) similar to carcinomas. Calcified fibroadenomas display strong shadowing and may mimic scirrhous carcinomas at ultrasonography (Fig. 12.19). However, these lesions can be differentiated easily on mammography due to the pathognomonic coarse macrocalcifications of fibroadenoma, not present in carcinoma.

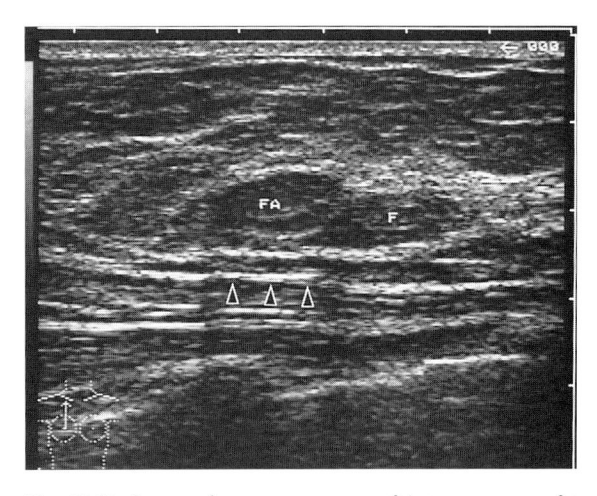

Fig. 12.17. Isomorphous appearance of intramammary fat lobule (*F*) and fibroadenoma (*FA*). Differentiation was possible by analysis of time-of-flight artifact at the flat surface of the pectoral muscle: there is a "positive" step (*arrowheads*) behind the fibroadenoma caused by speeding up the sound velocity and a "negative" step dorsal to the fat lobule (slow-down of velocity)

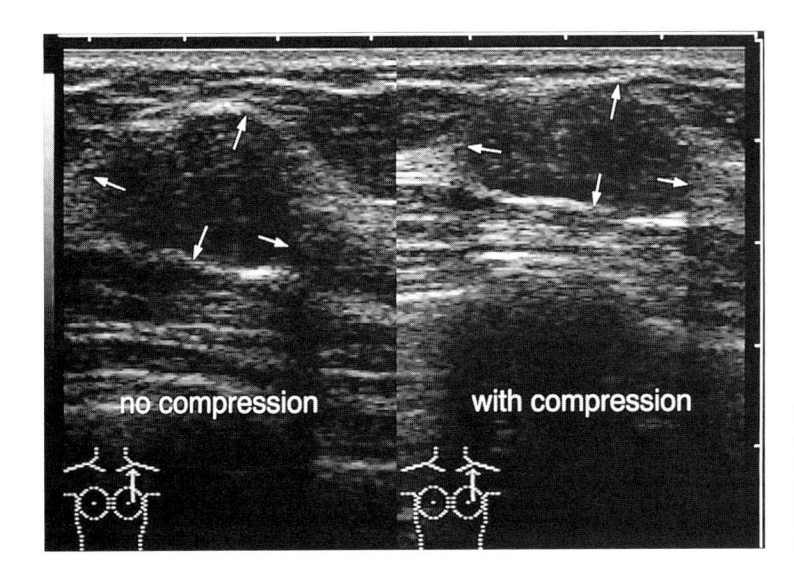

Fig. 12.16. Elastic macrolobulated fibroadenoma with benign features: D/W ≪ 1, elasticity ~20%, harmonic displacement of surrounding tissue (no disruption of architecture), and capsulated smooth margin

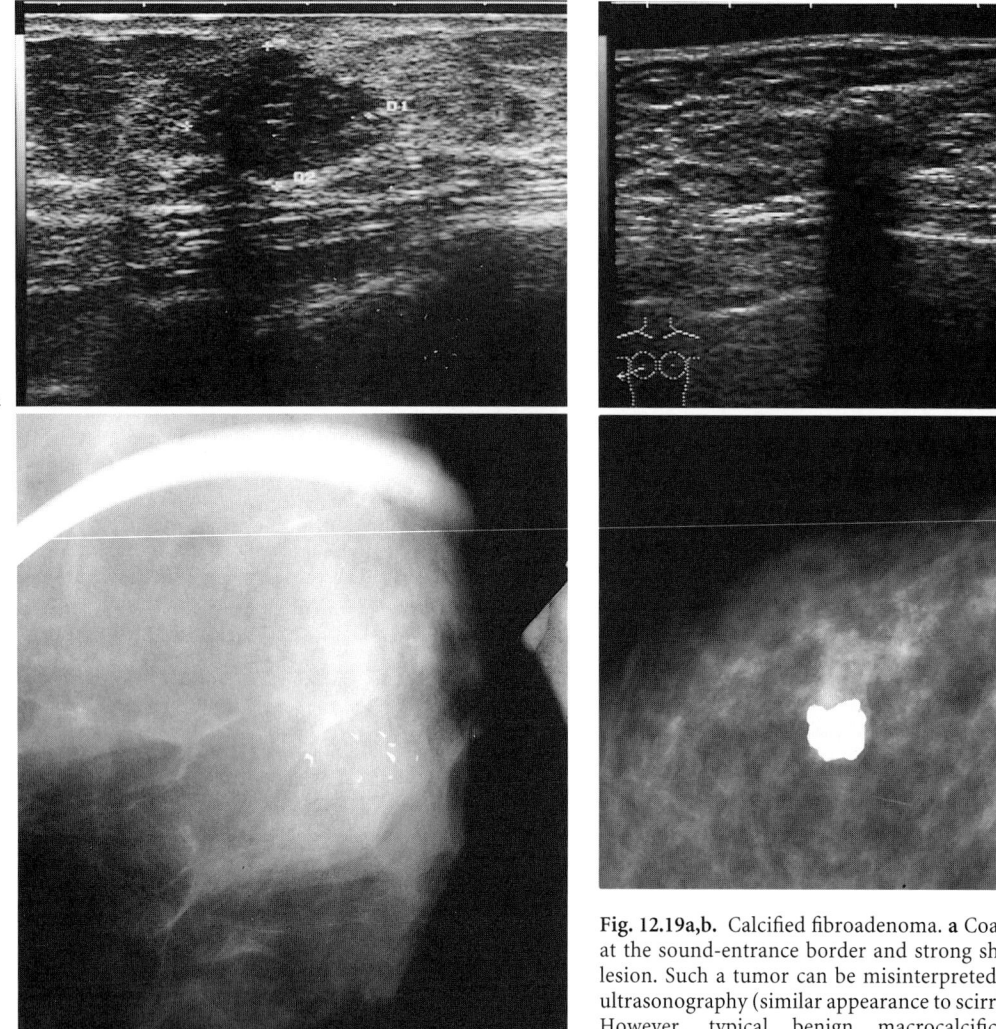

Fig. 12.18a,b. Sclerosing fibroadenoma. a Ultrasonography revealed an irregularly marginated lesion with an inhomogeneous internal echo pattern (false-positive findings). A smooth-marginated lesion with nonsuspicious macrocalcifications and a "benign" halo sign was seen on the mammogram (b)

Fig. 12.19a,b. Calcified fibroadenoma. a Coarse bright echoes at the sound-entrance border and strong shadow behind the lesion. Such a tumor can be misinterpreted as malignant on ultrasonography (similar appearance to scirrhous carcinoma). However, typical benign macrocalcifications on the mammogram clearly establish the diagnosis (b)

12.10.2 Hamartomas

Hamartomas are circumscribed masses which can contain all tissue components of the breast parenchyma. They are separated from the neighboring tissue by a pseudocapsule. On the mammogram they present a pathognomonic "cotton-wool" or cauliflower pattern (KRONSBEIN et al. 1983). Depending on the individual tissue composition they may be hypoechoic (fibroadenoma-like) or more hyperechoic (glandular-like). Due to their high elasticity they can be easily distinguished from solid tumors. In dense mastopathic breasts, detection may be difficult. Even when these lesions present with palpable masses open biopsy can be avoided because of their pathognomonic benign mammographic as well as ultrasographic (high elastic) appearance.

12.10.3 Adenomas

Tubular adenomas are of particular interest. They are highly elastic (compressibility >40%) and are usually interlaced with septa; on ultrasonography they have similar appearances to that of fatty islets. These generally impalpable masses are usually detected during mammographic screening and present as well-demarcated oval opacities of fairly low density (there is "discrepancy of size and density"). The solid nature of the lesion is easily demonstrated by ultrasonography. Aspiration is unnecessary because the high degree of elasticity can be considered as a highly reliable sign of benignancy (WALZ et al. 1994).

12.10.4 Lipomas

Lipomas are generally observed by clinical examination as taut elastic superficial masses. They are usually located in the subcutaneous fat, but may also occur in the glandular tissue or in the retromammary space. Characteristically they are encapsulated and smooth marginated, of flat oval shape, and easily compressible. The internal texture is homogeneous. Both hypo- and hyperechoic variants exist, probably due to different degrees of fibrosis or to edema in cases of inflammation (Fig. 12.20). The mammographic appearance of lipoma is pathognomonic benign.

12.10.5 Abscesses

Abscesses can cause problems in differential diagnosis as they often present with "malignant" sonographic characteristics. The purulent center (inhomogeneous low echoes) is usually geographically circumscribed and surrounded by a hyperechoic rim (demarcation zone and edema). By sonopalpation slight central turbulence of semiliquid abscess contents may be induced, which can be visualized on the B-mode image. Hence discrimination between abscesses and solid lesions may be possible without aspiration (Fig. 12.21).

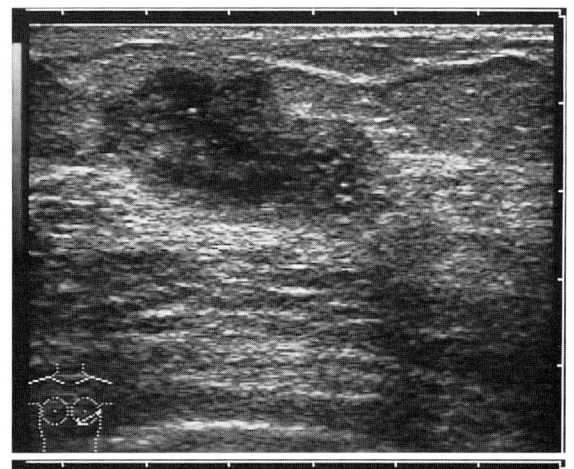

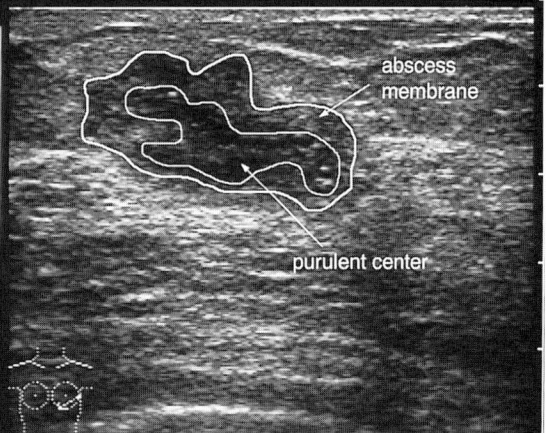

Fig. 12.21a,b. Abscess: irregularly marginated hypoechoic lesion with purulent center (outlined in b) (viscous fluctuations on palpation)

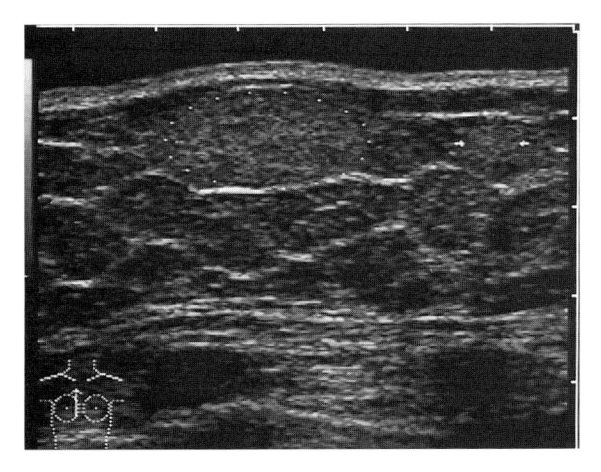

Fig. 12.20. Typical subcutaneous lipoma. Clinically there was taut elastic smooth resistance. The easily deformable smooth-marginated echogenic lesion caused protrusion of the skin

12.10.6 Chronic or Interstitial Mastitis

In chronic or interstitial mastitis without abscess formation only an increase in the echointensity is observed, often accompanied by increased attenuation. The anatomical borderlines are obscured, whereas the elasticity of the breast structures is not affected, so that these conditions do not appear suspicious. Similar diffuse changes are observed in the postirradiated breast (KINDINGER et al. 1994). All these changes are caused by the accompanying edema, which also may produce some skin thickening and dilatation of subcutaneous lymphatic spaces (see also Sect. 12.11.6, Fig. 12.37).

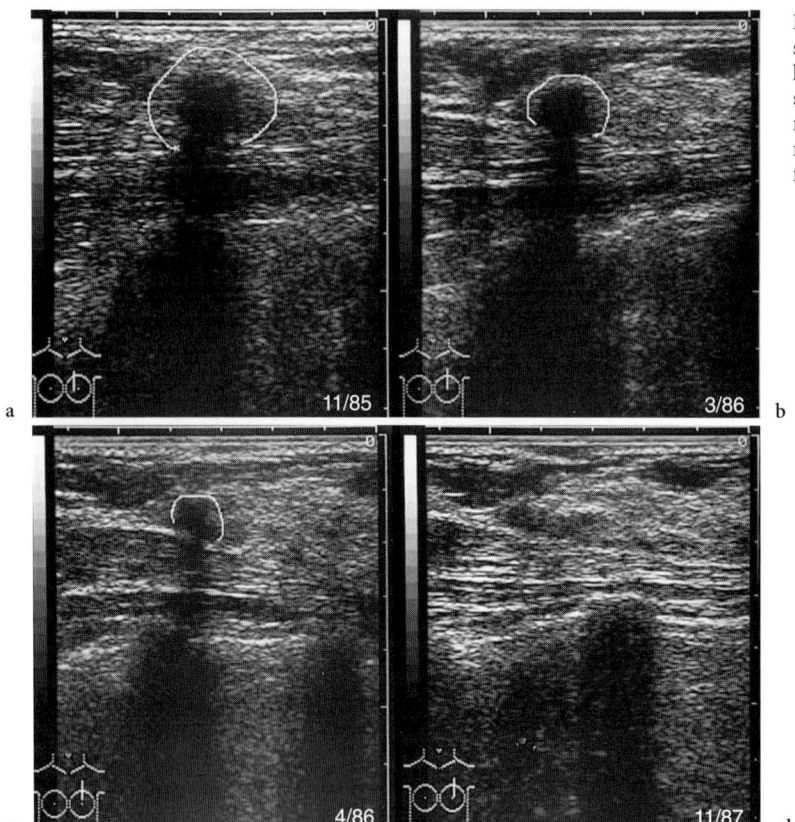

Fig. 12.22a–d. Follow-up examination of scar tissue. **a** Initially suspicious appearing lesion with echogenic border sign and shadowing (1 month post surgery). Diminution was evident after **b** 4 and **c** 6 months. **d** Two years later a nearly normal finding was obtained

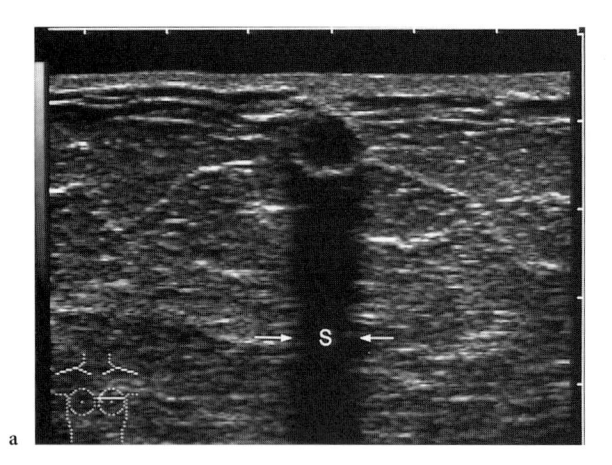

Fig. 12.23a,b. Calcified oil cyst 4 years after biopsy. **a** Ultrasonography revealed an encapsulated lesion with strong shadowing (nondiagnostic). **b** Mammography clearly demonstrated the cyst

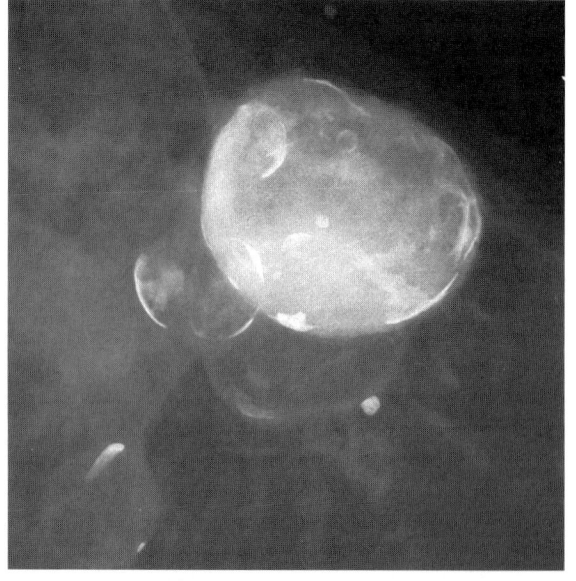

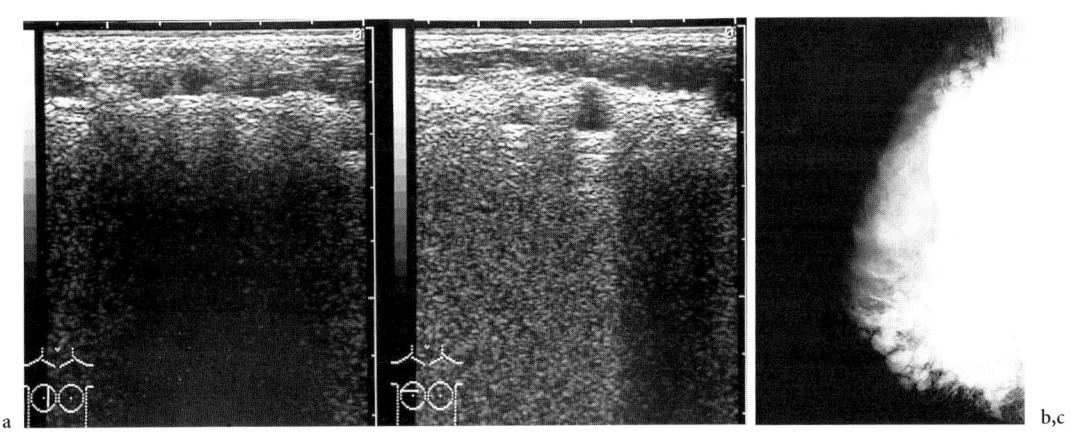

Fig. 12.24a–c. Silicone granuloma. **a,b** Typical snowstorm pattern (diffuse sound scattering at silicone-to-fibrous interfaces) and shadowing phenomena. A triangular cystic-like hypoechoic lesion is demonstrated (D/W >>1) caused by negative time-of-flight artifact). **c** Mammographic appearance

12.10.7 Scars

Fresh postoperative scars are characterized by a poorly demarcated hypoechoic center (due to the irregular resection margin, formation of serous fluid collections or hematoma or fat colliquations). According to the tissue damage, the contours of intramammary structures may be interrupted. With increasing reactive or reparative fibrosis, attenuation phenomena may occur. The latter depend on the tissue compression applied with the transducer and may disappear completely if there is enough residual elasticity of the tissue.

12.10.8 Fat Necrosis

It may be impossible to differentiate fixed partially fibrotic fat necrosis from carcinoma (inhomogeneous hypoechoic center with echogenic lateral shadowing). In doubtful cases, clarification must be obtained by mammographic demonstration of oil cyst(s) or if this feature is not present, by fine-needle aspiration, core biopsy or magnetic resonance imaging of the lesion. In patient with breast conservation therapy, early postoperative mammographic and sonographic examination of the scar is advisable in order to monitor changes of the lesion on follow-up examinations, which should be performed in the first 2 postoperative years at intervals of 4–6 months. Usually gradual regression of the "suspicious" ROI can then be observed (Fig. 12.22).

12.10.9 Oil Cysts

Fat necrosis and post-traumatic oil cysts often become calcified after 1–3 years. As in calcified fibroadenoma, their appearance can vary, with either jagged borders surrounded by a hyperechoic rim or capsule-like demarcation. Reliable benign diagnosis is usually only achieved by mammography (Fig. 12.23).

12.10.10 Lesions Following Breast Augmentation Mammoplasty

After breast augmentation mammoplasty the changes in the breast parenchyma resemble those seen after excisional biopsy. Because of diagnostic problems with mammography in patients with breast implants, ultrasonography is a valuable complementary examination technique for these patients. On the other hand, breast tissue is very difficult to evaluated sonographically after injection of free silicone: the acoustic interference caused by the numerous tiny drops of freely dispersed silicone and the mesh of ingrowing connective tissue fibers (extremely inhomogeneous tissue composition!) results in diffuse acoustic scattering since the sound velocity of silicone gel is only about half that of normal soft tissue. The sonogram then shows a typical "snow-storm" pattern (BARLOW 1980) and hypoechoic cyst-like triangular-shaped (D/W >1) *silicone granuloma* (Fig. 12.24). Focal collections of free silicone have a fairly consistent appearance and the above-mentioned phenomena are quite characteristic of silicone leakage from damaged inlays (PALMON et al. 1994).

12.11 Malignant Diseases

Breast carcinomas present with a variety of morphological appearances and different macroscopic growth patterns (BÄSSLER 1984). In order to understand the diagnostic potential of ultrasonography, full knowledge of the various mammographic and sonographic appearances of malignancy is essential (BARTH 1979; TEUBNER et al. 1993). Therefore, in the following some histopathological and sonographic characteristics are correlated, giving consideration to specific acoustic properties of different tissue compositions, as mentioned above. The following tumor types will be considered:

1. Intraductal carcinoma
2. Invasive ductal carcinoma
3. Stellate carcinoma
4. Circumscribed carcinoma
5. Diffusely infiltrating carcinoma
6. Inflammatory carcinoma

12.11.1 Intraductal Carcinoma

In noninvasive tumors, the intraductal neoplastic epithelial proliferations do not penetrate the basement membrane. The histological pattern may present micro-papillary, cribriform, or solid with

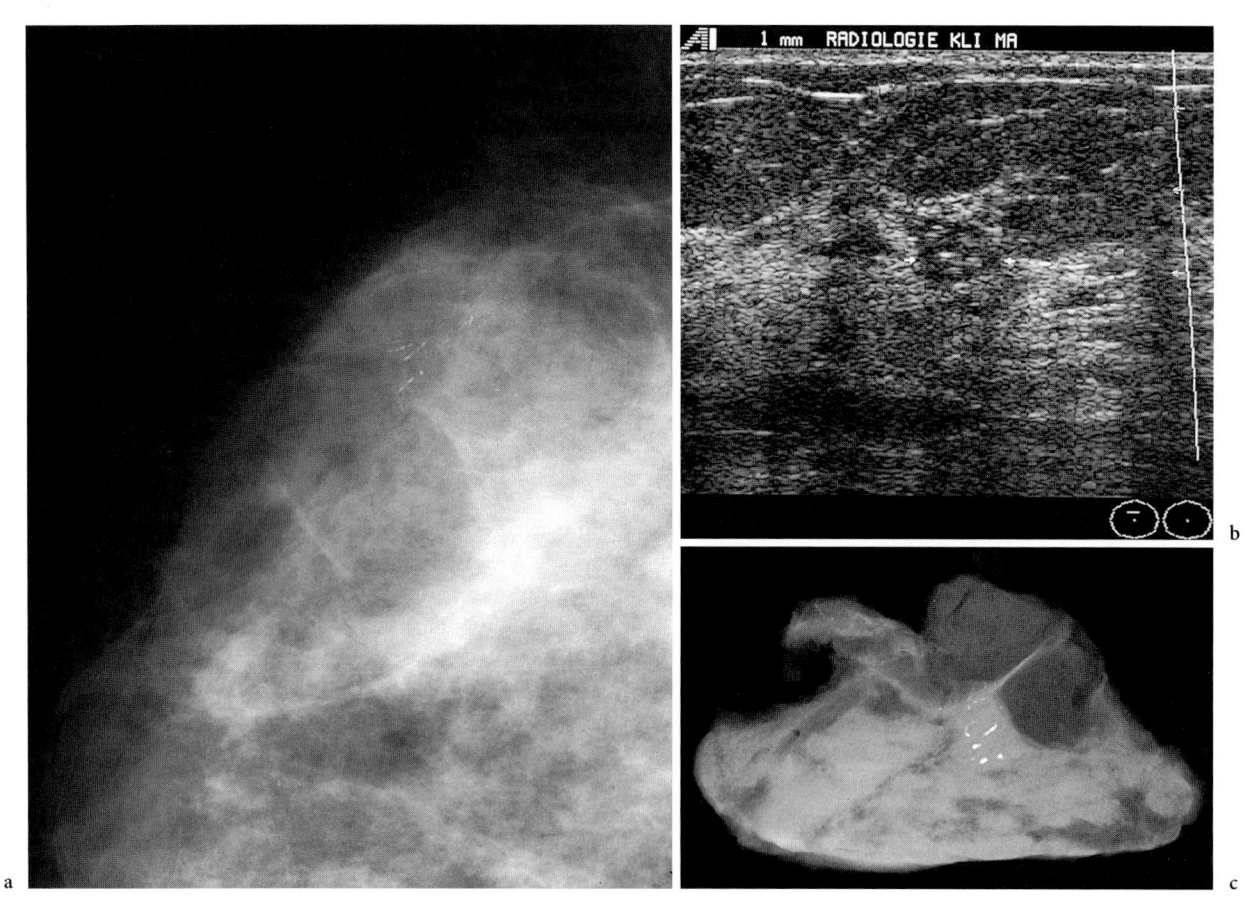

Fig. 12.25a–c. Ductal carcinoma in situ detected by screening mammography. No sonographic "microcalcification correlate" is visible. **a** Full-size magnification view of tiny microcalcifications. **b** Even under movement of the needle tip, no clear change in echogenicity of the clustered microcalcifications was demonstrable. **c** Correlative specimen radiograph

central necrosis (comedo type), accompanied by microcalcifications within the lumen of the ducts, which are generally clearly demonstrable by mammography. The size of these microcalcifications is usually smaller than the ultrasonic beam width, resulting in medium echo strengths only. This explains why these tiny calcifications cannot be detected by ultrasonography, insofar as the echogenic background pattern of the surrounding glandular tissue obscures the tumor's own echoes, unless there is very extensive intraductal proliferation (Fig. 12.25). Therefore mammography is superior at early tumor stages of intraductal carcinoma: among ten of our own patients with noninvasive intraductal carcinoma (without palpatory findings), no "microcalcification correlate" was perceived by ultrasonography (TEUBNER et al. 1990); these clinically occult early carcinomas were exclusively detectable by mammography!

The same holds true in minimally invasive ductal carcinomas with a predominant intraductal component. These tumors may spread a long distance within ductal segments. Since the invasion into the surrounding glandular tissue is only minimal, the acoustic matrix is preserved, resulting in a similar echo pattern as in "normal" glandular tissue. Therefore, again, these entities are sonographically occult in about 50% of all cases (TEUBNER et al. 1985a,c).

In more advanced stages, corkscrew-like deformed and widened lactiferous ducts can be demonstrate by high-resolution (>10 MHz) ultrasonography (Fig. 12.26), particularly with when performing radial scans along the branches of the ductal network (TEBOUL 1991). Recently KAMIO et al. (1994) reported on 198 cases with dilated ducts (60 with "regular type" and 138 with "irregular type II" wall contours). Ninety-five percent of patients with regularly dilated ducts did not have intraductal carcinoma, while 92% with irregular wall contours had malignant disease.

It has been reported anecdotally that using the "radial scanning technique," ultrasonography can

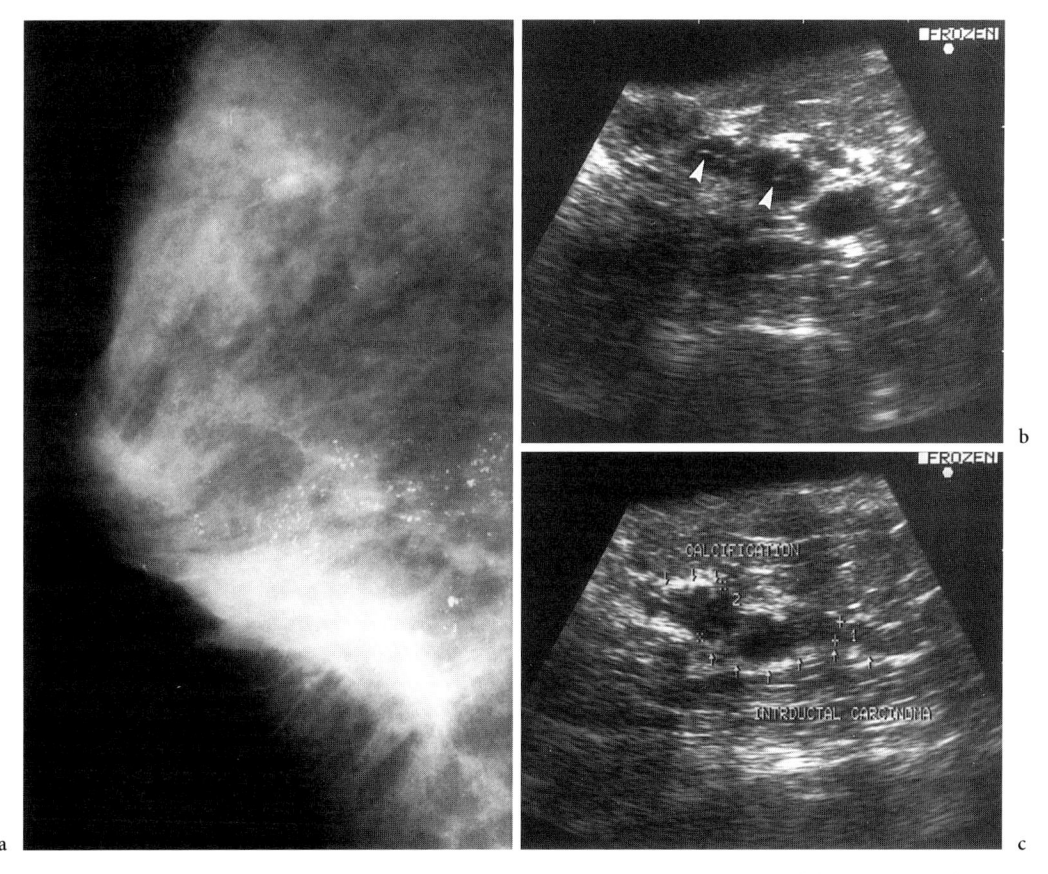

Fig. 12.26. a Advanced intraductal spreading carcinoma with multiple linear/segmentally arranged microcalcifications (diameter: 0.2–1.0 mm) is observed on the mammogram. **b,c** High-resolution ultrasonography (13 MHz, radial scanning planes) demonstrates corkscrew-like deformed and widened ducts. (diameter 1.4–4.0 mm). Some of the intraductal calcifications (>300 μm) are perceptible in the central lumen of the thickened hypoechoic ducts (*arrowheads*)

detect thickened duct segments in noninvasive or minimally invasive tumors *without* calcifications (TEUBNER et al. 1993). Therefore, in all cases with substantial segmental ductal dilations and slight wall irregularities, intraductal carcinomas must be considered in the differential diagnosis.

In some rare cases intraductal tumor spread may involve a complete breast segment. Even if the tumor remains "in situ," a segmental diffusely decreased echo pattern can be recognized if the necrotic debris of comedo DCIS is the predominant tissue component (Fig. 12.27). Special attention must be paid to this subtle sign by carefully comparing the different echogenicity in neighboring segments or quadrants.

Large invasive tumors usually present with the typical sonographic characteristics of invasive ductal carcinoma. In these cases, microcalcifications demonstrated on mammograms usually will also be visualized by ultrasonography, since the hypoechoic background pattern of the tumor mass good contrast

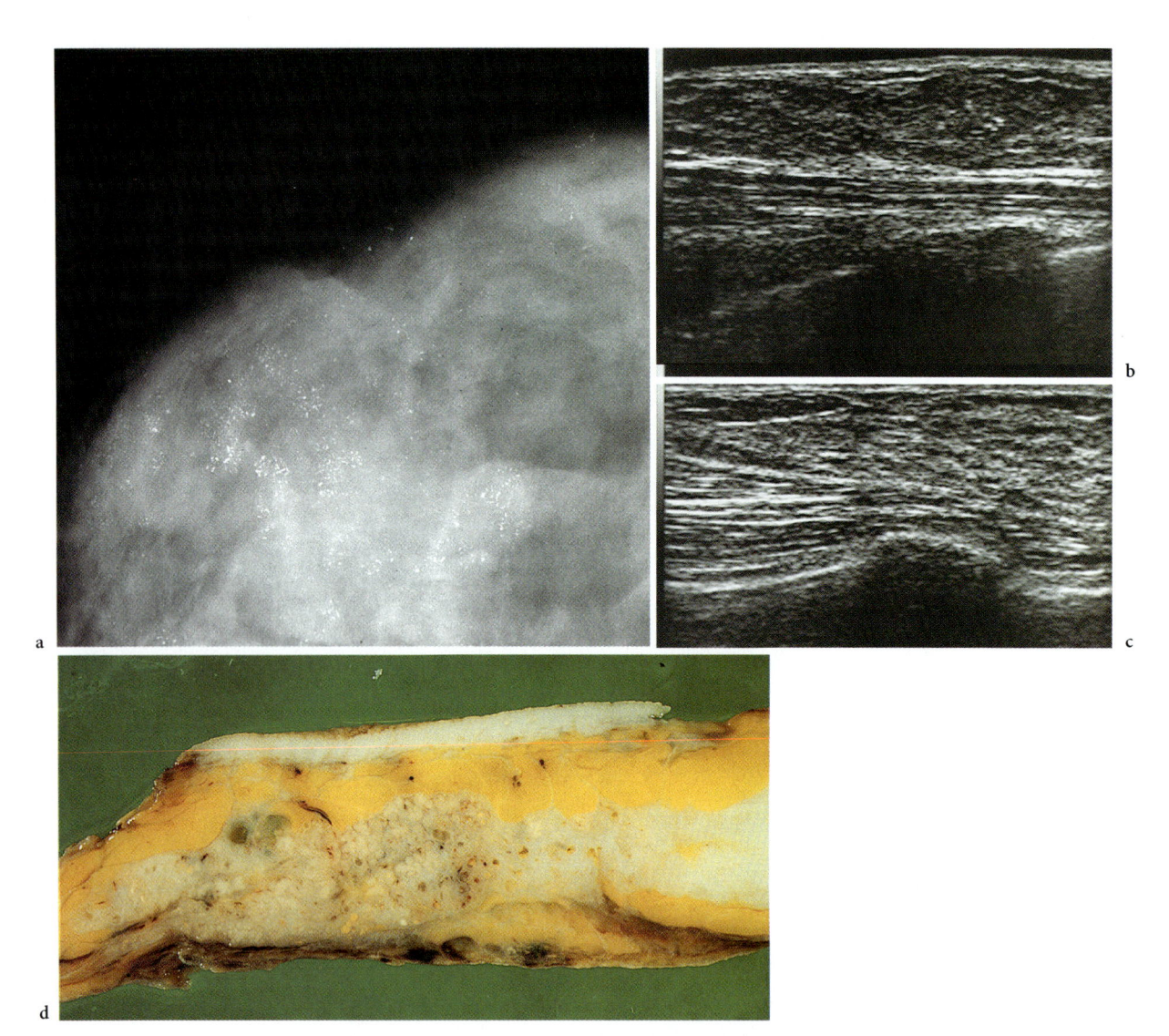

Fig. 12.27a–c. Thirty-five year old patient with unspecific itching in her left breast without any suspicious palpatory finding. Histology: 4-cm-diameter noninvasive comedo carcinoma **a.** Mammography demonstrates multiple clustered polymorphous microcalcifications scattered over the whole outer upper quadrant. **b** Ultrasonography reveals a diffuse decrease in echogenicity in the 1–2 o'clock segment as compared with the "normal" echo pattern at the 11–12 o'clock segment (**c**). Within the hypoechoic background some bright microcalcifications are visible. **d** Macroscopic gross slice reveals advanced comedo DCIS, clearly demarcated from unaffected glandular tissue. The necrotic debris of enlarged tumorous transformed ducts is melting together, resulting in a "homogeneous" tissue composition with few acoustic interfaces. This gives a "hypoechoic" background pattern, making the sonographic demonstration of intraductal microcalcifications possible

against bright speckles deriving from any calcification (Fig. 12.28).

12.11.2 Invasive Ductal Carcinoma

The most common type of breast cancer is invasive ductal carcinoma, with a prevalence of 75%. The macroscopic growth pattern of this tumor type is generally mixed (circumscribed and stellate), resulting in a variety of appearances. In former literature, these tumors were classified into further subgroups (depending on the relation of cells to stroma) which are also important for the sonographic appearance (carcinoma solidum simplex/solidum scirrhosum/solidum medullare).

On the sonogram the tumor shape is generally irregular and ill defined (as with mammography) (Fig. 12.29), the adjacent architecture is disrupted, and the depth-to-width ratio often exceeds 1. Typically, the center of the tumor is hypoechoic, surrounded by a hyperreflective halo ("echogenic border sign," see Fig. 12.31a) (TEUBNER 1985; TAKEHARA et al. 1983). The hyperreflective periphery is compounded with the hypoechoic center but can show an echogenicity comparable to that of the adjacent glandular tissue. Due to isoechoicity with adjacent glandular tissue, this important phenomenon may only be recognized during dynamic real-time examination if the tumor area is evaluated under differing compression and simultaneous palpation ("sonopalpation"): following this procedure,

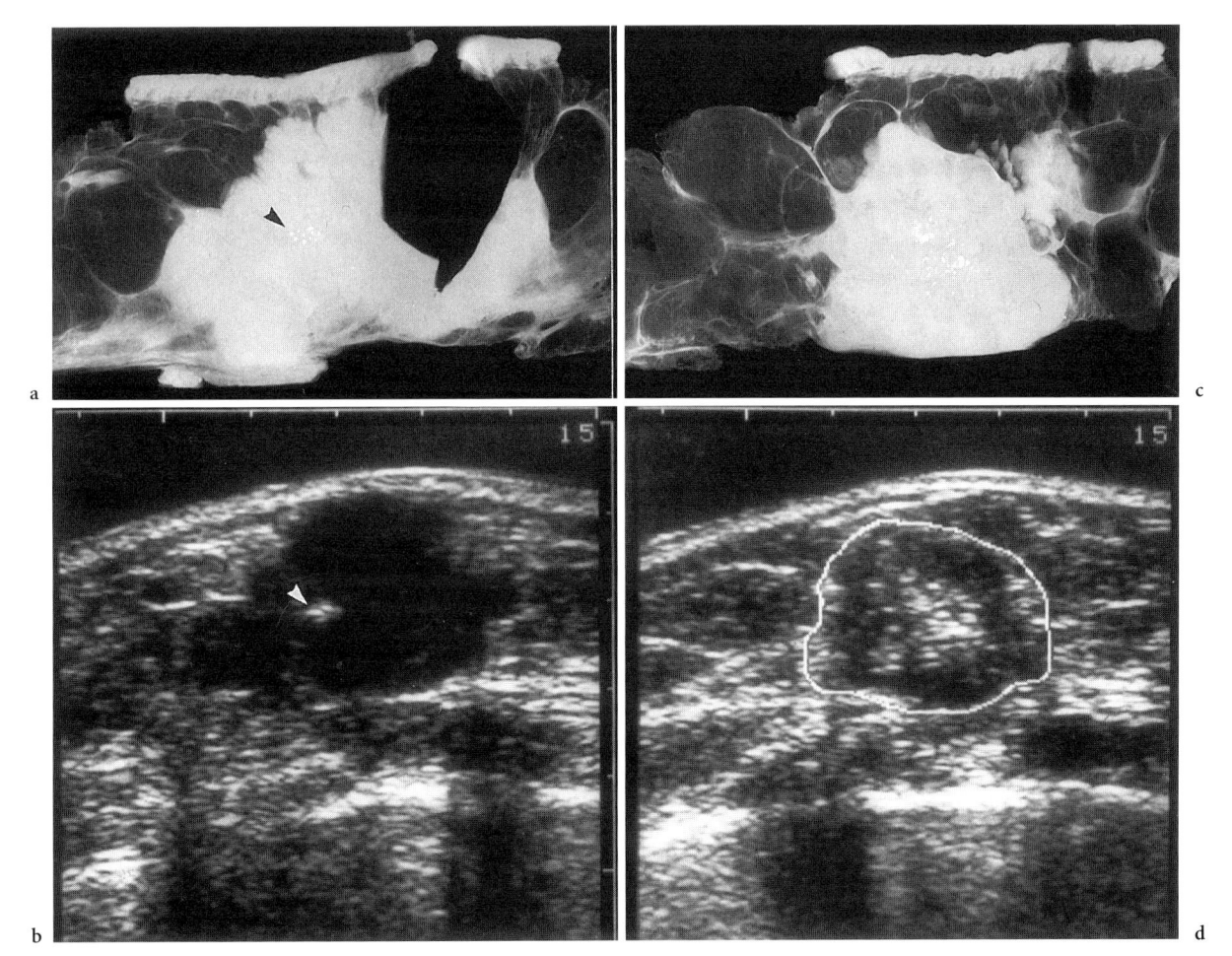

Fig. 12.28a–d. Comparison of ultrasonography and mammography in the demonstration of microcalcifications (4-cm-diameter ductal invasive carcinoma with central calcifications). **a** Specimen radiograph of central parts of the tumor: solid, rediodense lesion without fat inclusions. A few clustered microcalcifications are seen within a 3-mm-diameter area (*arrowhead*). **b** Corresponding sonogram (in vivo): lobulated tumor (*arrowhead*) appearing homogeneously hypoechoic with some bright reflexes caused by mammographically demonstrated microcalcifications. **c** Upper part of the tumor with multiple expanding microcalcifications. **d** Corresponding sonogram: centrally echodense tumor (microcalcification correlate). Note: similar echogenicity of microcalcifications as compared with adjacent unaffected ("normal") glandular tissue

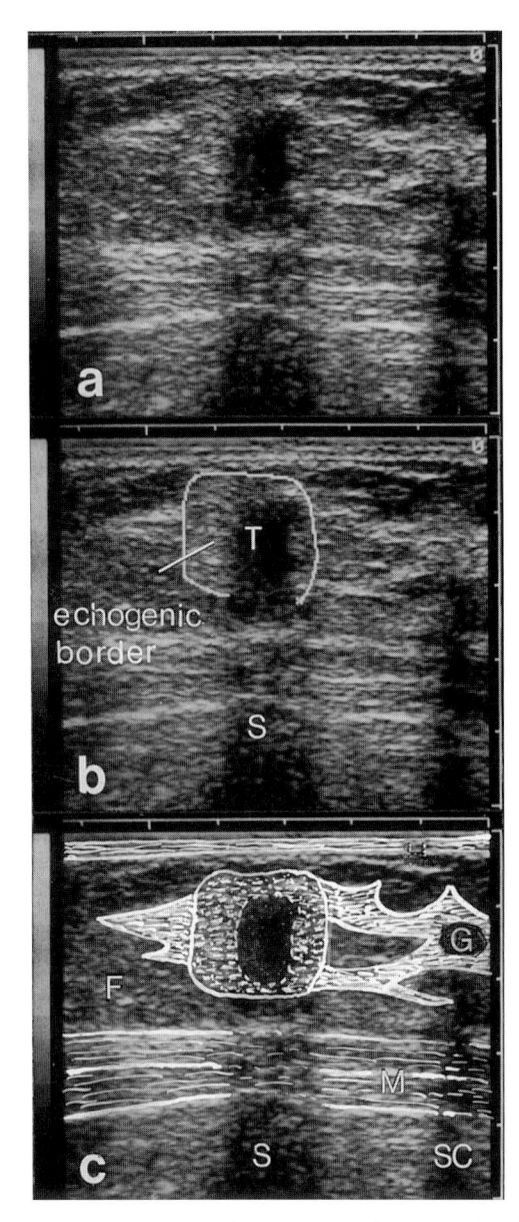

tissue stainings, which were evaluated at medium- and low-power magnifications (TEUBNER et al. 1994). The main differences in the periphery and at the center of the tumor concerned the amount and distribution of fat cells and fibrous structures, respectively (Fig. 12.30).

The histological cut surface of this tumor entity typically shows a target-like pattern with different tissue compositions in the center and the periphery: The central tumor parts are almost always characterized by predominant fibrohyalinosis with sparsely interpersed remaining tumor cells, necrotic zones, and only a few residual ductal elements; therefore, central area must be hypoechoic since there is only one prevalent tissue component. On the other hand, the echogenic periphery can be visualized since the firm echogenic border (compounded with the hypoechoic center) and the elastic glandular tissue slide against one another.

In order to understand the bioacoustic nature of this phenomenon, we correlated the sonograms of 22 carcinomas showing an "echogenic border" with histological whole mount sections in special connective

Fig. 12.29a–c. Typical appearance of invasive ductal carcinoma: irregularly marginated hypoechoic tumor (*T*) with D/W > 1, disruption of architecture, and dorsal shadowing (*S*). Marked echogenic border, recognizable during dynamic real-time examination by "sonopalpation". *G*, Unaffected glandular tissue; *M*, pectoral muscle; *SC*, shadowing behind Cooper's ligament

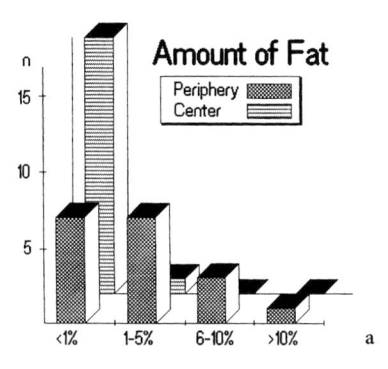

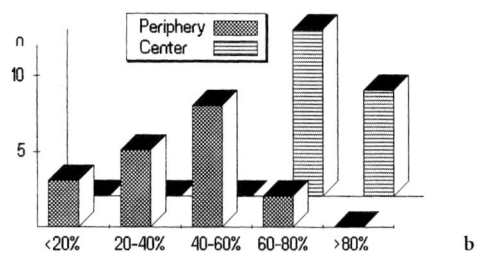

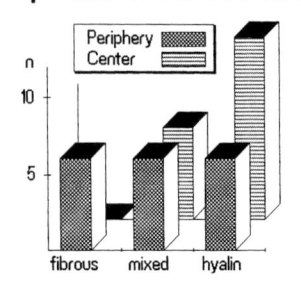

Fig. 12.30a–e. Histological aspects of the tissue composition at the periphery of the tumor as compared with the center. Major differences exist in the amount of fat cells and the fibrotic architecture (TEUBNER et al. 1994)

Alignment of Fibrous Filaments

d

Thickness of Fibrous Filaments

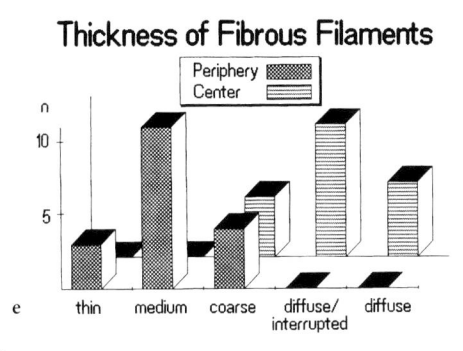

e

Fig. 12.30d,e

the periphery displays side by side strands of collagen fibers (desmoplastic reaction), proliferating tumor cells, and some fatty inclusions; this mixture of tissue components is responsible for the high echogenicity (Fig. 12.31). Therefore the echogenic border must be included in the measurement that determines the preoperative tumor size (Fig. 12.32); if only the hypoechoic center is considered, tumor size may be underestimated (ERNST et al. 1990; NISHIMURA et al. 1987).

About 30% of invasive ductal carcinomas present with increased sound absorption (shadowing). Two possible mechanisms have been suggested: the high content of collagen (KOBAYASHI 1979) and the spiculated surface (TEUBNER et al. 1983; UENO et al. 1985).

12.11.3 Spiculated Carcinoma

Spiculated tumors comprise several histological entities, but present with comparatively similar morphological appearances at ultrasonography. The spiculated surface (strands of productive fibrosis) leads to diffuse refraction of the incident sound waves, resulting in a hyperreflective corona ("halo") followed by a shadow zone (TEUBNER et al. 1983; UENO et al. 1985). The casting shadow prevents the assessment of the "true" internal echo texture, which therefore generally appears hypoechoic due to lost insonated energy. At the posterior margin the same refractive effects can appear, enhancing the shadowing phenomenon once again (Fig. 12.33).

The following tumor entities can present with a spiculated growth pattern (BÄSSLER 1984):

a) Invasive ductal carcinoma (scirrhous type),
b) Tubular carcinoma (typical),
c) Invasive lobular carcinoma (atypical)

ad a): In *invassive ductal carcinoma* with a scirrhous growth pattern, the tumor cells are closely aligned in rows and are separated by strands of stroma. Both the center and the periphery are domi-

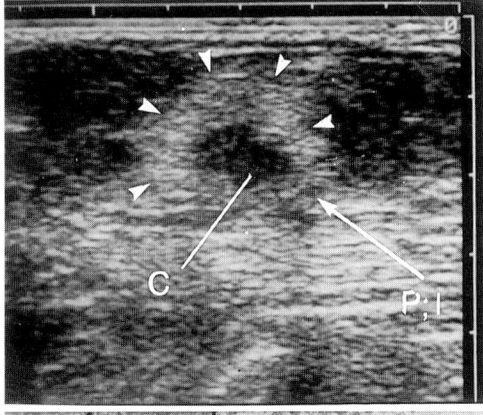

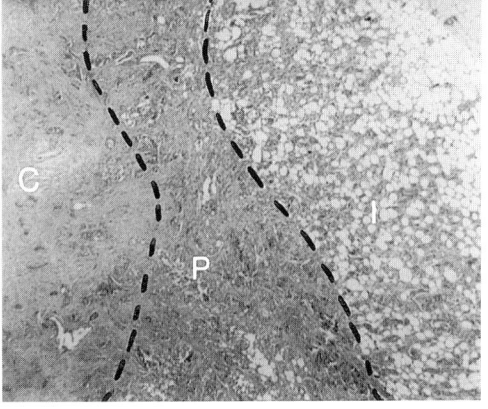

Fig. 12.31a,b. Sonographic-histomorphological analysis of the "echogenic border sign" (ductal invasive carcinoma, max. diameter 2.1 cm). a The sonogram demonstrates a centrally hypoechoic-appearing lesion (9 × 14 mm), surrounded by a clearly visible 8-mm-thick halo. b Histomorphology reveals, at 14-fold magnification, a different tissue composition at the periphery and at the center of the tumor: homogeneous hyalinosis is observed in the central portion of the tumor (*C*), while a mixture of tumor cells and net-like arranged fibrotic filaments is seen at the echogenic periphery (*P*), with fat inclusions (>30%) within the infiltration zone (*I*)

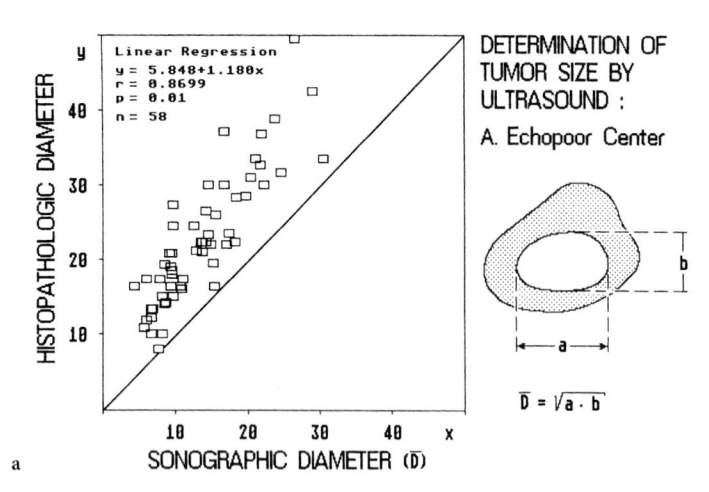

Fig. 12.32. Comparison of sonographically assessed tumor size and pathological measurements of 58 excised breast carcinomas with halo sign. The importance of "echogenic border" in tumor size determinations is clearly demonstrated

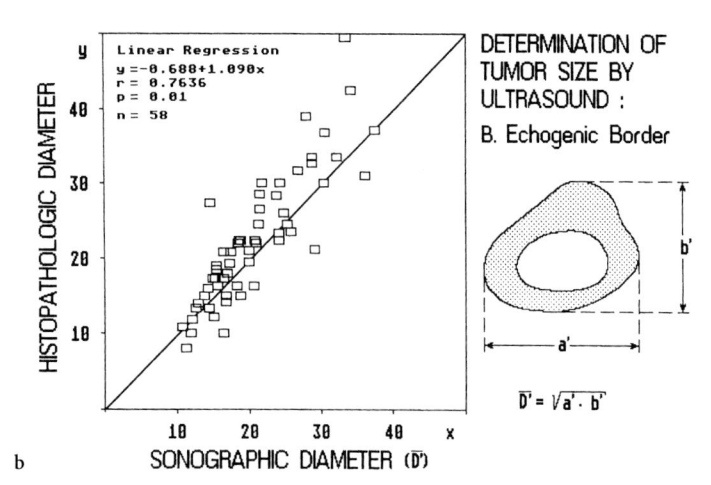

nated by the productive fibrosis and accommodate only a few tumor cell clusters.

ad b): In *tubular carcinoma,* the tumor cells typically show tubular differentiation and are embedded in loose or partly hyalinized connective tissue.

These two tumor types are characterized by a close interposition of connective tissue and epithelial structures, which are usually found at the periphery of ductal invasive carcinomas. Depending on the space between the fibrotic and epithelial strands as well as on the presence of fatty inclusions, these masses can present with more or less pronounced echogenic appearances. Especially tumors with a high fat content, which are mammographically somewhat transparent, generally appear isoechogenic to normal glandular tissue.

The phenomenon of echogenic carcinoma accompanied by a strong shadow zone has very rarely been described in the literature. This is explained because the shadow zone behind the tumor is much more conspicuous and therefore usually leads to the misinterpretation of a (nonexistent) hypoechoic tumor (Fig. 12.34). The correct image interpretation is only possible during dynamic scanning with varying tissue compression!

ad c): Invasive lobular carcinomas typically present with a diffuse growth pattern with minimal disruption of normal breast architecture in early stages (these tumors are sonographically and mammographically occult in many cases). Some tumors of this entity, however, present with a localized scirrhous pattern (similar to invasive ductal carcinoma); these cases are important representatives of *"echogenic carcinomas,"* sometimes accompanied by a shadow zone (Fig. 12.35).

12.11.4 Circumscribed Carcinoma

Circumscribed carcinomas include medullary carcinoma, mucinous carcinoma, and intracystic

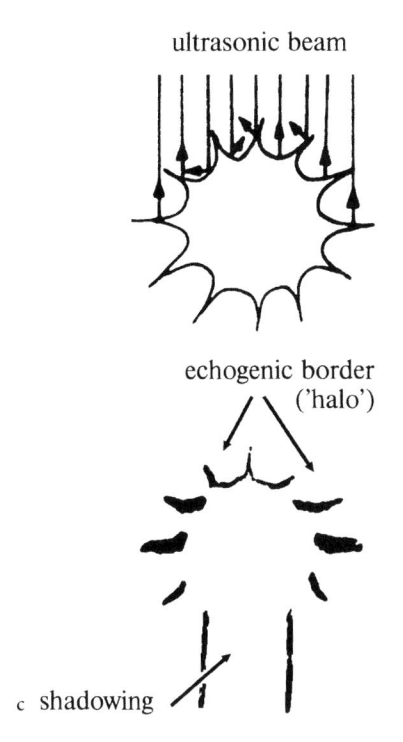

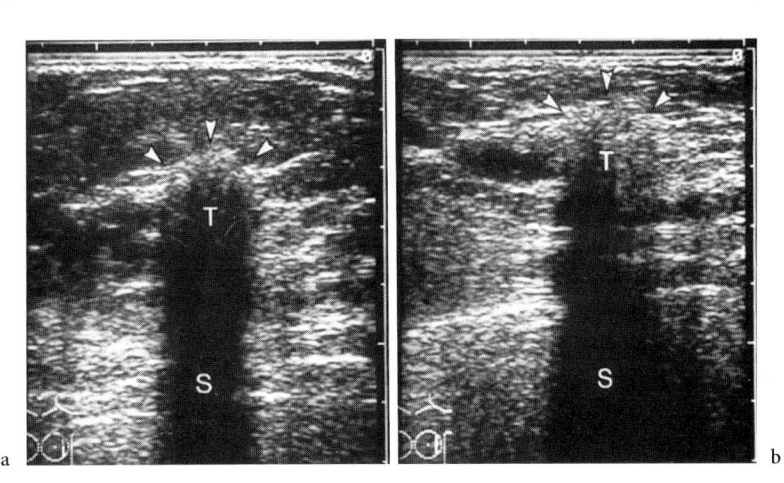

Fig. 12.33a–c. Sonographic evaluation of scirrhous carcinoma (2 cm diameter) with differing compression. a No compression: An irregularly marginated tumor (*T*) is observed. The internal echotexture is lost due to strong absorption (*S*) at the front of the tumor. b Even under higher compression shadowing is clearly demonstrable, but under this condition there is increasing central echodensity (artificially hypoechoic tumor without compression?). c Explanation of the origin of shadowing phenomena in scirrhous carcinoma: refractive effect at the spiculated surface (according to UENO et al. 1985)

papillary carcinoma. Since intracystic carcinoma have a true capsule, they may be misdiagnosed at sonography as smooth-marginated benign lesions.

Medullary carcinomas are mainly composed of tumor cells with only a small amount of connective tissue. Typically, these masses are hypoechoic. Depending on the fibrous content, however, they may appear more reflective than subcutaneous fatty tissue. In some cases the surface shows a fine lobular outline which may lead to a narrow (1–3 mm) echogenic border. Larger tumors present with perifocal edema (see as perifocal reticular patterns on mammography and as increased echoes from the adjacent fatty tissue on ultrasonography).

Mucinous (Colloid) carcinomas show a round or oval circumscribed growth pattern. In the inner part, relatively sparse collections of tumor cells are surrounded by mucin, which mainly constitutes the tissue content. These tumors are generally hypoechoic. More echogenic types usually show a heterogeneous pattern (TEUBNER et al. 1993).

Intracystic papillary carcinomas present with smooth margins mammographically. However, intracystic proliferations can be clearly identified by ultrasonography. Sometimes sedimentation phenomena lead to the diagnosis ("fluid-fluid level") (TSUNODA et al. 1990). Since benign papillomas cannot be distinguished from intracystic papillary carcinomas, all cysts with intracystic luminal masses or irregularities should be removed by open biopsy.

12.11.5 Diffusely Infiltrating Carcinoma

Infiltrating lobular carcinoma typically presents as diffusely infiltrating malignancy. This entity presents with a diffuse growth pattern with small linear, "Indian file" tumor infiltrates through the adjacent tissue or a "target-like" pattern around the ducts without extensive disruption of the normal breast architecture. Even in advanced stages the preexisting matrix of the gland may remain almost unaffected and the lesion may be difficult to diagnose on the mammogram. These cancers are often seen on only one mammographic view, presenting as an nonspecific density. Clinically the only finding may be the induration caused by the desmoplastic stroma reaction.

From a physical point of view it is obvious that the morphological alterations of echo texture caused by such slight changes in the tissue structure are only minimal. Usually only slight architectural disruption of the tissue structure or less elastic echogenic tissue

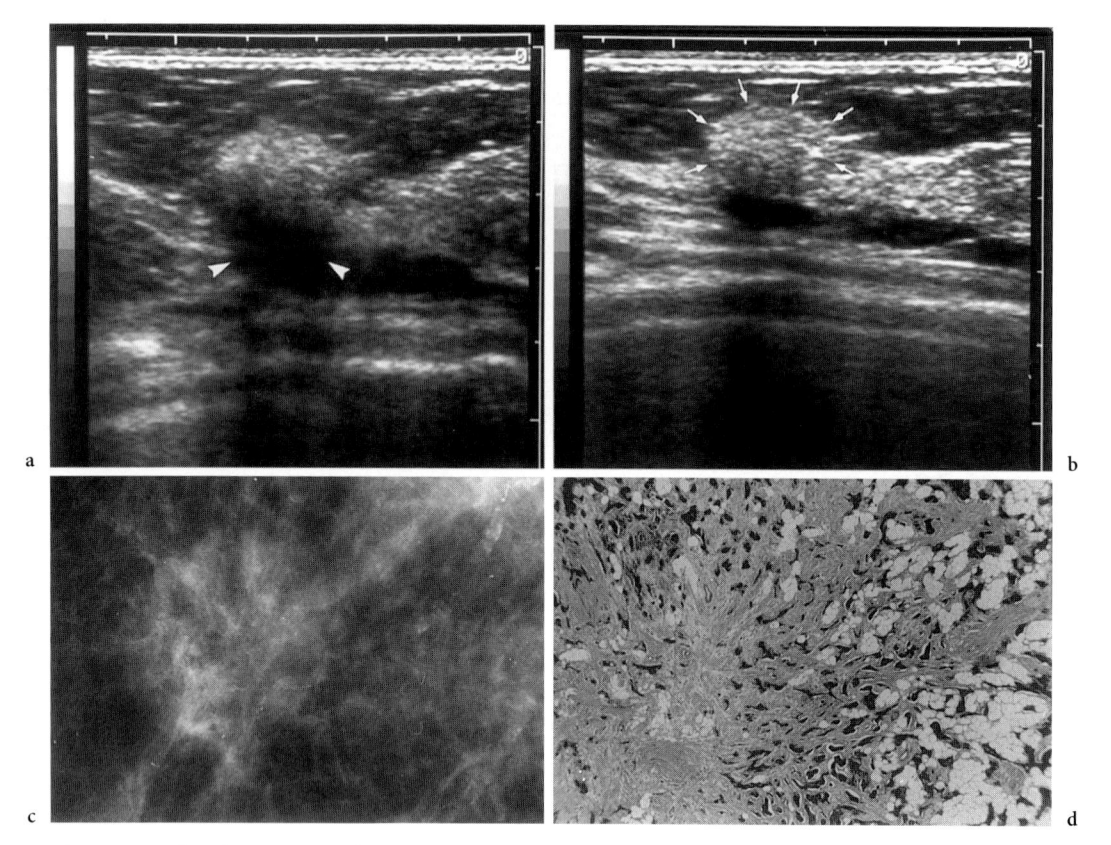

Fig. 12.34a–d. Echogenic scirrhous carcinoma (ductal invasive without central hyalinosis). **a** In the event of insufficient tissue compression there is simulation of a hypoechoic tumor, with artificial development of a hypoechoic area (*arrowheads*) dorsal to the echogenic carcinoma (induced by the absorption zone in the hypoechoic prepectoral fatty tissue). **b** Under compression there is no change in the demonstration of the echogenic tumor (*arrows*), but the hypoechoic area behind the carcinoma tends to disappear. **c** Magnification view of spiculated mass with translucent center. **d** Ductal invasive scirrhous carcinoma: isotropic tissue composition consisting of fibrous stroma, tumor epithelia, and subtle fatty inclusions (causing multiple acoustic interfaces responsible for the high echogenicity!)

areas are observed during dynamic real-time ultrasonography. Occasionally the breast structure may be obscured due to reactive edema (Fig. 12.36). When performing a core biopsy for histological examination on these lesions, care must be taken to preferentially sample the hyperechoic areas rather than the hypoechoic zones, which may represent artifactual shadow zones.

12.11.6 Inflammatory Carcinoma

In patients with inflammatory breast carcinoma, the obstruction of lymph vessels by infiltrating tumor cells causes an increase in the interstitial fluid content, and precise mammographic localization of the individual tumor manifestations may be difficult. The skin edema (increased thickness of the skin) can be clearly seen on ultrasonography (as on mammography), and fluid collections may be observed along the interstitial septa surrounding fat lobules (Fig. 12.37). Circumscribed infiltrating foci present as hypoechoic areas which can be aspirated with fine needles under sonographic guidance.

12.12 Diagnostic Value of Ultrasonography Breast Cancer Diagnosis

Knowledge of the varying sonographic appearance of breast carcinomas is very important in understanding the value of ultrasonography in breast cancer diagnosis. It is often possible to predict the sonographic characteristics from the mammographic appearance of a lesion: ill-defined tumors with a mottled radiolucent center are often imaged by ultrasonography as hyperreflective tumors, whereas mammographically dense lesions

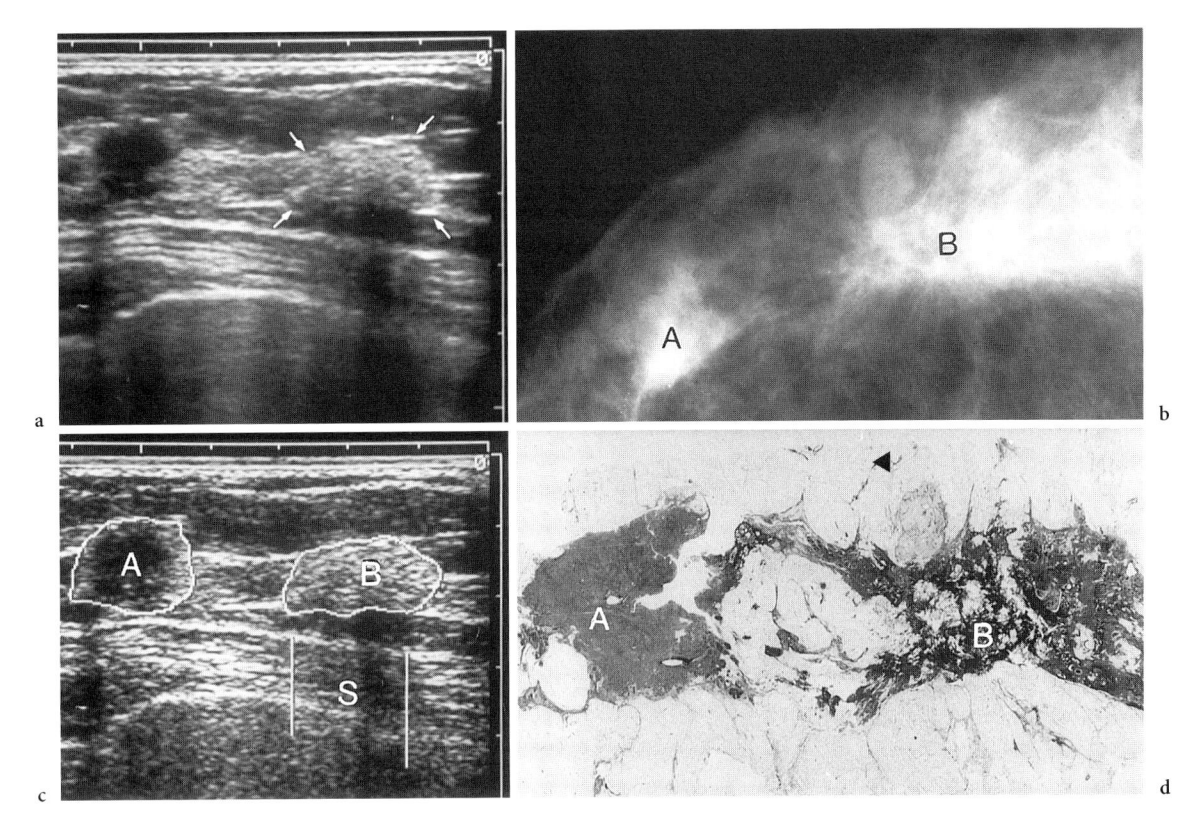

Fig. 12.35a–d. Two adjacent multifocal carcinomas with distinct morphological appearances on ultrasonography: a hypoechoic invasive ductal (tubuloductal) carcinoma with a thin echogenic border (*A*) and an echogenic invasive lobular carcinoma (*B*) with a stellate growing pattern, shadowing (*S*), and disruption of the anatomical architecture (*arrows*). A small fibroadenoma (*arrowheads*) in front of the lobular carcinoma was not detected by ultrasonography (same echo pattern as fatty tissue). The histomorphological analysis of the hypoechoic lesion (**d**) revealed central necrosis of the tumor with a narrow infiltration zone at the periphery (echogenic border); the echogenic lobular carcinoma consists of different tissue components with a distinct acoustic impedance (fat inclusions, productive fibrosis, tumor cells, preserved/minimally affected glandular tissue), responsible for the strong echogenicity

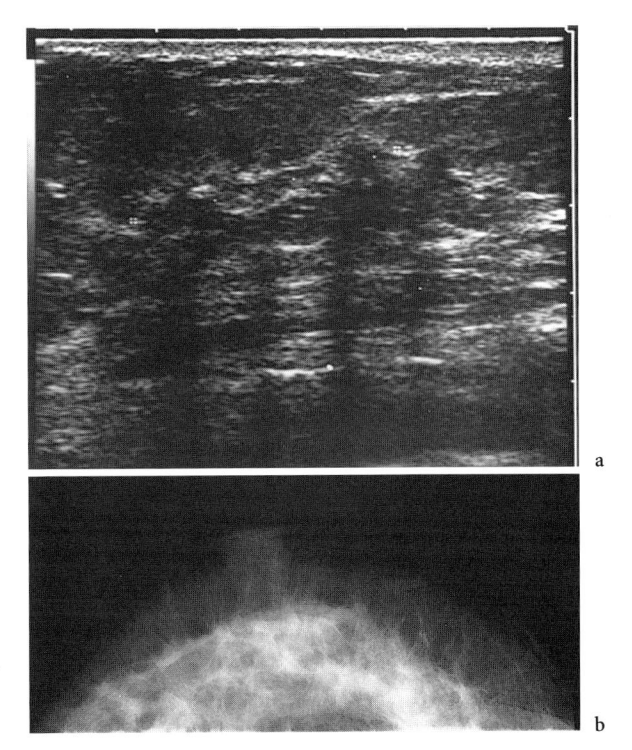

Fig. 12.36a,b. Diffuse lobular carcinoma in a 46-year-old patient, 5 years after breast-conserving therapy. Within 9 months there had been advanced shrinkage of the whole breast. **a** Ultrasonography shows an unsharp glandular-to-fat demarcation with diffuse shadowing artifacts but no tumor mass. **b** Mammography demonstrates thickened Cooper's ligaments and a swab-like inhomogeneous increase in radiographic density. Ultrasonography-guided core-cut biopsy of echogenic tissue areas confirmed the diagnosis prior to mastectomy

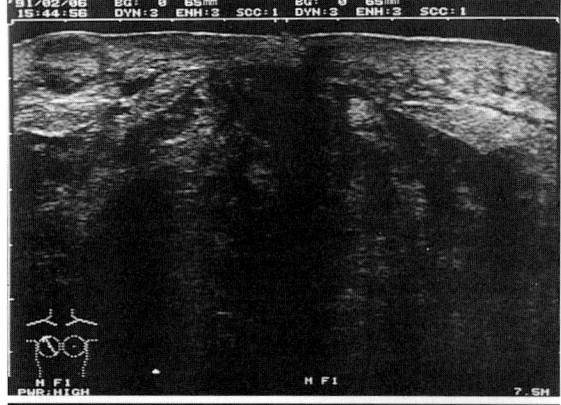

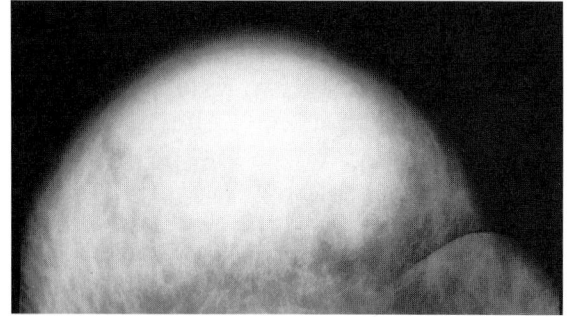

Fig. 12.37a,b. Inflammatory breast carcinoma. a Ultrasonography showing skin thickening and widened lymphatic spaces of the subcutaneous layer. A giant tumor mass is involving the whole gland. Ultrasonography-guided core-cut biopsy of the hypoechoic tumor center confirmed the diagnosis prior to primary chemotherapy. b Opaque density of the whole breast

usually have a hypoechoic central core on sonograms.

The widespread assumption that carcinomas are hypoechoic is only partly true. In the most common type of carcinoma, the infiltrating ductal carcinoma, the hypoechoic center may be obvious, but this center is almost always surrounded by a wide hyperechoic rim (zone of tumor infiltration). If there is no central hyalinosis, even these tumors may exceptionally be purely hyperechoic.

The phenomenon of the echogenic border (also termed "halo" or "hyperechoic rim") is one of the most reliable criteria of malignancy. It occurs in less than 9% of all benign lesions, mainly in the context of post-traumatic changes or in cases of scarring, inflammation, or peripheral calcific deposits in fibroadenoma. If these several causes can be excluded by clinical or mammographic examination in a specific case, the lesion is most probably malignant when a hyperechoic rim is present on ultrasonography. Another very important sign of infiltrating tumor growth is an abrupt disruption of the pre-existing intramammary tissue strands along the border of the lesion as well as a vertical orientation of the main tumor axis (D/W >1; D = depth, W = width).

Hyperreflective noncompressible lesions must be distinguished sonographically from mastopathic nodules. Differentiation of these entities can only be achieved through sonopalpation. Defined hyperechoic nodules should be biopsied with fine-needle aspiration or core biopsy under sonographic guidance in order to exclude diffuse infiltrating (e.g., lobular) carcinoma if they fail to regress under antimastopathic therapy.

About 9% of all carcinomas are *mainly* hyperechoic or *completely* hyperreflective in the absence of central hyalinosis. This phenomenon is largely unknown and has as yet not been systematically analyzed, possibly because these tumors in particular often display a higher sound absorption and their posterior shadowing may be misinterpreted as the center of the tumor. In these cases dynamic scanning techniques are again extremely important: by varying the compression with the transducer it can be demonstrated that the "suspicious" area is only a sound artifact (see Fig. 12.34).

Invasive ductal carcinomas with a predominant intraductal component are usually sonographically occult but can be detected early on mammograms on the basis of accompanying pathognomonic pleomorphic microcalcifications. Hence sonographic exclusion of DCIS or minimal invasive intraductal carcinoma in patients with mastopathic hardness should only be considered if no microcalcifications suspicious for intraductal carcinoma are demonstrated the mammograms.

Mammography is clearly superior to ultrasonography in primarily fatty breasts and in the detection of tiny microcalcifications, which occur in about 30% of all cancers. The facts that microcalcifications are not consistently demonstrable by ultrasonography unless they are within a hypoechoic mass and the better tissue-to-tumor contrast in fatty involutional breasts at mammography are the reasons that ultrasonography plays no considerable role in breast mass screening.

On the other hand, ultrasonography has proven advantages over mammography in cancer diagnosis that apply to some women with radiodense breasts (Fig. 12.38) and in the detection of lesions very close to the chest wall (Fig. 12.39), or at the breast periphery (Frazier et al. 1985; Gordon and Goldenberg 1995; Jackson et al. 1993; Lambie et

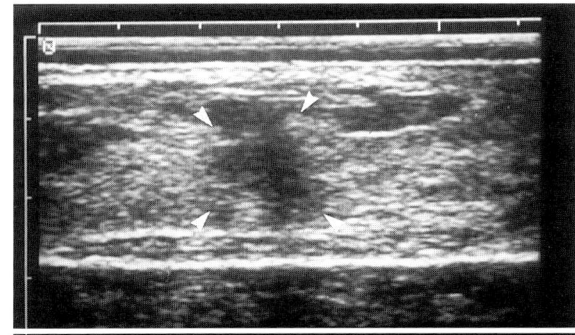

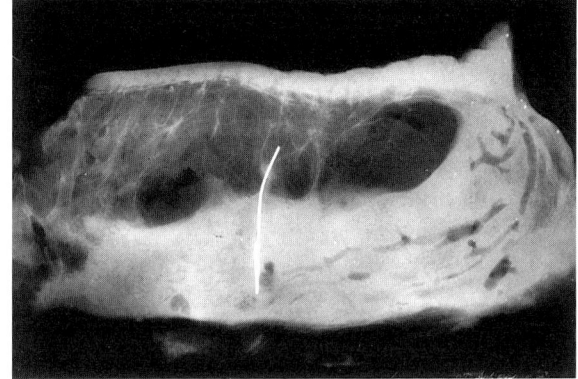

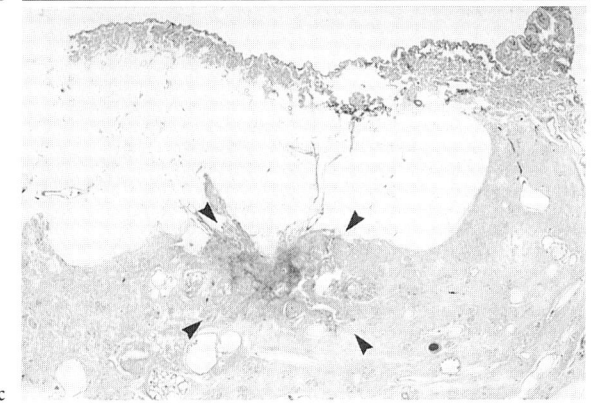

Fig. 12.38a–c. 1.5 cm tubuloductal invasive carcinoma exclusively detected by ultrasonography. **a** Specimen sonogram with irregularly marginated hypoechoic lesion (arrowheads). **b** Specimen radiograph after ultrasonography-guided needle localization of the suspicious appearing lesion: no mammographic correlate! (False-negative mammographic diagnosis since tumorous and dense glandular tissues have the same radiographic absorption characteristics.) **c** Histologic whole mount section

al. 1983, TEUBNER et al. 1985c). According to the author's daily experience and in agreement with other studies (GORDON and GOLDENBERG 1996; MADJAR 1994) it can be assumed that with dynamic scanning techniques using real-time high-resolution ultrasonography and state-of-the-art equipment ($\geq$7.5 MHz) ultrasonography is as reliable as mammography in the detection of infiltrating carcinoma equal or larger than 8 to 10 mm in diameter. It may be actually superior to mammography in the diagnosis of carcinomas larger than 1.5 cm in diameter (TEUBNER et al. 1990).

In the differential diagnosis of smoothly margined mammographic opacities the main advantage of ultrasonography lies in the differentiation into cystic and solid lesions. Within the group of solid masses, however, the additional diagnostic information for further specification is limited since both carcinomas and benign tumors may present as sharply defined lesions with "benign" criteria on sonography and mammography. Therefore consideration of the case history, the course of the disease, and the patients age is sometimes more appropriate for determination of the a priori cancer probability of a certain lesion than the detailed analysis of mammographic or sonographic morphological criteria.

The compressibility of a smoothly marginated lesion, however, as observed during sonopalpation, can be viewed as a highly reliable criterion of benignancy. Thus the author could not find any single compressible carcinoma (i.e., alteration in thickness >10% by variation of applied transducer pressure to the tissue), within a subgroup of more than one hundred evaluated breast cancers with *well-defined* tumor margins. In contrast to this, benign lesions were compressible in 30% of cases (alteration in thickness >20%) (WALZ et al. 1994). Histological clarification of sonographically probably benign lesions is not generally necessary; it is, however, indicated in all doubtful cases (STAVROS et al. 1995). In general circumscribed solid mass should be managed with periodic sonographic and/or mammographic surveillance.

Several studies now agree that breast sonography is superior to mammography in the differential diagnosis of *palpable* findings. Nevertheless, in cases of suspicious palpable lesions with uncharacteristic or equivocal sonographic appearance core biopsy should be carried out. Especially in the demonstration and assessment of carcinomas in dense breasts with more than 10% mammographically negative diagnoses or only minimal mammographic signs of malignancy ultrasonography may be advantageous (TEUBNER 1993). Therefore, ultrasonography should not only be used to differentiate cystic from solid lesions but also in selected equivocal cases where mammography fails to yield a reliable diagnosis. All additional diagnostic information yielded by

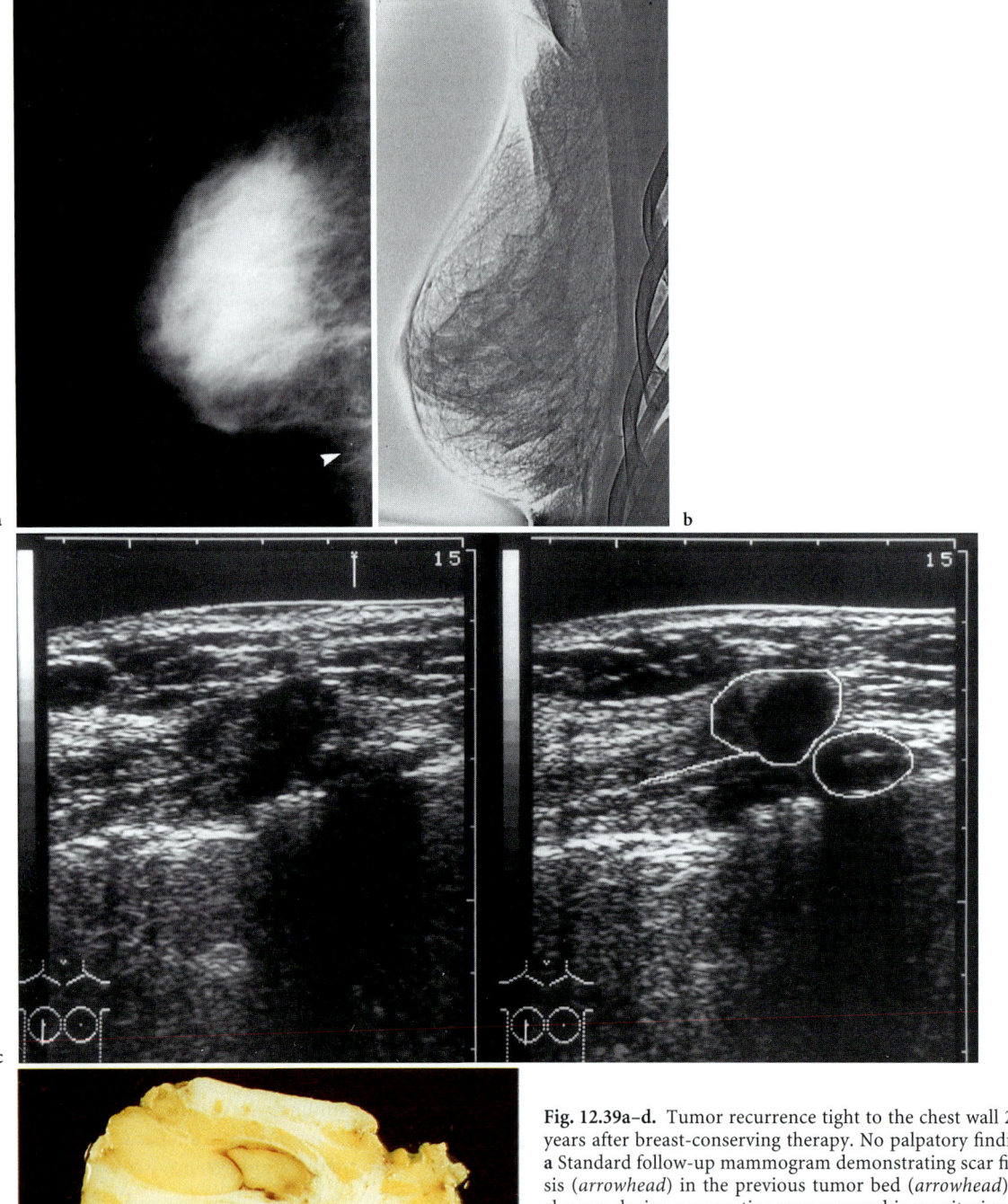

Fig. 12.39a–d. Tumor recurrence tight to the chest wall 2 1/2 years after breast-conserving therapy. No palpatory findings. **a** Standard follow-up mammogram demonstrating scar fibrosis (*arrowhead*) in the previous tumor bed (*arrowhead*). No changes during consecutive mammographic monitoring (every 6 months). **b** Xeroradiography of the same breast is unable to demonstrate any lesions close to the chest wall (unjustified security since only parts of the thoracic wall are imaged tangentially). **c** Irregularly marginated hypoechoic lesion exclusively detected by ultrasonography Infiltration of intercostal muscle. Ultrasonography-guided core-cut biopsy confirmed the diagnosis prior to primary resection of intercostal muscle and fifth rib. **d** Gross slice section of resected tissue reveals a 1.5-cm recurrent tumor originating dorsal to the fibrotic scar

Table 12.3. Additional diagnostic information provided by ultrasonography, as compared with mammography

A. *Cross-sectional imaging process*
- Better contour analysis of lesions in dense breasts: boundaries of a tumor are not masked by superimposing anatomical structures
- Texture analysis of internal tissue composition of the tumor
- Demonstration of lesions near to the chest wall and evaluation of infiltration into the breast muscle
- Examination of deep axillary and internal mammary regions behind the ribs

B. *Other physical tissue information*
- Tissue echogenicity dependent on microscopic mechanical tissue composition, which is independent of summed x-ray absorption ($\sim\rho\cdot z^3$)
- Better tissue contrast between tumorous (hypoechoic) and glandular (hyperechoic) tissue in mastopathic breasts (no differences in x-ray absorption of tumorous vs dense glandular tissue)
- Analysis of internal tissue composition

C. *Dynamic tests*
- Analysis of elasticity and movability of a lesion
- Pseudo 3D aspect of anatomical tissue arrangement by continuous real-time imaging (better perception of architectural distortions

Table 12.4. Indications for breast ultrasonography

A. *Diagnostic*	
Palpable abnormalities:	– Differentiation between cystic and solid lesions
	– Differential diagnosis by dynamic tests: elasticity, deformability, mobility
	– Contour analysis of mammographically nonspecific masses (visualization affected by superimposed glandular tissue)
	– Exclusion of masses in nondiagnostic dense breasts without pathological findings on the mammogram)
Nonpalpable lesions (detected on mammogram):	– Same indications as with palpable abnormalities except that exclusion of a mammographically detected lesion is not possible (additional close-up views/other projections are required)
B. *Perioperative*	
Preoperative tumor staging (especially in breast-conserving therapy:	– Tumor size, multicentric growth pattern, intraductal spreading
	– Exclusion of contralateral tumor
	– Axillary lymph nodes (if sonographically demonstrable, then highly suspicious)
	– Cyst aspiration (nonpalpable, equivocal on mammogram)
Interventional:	– Ultrasonography-guided fine-needle aspiration and core-cut biopsy
	– Preoperative needle localization of nonpalpable tumors
	– Specimen sonogram for evaluation of tumor-free resection space
Postoperative	
After breast-conserving therapy:	– Monitoring of scar
	– Early diagnosis of recurrences or second carcinoma
Inlay:	– Exclusion of rupture/silicone bleeding
	– Exclusion of recurrences

ultrasonography, as compared with mammography, is a result of the different imaging processes and other physical tissue information (Table 12.3). These features from the basis for the most important indications for breast ultrasonography, as summarized in Table 12.4.

Except in very few instances, sonography should not be considered as an independent imaging modality but should rather be seen as a procedure used tu supplement mammography and clinical breast examination. Sensible combination of these methods increases the sensitivity and specificity of breast diagnosis.

References

Barth V (1979) Feinstruktur der Brustdrüse im Röntgenbild. Thieme, Stuttgart

Barlow RE, Torees WE, Sones PJ, Someren A (1980) Sonographic demonstration of migrating silicone. AJR 135:170–171

Bassett LW, Kimme-Smith C, Sutherland LK, Gold RH, Sarti D, King W (1987) Automated and hand-held breast ultrasound: effect on patient management. Radiology 165:103–108

Bässler R (1984) Mammakarzinom. In: Remmele W (ed) Pathologie 3. Springer, Berlin Heidelberg New York, pp 351–390

Cole-Beuglet C, Beique RA (1975) Continuous ultrasound B-scanning of palpable breast masses. Radiology 117:123–128

Cole-Beuglet C, Kurtz AB, Rubin CS, Goldberg BB (1980) Ultrasound mammography. Radiol Clin North Am 18:133–143

Cole-Beuglet C, Soriano RZ, Kurtz AB, Goldberg BB (1983a) Ultrasound analysis of 104 primary breast carcinomas classified according to histopathologic type. Radiology 147:191–196

Cole-Beuglet C, Soriano RZ, Pasto M, Baltorowich O, Rifkin M, Kurtz AB, Goldberg BB (1983b) Solid breast mass lesions: can ultrasound differentiate benign and malignant? In: Jellins J, Kobayashi T (eds) Ultrasonic examination of the breast. Wiiley, New York, pp 45–55

Cole-Beuglet C, Soriano RZ, Kurtz AB, Goldberg BB (1983c) Fibroadenoma of the breast: sonomammography correlated with pathology in 122 patients. AJR 140:369–375

Dale G, Gairard B, Gros CM (1975) Caractere Echographique des Epitheliomas mammaires. J Radiol Electrol 57:576–578

Dale G, Gros CM (1977) 'Echotomographie mammaire par balayge rapide. Senologia 2(2):3–9

Dempsey PJ (1988) Breast sonography: historical perspective, clinical application, and image interpretation. Ultrasound Q 6:69–90

Egan RL, Egan KL (1984) Detection of breast carcinoma: comparison of automated water-path whole-breast sonography, mammography, and physical examination. AJR 143:493–497

Ernst R, Weber A, Bauer KH, Friemann J, Zumtobel V (1990) Bedeutung der Sonographie der Brustdrüse für die operative Therapie des Mammakarzinoms. Chirurg 61:518–525

Feig SA (1989) The role of ultrasound in a breast imaging center. Semin Ultrasound CT MR 10:90–105

Fields S, Dunn F (1973) Correlation of echographic visualizability of tissue with biological composition and physiological state. J Acoust Soc Am 54:809–812

Filipczynski L, Lypacewicz G (1984) Capability of echo and shadow detection of calcifications in breast tissue by means of ultrasonics. Proc 5th Euroson'84, Strasbourg. Abstract 010

Fleischer AC, Muhletaler CA, Reynolds VH, et al. (1983) Palpable breast masses: evaluation by high frequency, handheld real-time sonography and xeromammography. Radiology 148:813–817

Fleischer AC, Thieme GA, Winfield AC, Reynolds VH, Kaufman AJ, Baxter JW (1985) Breast sonotomography and high-frequency, hand-held, real-time sonography: a clinical comparison. J Ultrasound Med 4:577–581

Frazier TG, Murphy JT, Furdong A (1985) The selected use of ultrasound mammography to improve diagnostic accuracy in carcinoma of the breast. J Surg Oncol 29:231–232

Fornage BD, Lorigan JG, Andry E (1989) Fibroadenoma of the breast: sonographic appearance. Radiology 172:671–675

Fornage BD, Sneige N, Faroux MJ, Andry E (1990) Sonographic appearance and ultrasound-guided fine-needle aspiration biopsy of breast carcinomas smaller than 1 cm^3. J Ultrasound Med 9:559–568

Friedrich M (1980) Ultraschalluntersuchung der Brust mit einem hochauflösenden "Real-Time" Gerät. Radiologe 20:209–225

Friedrich M, Kroll U (1981) Ultraschalldiagnostik am Weichteilmantel – Erfahrungen mit einem real-time-Nahbereichsscanner. RöFo 135:73–79

Friedrich M (1987) Einfach Vorlaufstrecke für die Nahbereichssonographie. RöFo 146:102–110

Gordon PB (1995) US for problem solving in breast imaging: tricks of the trade. RSNA Syllabus: Categorical Course in Breast Imaging, pp 121–131

Gordon PB, Goldenberg SL (1995) Malignant breast masses detected only by ultrasound: a retrospective study. Cancer 76(4):626–630

Gordon PB, Goldenberg SL (1996) Author reply, Cancer 77(1):209

Gros ChM, Dale G, Gairard B (1977) Echographie mammaire: critères de malignite. Senologia 2(4):47–57

Harper AP, Kelly-Fry E, Noe JS, Bies JR, Jackson VP (1983) Ultrasound in the evaluation of solid breast masses Radiology 146:731–736

Harper AP (1994) Ultrasound evaluation of asymptomatic patients as an adjunct to X-ray mammography in dense breasts. In: Madjar H, Teubner J, Hackelöer BJ (eds) Breast ultrasound update. Karger, Basel, pp 26–31

Heywang SH, Lipsit ER, Glassman LM (1984) Specificity of ultrasonography in the diagnosis of benign breast masses. J Ultrasound Med 3:453–461

Hirst C (1994) Sonographic appearance of breast cancer 10 mm or less in diameter. In: Madjar H, Teubner J, Hackelöer BJ (eds) Breast ultrasound update. Karger, Basel, pp 127–139

Howry DH, Stott DA, Bliss WR (1954) The ultrasonic visualisation of the breast and other soft tissue structures. Cancer 7:354–358

Jackson VP, Rothschild PA, Kreipke DL, Mail JT, Holden RW (1986) The spectrum of sonographic findings of fibroadenoma of the breast. Invest Radiol 21:34–40

Jackson VP, Kelly-Fry E, Rothschild PA, Holden RW, Steven AC (1986) Automated breast sonography using a 7.5 MHz PVDF transducer. Radiology 159:679–684

Jackson VP (1990) The role of ultrasound in breast imaging. Radiology 177:305–311

Jackson VP, Hendrick RE, Feig SA, Kopans DB (1993) Imaging the radiographically dense breast. Radiology 188:297–301

Jackson VP (1994) Present and future role of ultrasound in breast imaging. RSNA Syllabus: Categorical Course in Physics, pp 247–253

Jackson VP (1995) The current role of ultrasonography in breast imaging. Radiol Clin North Am 33/6:1161–1170

Jellins J, Kossoff G, Buddee FW, Reeve TS (1971) Ultrasonic visualization of the breast. Med J Aust 1:105–107

Jellins J, Reeve TS, Kossoff G, Griffiths K (1982) The ultrasonic characterization of breast malignancies. In: Levi S (ed) Ultrasound and cancer. Excerpta medica, Amsterdam

van Kaick G, Schmidt W, Teubner J, Lorenz D, Lorenz A, Müller A (1980) Echomammographie mit verschiedenen Gerätetypen bei herdförmigen Läsionen. Tumordiagnostik 1:179–186

Kamio T, Hamano K, Kameoka S, Kimura T (1992) Ductal echography. In: Ioannidou-Mouzaka L, Agnantis NJ, Karydas I (eds) Senology. Excerpta Medica, Amsterdam, pp 109–112

Kamio T, Kameoka S, Mamano K (1994) Dutcal echography: classification of ducts. In: Madjar H, Teubner J, Hackelöer BJ (eds) Breast ultrasound update. Karger, Basel, pp 91–98

Kasumi F, Tanaka H (1983) Detection of microcalcifications in breast carcinoma by ultrasound. In: Jellins J, Kobayashi T (eds) Ultrasonic examination of the breast. Wiley, Chichester, pp 89–97

Kasumi F, Fukami A, Kuno K, Kajitani T (1982) Characteristic echographic features of circumscribed cancer. Ultrasound Med Biol 8:369–375

Kasumi F (1988) Can microcalcifications located within breast carcinomas be detected by ultrasound/imaging? Ultrasound Med Biol 14 (Suppl 1):175–182

Kasumi F (1991) The diagnostic criteria of breast lesions of the Japan Society of Ultrasonics in Medicine and topical issues in the field of breast ultrasonography in Japan. In: Kasumi F, Ueno E (eds) Topics in breast ultrasound. Shinohara, Tokyo, pp 19–26

Kasumi F, Sakuma H (1994) Ultrasonic image of intracystic tumor. In: Madjar H, Teubner J, Hackelöer BJ (eds) Breast ultrasound update. Karger, Basel, pp 168–173

Kelly-Fry E, Morris ST, Holden RW, Jackson VP, Sanghvi NT (1987) Potential of automatic control frequency, image, contrast and received bandwidth for image characterization of solid breast masses. Ultrasound Med Biol 14 (Suppl 1):143–161

Kindinger R, Teubner J, Diezler P, Georgi M (1994) Long-term follow-up using sono- and mammography to evaluate posttherapeutic alterations in breast cancer tissue treated conservatively. In: Madjar H, Teubner J, Hackelöer BJ (eds) Breast ultrasound update. Karger, Basel, pp 240–252

Kobayashi T (1977) Gray-scale echography for breast cancer Radiology 122:207–214

Kobayashi T (1979) Diagnostic ultrasound in breast cancer: analysis of retrotumorous echo patterns correlated with sonic attenuation by cancerous connective tissue. J Clin Ultrasound 7:471–479

Kopans DB (1984) "Early" breast cancer detection using techniques other than mammography. AJR 143:465–468

Kopans DB, Meyer JE, Steinbock RT (1982) Breast cancer: the appearance as delineated by whole breast-path ultrasound scanning. J Clin Ultrasound 10:313–322

Kossoff G (1972) Improved techniques in ultrasonic cross-sectional echography. Ultrasonics 10:221–227

Kossoff G (1988) Causes of shadowing in breast sonography. Ultrasound Med Biol 14 (Suppl 1):211–215

Kossoff G, Garrett WJ, Carpenter DA, Jellins J, Dadd MJ (1976) Principles and classification of soft tissues by gray scale echography. Ultrasound Med Biol 2:89–105

Kronsbein H, Bässler R, von Daniels H (1983) Das Hamartom der Mamma. Vergleichende mammographische und histopathologische Untersuchungen. RöFo 138:613–619

Lambie RW, Hodgen D, Herman EM, Kopperman M (1983) Sonomammographic detection of lobular carcinoma not demonstrated on xeromammography. J Clin Ultrasound 11:495–497

Lees WR (1981) Real-time compression studies: application in symptomatic women and in screening. In: Proc 2nd Int Congress on the Ultrasonic Examination of the Breast. London, June 1981, Abstract 46

Leucht WJ, Rabe DR, Humbert KD (1988) Diagnostic value of different interpretative criteria in real-time sonography of the breast. Ultrasound Med Biol 14 (Suppl):59–73

Madjar H, Makowiec U, Mundinger A, Du Bois A, Kommoss F, Schillinger H (1994) Einsatz der hochauflösenden Sonographie in der Brustkrebsvorsorge. Ultraschall Med 15:20–23

Majewski A, Rosenthal H, Wagner HH (1986) Results of real-time sonography and raster mammography of 200 breast cancers. RöFo 144:343–350

Maslak SH (1985) Computed sonography. In: Sanders RC, Hill MC (eds) Ultrasound annual 1985. Raven, New York, pp 1–16

Nishimura S, Matsusue S, Koizumi S, Kashihara S (1987) Tumor size of breast cancer measured by ultrasonography and resected specimen. Ultrasound Med Biol 14 (Suppl 1):139–142

Palmon LU, Forshager MC, Everson LI, Cunningham BL (1994) US of ruptured breast implants: sensitivity of snowstorm appearance (abstract). Radiology 193(P):177

Pamilo M, Soiva M, Anttinen I, Roiha M, Suramo I (1991) Ultrasonography of breast lesions detected in mammography screening. Acta Radiol 32:220–225

Salvador M, Salvador R, Olona M (1994) Tumor hardness: ultrasonic signs in breast pathology. In: Madjar H, Teubner J, Hackelöer BJ (eds) Breast ultrasound update. Karger, Basel, pp 99–109

Sickles EA, Filly RA, Callen PW (1983) Breast cancer detection with sonography and mammography: comparison using state-of-the-art equipment. AJR 140:843–845

Smallwood JA, Guyer P, Dewbury K, Mengatti S, Herbert A, Royle GT, Taylor I (1986) The accuracy of ultrasound in the diagnosis of breast disease. Ann Coll Surg Engl 68:19–22

Stavros AT, Thickman D, Rapp CL, Dennis MA, Parker SH, Sisney GA (1995) Solid breast nodules: use of ultrasound to distinguish between benign and malignant lesions. Radiology 196:123–134

Tabar L, Dean PB (1985) Lehratlas der Mammographie. Thieme, Stuttgart

Takehara Y, Hisada Y and Yamada K (1983) Ultrasonic diagnosis of breast carcinoma – advantages of high frequency transducer. In: Jellins J, Kobayashi T (eds) Ultrasonic examination of the breast. Wiley, New York, pp 83–88

Teboul M (1991) Ductal echography – a new ultrasonic and sampling technic for breast malignancies. In: Kasumi F, Ueno E (eds) Topics in breast ultrasound. Shinohara, Tokyo, pp 48–57

Teixidor H, Kazam E (1977) Combined mammographic-sonographic evaluation of breast masses. AJR 128:409–417

Teubner J, van Kaick G, Schmidt W, Kubli F (1981) Echomammography with different scanning units. In: Proc 2nd Int Congress on the Ultrasonic Examination of the Breast. London, June 1981, Abstract 53

Teubner J, van Kaick G, Pickenhan L, Schmidt W (1982) Vergleichende Untersuchungen mit verschiedenen echomammographischen Verfahren. Ultraschall 3:109–118

Teubner J, Müller A, Pickenhan L, van Kaick G (1983) Sonographic morphology of the breast. In: Lerski RA, Morley P (eds) Ultrasound' 82. Pergamon, Oxford, pp 397–405

Teubner J (1985) The "echogenic border": An important diagnostic criterion in tumor diagnosis of the breast. In: Gill RW, Dadd MJ (eds) Proc 4th International Meeting of the WFUMB 85, Sydney, Australia. Pergamon, Sydney, p 342

Teubner J, van Kaick G, Junkermann H, et al. (1985) 5 MHz realtime-sonographie of the breast: examination technique and diagnostic value. Radiologe 25:457–467

Teubner J, van Kaick G, Georgi M (1985b) Compression of breast tissue: a criterion for mammasonography. In: Gill RW, Dadd MJ (eds) Proc 4th international Meet of the WFUMB'85, Sydney, Australia. Pergamon, Sydney, p 348

Teubner J, Junkermann H, van Kaick G, Piokenhan L (1985c) Diagnosis of breast cancer: comparison of clinical examination, mammography and 5 MHz realtime sonography. In: Jellins J, Kossoff G, Croll J (eds) Proc 4th International Congress on the Ultrasonic Examination of the Breast. Witton, Sydney, pp 125–133

Teubner J, Lenk JZ, Wentz KU, Georgi M (1987) Vergrößerungsmammographie mit 0.1 mm Mikrofokus: Vergleich von Raster- und Ver-größerungstechnik bei Zielaufnahmen. Radiologe 27:155–164

Teubner J, Heuser-Stein O, Simon R, Bohrer M, Intraphuvasak J, Saeger HD, Georgi M (1990) Mammographie-Screening mit oder ohne Ultraschall? In: Gebhardt J, Hackelöer BJ, Klinggräff G, Seitz K (eds) Ultraschalldiagnostik '89. Springer, Berlin Hoidelberg New York, pp 40-46

Teubner J (1993) Experimentelle, histomorphologische und klinische Untersuchungen zur diagnostischen Wertigkeit der Real-Time Sonographie der Brustdrüse im Vergleich zur Mammographie. Habilitationsschrift, Fakultät für Klinische Medizin Mannheim, Universität Heidelberg

Teubner J, Bohrer M, van Kaick G, Georgi M (1993) Echomorphologie des Mammakarzinoms. Radiologe 33:277-286

Teubner J, Bohrer M, van Kaick G, Georgi M (1994) Correlation between histopethology and echomorphology in breast cancer. In: Madjar H, Teubner J, Hackelöer BJ (eds) Breast ultrasound update. Karger, Basel, pp 63-74

Thijssen JM, Oosterveld BJ (1990) Texture in tissue echograms: speckle or information? J Ultrasound Med 9: 215-229

Thono E, Cosgrove DO, Sloane JP (1994) Ultrasound diagnosis of the breast. Churchill Livingstone, London

Tsunoda HS, Ueno E, Tohno E, Akisada M (1990) Echogram of ductal spreading breast carcinoma. Jpn J Med Ultrasonics 17:44-49

Ueno E, Tohno E, Itoh K, Assoka Y (1985) Multivariate statistic analysis of ultrasound mammogram. In: Gill RW, Dadd MJ (eds) Proc 4th International Meeting of the WFUMB '85, Sydney. Pergamon, Sydney

Ueno E, Tohno E, Ithe K (1986) Classification and diagnostic criteria in breast echography. Jpn J Med Ultrasonics 13:19-31

Ueno F, Tohno F, Soeda S, Asaoka Y, Itho K, Bamber JC, Blaszzvk M, Davev J, McKinna JA (1988) Dynamic tests in real-time breast echography. Ultrasound Med Biol 14 (Suppl 1):53-57

Vilare M, Kurtz AB, Needleman L, Fleischer AC, Mitchell DG, Rosenberg A, Miller C, Rifkin MD, Pennell R, Baltarowich O, Goldberg BB (1989) Hand-held and automated sonomammography: clinical role relative to x-ray mammography. J Ultrasound Med 8:95-100

Walz M, Teubner J, Georgi M (1994) Elasticity of benign and malignant breast lesions. In: Madjar H, Teubner J, Hackelöer BJ (eds) Breast ultrasound update. Karger, Basel, pp 91-98

Weiss L, Rosner D, Glenn WE (1978) Visualization of breast lesions with an advanced ultrasonic device: results of a pilot study. J Surg Oncol 10:251-271

Wild JJ, Reid JM (1952) Further pilot echographic studies on the histological structure of tumors of the living intact human breast. Ann J Pathol 28:839-854

Wild JJ, Reid JM (1954) Echographic visualisation of lesions of the living human breast. Cancer Res 14:277-283

13 Doppler Sonography of Breast Tumors

S. Delorme

CONTENTS

13.1	Introduction	221
13.2	Techniques and Clinical Results	221
13.2.1	Continuous-Wave Doppler	221
13.2.2	Duplex Doppler	222
13.2.3	Color Doppler	223
13.3	Current Status	225
13.3.1	Tumor Detection	226
13.3.2	Differential Diagnosis	226
13.3.3	Prognostic Assessment and Therapy Monitoring	226
13.4	Future Aspects	227
13.4.1	Technical Innovations	227
13.4.2	Intravascular Ultrasound Contrast Agents	227
	References	228

13.1 Introduction

The blood supply of tumors is drawn from vessels which are generated by the surrounding host tissue upon stimulation by angiogenetic factors produced by the tumor (Folkman 1985). The tumor's proliferation rate as well as its ability to produce angiogenetic factors determine whether the angiogenesis compensates for the increased oxygen demand of the growing neoplasm and also the degree of differentiation of the resulting vascular architecture. When compared with normal vessel architecture, tumor vasculature is rather primitive (Less et al. 1991), with the following features:

1. Inadequate reduction in diameter and segment length with ascending hierachic order in the capillary bed.
2. Trifurcations and vascular rings.
3. Incomplete vessel walls: Tumor vessels lack any autoregulatory capabilities due to a missing muscular layer. The endothelium is often defective, enabling direct tumor–blood contact as well as increased capillary permeability.

S. Delorme, MD, Department of Radiological Diagnostics and Therapy, Deutsches Krebsforschungszentrum, Im Neuenheimer Feld 280, 69120 Heidelberg, Germany

4. Development of large sinusoids and arteriovenous shunts.

The degree of hypervascularity and the extent of architectural abnormalities of newly formed vessels are unpredictable in an individual case. Tumor blood flow is further determined by physiologic factors such as intralesional pressure, which influences peripheral vascular resistance.

In most cases of breast cancer, the tumor appears to contain more vessels than the surrounding fatty and glandular tissue, as shown by x-ray angiography (Fuchs and Strigl 1985). With high-frequency transducers, Doppler sonography is capable of demonstrating intratumoral blood flow. In the healthy breast, Doppler sonography will commonly detect only large, supplying vessels or the periareolar vasculature (Burns et al. 1982).

Studies with Doppler sonography carried out in breast tumors are mainly concerned with the differential diagnosis of benign and malignant lesions (Belcaro et al. 1988; Britton and Coulden 1990; Cosgrove et al. 1990, 1993; Madjar et al. 1986, 1990, 1993b; Jellins 1988; Srivastava et al. 1988; Huber et al. 1994a,b; Schoenberger et al. 1988; Fournier et al. 1993; Konishi et al. 1993; Burns et al. 1982). However, Doppler sonographic assessment of tumor vascularity also is potentially applicable for prognostic assessment (Weidner et al. 1991) and prediction of therapy response. Only one continuous-wave (CW) Doppler study has yet addressed prognostic aspects of tumor vascularity (Madjar et al. 1988).

13.2 Techniques and Clinical Results

13.2.1 Continuous-Wave Doppler

Continuous-wave Doppler permits use of frequencies as high as 8 or 10 MHz without serious artifacts, thereby allowing for detection of low flow velocities. However, there is no B-mode guidance. Because its depth resolution is entirely determined by the physical penetration of the ultrasound beam, and because of the lack of B-mode guidance, CW Doppler has serious limitations: Since the source of the signal cannot be determined, CW Doppler is only applicable to palpable lesions. Furthermore, due to poor spatial resolution, the examiner may easily measure parameters twice in a single location or miss another vessel. CW Doppler measures frequency shifts, not flow velocities, because no angle correction is possible. The first studies with CW Doppler in breast tumors were reported by BURNS et al. in 1982. Despite the unpredictable impact of the Doppler angle, MADJAR et al. (1990) found a 1450-Hz frequency shift in healthy breasts (SD, 370 Hz), and a 2630-Hz frequency shift in breast cancers (SD, 1250 Hz). Vessels were also found in most benign tumors, but the number of vessels in malignancies, as far as could be reliably determined by this method, was higher than 2, whereas benign lesions showed lower vessel counts. The results reported by SRIVASTAVA et al. (1988) are comparable, with higher standard deviations.

Because of the variations caused by the unknown Doppler angle, some authors have evaluated derived values, such as the resistance index or the pulsatility index. These values are angle-independent and reflect intratumoral flow resistance. However, the results are contradictory (SOHN et al. 1992; FOURNIER et al. 1993; KONISHI et al. 1993; BURNS et al. 1982). It is therefore unlikely that there is any tumor-specific flow pattern which permits lesion characterization by assessment of the flow curve alone. CW Doppler has only rarely been applied for prognostic assessment. In small series, high-frequency shifts were likely to be found in tumors with rapid local or systemic progression, with nodal metastasis, or with negative estrogen and progesterone receptors (MADJAR et al. 1988).

13.2.2 Duplex Doppler

Duplex Doppler is a pulsed Doppler system and uses B-mode guidance (Fig. 13.1). Therefore, it permits sampling of Doppler signals from a selected depth in a known location, and thereby the examination of impalpable tumors. However, it is more susceptible to artifacts than CW Doppler, limiting the transmitted frequency to 5–7 MHz and thereby reducing its sensitivity to slow blood flow. As a result, BRITTON and COULDEN (1990) found vessels in only 10% of benign lesions using duplex Doppler. Unless the direction of the small tumor vessels is visible in B-mode, again, there is no angle correction with duplex Doppler, imposing the same limitations as with CW Doppler. In a preliminary study by SCHOENBERGER

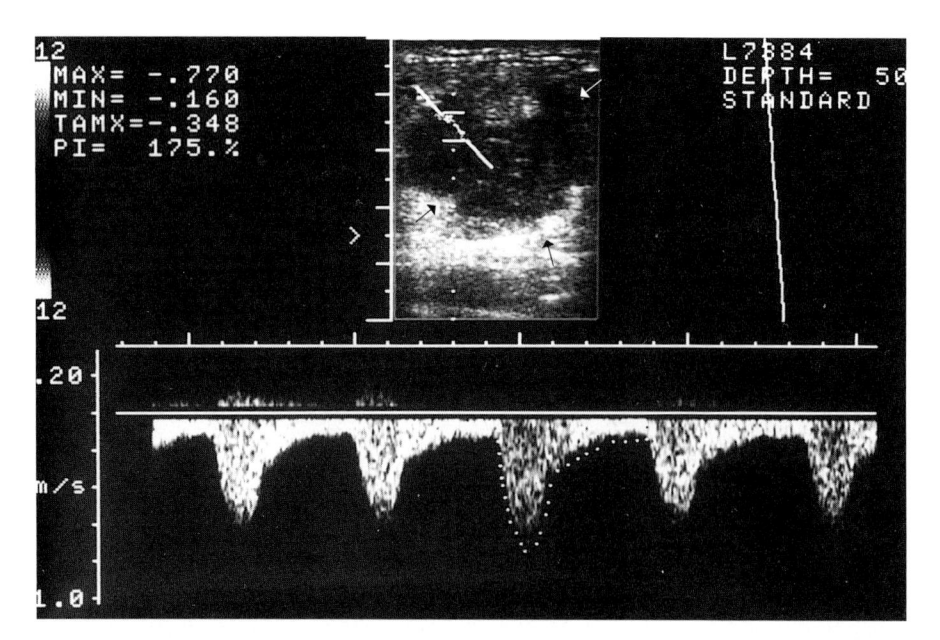

Fig. 13.1. Duplex Doppler. The B-mode image at the top shows an invasive ductal carcinoma (*arrows*) and the position of the Doppler sample volume (indicated by the gap between *two short dashes on the dotted line*). The resulting Doppler spectrum is displayed at the *bottom*. Since in this case the reference image at the top was color coded (not depictable on this black and white reproduction), the flow direction could be accounted for (indicated by *diagonal lines*), thus allowing the calculation of true flow velocities

et al. (1988), blood flow could be demonstrated in all 12 patients with breast cancer, using a 3.5-MHz probe, whereas none of 26 benign tumors showed detectable vessels.

13.2.3 Color Doppler

Like duplex Doppler, Color Doppler uses pulsed ultrasound transmission and gated signal reception, enabling localization of the source of a signal to a voxel as small as $1 \times 1 \text{mm}^2$ in the ultrasound plane. Using a line-by-line interrogation of the tissue, it generates a map of recorded frequency shifts which is color coded and superimposed on the B-mode image. The result is a color-coded image of the vessel in its original location, displayed in real-time, with the colors coding for the frequency shift and the flow direction (Figs. 13.2, 13.3). The advantages of color Doppler are:

1. An angle correction is possible, even if the vessel is not visible in B-mode. This permits measurement of flow velocities instead of frequency shifts.
2. It is less likely to miss a vessel, since it shows the entire tumor cross-section.
3. Double counts or missed vessels are less likely to occur.
4. The examiner obtains a subjective impression of the vascular density inside the tumor.

Like duplex Doppler, this method suffers from artifacts, limiting the transmitter frequency. Only

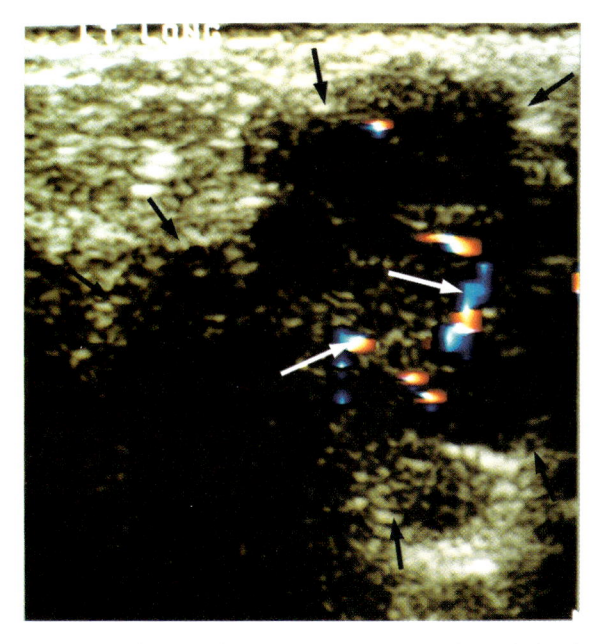

Fig. 13.2. Color Doppler. Doppler signals are color coded and superimposed on the B-mode image. The color (e.g., blue or red) codes for the flow direction (towards or away from the transducer), while the color hue (e.g., dark or bright red) codes for the flow velocity. The maximal flow velocity displayed without aliasing is indicated at the top and bottom of a color palette bar. Since an angle correction is impossible with this modality, the color code assumes a Doppler angle of 0°. The true flow velocities are higher because only a few vessels lead directly towards or away from the transducer. This image shows vessels (*large arrows*) in a breast tumor (*small arrows*). Since the B-mode features of this tumor (irregular, blurred margins, echogenic rim, distal shadowing) are highly suggestive of malignancy, color Doppler added no relevant information. Histology showed infiltrating ductal carcinoma

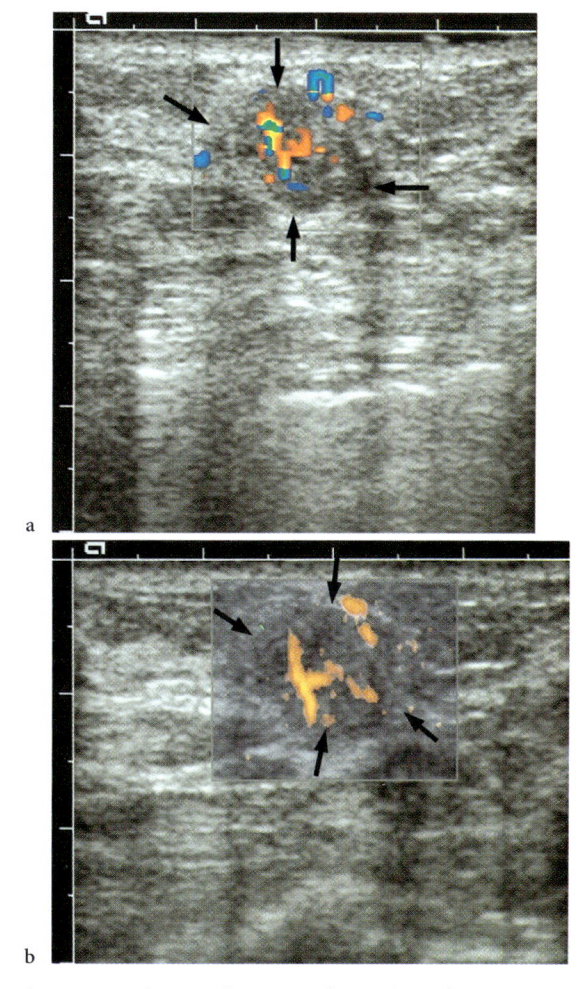

Fig. 13.3. a Color Doppler image of a suspicious breast tumor. Despite the circumscribed margins of this lesion (*arrows*), the high degree of detected vascularity is not typical of a benign tumor and should prompt excisional biopsy. **b** In Doppler amplitude imaging mode, vessels are encoded by a single color with varying degrees of brightness. In this case, this mode did not enable the depiction of more vessels than did conventional color Doppler. However, the vessel architecture appears somewhat clearer because the image is free of aliasing

recently, highly sophisticated units have been developed to work with 7 or 7.5 MHz, producing excellent results. The even higher frequencies implemented by some manufacturers appear to require such strong artifact suppression that we have not found these systems superior to those using 7 MHz.

Color Doppler may be applied to guide spectral Doppler measurements for correct sample volume placement and adequate angle correction or to count detctable vessels. In a study on 37 patients with breast carcinoma carried out at the German Cancer Research Center, we found:

1. A wide spectrum of flow velocities, pulsatility and resistance indices, and number of intratumoral vessels.
2. No correlation of these parameters with tumor size or nodal status. There was a weak correlation of maximal flow velocity with the calculated tumor volume.
3. Lack of detectability of feeding vessels (leading into the tumor from the adjacent tissue) in five cases (14%), and absence of strictly intratumoral vessels in eight cases (21%). In four patients (10%), the tumor was devoid of any detectable Doppler signal (DELORME et al. 1993).

The validity of studies carried out with spectral Doppler (with duplex technique or with color Doppler guidance) is limited because most tumors are inhomogeneous. Therefore, it is unclear whether the vessel from which signals are collected is representative for the entire lesion. Vessels in the tumor periphery and in the tumor center may have entirely different hemodynamic properties. To overcome this problem, MADJAR et al. (1994) evaluated *every de-*

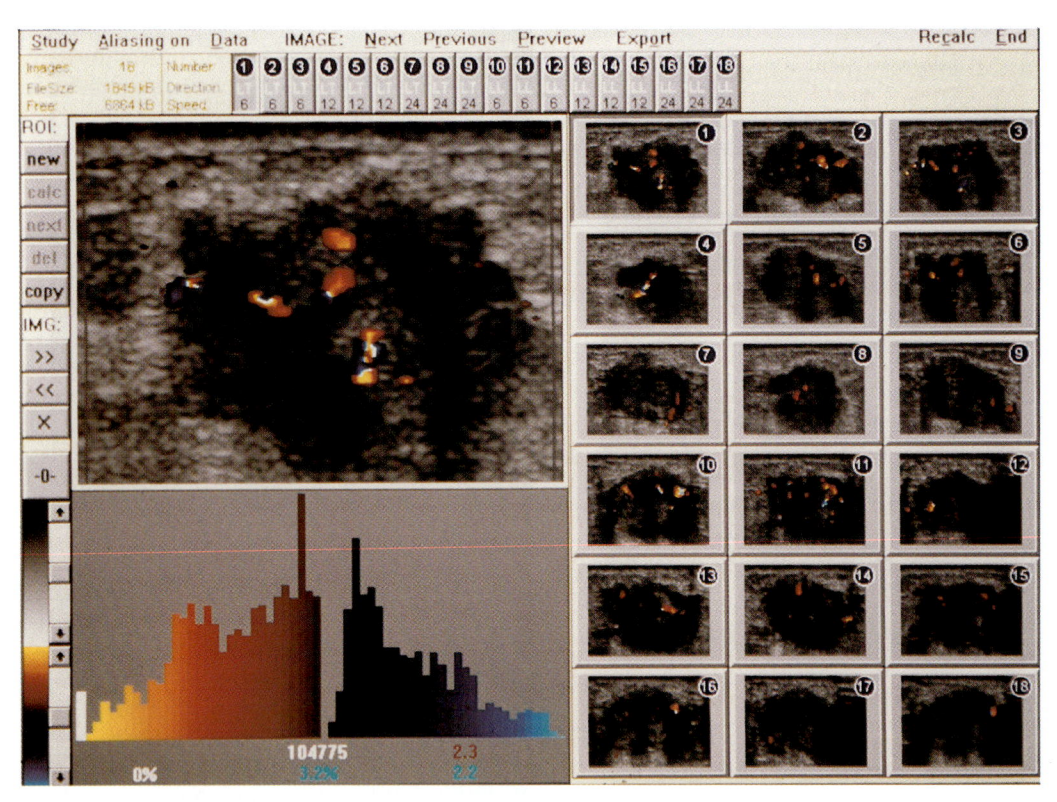

Fig. 13.4. Computer-assisted image analysis of color Doppler images. A digitized color Doppler image is recalled for evaluation. The working window (*top left*) shows the image being processed. The examiner delineates an ROI, which is indicated by a green polygon. The color of a pixel is characterized by a "color value" determined by the location of this color on the color palette bar. First-order statistics of the color values in the ROI are calculated by the program, and the distribution of color values is displayed at the *bottom left* of the window. Upon confirmation of the ROI, the system stores the first-order statistics of color values, together with the percentage of color pixels in the ROI (color pixel density). These values are then available for further analysis. This analysis mostly uses the color pixel density and the average color value in the ROI (mean color value). [From HUBER et al. (1994) Breast tumors: computer-assisted quantitative assessment with color Doppler US. Radiology 192:797–801]

tectable vessel in breast tumors, adding all measured flow velocities. The resulting sums of flow velocities were significantly different in benign and malignant lesions. However, this method is extremely tedious and hardly suitable for clinical application.

Since the color Doppler image already contains information on vessel density (the amount of color pixels in the image) as well as flow velocities (encoded by the color hue), it is possible to extract quantitative parameters from the image itself. The advantage of this approach is that all vessels in the tumor cross-section are included in the analysis and that errors or observer bias occur only through the selection of the imaging plane and variations in the cardiac cycle. Its disadvantage is the lack of any angle correction. Furthermore, it cannot be done simply by subjective assessment. An objective evaluation of color Doppler images is tedious if carried out without computer assistance. COSGROVE and co-workers applied a method of "pixel counting" derived from techniques applied to histopathologic sections and found significantly more color pixels in carcinomas than in benign lesions (Cosgrove et al. 1990, 1993).

A computer-assisted image analysis system dedicated to the evaluation of color Doppler images was developed at the German Cancer Research Center. It collects a set of cross-sections though the tumor. Upon the delineation of a region of interest (ROI), which contains the tumor and serves to define the cross-section area as well as to exclude extratumoral vessels from evaluation, the system calculates the percentage of color pixels in the ROI as well as first-order statistics of the distribution of color hues ("color values") (Figs. 13.4, 13.5). These color values numerically describe the location where the color of a given pixel is located on the color palette bar shown in the image and are thereby influenced by flow velocity. A recalculation of true flow velocities is not possible, since the color values do not account for the Doppler angle and are influenced by several physical and instrumental factors. A study on 57 patients with benign and malignant breast tumors found higher mean color values and a higher percentage of color pixels in the images for malignant tumors than in those for benign lesions (Fig. 13.5). The color values appeared to be more valid for differentiation of benign and malignant disease than the percentage of color pixels (i.e., the "amount" of color in the image). The sensitivity thus achieved was 92%, and the specificity, 78% (HUBER et al. 1994a).

13.3 Current Status

In the clinical setting, Doppler sonography may find a role in selected cases:

1. To facilitate tumor detection.
2. As an aid to the differential diagnosis of an already detected lesion.
3. For prognostic assessment in patients with known breast cancer. The degree of hypervascularity is positively correlated with the risk of distant metastases, as demonstrated in a histologically controlled study by WEIDNER et al. (1991).
4. For monitoring of nonsurgical therapy, such as preoperative chemotherapy, radiotherapy, regional chemotherapy, or local hyperthermia of recurrences. Assessment of tumor vascularity might also help to predict the efficacy of these therapy modalities. The response to chemotherapy and radiotherapy is partially dependent on the blood supply of a tumor, enabling the local delivery of the drug and good tissue oxygenation. Local hyperthermia is more suitable for poorly vascularized lesions, since blood flow causes rapid dissipation of the applied heat.

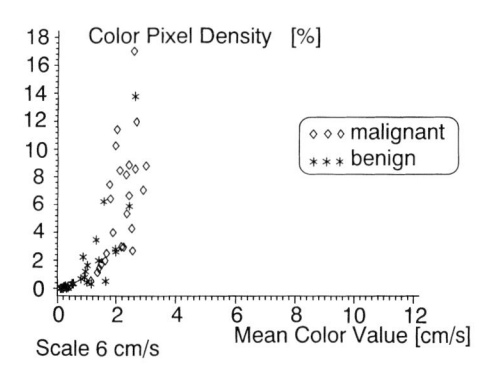

Fig. 13.5. A color Doppler image can be characterized by the percentage of color pixels in an ROI (color pixel density) and by the mean color value, which is a numerical descriptor of the color hues found in an image. This figure is a scatter diagram of mean color values (x-axis) and color pixel densities (y-axis) obtained with a scale maximum of 6 cm/s on an Acuson 128 XP 10. Each *dot* represents six averaged measurements from a single patient with either breast cancer or a benign focal lesion of the breast. The diagram shows that the color pixel density and the mean color value are positively correlated, i.e., that lesions with a high amount of color also have brighter color hues, indicating higher flow velocities. Color pixel density and mean color value are both higher in malignant tumors than in benign lesions, yielding a sensitivity of 92% and a specificity of 78% for the diagnosis of breast cancer. [From HUBER et al. (1994) Breast tumors: computer-assisted quantitative assessment with color Doppler US. Radiology 192:797–801]

Criteria to characterize the Doppler findings in a tumor are (a) the number of vessels, (b) flow velocities or frequency shifts, (c) pulsatility or resistance indices, and (d) parameters derived from color Doppler image analysis. These are the available "tools" to facilitate tumor detection, to assist differential diagnosis, for prognostic assessment, and for therapy monitoring, which were the abovementioned possible applications of this imaging modality.

13.3.1 Tumor Detection

For a lesion clearly visible in B-mode, a meticulous examination technique is required to achieve a clear display of blood flow. Any rapid movements will cause flashing artifacts. It is not possible to scan the entire breast for blood flow. Therefore, Doppler sonography cannot be expected to be more sensitive than B-mode sonography.

13.3.2 Differential Diagnosis

Irrespective of the technique applied, the cited studies unanimously show that a high vessel density and high blood flow velocities are suggestive but not diagnostic of malignancy (BELCARO et al. 1988; BRITTON and COULDEN 1990; COSGROVE et al. 1990, 1993; MADJAR et al. 1986, 1990, 1993b; JELLINS 1988; SRIVASTAVA et al. 1988; HUBER et al. 1994a,b; SCHOENBERGER et al. 1988; FOURNIER et al. 1993; KONISHI et al. 1993; BURNS et al. 1982). Despite the influence of the Doppler angle, the studies by MADJAR and SRIVASTAVA using CW Doppler showed significant differences between benign and malignant changes though there was a broad overlap (MADJAR et al. 1990, 1993b; SRIVASTAVA et al. 1988). The angle-independent parameters such as the resistance or pulsatility index do not appear to convey any information of diagnostic value because the findings in malignant tumors are too variable (SOHN et al. 1992; FOURNIER et al. 1993; KONISHI et al. 1993).

A vessel count should only be carried out with color Doppler because it is most likely to detect even small vessels and to ensure that the evaluated vessel is in fact associated with the tumor. The importance of good signal localization was illustrated by SRIVASTAVA et al. (1988), who reported CW Doppler signals from cysts. Obviously, these signals originated from the adjacent breast tissue and not from the cysts themselves.

In brest carcinomas, the vascularity is extremely variable because it is determined by multiple, unpredictable factors. The findings of SCHOENBERGER et al. (1988), who reported a 100% sensitivity and specificity, could not be confirmed by any other author. It rather appears that there remains a subset of 5%–10% of lesions which show no or very little detectable blood flow. This accounts for those carcinomas which are indistiguishable from benign disease with Doppler ultrasound, irrespective of the method and equipment applied. Therefore, Doppler sonography is of no clinical value when open surgical biopsy is the procedure of choice for a given suspicious lesion. However, for those cases where no biopsy is planned (e.g., because of the patient's preference or in probably benign lesions), Doppler sonography may be performed by the experienced examiner, because a high degree of vascularity may be the only sign of malignancy in an otherwise unsuspicious lesion. One must add the proviso that since probably benign lesions are only rarely found to be malignant, the relatively low yield of Doppler imaging successes must be weighed against the cost of the procedure.

13.3.3 Prognostic Assessment and Therapy Monitoring

It has not been proven that Doppler signals are correlated with capillary blood flow (which is not detectable with Doppler) and thereby with nutritive perfusion. Indeed, comparison with a vessel density score using an immunohistochemical endothelium stain has shown that the Doppler signal yield may not be correlated with the capillary density but rather with the presence of larger (i.e., detectable) vessels (LAGALLA et al. 1994). Because of their high flow velocities and volumes, arteriovenous shunts may significantly contribute to the Doppler signals but bypass the capillaries. With these limitations in mind, assessment of vascularity for the identification of high-risk patients or for therapy monitoring requires a *reliable quantification of Doppler findings* by a few, easy-to-handle parameters. Flow velocities as determined by spectral Doppler measurements are a possible approach, but may be dependent on the location where the signal is acquired. This location (i.e., in the tumor center or the periphery) may depend on where a signal is detectable in a particular instance but also on the examiner's preference. The method of including *all* detectable vessels as described by MADJAR et al. (1994) is an attempt to overcome this limitation but, as already mentioned, is certainly too tedious for clinical application.

Though the Doppler image itself contains information on flow velocities and vessel density, it is too complex to be quantitatively characterized by description alone. Computer-assisted quantitative image analysis is an objective and more reproducible approach that merits further evaluation, because the image information can be condensed to a few numerical parameters (Huber et al. 1994a).

13.4 Future Aspects

13.4.1 Technical Innovations

Recent developents in color Doppler technology have resulted in improved detection of low-velocity blood flow by higher transmitter frequencies or a higher signal-to-noise ratio of the system or modified algorithms such as cross-correlation methods or the "maximum entropy method." An entirely different approach is to code the Doppler signal amplitude instead of the frequency shift. This Doppler amplitude imaging technique, which is offered by several manufacturers as "color Doppler energy", "ultrasound angiography," or "power Doppler", generates an image where blood flow is displayed independently of flow velocity or direction. This method is highly sensitive to low velocity and volume flow and will often detect a signal even in vessels insonated at 90°. The price paid for elimination of problems arising from aliasing or rectangular insonation is the loss of any information on flow velocities or directions (Fig. 13.3).

All developments have in common that highly sophisticated, "intelligent" algorithms are required to eliminate artifacts due to tissue motion, such as transmitted cardiac pulsations. Furthermore, they have brought about improved detection of blood flow not only in malignant tumors but also in benign conditions, thereby creating problems in characterizing a lesion. As far as Doppler amplitude imaging is concerned, no study has addressed the value of this method for the assessment of breast tumors. It is as yet unknown which are the physiologic determinants of the signal amplitude in a particular vessel. However, one may assume that Doppler amplitude imaging is a suitable method to assess the degree of signal enhancement after the administration of intravascular ultrasound contrast agents, once they are approved for use in investigating breast tumors.

13.4.2 Intravascular Ultrasound Contrast Agents

Most ultrasound contrast agents consist of galactose particles which carry on their surface microbubbles of air adsorbed from the solvent fluid. Hitherto, they have been suitable only for echocardiography because of complete degradation during the first lung passage. Newly developed agents which are stabilized by a palmitate coating or are albumin-based, surviving the lung passage and circulating for several minutes, are undergoing phase III clinical trials. By increasing the signal amplitude, such agents achieve an improved detection of small vessels which escape unenhanced Doppler imaging because of their poor flow volume. In preliminary studies, they have been shown to improve the detection of vessels initially missed with unenhanced Doppler and to increase the overall amount of color displayed in the tumor cross-section (Spreafico et al. 1994; Madjar et al. 1993a). The use of contrast medium may possibly permit a more valid assessment of the blood flow in very small vessels. Alternatively, the degree and kinetics of contrast enhancement itself may help to characterize a tumor or to quantify its vascularity. For the latter approach, Doppler amplitude imaging will probably be a valuable evaluation tool, because the arrival of contrast medium in the tumor leads to a signal amplification which is directly encoded by this technique. However, it has not yet been demonstrated that the use of ultrasound contrast media does improve the characterization of breast lesions, nor have these agents been applied to the prognostic assessment of breast cancer.

Harmonic imaging relies on nonlinear backscattering properties of ultrasound contrast media, causing resonance phenomena at the transmitted frequency and at the upper or lower harmonics (e.g., half or double the transmitted frequency). Due to this resonance, an echo will also be recorded when the spectrum of received frequencies is restricted to a small window around the first lower or upper harmonics. Since the above backscattering properties are not shared by soft tissue, these harmonics will be mainly received from locations where resonating microbubbles are present, improving the ratio of blood echo intensity to tissue echo intensity (signal-to-clutter ratio). Since the signals in harmonic imaging will depend solely on the presence of contrast media, and not on flow velocities, this technique might possibly allow assessment of contrast enhancement even in the capillary bed, similarly to the contrast enhancement depicted with CT. However, this technique is still at an experimental stage and has mainly been applied in phantom studies, in major vessels, and in animal studies. Experiences in respect of tumor perfusion have not yet been reported (BURNS 1994; SCHROPE and NEWHOUSE 1993).

References

Belcaro G, Laurora G, Ricci A, Gianchetti E, Legnini M, Napolitano AM (1988) Evaluation of flow in nodular tumors of the breast by Doppler and duplex scanning. Acta Chir Belg 88:323-327

Britton PD, Coulden RA (1990) The use of duplex Doppler ultrasound in the diagnosis of breast cancer. Clin Radiol 42:399-401

Burns PN (1994) Ultrasound contrast agents in radiological diagnosis. Radiol Med (Torino) 87:71-82

Burns PN, Halliwell M, Wells PNT, Webb AJ (1982) Ultrasonic Doppler studies of the breast. Ultrasound Med Biol 8:127-143

Cosgrove D, Bamber JC, Davey JB, McKinna JA, Sinnet HD (1990) Color Doppler signals from breast tumors. Radiology 176:175

Cosgrove D, Kedar RP, Bamber JC, et al. (1993) Breast diseases: color Doppler US in differential diagnosis. Radiology 189:99-104

Delorme S, Anton HW, Knopp MV, et al. (1993) Breast cancer: assessment of vascularity by color Doppler. Eur Radiol 3:253-257

Folkman J (1985) Tumor angiogenesis. Adv Cancer Res 43:185-203

Fournier D, Dreyer JL, Hessler C, Motateanu M, Chapuis L (1993) Color Doppler sonography in breast diseases. Is the so-called tumoral flow specific? Imaging 60 (Suppl 2):52 (abstract)

Fuchs HD, Strigl R (1985) Diagnose und Differentialdiagnose des Mammakarzinoms mittels intravenöser DSA. Fortschr Röntgenstr 142:314-320

Huber S, Delorme S, Knopp MV, et al. (1994a) Breast tumors: computer-assisted quantitative assessment with color Doppler US. Radiology 192:797-801

Huber S, Delorme S, Knopp MV, Junkermann H, Zuna I, von Fournier D, van Kaick G (1994b) Computer-assisted image analysis: a new diagnostic aid for quantitation of color Doppler information in breast tumors. In: Madjar H, Teubner J, Hackelöer BJ (eds) Breast ultrasound update. Karger, Freiburg, pp 308-312

Jellins J (1988) Combining imaging and vascularity assessment of breast lesions. Ultrasound Med Biol 14 (Suppl 1):121-130

Konishi Y, Hamada M, Shimada K, Okuno T, Hashimoto T, Kajiwara T (1993) Doppler spectral analysis of the intratumoral waveform in breast diseases. Imaging 60 (Suppl 2):18 (abstract)

Lagalla R, Caruso G, Marasa L, D'Angelo I, Cardinale AE (1994) Capacità angiogenetica delle neoplasie mammarie e correlazione con le semeiotica color Doppler. Radiol Med 88:392-395

Less JR, Skalak TC, Sevick EM, Jain RK (1991) Microvascular architecture in a mammary carcinoma: branching patterns and vessel dimensions. Cancer Res 51:265-273

Madjar H, Jellins J, Schillinger H, Hillemanns HG (1986) Differenzierung von mammakarzinomen durch CW-Doppler-Ultraschall. Ultraschall Med 7:183-184

Madjar H, Giese E, Schillinger H (1988) Durchblutungsmessungen an mammatumoren. Vergleich mit prognosefaktoren. Arch Gynecol Obstet 245:697-698

Madjar H, Münch S, Sauerbrei W, Bauer M, Schillinger H (1990) Differenzierte Mammadiagnostik durch CW-Doppler-Ultraschall. Radiologe 30:193-197

Madjar H, Prompeler H, Schurmann R, Goppinger A, Breckwoldt M, Pfleiderer A (1993a) Verbesserung der diagnostik der blutversorgung von mammatumoren durch Ultraschall-Kontrastmittel. Geburtshilfe Frauenheilkd 53:866-869

Madjar H, Sauerbrei W, Wolfarth R, Prömpeler H, Bauknecht T, Pfleiderer A (1993b) Color Doppler imaging and duplex measurements for determination of abnormal breast vascularity. Imaging 60 (Suppl 2):17 (abstract)

Madjar H, Prömpeler R, Wolfahrt R, Bauknecht T, Pfleiderer A (1994) Farbdopplerflussdaten von Mammatumoren. Ultraschall Med 15:69-76

Schoenberger SG, Sutherland CM, Robinson AE (1988) Breast neoplasms: duplex sonographic imaging as an adjunct in diagnosis. Radiology 168:665-668

Schrope BA, Newhouse VL (1993) Second harmonic ultrasonic blood perfusion measurement. Ultrasound Med Biol 19:567-579

Sohn C, Stolz W, Grischke EM, Wallwiener D, Bastert G, von Fournier D (1992) Die dopplersonographische Untersuchung von Mammatumoren mit Hilfe der Farbdopplersonographie, der Duplexsonographie und des CW-Dopplers. Zentralbl Gynäkol 114:249-253

Spreafico C, Lanocita R, Frigerio LF, et al. (1994) The Italian experience with SH U 508 A (Levovist) in breast disease. Radiol Med (Torino) 87:59-64

Srivastava A, Webster DJT, Woodcock JP, Shrotria S, Mansel RE, Hughes LE (1988) Role of Doppler ultrasound flowmetry in the diagnosis of breast lumps. Br J Surg 75:851-853

Weidner NR, Semple JP, Welch WR (1991) Tumor angiogenesis and metastasis: correlation in invasive breast carcinoma. N Engl J Med 324:1

14 Magnetic Resonance Imaging of the Breast

M. Friedrich

CONTENTS

14.1 Basic Principles of MRI 229
14.2 Technical Equipment 229
14.2.1 Contrast Agents 230
14.2.2 Imaging Sequences 231
14.3 The Procedure for MR Examination
 of the Breast 231
14.3.1 Contrast Medium Administration 231
14.3.2 Choice of Pulse Sequence 232
14.3.3 Diagnostic Criteria and Methods
 of Image Evaluation 232
14.4 Clinical Results 234
14.4.1 Benign Entities 234
14.4.2 Carcinoma 254
14.4.3 Postoperative Status 266
14.5 MR-Guided Biopsy 271
14.6 Diagnostic Value and Established
 Indications for MR of the Breast 273
 References 278

14.1 Basic Principles of MRI

Medical magnetic resonance imaging (MRI) uses radiofrequency (rf) waves to extract cross-sectional image information from the human body through the interaction of these waves with the magnetic properties (nuclear magnetic spins) of atomic nuclei, mainly hydrogen nuclei (protons), according to their varying density and chemical binding in the tissues. In a strong magnetic field, as in a superconducting magnet, the normally randomly oriented magnetic dipoles of the protons are preferentially aligned parallel to the external magnetic field. By application of an rf pulse to the sample in a transverse direction with an appropriate strength and frequency (the resonance or Larmor frequency of the protons, depending on the field strength), the magnetic spins can be tilted into a rotational movement around the original spin axis of the protons (precession) perpendicular to the magnetic field.

Within a certain time (the transverse or spin-lattice relaxation time constant T1 ~ 0.5–2 s) the preceding spins are gradually realigned into the original orientation of the main magnetic field. During this realignment process the electromagnetic energy absorbed during the original rf pulse by the nuclei is emitted from the sample as an electromagnetic signal, the MR signal, which can be detected with an antenna, the MR coil.

The rf pulse applied to the tissue also tends to align the spin axes in the direction of the rf pulse. The angle of the spin axes is called the "phase." When the rf pulse ceases, the individual spins immediately begin to go out of phase. This dephasing process (the spin-spin relaxation) is characterized by the T2 relaxation time constant (10–200 ms). For more information the reader is referred to the more detailed literature (Stark et al. 1988).

14.2 Technical Equipment

Today MRI of the breast is mainly carried out with superconducting high-field magnets (1–1.5 T). Recent investigations (Kuhl et al. 1995a) have shown that field strength is not the decisive factor in differentiating benign from malignant tissue of the breast by dynamic contrast-enhanced MRI; the choice of a contrast medium-sensitive imaging sequence (e.g., 2D gradient or 3D acquisition) is probably more important than field strength or quantity of contrast medium. Experience with low-field equipment is too limited to allow reliable conclusions.

In order to improve the signal-to-noise ratio and thus image quality, a dedicated surface coil (double breast coil) is used; this surrounds each breast with the patient in the prone position. The breasts are also immobilized by this measure (Kaiser and Kess 1989; Fig. 14.1).

M. Friedrich, MD, Professor, Abteilung für Radiologie und Nuklearmedizin, Krankenhaus Am Urban, Dieffenbachstraße 1, 10967 Berlin, Germany

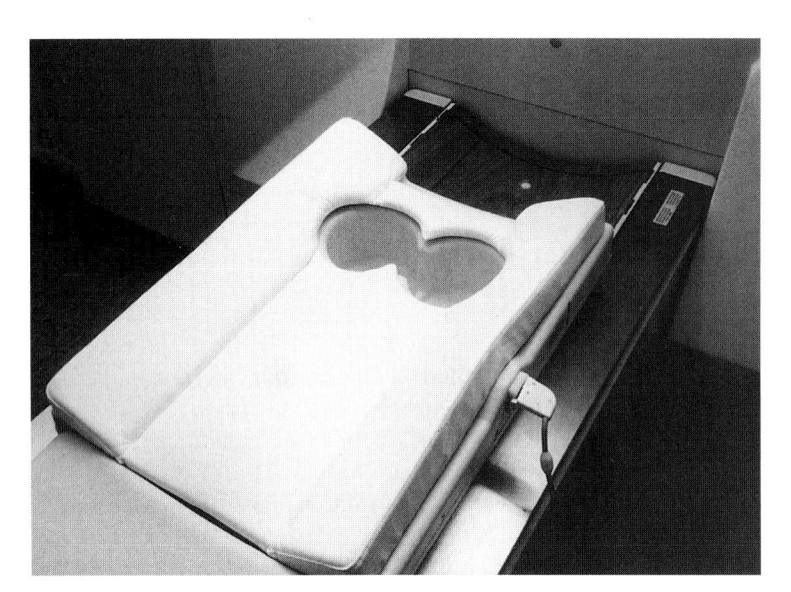

Fig. 14.1. Double breast coil for use with the patient in the prone position

14.2.1 Contrast Agents

In the early MR studies on breast disease (El Yousef et al. 1984; Dash et al. 1986; Friedrich and Semmler 1987) it was apparent that MRI without contrast enhancement had no major advantages over conventional methods. Only since the introduction of contrast agents, and especially gadopentetate dimeglumine (Gd-DTPA, Magnevist, Schering AG, Berlin), into clinical practice has the potential role of contrast-enhanced MRI in breast cancer diagnosis been addressed in numerous papers (Bradley Pierce et al. 1991; Fischer et al. 1993; Harms et al. 1993; Heywang-Köbrunner 1993, 1994; Heywang-Köbrunner et al. 1988, 1989, 1990, 1993a,b, 1994; Kaiser 1989, 1990, 1992, 1993; Kaiser and Deimling 1990; Kaiser and Hahn 1995; Kaiser and Kess 1989; Kaiser and Reiser 1992; Kaiser and Zeitler 1986a,b, 1989). The contrast agent mainly used in MRI of the breast belongs to the class of paramagnetic substances (ions) which have a magnetic dipole moment approximately 1000 times that of protons. They shorten the relaxation times T1 and T2 of the water protons in their immediate vicinity. In a spin-echo sequence a shortening of T1 leads to an increase in signal intensity, while a shortening of T2 leads to a decrease in signal intensity. The net effect, then, of the contrast medium is determined by the T1/T2 dependence of the pulse sequence used. At low concentrations of Gd-DTPA signal enhancement based on shortening of T1 predominates whereas at high concentrations a decrease in signal intensity prevails due to the shortening of T2. Thus, a T1-weighted pulse sequence is particularly favorable for signal enhancement by this T1 contrast agent. Because of the high toxicity of the free Gd^{3+} ion it has to be complexed with a chelating agent, DTPA (diethylene triamine penta-acetic acid), thereby improving osmolarity and water solubility for more rapid renal elimination of the contrast agent.

Owing to its hydrophilia and high molecular weight, Gd-DTPA is distributed exclusively in the intravascular and extracellular space and is rapidly excreted by the kidneys. The usual dose for MRI of the breast is 0.1–0.16 mmol/kg body weight. The rate of intolerance reactions such as nausea and vomiting is less than 1%. There is no significant volume load to the cardiovascular system.

The optimal dosage of the contrast agent is still controversial. Whereas most authors favor a rapid injection of 0.1 mmol Gd-DTPA/kg body weight, some investigators report an improved sensitivity in the detection of carcinomas and a better differentiation between benign and malignant processes using 0.16 or even 0.2 mmol Gd-DTPA/kg (Heywang-Köbrunner et al. 1994).

New macromolecular paramagnetic Gd compounds have recently been developed as blood pool markers. By measuring the increased permeation of the substance through small tumor vessels into the extracellular space and its elimination from here, which is prolonged in tumors in comparison with normal tissue, an additional dynamic parameter to differentiate benign from malignant tissue may be found (Adam et al. 1995).

14.2.2 Imaging Sequences

By modifying the amplitude and duration of the rf pulse, the MR signal generated by the relaxation process can be caused to vary greatly. The recorded MR signal is mainly influenced by the number of excited protons (proton density), the pulse repetition time (TR) between the individual excitation pulses, the delay or echo time (TE) after which the MR signal is recorded, and the relaxation times T1 and T2 of the tissue. Depending on the varying relation between TR and TE and the relaxation times T1 and Tl of the sample, T1- and T2- or proton density-weighted images can be obtained. The most important pulse techniques in MRI of the breast are spin-echo and gradient-echo sequences. Spin-echo images with TR <700 ms and TE <20 ms are described as T1 weighted, sequences with long TR (>1500 ms) and long TE (>90 ms) are T2 weighted, and images generated with long TR and short TE are termed proton density weighted. Tissues with a short T1, such as fat, appear bright on T1-weighted images, while tissues with a long T2, e.g., cysts, have a high signal intensity on T2-weighted images.

Gradient-echo sequences generally use short repetition and echo times (e.g., 100/6 ms), reduced excitation angles (e.g., 80°), and echo generation by gradient reversal. They have been described in the literature as FLASH (HAASE et al. 1986), FISP (OPPELT et al. 1986), RARE (HENNIG et al. 1984), fast-field echo (FFE) (VAN MEULEN et al. 1985), and GRASS (UTZ et al. 1986). The main advantages of gradient-echo sequences are a greater number of slices for a given repetition time, reduction of total imaging time, a higher signal-to-noise ratio, and much higher sensitivity to paramagnetic contrast agents (see Sect. 14.2.1) compared with the spin-echo technique.

Recently FLASH 3D sequences for breast imaging have been developed (HEYWANG-KÖBRUNNER 1993; MÜLLER-SCHIMPFLE et al. 1995a; KESSLER et al. 1995). These use very short TR and TE times (e.g., 9/3 ms) and medium excitation angles (e.g., 30–50°). This technique yields rapid acquisition (1–2 min) of a large number (32/64) of contiguous thin-slice (2/4 mm) T1-weighted sections for dynamic studies with total volume rendering of both breasts. A further advantage of this technique is the linear relationship between signal increase and tissue concentration of the contrast medium, thus yielding a better differentiation of carcinoma from benign entities in the dynamic enhancement profile (KUHL et al. 1995a). One disadvantage is the lower signal-to-noise ratio and the limited in-plane spatial resolution of 3D acquisition compared with 2D gradient-echo sequences.

There have been some reports on fat suppression techniques in breast MRI. The aim is to suppress the strong signal of fat tissue and thereby render more conspicuous the breast tissue enhancement, especially at the borderline with fat. The following techniques have been reported: RODEO ("rotating delivery of excitation off-resonance imaging"), phase difference (Dixon technique), STIR (short T1 inversion recovery), and FATSAT (HARMS et al. 1993), using a preparation pulse. The main problem with these techniques is that it is difficult to suppress the fat signal homogeneously in the whole image plane in order to guarantee correct evaluation of contrast enhancement dynamics at any point in the image; often the enhancement effect cannot be evaluated quantitatively. Sequences which use magnetization transfer from protein molecules to water molecules (BRADLEY PIERCE et al. 1991; SCHREIBER et al. 1995) as contrast-enhancing factor have been investigated, but so far have not found any clinical application.

14.3 The Procedure for MR Examination of the Breast

Exact fulfillment of a number of technical factors during an MR examination of the breast is essential in order to achieve reproducible and reliable results which can be evaluated correctly.

The examination should be carried out preferentially between the 5th and the 15th day of the menstrual cycle in order to avoid false-positive tissue enhancement. An interval of at least 3 months after a breast operation should be observed. After radiation therapy of the breast at least 6 months should elapse before an MR examination is carried out. All previous breast imaging information (e.g., mammograms, sonograms) as well as the complete history of the patient must be available at the beginning of the examination.

14.3.1 Contrast Medium Administration

A flexible cannula is inserted in a cubital vein and connected to a plastic tube. The patient is brought into a prone position with her breasts hanging into the double breast coil (Fig. 14.1). The arm with the inserted needle is placed in a relaxed position parallel to the body, in order to avoid any obstruction of the venous outflow from the arm into the thorax. An amount of 0.1 (or 0.16) mmol/kg Gd-DTPA is administered through the plastic tube and needle in a bolus injection no longer than 10 s, followed by a flush injection of physiological saline or glucose solution in order to empty the plastic tube and complete the administration of the total Gd-DTPA dose.

14.3.2 Choice of Pulse Sequence

After initial localizer scans in various planes, an axial multiecho spin-echo sequence encompassing both breasts is started, yielding proton density- and T2-weighted images. This sequence is considered necessary for easy identification of cysts and the evaluation of colloid and myxomatous tumors as well as hemorrhagic processes (fresh or older bleeding). Thereafter the actual MR examination is started, selecting a 2D gradient-echo or 3D acquisition sequence which reliably encompasses both breasts in contiguous axial slices not thicker than 5 mm. The sequence should be highly contrast sensitive. An approximately linear relationship between signal increase and contrast medium concentration should be established in previous measurements. The total acquisition time for one measurement should not surpass 1 min in order to guarantee sufficient temporal resolution for dynamic evaluation. The field of view and the matrix size are selected so as to yield an in-plane resolution of less than 1.5 mm. Care is taken to set an adequate echo time TE in order to avoid opposed phases of water and fat protons. The automatic radiofrequency tuning is switched off to ensure constant signal amplification of all pre- and postcontrast measurements. At our institution we prefer a sequence of one precontrast and four postcontrast measurements at 1-min intervals and one delayed measurement 8 min after contrast administration.

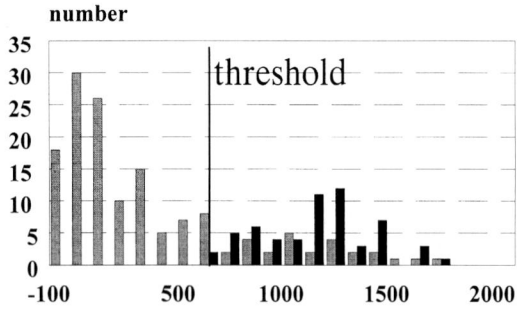

14.3.3 Diagnostic Criteria and Methods of Image Evaluation

14.3.3.1 Diagnostic Criteria

14.3.3.1.1 Contrast Enhancement. The new information gained with contrast-enhanced MRI of the breast is represented by a dynamic signal intensity increase among the various pathological entities of the breast after bolus administration of a standardized quantity of T1 contrast medium such as Gd-DTPA.

Before the advent of rapid volume acquisition techniques, only the relative increase of signal intensity after a time lapse of 5 min following contrast administration could be measured, and its morphological pattern of uptake evaluated (HEYWANG-KÖBRUNNER et al. 1988; HEYWANG-KÖBRUNNER 1993). Normalized units of contrast enhancement relative to surrounding breast tissue and a threshold were defined above which all lesions were to be regarded as malignant. Unfortunately a large number of benign entities also showed the same degree of delayed signal enhancement as the carcinomas and a high rate of false-positive results was obtained (~30%, HEYWANG-KÖBRUNNER et al. 1988; HEYWANG-KÖBRUNNER 1933). Nevertheless, in the latter study carcinoma could be excluded with a high negative predictive value if lesions displayed an overall contrast uptake below the threshold level (Fig. 14.2). MR examination therefore could be used to rule out contrast enhancement beyond the threshold level and thus exclude carcinoma in cases which are difficult to judge by mammography and ultrasonography.

Only when rapid acquisition techniques (fast 2D gradient-echo sequences: FLASH, FFE, GRASS) became available could the various phases of contrast uptake in the breast be analyzed (KAISER and ZEITLER 1989). The initial phase of rapid contrast

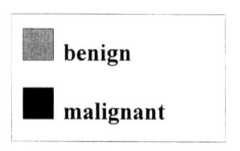

Fig. 14.2. Signal increase in static contrast-enhanced MRI (FLASH 3-D, 0.3–0.4 ml/kg body weight) (data from HEYWANG-KOEBRUNNER 1993)

uptake, especially during the first 2–3 min proved to contain valuable new information which improved differentiation between benign and malignant lesions. KAISER (1990, 1992) and STACK et al. (1990) reported a 90% signal intensity increase during the first minute after bolus injection of 0.1 mmol Gd-DTPA/kg using a special 2D gradient-echo sequence (Fig. 14.16, Sect. 14.4.2.1). The validity of this criterion was, however, questioned by FLICKINGER et al. (1992) and other investigators who often found an even higher signal increase in fibroadenomas than in carcinoma, although the latter did show a higher increase than mastopathy. Numerous authors (FISCHER et al. 1993) confirmed that the initial signal increase was valuable additional information for differential diagnosis, but basically insufficient to separate carcinoma from benign entities with the required certainty. Onther dynamic criteria such as an early signal intensity maximum within the first 5 min, and a signal intensity plateau or even contrast medium wash-out following the maximum, were defined as suspicious for carcinoma. In the course of these studies, however, it was also found that a certain number of infiltrating carcinomas (5%–10%) showed only weak contrast enhancement either in the initial or in the late phase (HEYWANG-KÖBRUNNER 1994).

14.3.3.1.2 Morphological Criteria. As it became apparent that the criteria of dynamic contrast enhancement were not absolutely reliable, morphological criteria of the contrast uptake were also included in image analysis. The inhomogeneous interior structure of carcinomas could be better discerned after contrast administration. Ring enhancement was also often found in malignant lesions with central tissue necrosis (FISCHER et al. 1993), although, as is to be expected, this occurs in inflammatory processes with abscess formation as well.

In conclusion, all the above-mentioned diagnostic criteria of contrast enhancement have been proven to be highly sensitive in the detection of lesions of any kind in the breast, but are, as will be discussed in more detail later, nonspecific and unreliable in the differential diagnosis of benign and malignant entities.

14.3.3.2 Methods of Image Evaluation

14.3.3.2.1 Visual Evaluation of Static Enhancement; the Subtraction Technique. After image reconstruction the precontrast and the first two postcontrast series are viewed at the viewing console in order to check any possible technical error such as incomplete contrast injection (no bolus enhancement in the heart), motion artifacts, or incomplete volume rendering of both breasts. Subtraction images from precontrast and the postcontrast series 4 and 8 min after bolus injection are routinely calculated and documented on monitor camera film together with all other pre- and postcontrast images. This may amount to some 150 images, from which it may be a problem to extract the diagnostically relevant information. Motion artifacts may simulate areas of focal enhancement in subtraction images, and must be identified as such by comparison with the original images. Flow artifacts and areas of hemorrhage must be recognized as such because they may simulate zones of contrast enhancement.

14.3.3.2.2 Evaluation of Dynamic Enhancement over a Region of Interest. The most commonly used method is to manually define a region of interest (ROI) over an area of focal enhancement and have a time-signal intensity profile calculated. The curve is then evaluated according to the established dynamic criteria of contrast enhancement. (see Sect. 14.3.3.1.1).

The definition of the size, shape, and location of the ROI critically influences the shape of the time-intensity profile, as partial volume effects of nonenhancing parts of the tissue may be inadvertently included in the ROI and flatten the signal intensity curve. Considerable variations in early uptake values, the occurrence of a signal maximum, and the amount of contrast enhancement were found using different methods of ROI definition (size and shape of ROI, pixel definition, definition from subtraction images) (STROHMAIER et al. 1995)

14.3.3.2.3 Computer-Assisted Image Evaluation. The detection of small and numerous focal enhancing lesions may be time-consuming and dependent on the individual observer. Dynamic visualization of the contrast uptake in one slice position over time in a cine-loop may be very helpful in localizing lesions (TEUBNER et al. 1995). Besides mere detection of a lesion, the dynamic criteria of contrast uptake and wash-out of a lesion must be analyzed. This can be done through computer analysis of the different dynamic parameters (initial signal increase, signal maximum, and wash-out). The computer can be programmed to identify only those lesions with dynamic criteria judged to be suspicious for malignancy. Various parameters [incremental contrast uptake (KUHL et al. 1995d), speed of initial contrast uptake (STROHMAIER et al. 1995), and other pharmacokinetic data (HESS et al. 1993)] have been evaluated. On a computer workstation these parametric images can also be visualized dynamically in a cine-loop mode (TEUBNER et al. 1995).

14.4 Clinical Results

14.4.1 Benign Entities

14.4.1.1 Fibrocystic Disease (Proliferative and Atypical Ductal Hyperplasia)

An increased amount of radiodense fibrous and adenomatous tissue may pose a diagnostic problem

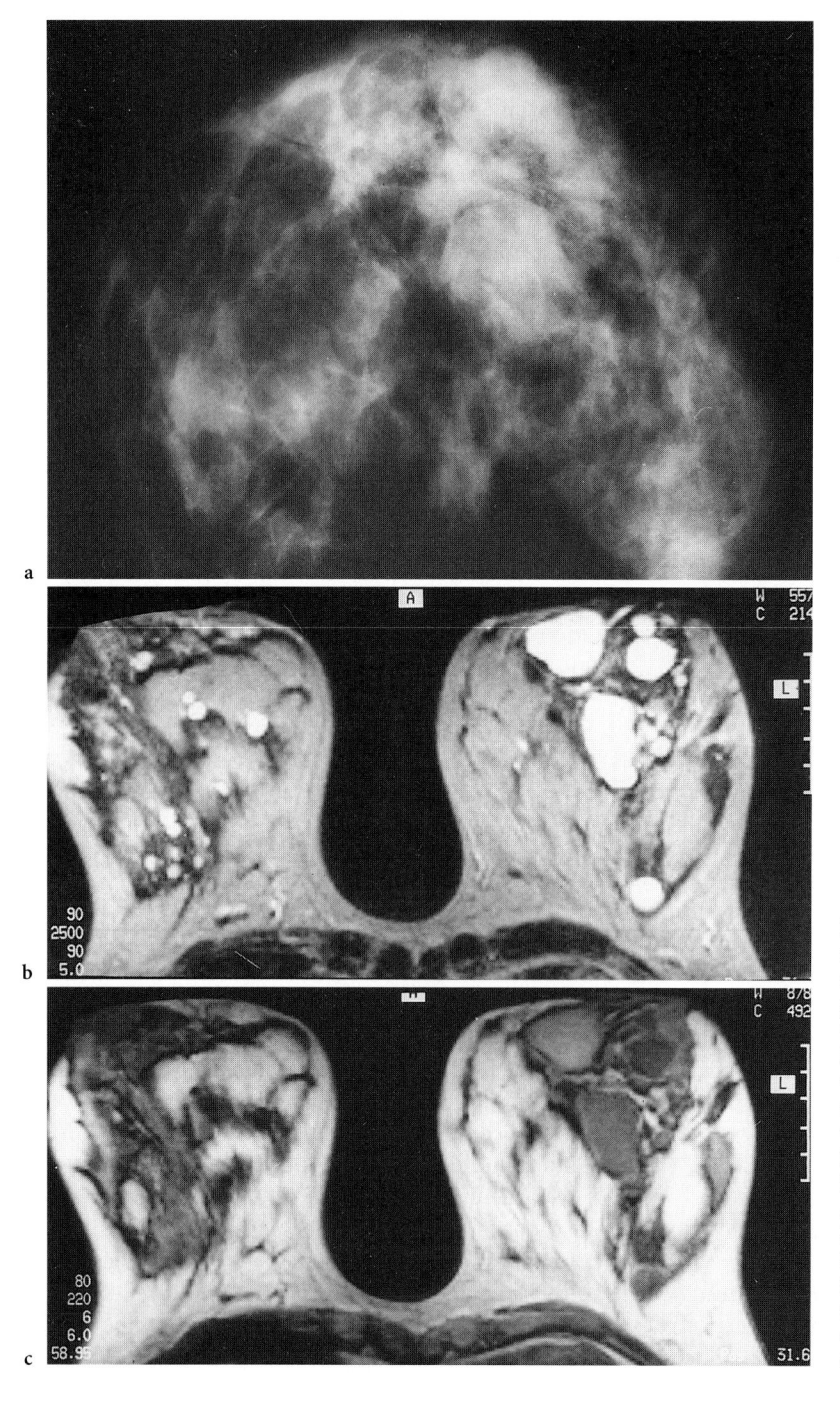

Fig. 14.3. a Left craniocaudal mammogram with multiple round opacities in the central subareolar region. b Axial T2-weighted SE image (2500/90 ms) with multiple fluid-filled high-intensity cysts with smooth inner walls. c Axial T1-weighted gradient-echo FLASH image (80°/220/6 ms) with varying signal intensity in the cysts indicating different proteinaceous/hemorrhagic contents of cyst fluid. d Axial T1-weighted FLASH image (80°/220/6 ms) after 0.1 mmol Gd-DTPA/kg i.v. shows ring-shaped enhancement in the wall of a small inflamed cyst on the right side e Subtraction image from d minus c, showing no substantial enhancement in most simple cysts

Fig. 14.3d,e

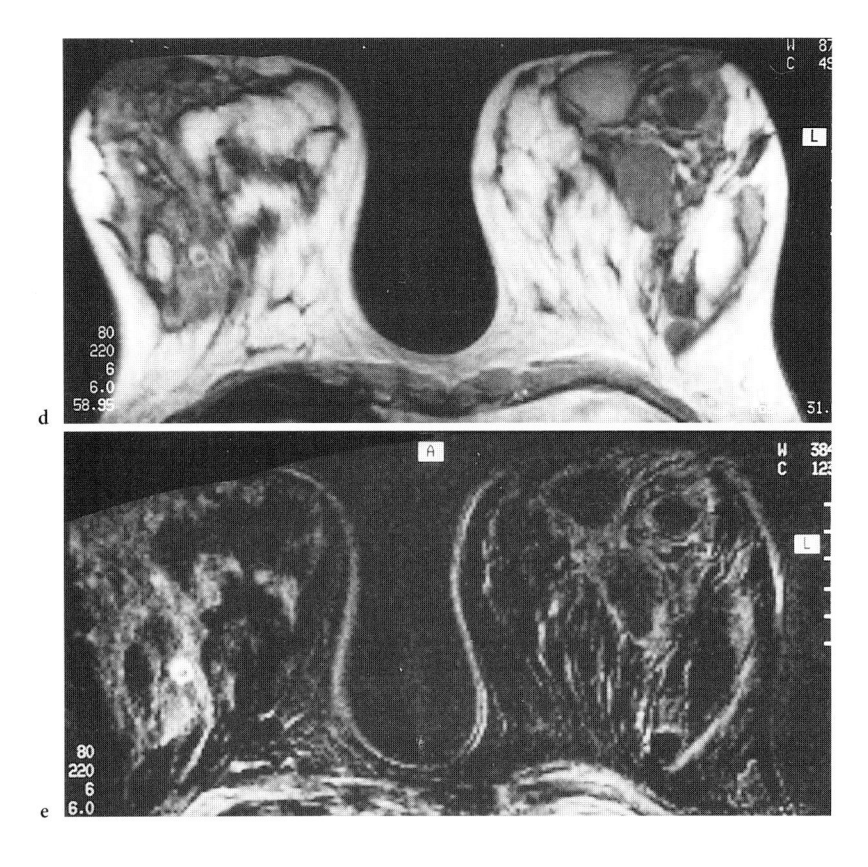

for mammography. A number of carcinomas are overlooked or are undetectable in radiodense breasts. Ultrasonography is a valuable complementary procedure to detect a considerable number of these lesions. Nevertheless, it is a well-known fact that one may fail to diagnose a carcinoma even using mammography and ultrasonography in combination. One initial perspective of the diagnostic potential of MRI of the breast was therefore to exclude and/or hopefully to detect malignancy in dense breasts with a higher degree of certainty than was possible with conventional methods. If, in cases of nodular fibrosis, no focal or intense diffuse contrast enhancement is found during dynamic MR examination, no suspicious microcalcifications are detected on the mammogram, and no shadowing lesion is found during ultrasonography, carcinoma can indeed be excluded with sufficient certainty for practical purposes (Heywang-Koebrunner 1993) If, however, as in about 30% of these diagnostically difficult cases (Heywang-Köbrunner 1993), multifocal or multinodular contrast enhancement is present, it may be impossible to exclude carcinoma.

Kuhl et al. (1995c) determined the variability of focal and diffuse areas of contrast uptake in healthy women in relation to the menstrual cycle. Of the areas of focal uptake found, 72% were transient. Between 30% and 50% of lesions displayed an initial contrast uptake of more than 80% in the first minute, at least once during the study. Kuhl et al. concluded that such lesions may be a normal finding and must be correlated with the other clinical and imaging data.

In cases of macrocystic disease, MRI may yield some additional information concerning the cyst contents (proteinaceous, hemorrhagic) and the status of the cyst wall (inflammatory changes, ring enhancement, Fig. 14.3d,e). In rare cases we have detected enhancing intracystic vegetations not found on the sonogram.

In cases of dense fibrocystic changes it is not possible to predict the degree of intraductal proliferation, nor even to estimate the ratio of ductal tissue versus interstitial fibrosis on the basis of mammographic or ultrasonographic signs. Some authors have claimed that these parameters can be assessed with contrast-enhanced MRI (Kaiser 1993; Heywang-Köbrunner 1993). Both authors have published time-signal intensity curves showing a gradual signal increase over time proportional to the degree of intraductal proliferation, thus suggesting the possibility of gaining information about the can-

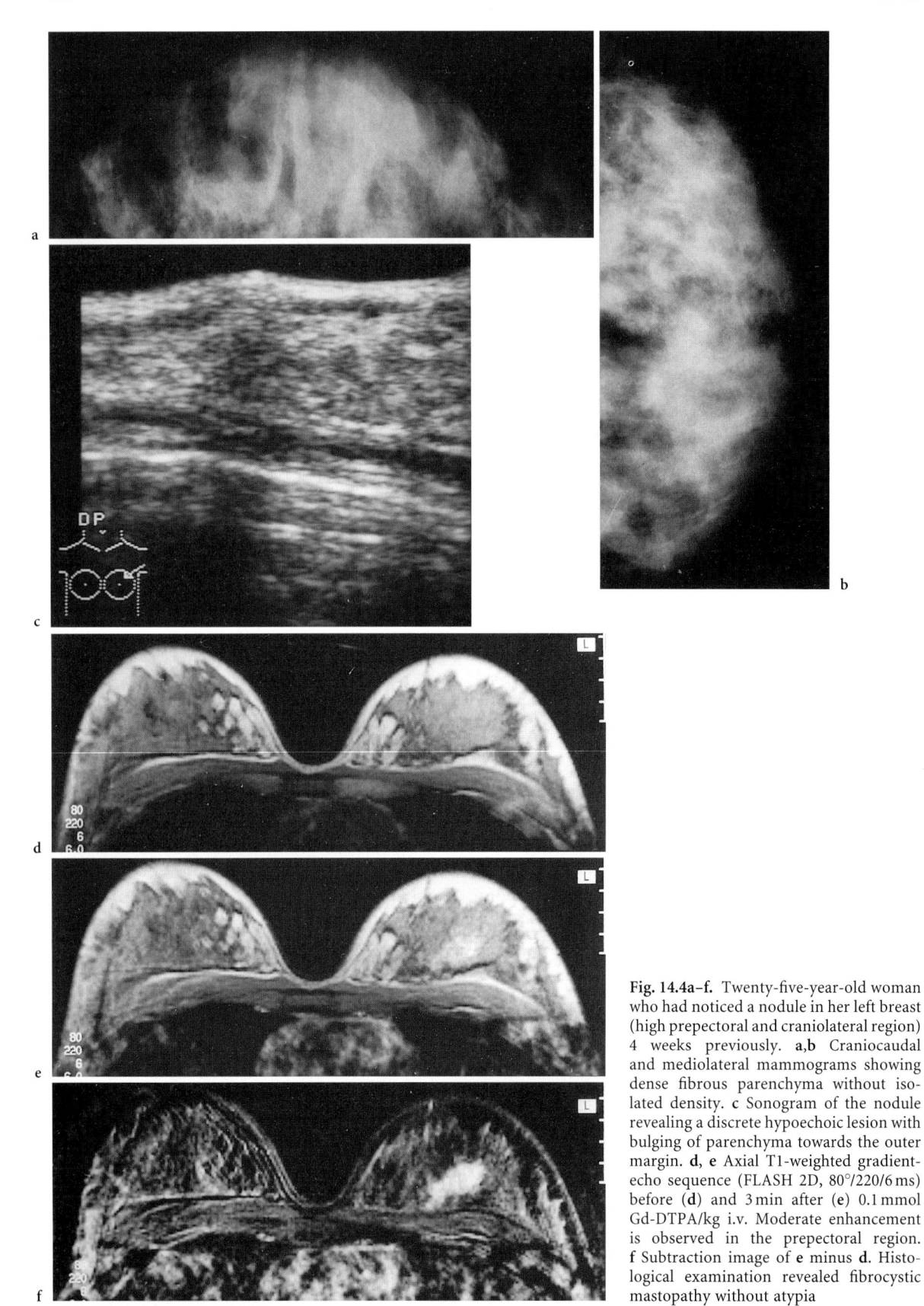

Fig. 14.4a-f. Twenty-five-year-old woman who had noticed a nodule in her left breast (high prepectoral and craniolateral region) 4 weeks previously. a,b Craniocaudal and mediolateral mammograms showing dense fibrous parenchyma without isolated density. c Sonogram of the nodule revealing a discrete hypoechoic lesion with bulging of parenchyma towards the outer margin. d, e Axial T1-weighted gradient-echo sequence (FLASH 2D, 80°/220/6 ms) before (d) and 3 min after (e) 0.1 mmol Gd-DTPA/kg i.v. Moderate enhancement is observed in the prepectoral region. f Subtraction image of e minus d. Histological examination revealed fibrocystic mastopathy without atypia

cer risk of the patient in a noninvasive way. These results could not, however, be fully confirmed in a recent study by SITTEK et al. (1995a), who found some proportional increase in enhancement between nonproliferative and proliferative dysplasia, but no correlation at all with atypical proliferative dysplasia. Nevertheless, enhancement seemed to correlate better with the progressive (adenomatous) than with the regressive (fibrocystic) form.

The enhancement in dysplastic breasts can be almost absent, or diffuse or multilobular or limited to certain areas, as in the case of Fig.14.4, where a palpable nodule in the left upper prepectoral region could be identified on the sonogram as a 1.5-cm, slightly hypoechoic thickening of the parenchyma. The contrast-enhanced MR image shows an asymmetric area of intermediate gradual contrast uptake without intensity maximum or wash-out effect. It corresponds to a focal zone of dysplasia with proliferation.

Also in cases of asymmetric radiodense tissue with an equivocal mammographic appearance and a complex ultrasonographic echo pattern (Fig. 14.5a–c) MRI can yield some additional information inasmuch as the area in the left upper medial quadrant displays only slight focal enhancement

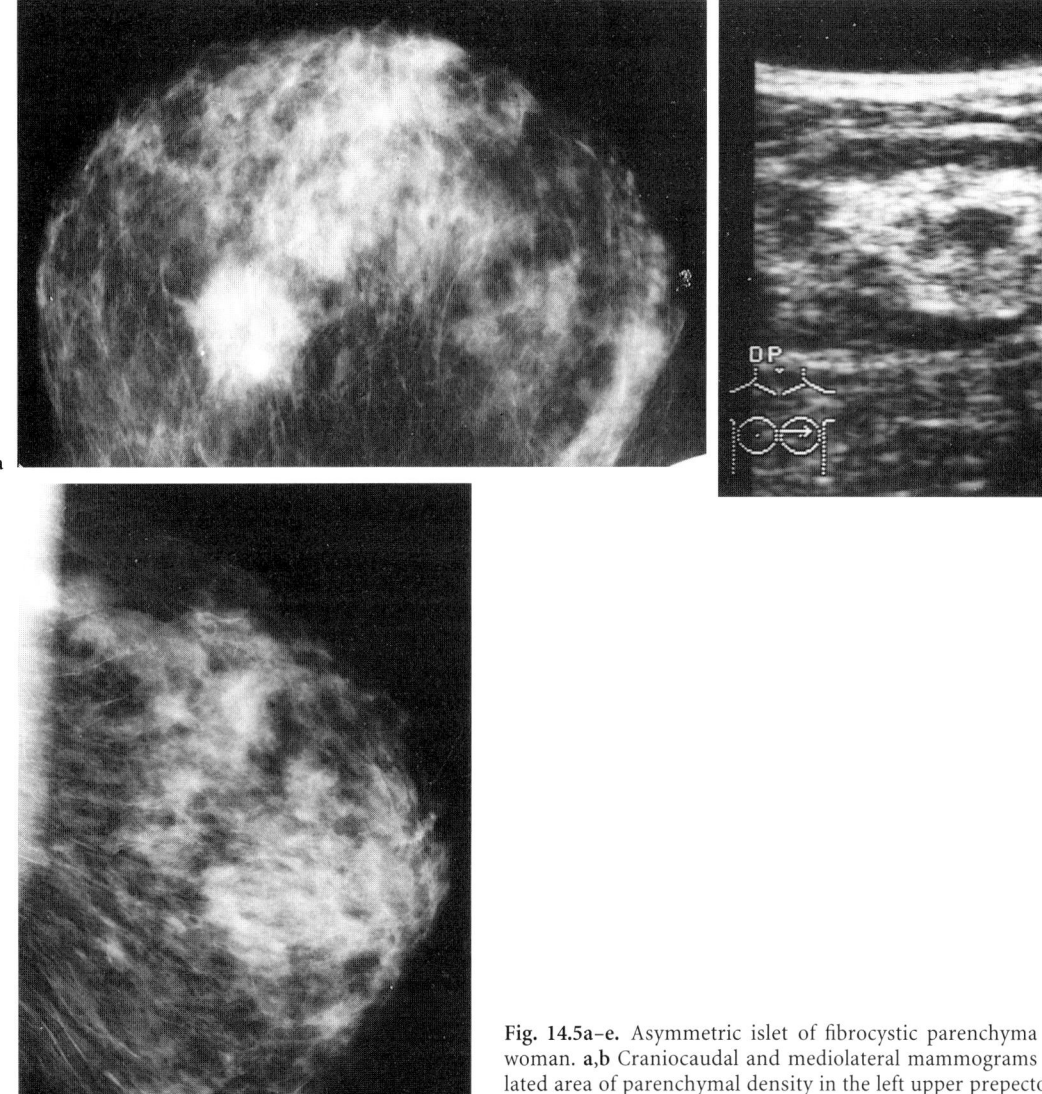

Fig. 14.5a–e. Asymmetric islet of fibrocystic parenchyma in a 45-year-old woman. a,b Craniocaudal and mediolateral mammograms revealing an isolated area of parenchymal density in the left upper prepectoral breast region with spiculated margins. c Sonogram of corresponding area shows pliable hyperechoic parenchyma with central hypoechoic fat inclusion. d,e Axial T1-weighted gradient-echo sequence (FLASH 2D, 80°/220/6 ms) before (d) and subtraction image after (e) contrast administration

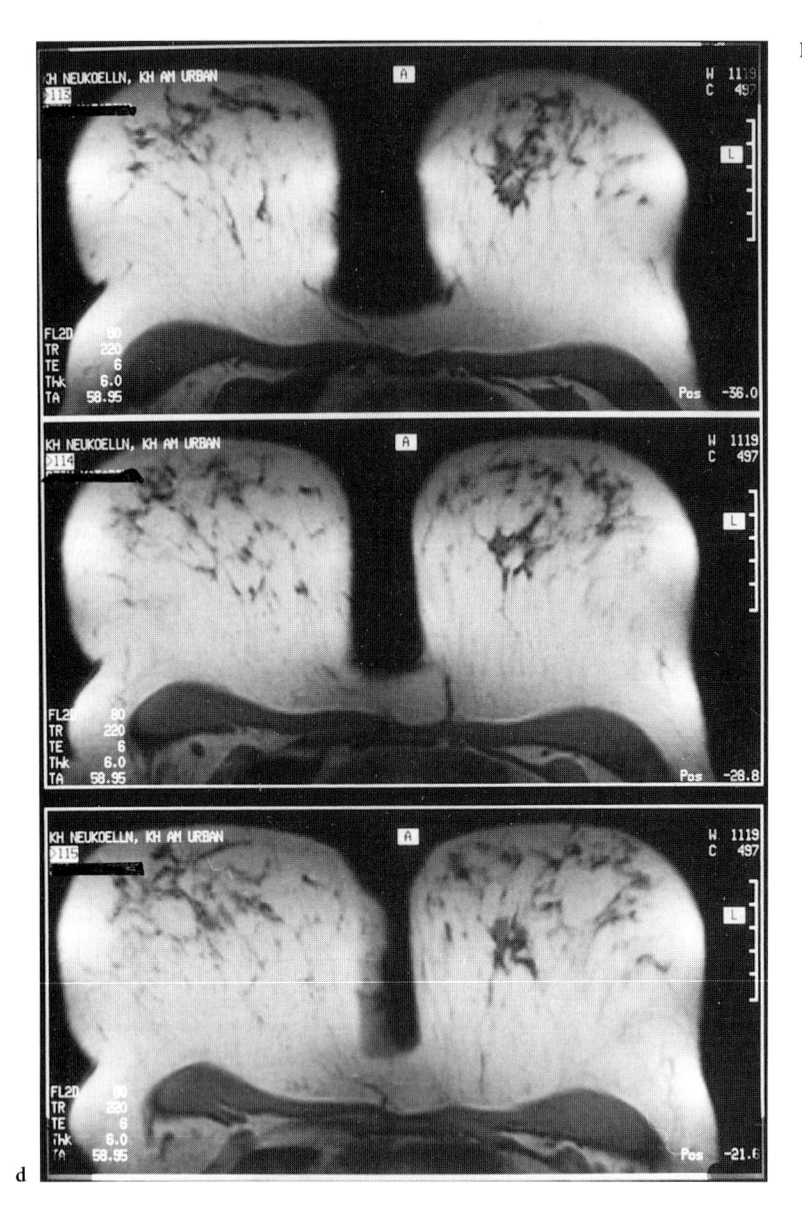

Fig. 14.5d

with a benign-appearing time-intensity profile, thus representing simple asymmetric breast parenchyma.

In 525 diagnostically difficult cases (mostly mastopathic), HEYWANG-KÖBRUNNER (1993) achieved an improvement in sensitivity through MRI from 60% with conventional methods (i.e., mammography ultrasonography) to 98.6% after MRI. Simultaneously specificity improved from 45% before to 65% after MRI.

On the other hand, MRI can provide only marginal help in cases of atypical ductal dysplasia, as in Fig. 14.6. A firm indistinct mass palpable in the right supra-areolar region could not be discerned on the mammogram and showed equivocal ultrasonographic signs. In the contrast-enhanced MR examination, multiple zones of intense focal enhancement were found in the retroareolar region, all but one with an unremarkable time-intensity profile. The one exception displayed the typical time-intensity curve of carcinoma (Fig. 14.6g) (see Sect. 14.4.2.1). Histological examination revealed atypical ductal hyperplasia, so that the contrast-enhanced MRI as well as the sonogram gave false-positive information indicating a probable carcinoma.

14.4.1.2 Fibroadenoma (Proliferating, Myxiod, Fibrous)

Fibroadenoma is the most common benign neoplasm of the female breast (~25%) and often poses a

Magnetic Resonance Imaging of the Breast 239

Fig. 14.5e

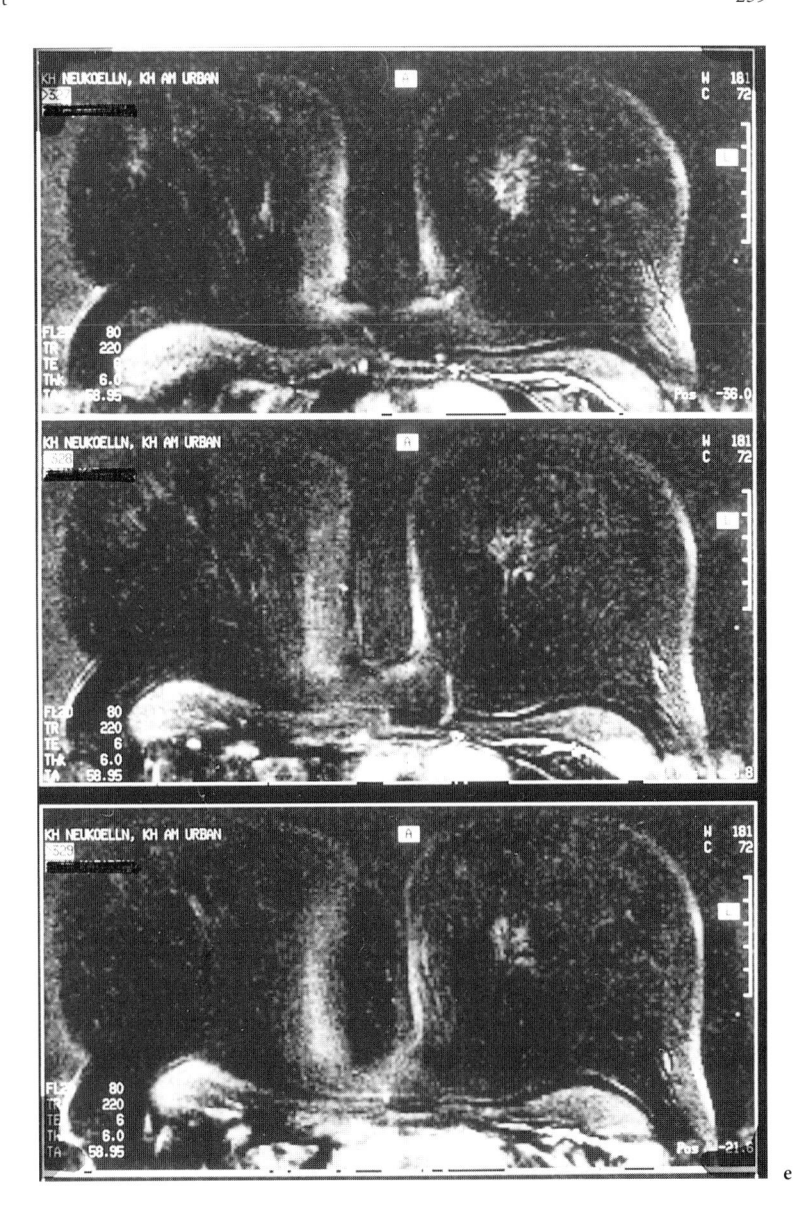

differential diagnostic problem. Depending on the age of the patient, it may contain mainly adenomatous proliferating tissue or show central myxoid degeneration (in younger women) or only fibrous components (in older patients). If the neoplasm is not typically calcified on the mammogram or is not known to be stable from previous follow-ups, it may be difficult or impossible to differentiate it from circumscribed medullary, solid, or myxoid carcinoma through mammographic or ultrasonographic examination. The literature mentions overlap of mammographic and ultrasonographic characteristics of fibroadenoma with circumscribed carcinoma in approximately 20% of cases (KASUMI 1991). As the visualization of and shape of fibroadenoma in MRI are identical with those on mammography and ultrasonography, theoretically it might be distinguished from carcinoma only through contrast enhancement characteristics. Unfortunately, however, neither the initial contrast uptake nor the nonexistence of a signal maximum or a wash-out phenomenon can distinguish it with sufficient certainty from carcinoma. In accordance with the histological composition, adenomatous (18/36, 50%: HEYWANG-KÖBRUNNER 1993) and myxoid fibroadenoma (10/10, 100%) may show strong contrast uptake, even higher than in carcinoma, whereas no contrast uptake may be seen in the fibrous types. Three out of 18 fibroadenomas showed strong initial enhancement during dynamic MRI (HEYWANG-

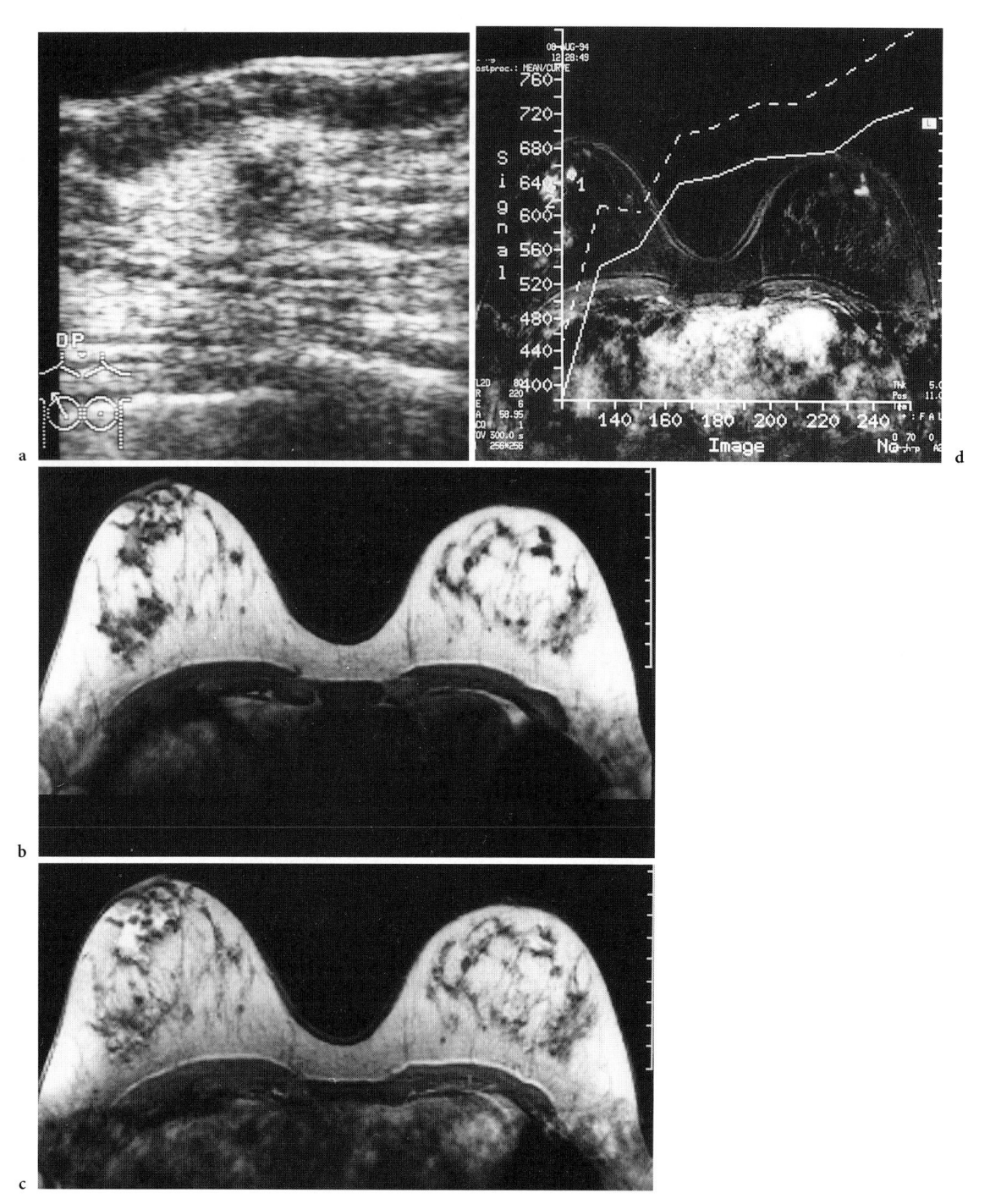

Fig. 14.6a–g. Mastopathy with atypical ductal hyperplasia. False-positive MR examination in a 54-year-old woman with bloody nipple discharge on the right side and numerous nodules bilaterally. **a** Right-sided sonogram shows a hypoechoic, unsharply marginated, shadowing lesion in right upper prepectoral region. **b–d** Axial T1-weighted gradient-echo sequence (FLASH 2D, 80°/220/6 ms) before (**b**) and after (**c**) 0.1 mmol Gd-DTPA/kg and subtraction image (**d**) with time-signal intensity curves over regions of focal enhancement: a gradual increase in signal was observed after administration of contrast medium. **e–g** Higher axial prepectoral sections (FLASH 2D, 80°/220/6 ms) without (**e**) or with (**f**) 0.1 mmol Gd-DTPA/kg and subtraction image (**g**) show initial peak enhancement with signal decrease after 3 min, suggestive of a malignant lesion. Histological examination revealed proliferative fibrocystic disease with atypical ductal hyperplasia

Fig. 14.6e–g

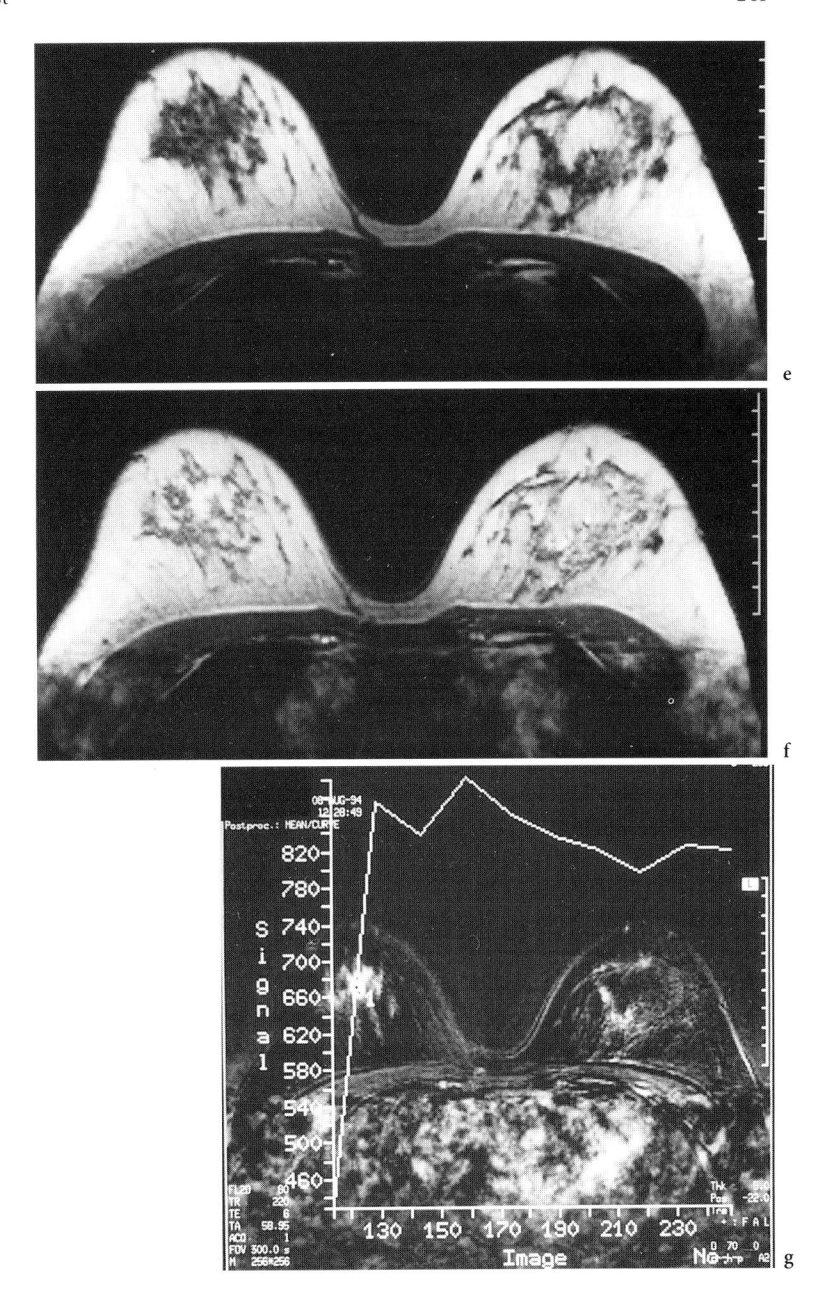

KÖBRUNNER 1993). Therefore a circumscribed equivocal mammographic density which has been shown to be solid by ultrasonography is not an indication for further diagnostic workup with MRI because it cannot be distinguished from a malignant lesion with certainty. Stereotaxically or ultrasonographically guided fine-needle or core biopsy yields the correct diagnosis in approximately 95%–98% of cases at a fraction of the cost of an MR examination (LIBERMAN et al. 1994).

Figure 14.7 shows a typical case of an adenomatous fibroadenoma in the left breast of a 37-year-old woman demonstrating benign morphology but an enhancement profile typical for carcinoma. Figure 14.8 gives an example of a large fibroadenoma with central necrosis and peripheral hemorrhage with indeterminate morphological and dynamic criteria. Figure 14.9 shows a small fibroadenoma with partial myxoid transformation and benign-appearing characteristics.

14.4.1.3 Papilloma

Papilloma is an intraductal or intracystic proliferation of epithelial cells which cause bloody nipple dis-

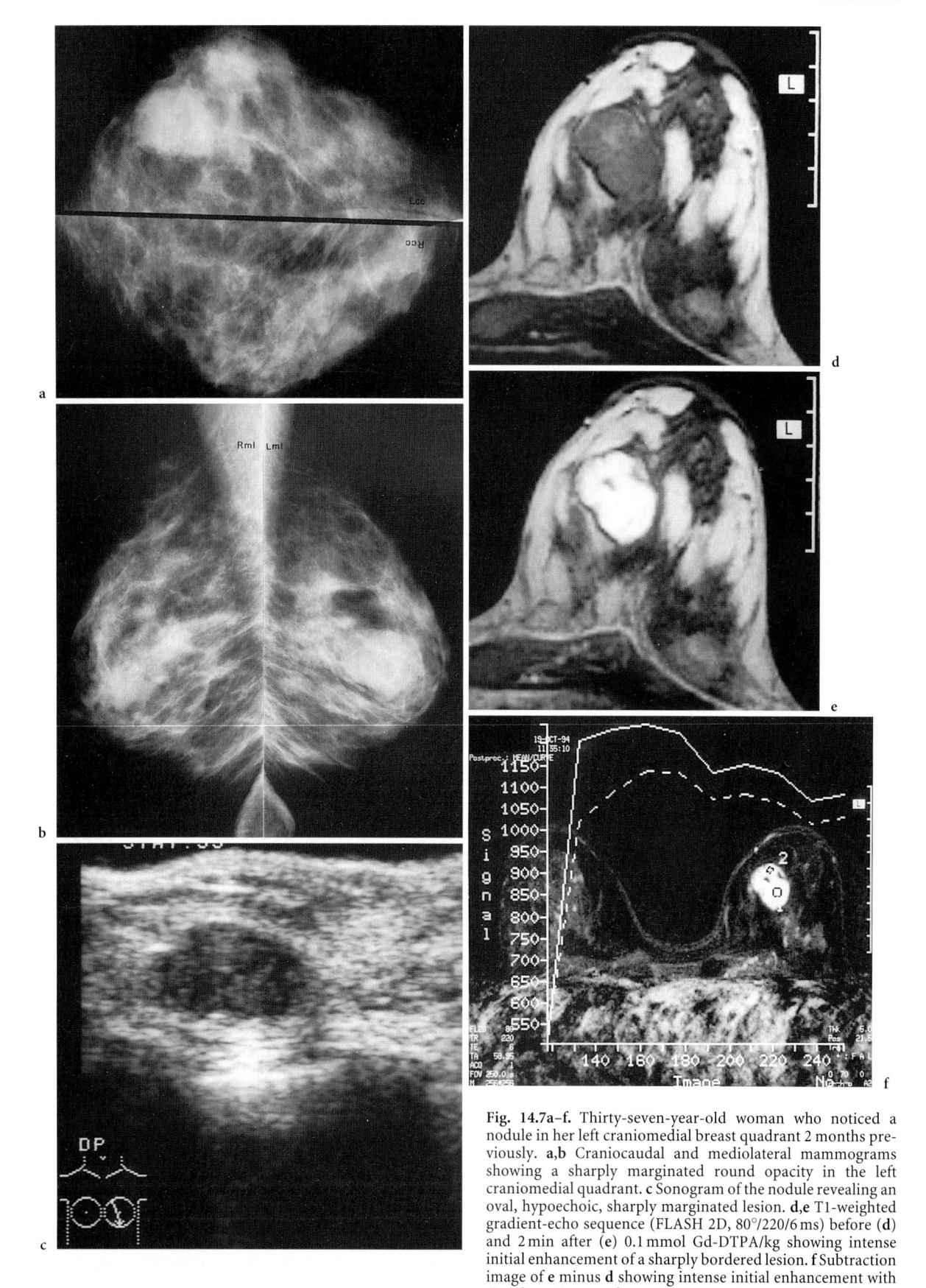

Fig. 14.7a–f. Thirty-seven-year-old woman who noticed a nodule in her left craniomedial breast quadrant 2 months previously. **a,b** Craniocaudal and mediolateral mammograms showing a sharply marginated round opacity in the left craniomedial quadrant. **c** Sonogram of the nodule revealing an oval, hypoechoic, sharply marginated lesion. **d,e** T1-weighted gradient-echo sequence (FLASH 2D, 80°/220/6 ms) before (**d**) and 2 min after (**e**) 0.1 mmol Gd-DTPA/kg showing intense initial enhancement of a sharply bordered lesion. **f** Subtraction image of **e** minus **d** showing intense initial enhancement with signal maximum after 2 min, suggesting a malignant lesion. Histological examination revealed a fibroadenoma

charge in cases of intraductal papillomatosis. Detection is difficult by mammography unless specific calcifications are present. Intraductal papillomatosis is easily demonstrated in galactography. Intracystic papilloma is usually detected through ultrasonography. Unfortunately, neither of these methods provides safe morphological signs of benignity. Though sensitive in detecting papilloma, MRI is also nonspecific in classification of benignity.

Figure 14.10a and b shows a 2-cm, sharply marginated opacity in the left breast of a 45-year-old woman which had developed over a period of 4 years. The intracystic nature of the lesion is obvious on the sonogram (Fig. 14.10c). The contrast-enhanced MR examination depicts the lesion with an enhancement profile typical of carcinoma. Histology proved the lesion to be an intracystic papilloma with atypical hyperplasia and not carcinoma.

Figure 14.11a and b shows a hypoechoic oval-shaped lesion in the medial central breast of a 51-year-old woman who had had a lumpectomy at the same site 20 years prior to examination. The lesion had grown markedly during the previous 10 months. The MR examination also demonstrates an oval, sharply marginated lesion with an enhancement profile typical of carcinoma. Histology revealed a moderately proliferating papilloma.

14.4.1.4 Postoperative and Intramammary Scars and Fat Necrosis (see also Chap. 17)

Intramammary retractive processes and stellate lesions have always been a diagnostic problem in mammography. In our opinion postoperative scarring following an operation not for carcinoma, how-

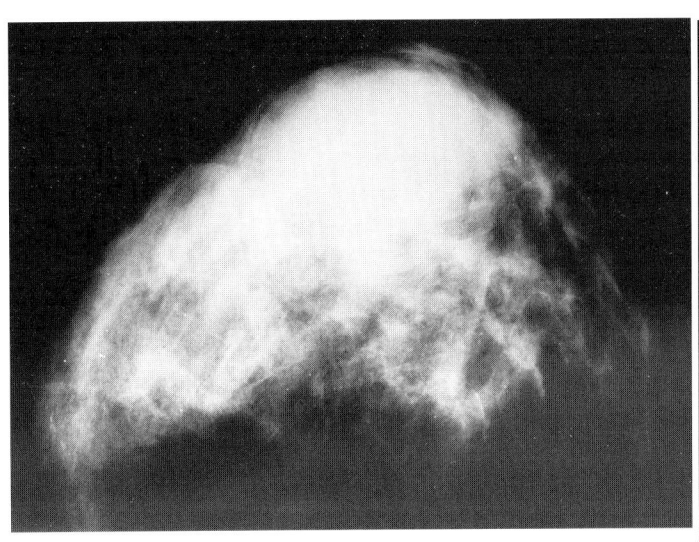

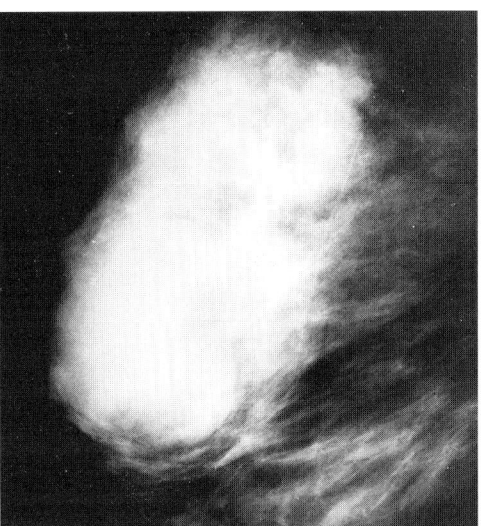

Fig. 14.8a–g. Forty-five-year-old woman who noticed recent growth of a long-existing nodule in her right breast. **a,b** Craniocaudal and mediotaleral mammograms revealing a large, partially sharply marginated density in the right retroareolar region. **c** Sonogram of a lobulated solid lesion with a hypoechoic, homogeneous echo pattern. **d,e** Proton density- and T2-weighted axial spin-echo sequence (SE 2500/20/90 ms) showing a solid tumor with a high fluid content and some peripheral hemorrhagic zones. **f,g** Same lesion; gradient-echo sequence (FLASH 2D, 80°/220/6 ms) after 0.1 mmol Gd-DTPA/kg i.v. showing peripheral enhancement with strong initial and further continuous signal intensity increase. Histological examination revealed a fibroadenoma with central necrosis and partially cystic transformation

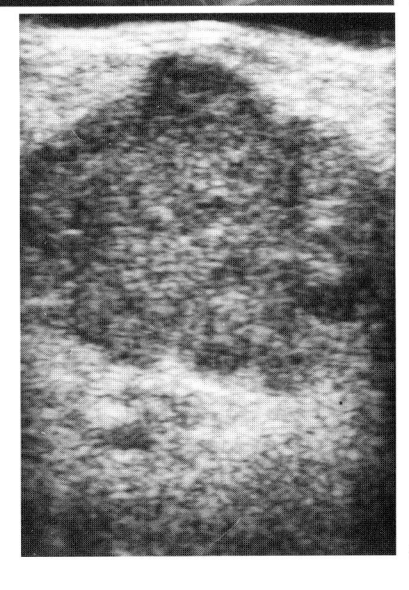

Fig. 14.8d–g

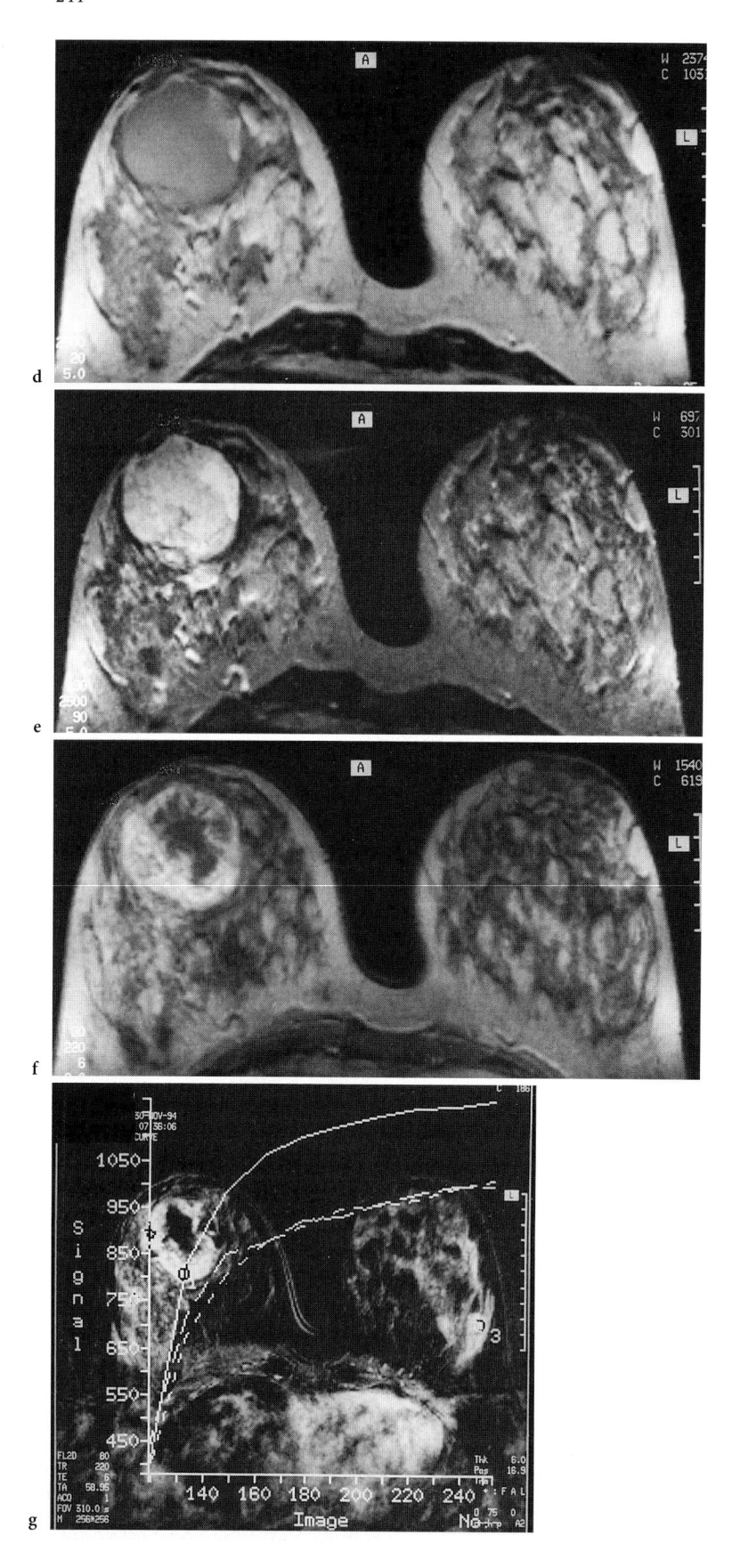

ever, does not pose such a problem as is often assumed, provided that preoperative mammograms are available for comparison. Many seemingly spiculated lesions are simply summation artifacts, which are not reproducible on a second view. Others can be easily shown to correspond to pliable and compressible hyperechoic parenchyma during ultrasonography. Nevertheless, many stellate lesions at mammography remain unclear even after imaging with complementary methods. The hypothesis that this problem can be solved by contrast-enhanced MRI presumes that scar tissue, if older than a few months, has few blood vessels and thus will display no or minimal contrast uptake during contrast-enhanced MRI, whereas all other processes, including scirrhous carcinoma, will show enhancement because of increased vascularization. The problem in clinical practice is that this hypothesis holds true for the majority of, but not all, equivocal spiculated densities. Unfortunately some scar tissue, such as spiculated fat necrosis, is in fact vascularized, whereas certain carcinomas present no remarkable neovascularization. Therefore one should not expect to differentiate these entities with absolute certainty by contrast-enhanced MR.

Nevertheless, in clinical practice contrast-enhanced MRI is an accepted procedure to classify spiculated lesions into hypo- and hypervascular entities, thus providing some assistance in refining the differential diagnosis. Figure 14.12a shows a stellate retraction of the upper prepectoral breast parenchyma 4 years after surgery. The sonogram (Fig. 14.12b) shows a hyperechoic disruption of architectural structure which was pliable during ultrasonography. No contrast uptake is seen in this avascular scar on the contrast-enhanced MRI (Fig. 14.12c,d).

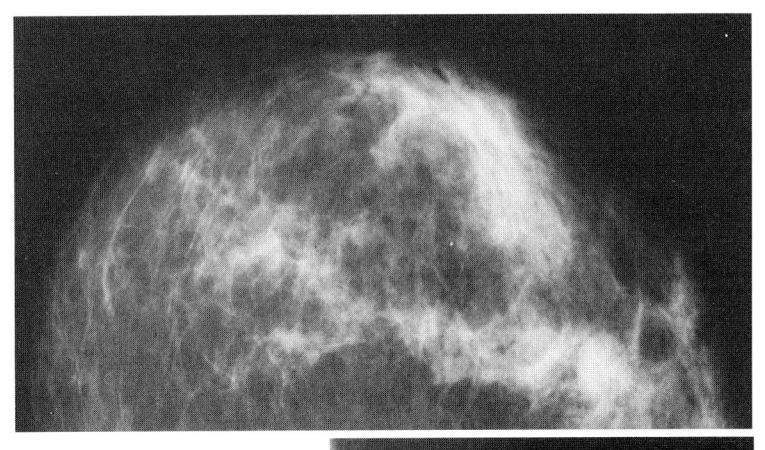

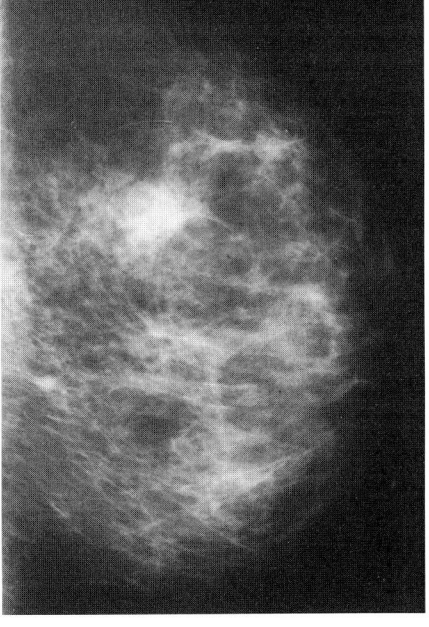

Fig. 14.9a–f. Myxomatous fibroadenoma in a 63-year-old woman with no physical findings. **a,b** Craniocaudal and mediolateral left-sided mammograms showing a sharply marginated opacity in the left upper outer quadrant. **c** Axial T2-weighted spin-echo image (SE 2500/90 ms) demonstrating intense signal intensity as in a lesion with a high fluid content. **d,e** T1-weighted gradient-echo sequence (FLASH 2D, 80°/220/6 ms) before (**d**) and 6 min after (**e**) 0.1 mmol Gd-DTPA/kg. **f** Subtraction image of **e** minus **d** showing gradual moderate contrast enhancement, characterizing the lesion as benign. Histological examination revealed a small fibroadenoma with myxomatous transformation

Fig. 14.9c–f

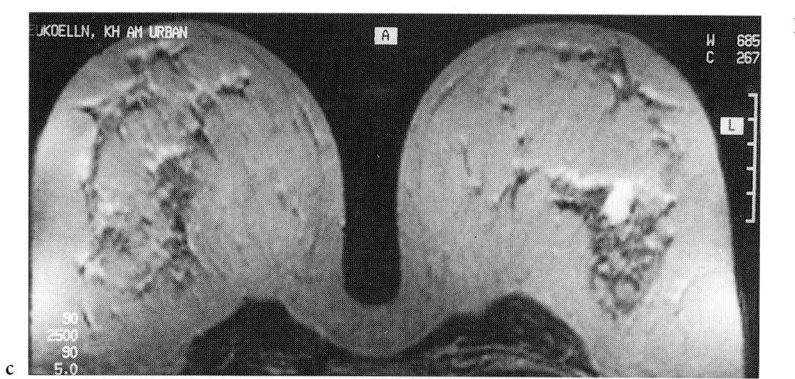

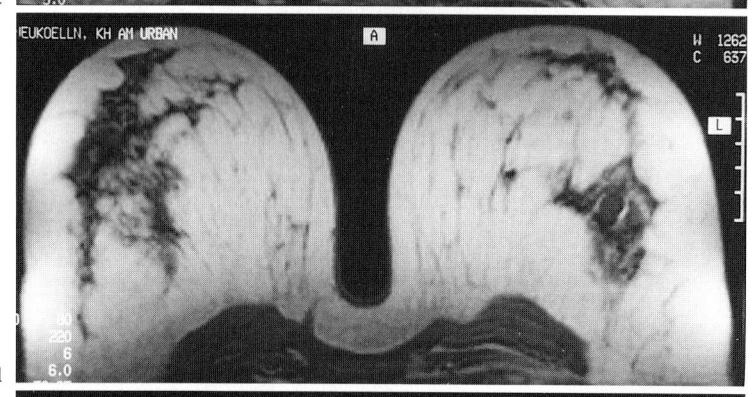

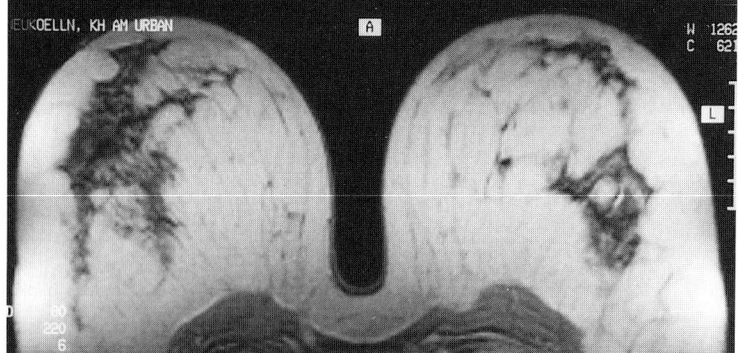

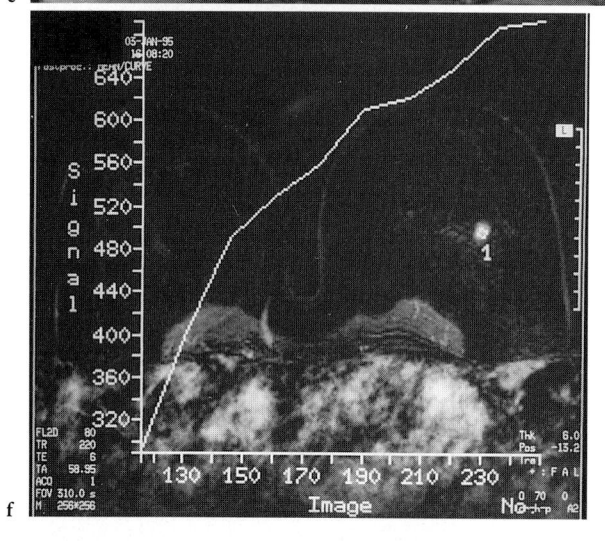

Magnetic Resonance Imaging of the Breast

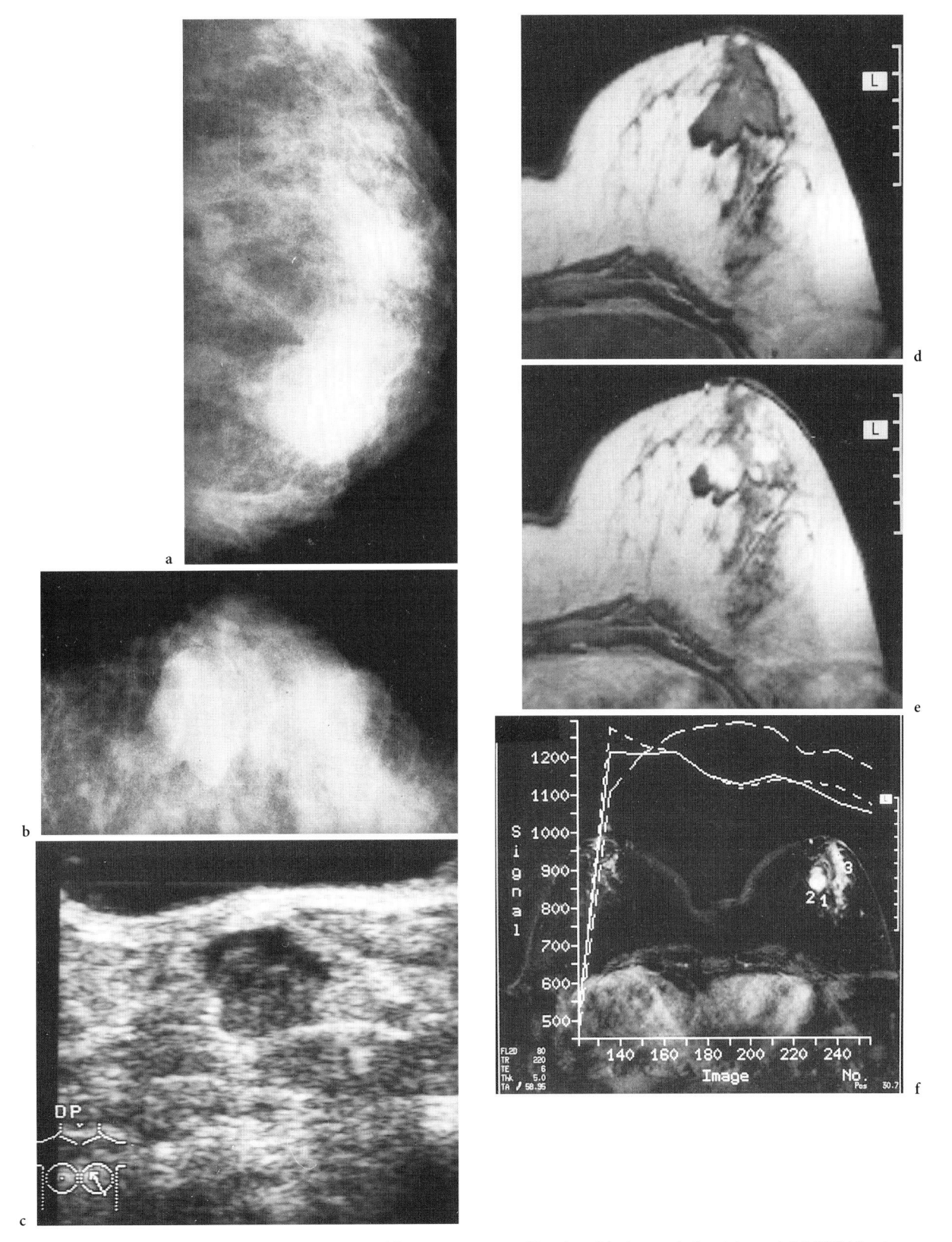

Fig. 14.10a–f. Intracystic papilloma in a 45-year-old woman. **a,b** Craniocaudal and mediolateral mammograms showing a lobular round opacity in the left retroareolar region; gradual growth for 6 years was documented by mammographic follow-up. **c** Sonogram revealing a partially cystic lesion with intracystic tumor. **d–f** Axial gradient-echo sequence (FLASH 2D, 80°/220/6 ms) before and after 0.1 mmol Gd-DTPA/kg i.v. There is strong enhancement of intracystic tumor, suggestive of intracystic carcinoma. Histological examination revealed an intracystic papilloma with atypical hyperplasia, but no carcinoma

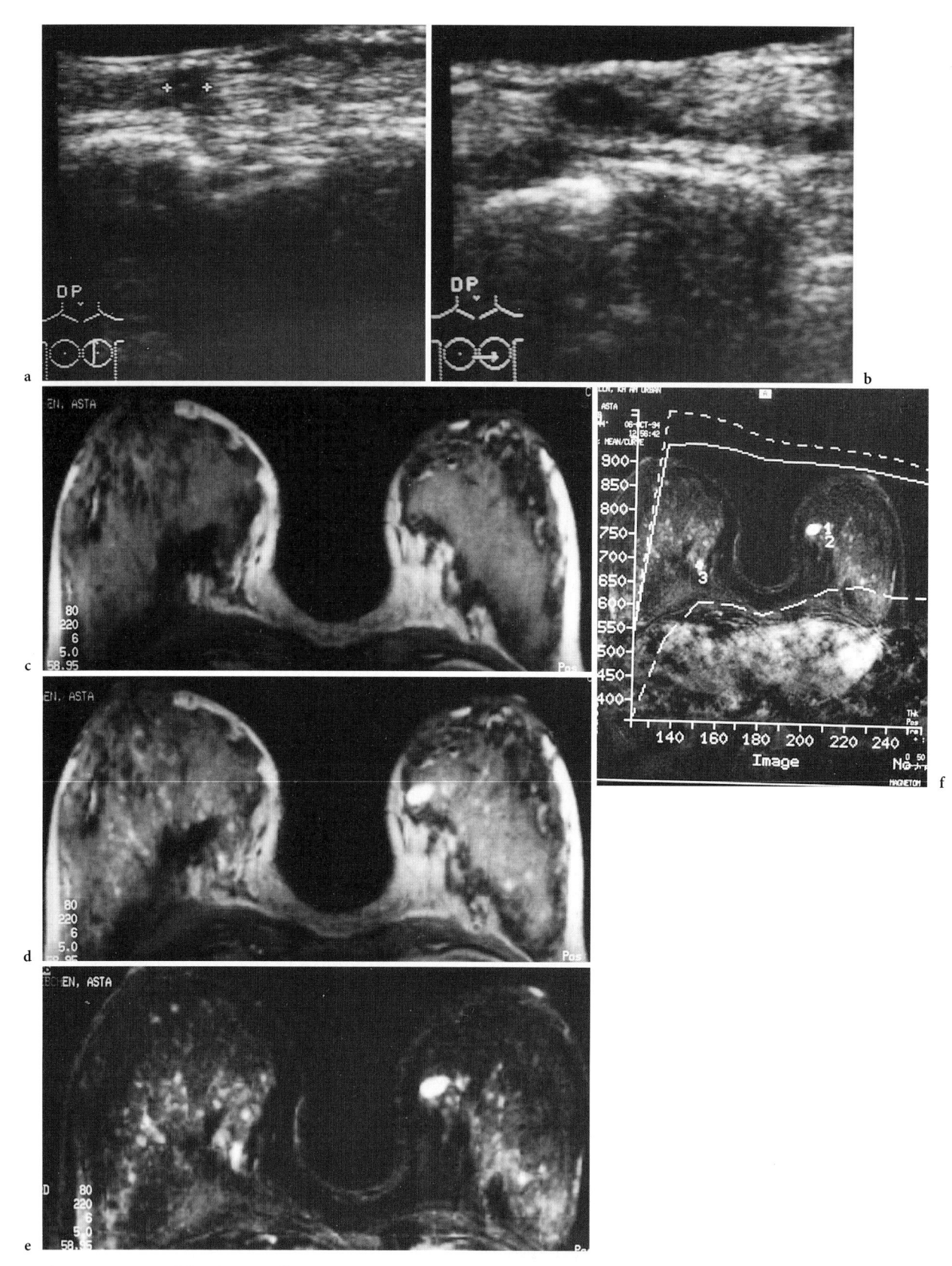

Fig. 14.11a–e. Proliferating papilloma in a 51-year-old woman. Twenty-two years following lumpectomy between the medial quadrants, the patient noticed a small nodule at the medial parasternal end of scar. **a,b** Ultrasonographic follow-up of the lesion from January to October 1994 with distinct growth of the lesion. **c** Axial gradient-echo sequence (FLASH 2D 80°/220/6 ms) before and after 0.1 mmol Gd-DTPA/kg i.v. There is strong enhancement of tumor, suggestive of carcinoma. Histological examination revealed a moderately proliferating papilloma

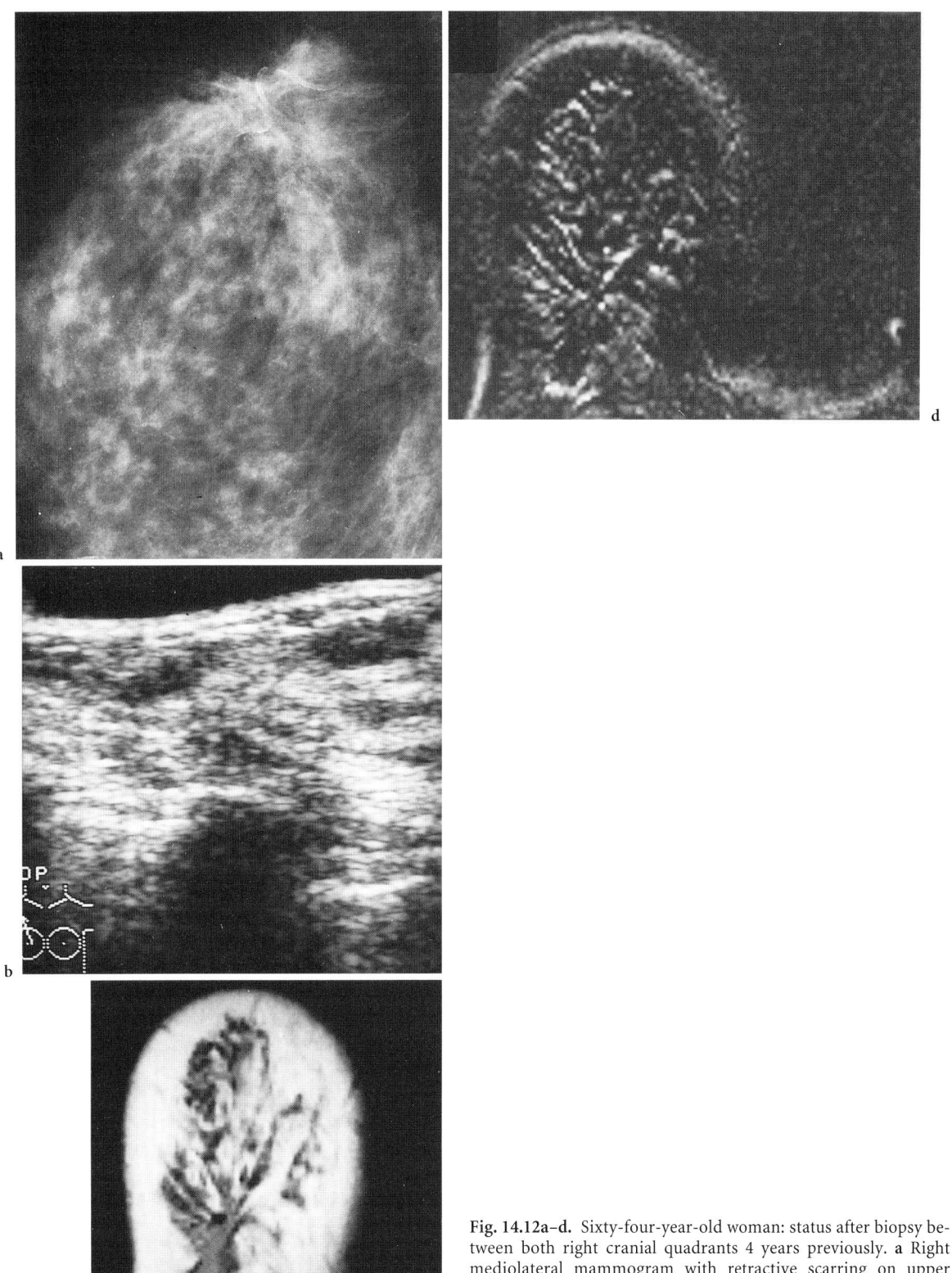

Fig. 14.12a–d. Sixty-four-year-old woman: status after biopsy between both right cranial quadrants 4 years previously. **a** Right mediolateral mammogram with retractive scarring on upper breast margin. **b** Sonogram showing hyperreflective disruption of the architectural pattern. **c** Axial gradient-echo sequence (FLASH 2D, 80°/220/6 ms) after 0.1 mmol Gd-DTPA/kg i.v. and **d** subtraction image. No contrast enhancement is observed in the scar

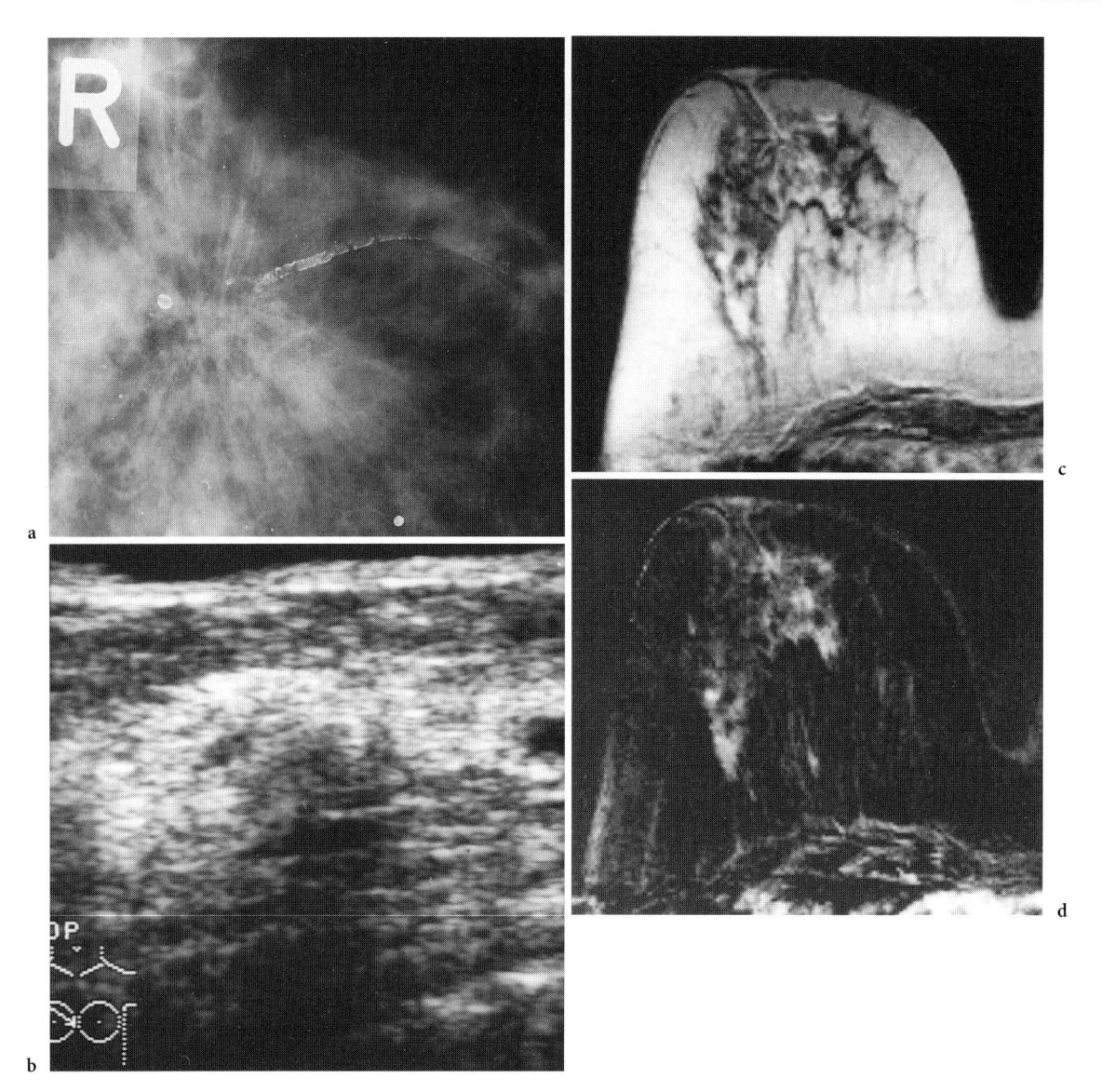

Fig. 14.13a–d. Intramammary scar in an 82-year-old woman Status post biopsy in left upper outer quadrant 32 years previously; unremarkable findings on the right side. **a** Craniocaudal mammogram showing a spiculated retractive mass in the right medial quadrant. **b** Sonogram revealing an indistinct region of shadowing with a broad peripheral echogenic rim. **c–e** Axial gradient-echo sequence (FLASH 2D, 80°/220/6 ms) before (**c**) and after (**d**) 0.1 mmol Gd-DTPA/kg i.v. and subtraction image (**e**) from **d** minus **c**. There is weak contrast enhancement. There was no histological proof of disease

In Fig. 14.13a the craniocaudal mammogram of an 82-year-old woman shows a stellate lesion with a radiolucent center in the right medial breast. During ultrasonography (Fig. 14.13b) an indistinct region of shadowing with a wide echogenic rim was found. On the contrast-enhanced MR examination (Fig. 14.13c,d) faint contrast uptake was noticed in a star-like retractive structure in the retroareolar region. The lesion was assumed to be an intramammary scar. Apart from follow-up no further diagnostic measures were considered necessary.

Figure 14.14a and b shows a star-like retraction on the craniocaudal and oblique mammograms of a 43-year-old woman with a slight skin dimpling in the lateral breast. There is no well-defined opacity at the center of the lesion. Axial contrast-enhanced MRI (Fig. 14.14c–f) depicts a retractive process at the outer border of the breast parenchyma with star-like focal contrast uptake. The time-intensity profile is indeterminate. Histology proved the lesion to be an intramammary scar within which a papilloma was found.

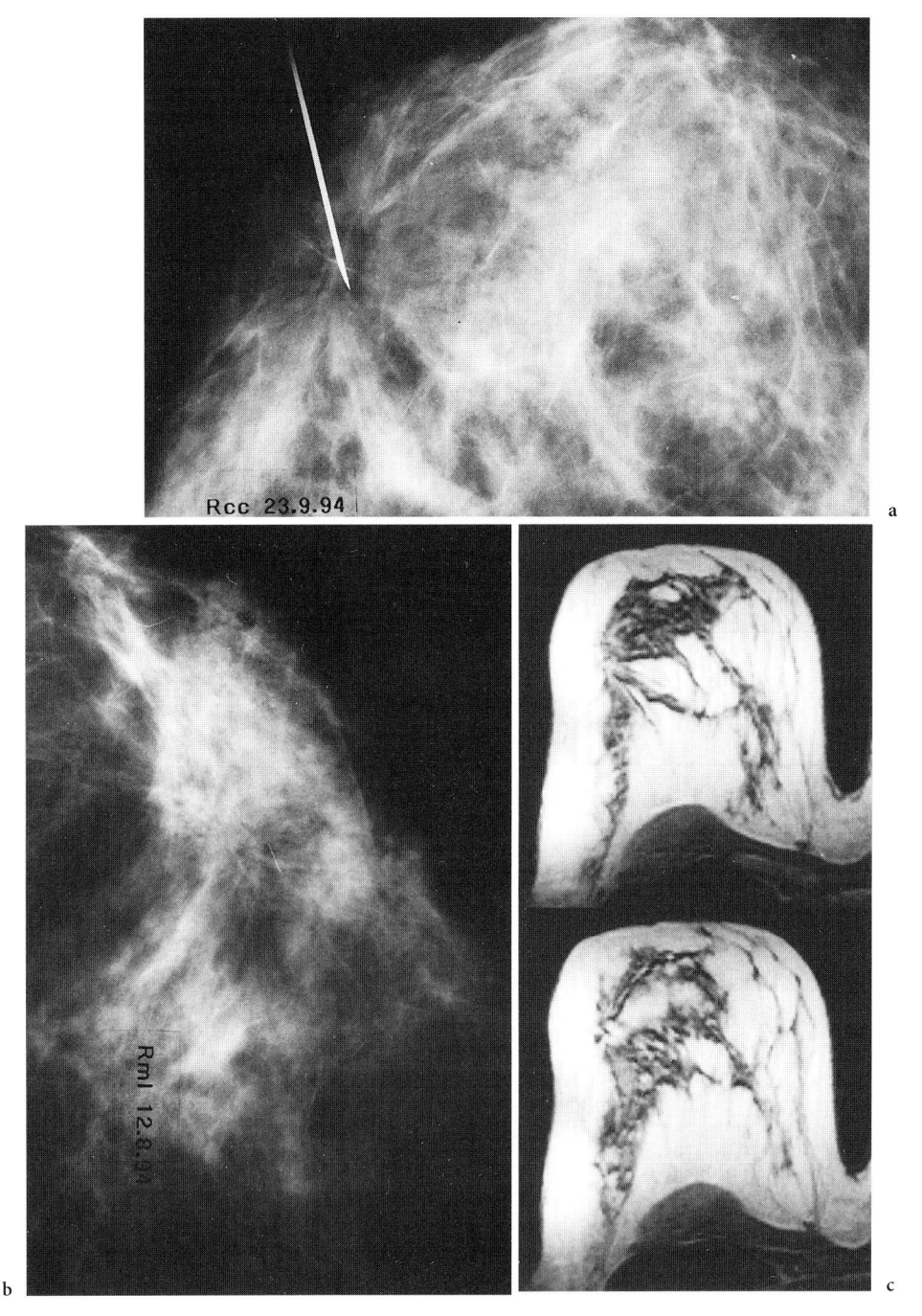

Fig. 14.14a–f. Intramammary scar and papilloma in a 43-year-old woman with a slight skin dimpling in the right outer breast quadrant. **a, b** Spiculated retraction in the right upper outer quadrant with radiolucent center. **c–e** Axial gradient-echo sequence (FLASH 2D, 80°/220/6 ms) before (**c**) and after (**d**) 0.1 mmol Gd-DTPA/kg i.v. and subtraction images (**e**): weak central contrast enhancement is present. **f** Time-intensity profile not suggestive of a malignant lesion. Histological examination revealed a radial scar with a fortuitous finding of a papilloma

Figure 14.15a and b shows the craniocaudal and oblique mammograms of a 60-year-old woman who had had a left retroareolar lumpectomy and postoperative radiotherapy for an infiltrating ductal carcinoma [pT2N1(1/12)] 2 years previously. Clinically there was nipple retraction and a firm indistinct mass in the left retroareolar region. A stellate mass with numerous peripheral spicules and a smoothly marginated radiolucent center is seen on the mammogram, suggesting postoperative fat necrosis

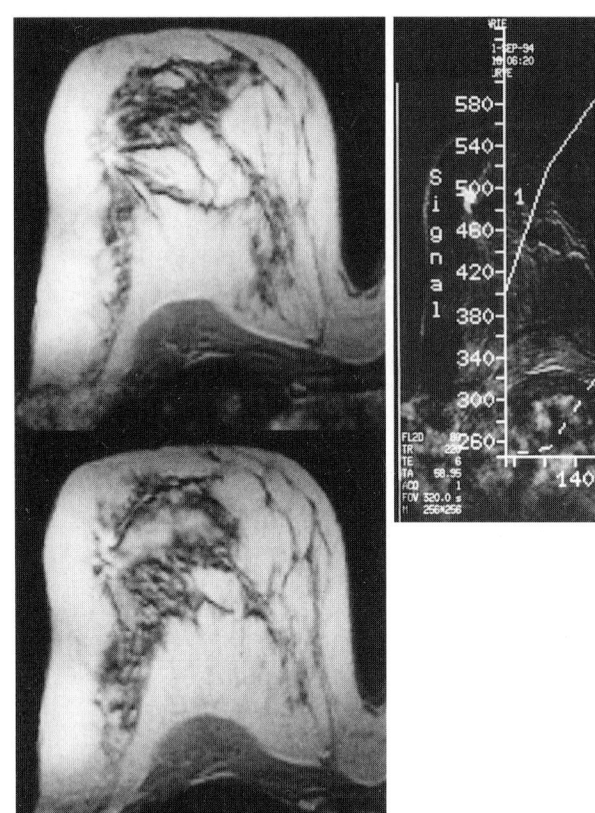

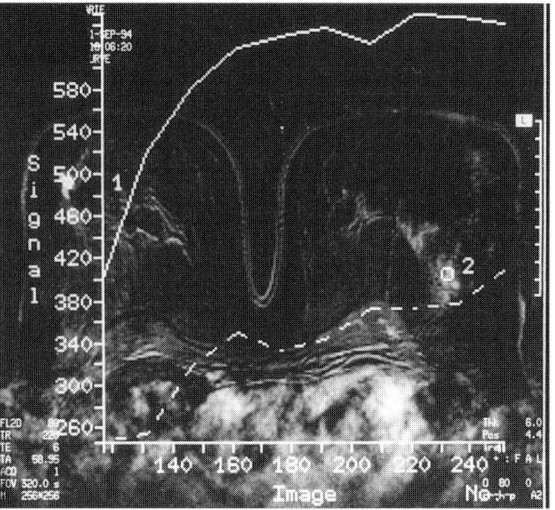

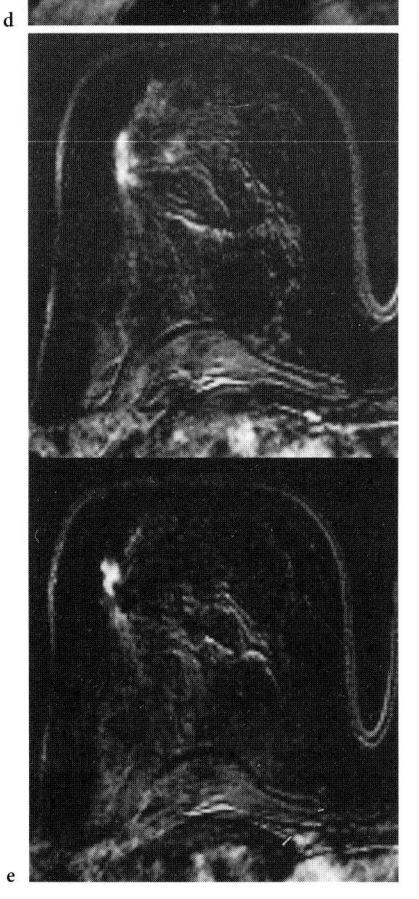

Fig. 14.14d–f

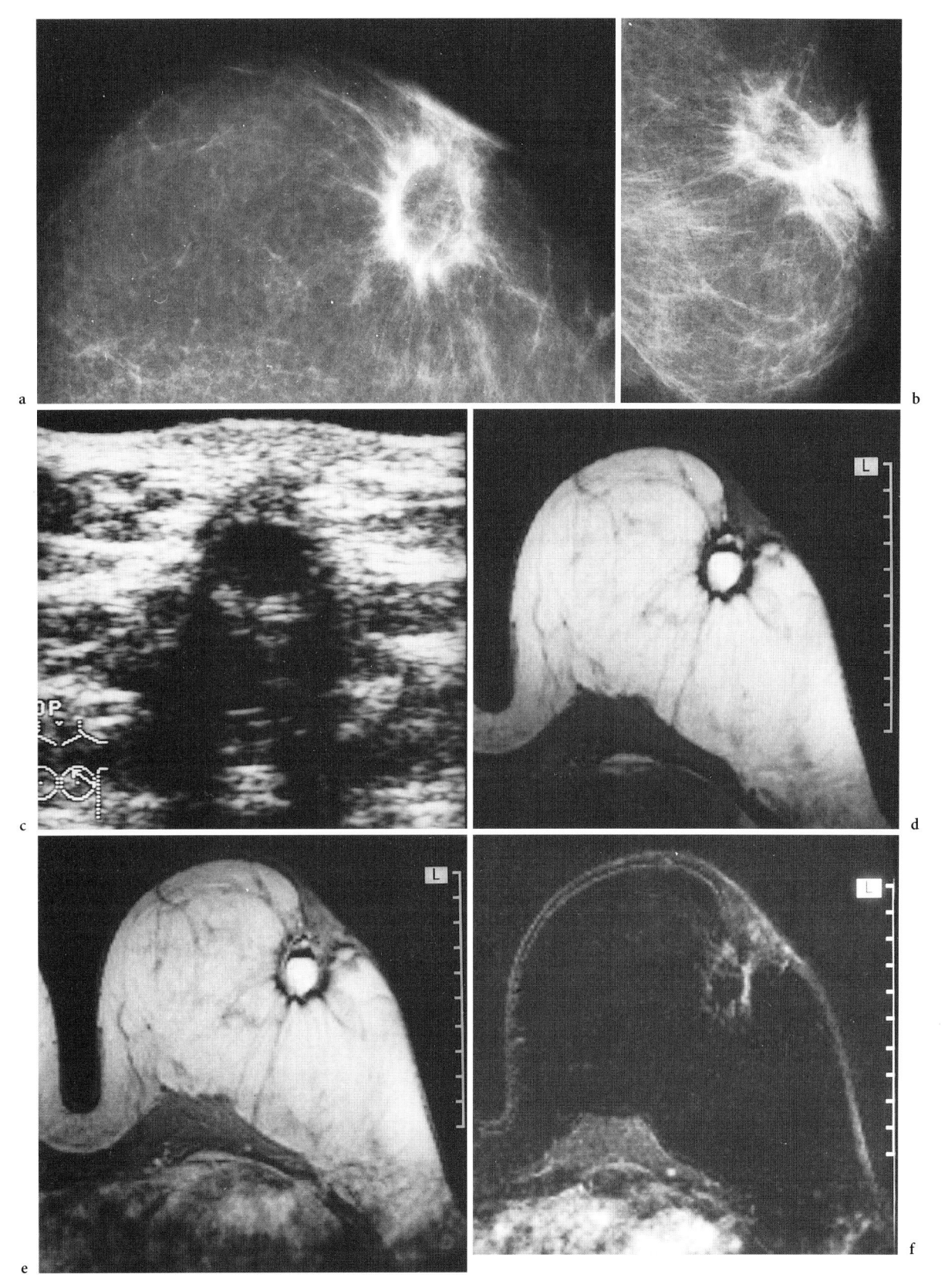

Fig. 14.15a–f. Postoperative oil (foreign body) granuloma in a 60-year-old woman who had undergone retroareolar lumpectomy [infiltrating ductal carcinoma, pT2N1(1/12)], postoperative radiotherapy, and polychemotherapy 2 years previously. Marked nipple retraction and scarring are present at the operative site. **a,b** Retroareolar mass with smoothly marginated fat-containing center and spiculated outline. **c** Sonogram showing a strongly attenuating anechoic mass, suggestive of an oil granuloma. **d–f** Axial gradient-echo sequence (FLASH 2D, 80°/220/6 ms) before (**d**) and after (**e**) 0.1 mmol Gd-DTPA/kg i.v. and subtraction image (**f**) showing weak ring-shaped enhancement in the granuloma wall and no contrast medium uptake in central fat necrosis, proven by open biopsy

with oil cyst. The sonogram (Fig. 14.15c) displays a strong attenuating anechoic mass with lateral refraction shadows. The MR examination confirms the mammographic finding of a lesion with central fat content with faint contrast uptake in the wall. Despite the imaging diagnosis of oil cyst the patient was operated on because of the suspicious clinical findings, and the diagnosis of oil-containing foreign body granuloma was confirmed; there were no histological signs of cancer recurrence.

14.4.2 Carcinoma

Breast carcinoma is a rather heterogeneous group of malignant tumors. It is commonly subdivided according to the histological site of its origin and main route of spread, into the noninvasive stages of ductal and lobular carcinoma (in situ stage) and the invasive stages of these subtypes. Besides these there are rare forms such as medullary and mucinous carcinoma. Additional histological classification refers to the varying grades of differentiation, the different cell types, and patterns of intraductal or intralobular growth, e.g., comedo-type, cribriform, micropapillary, papillary, tubular, or adenoid. Apart from these forms there is a poorly differentiated type of carcinoma which diffusely invades all histological structures, known as inflammatory carcinoma because of its clinical symptoms. The presumed advantage of contrast-enhanced MRI in breast cancer detection over existing imaging procedures such as mammography and ultrasonography lies in the ability to detect carcinomas through their generally increased vascularization, the possibly increased permeability of tumor capillaries to molecules of a certain size, and/or a larger extracellular space of most tumors compared with normal tissue.

The increased and often chaotic neovascularization of most malignant tumors has long been known to pathologists, oncologists, and diagnosticians. It is commonly explained by the secretion of so-called tumor angiogenetic factors by the tumor cells (FOLKMAN 1985; FOLKMAN and SHING 1992). Other procedures in breast cancer diagnosis, such as thermography, Doppler ultrasonography and contrast-enhanced computed tomography of the breast are also based on the principle of tumor neovascularization, but these procedures are not as sensitive as contrast-enhanced MRI.

On the other hand, it must be admitted that neovascularization is not specific for all malignant tumors or even tumors in general. It is seen in a number of benign entities of the breast (e.g., some fibroadenomas, proliferative mastopathy, and chronic inflammatory processes). Moreover the principle of tumor neovascularization is not univerally valid as there are a number of definitely hypovascular tumors. The increased extracellular space characteristic of malignant tumors is also present in several benign tumors. From these histopathological facts and the basic principles of the contrast media used so far in MRI, it cannot be assumed that contrast-enhanced MRI of the breast is a specific method for differentiating malignant from benign lesions, as was claimed in the first publications on the subject (KAISER 1989). The basic nonspecificity of MRI known from other clinical fields of application also holds for contrast-enhanced MRI of the breast. This has been confirmed by all later investigators in the field.

14.4.2.1 Infiltrating Carcinoma

The majority of infiltrating carcinomas are hypervascular and as such are detected with high sensitivity through MRI (~90%). The morphological features of a malignant mass on non-enhanced MR images are identical to those seen with mammography and ultrasonography.

KAISER and ZEITLER (1989) described the following dynamic criteria of contrast uptake suspicious for carcinoma, provided a T1-weighted 2D FLASH sequence (80°/100/5 ms) is used, starting immediately after a standardized bolus injection of 0.1 mmol Gd-DTPA/kg, and repeated at intervals of 1 min for 8 or 10 min:

1. An increase in signal intensity of more than 90% during the first minute after bolus injection
2. Signal intensity maximum between the first and second minutes after bolus injection
3. Signal intensity plateau or leveling off after the second minute following bolus injection (Fig. 14.16)

The dynamic criteria of a benign lesion are:

1. An increase in signal intensity of less than 90% during the first minute after bolus injection
2. Gradual increase in signal intensity up to the end of the measurement (Fig. 14.16)

The accepted morphological features of malignancy in contrast-enhanced MRI are an inhomogeneous internal contrast uptake and an irregular outline of the lesion, in approximately one-

Fig. 14.16. Signal enhancement in dynamic contrast-enhanced MRI (2D FLASH, 80°/100/5 ms; 0.1 mmol Gd-DTPA/kg body weight) (modified from KAISER 1993)

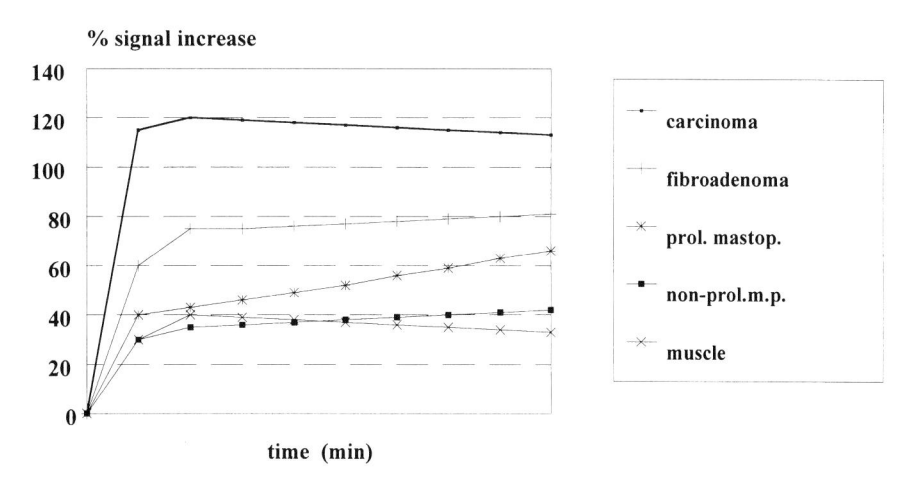

third of cases with rim enhancement [5 of 16 carcinomas in the study by GREENSTEIN OREL et al. (1994)].

In the Figs. 14.17–14.21 some typical examples of infiltrating carcinomas are demonstrated. Figure 14.17a and b shows the craniocaudal and oblique mammograms of a 60-year-old woman with a family history of breast carcinoma. In the lower outer quadrant a small spiculated density is observed which corresponds to a 1-cm, oval, centrally hypoechoic lesion with a broad echogenic rim on the sonogram (Fig. 14.17c). Intense contrast uptake with time-intensity profile typical for carcinoma is seen during contrast-enhanced MRI (Fig. 14.17d, e). An infiltrating lobular carcinoma [pT1bN0(0/15)M0G2] was found at surgery.

A typical example of infiltrating intraductal carcinoma with ring-shaped enhancement, jagged borders, and a characteristic time-intensity profile is depicted in Fig. 14.18.

Figure 14.19 shows the case of a 67-year-old woman who had had right-sided mastectomy 6 years previously. She had no clinical symptoms in her left breast. During ultrasonography (Fig. 14.19b) a very small shadowing lesion was detected in the medial left breast, suspicious for carcinoma. The craniocaudal compression view of the corresponding region, with a skin marker, did not show any abnormality. During MRI (Fig. 14.19c–e) an enhancing lesion with a suspicious uptake profile was observed near the border of the medial quadrant. Histology confirmed the diagnosis of carcinoma.

As already mentioned, a small number of carcinomas (5%–12%) fail to display intense early contrast uptake, and show only moderate enhancement after several minutes (FLICKINGER et al. 1992; SCHNALL et al. 1992; FISCHER et al. 1993). HEYWANG-KÖBRUNNER (1993) found delayed enhancement in 5 out of 27 infiltrating carcinomas (~20%) during dynamic MRI, as did GILLES et al. (1994a) in 2 out of 37 cases (~5%).

Figure 14.20 demonstrates a case of a 52-year-old woman who had noticed a nodule in her left lateral breast. The mammogram and sonogram depict a suspicious spiculated lesion at the corresponding site (Fig. 14.20a,b). Figure 14.20c–f demonstrates clearly the gradual contrast uptake which remains moderate even after 8 min, a feature typical for benign lesions. Histology proved a moderately differentiated infiltrating ductal carcinoma (pT1N0(0/14)G2).

Often MRI can demonstrate the actual extent of infiltrating carcinoma more clearly than other imaging methods. Figure 14.21 shows a case of diffusely infiltrating carcinoma which developed rapidly in the right breast of a 42-year-old woman. Clinically there was general hyperthermia of the right side and a large firm mass in the lower half of the right breast was palpable. The comparison of the latest right-sided mediolateral mammogram (Fig. 14.21b) with the previous mammogram (2 years previously; Fig. 14.21a) shows a diffuse, radiodense, infiltrative process with retraction in the lower half of the breast. The T2-weighted axial MR images depict a general coarsening of the interstitial structures and intense lymphedema in the lower half of the breast (Fig. 14.21c). Only after contrast administration (Fig. 14.21d–g) could the exact extent of the diffusely infiltrating carcinoma be recognized and distinguished from the accompanying interstitial edema.

14.4.2.2 Staging of Suspected Breast Cancer (Detection of Multifocality/Multicentricity)

Particularly when breast conservation therapy is intended it is very important to ascertain

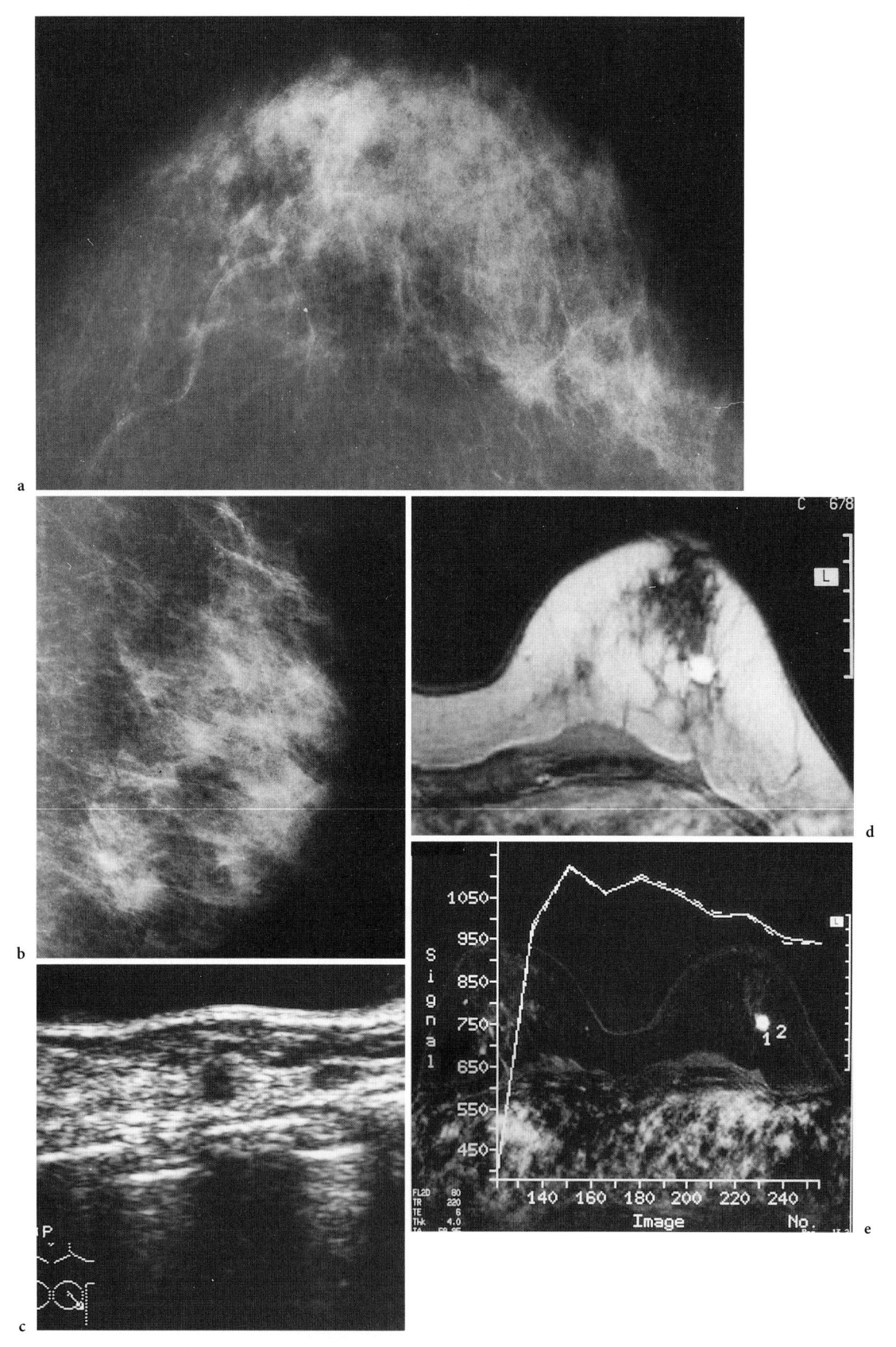

Fig. 14.17. a,b Craniocaudal and mediolateral mammograms showing a small spiculated density at the laterocaudal prepectoral margin of the left breast parenchyma. **c** Sonogram demonstrating an oval-shaped hypoechoic lesion with broad echogenic rim, suggestive of carcinoma. **d,e** Axial T1-weighted gradient-echo sequence (FLASH 2D, 80°/220/6 ms) 1 min after administration of 0.1 mmol Gd-DTPA/kg. There is intense contrast enhancement with typical dynamic criteria of a malignant lesion. Histological examination revealed an infiltrating lobular carcinoma pT1bN0(0/15)

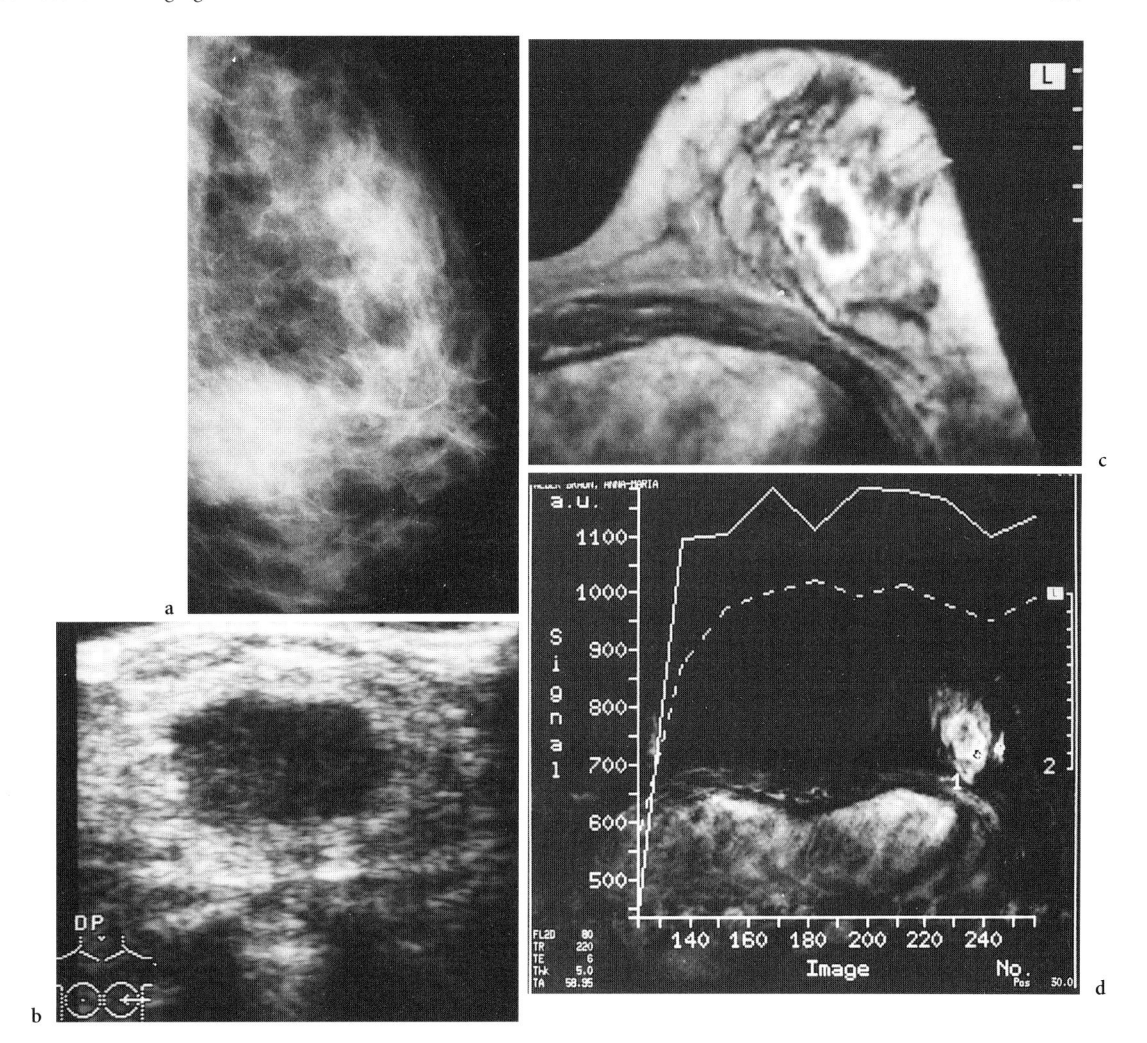

Fig. 14.18. a Left mediolateral mammogram showing an unsharp 3.5-cm opacity in the lower breast half. **b** Sonogram revealing a lobulated hypoechoic lesion with an inhomogeneous internal echo pattern. **c,d** Axial T1-weighted gradient-echo sequence (FLASH 2D, 80°/220/6 ms) demonstrating ring-shaped peripheral enhancement with dynamic criteria suggesting a malignant lesion. Histological examination revealed an intraductal carcinoma

preoperatively whether a detected carcinoma is unifocal, multifocal/multicentric, or even bilateral. The reported frequency of multifocality/multicentricity of breast carcinoma varies greatly (14%–60%). SCHWARTZ et al. (1980) reported a rate of 60% when serial sectioning of the whole mastectomy specimen was carried out. Whereas it may be difficult to localize the different foci of multifocal carcinoma with conventional methods, MRI appears to be much more sensitive in this respect. Because of the high detection rate of MRI for infiltrating carcinoma one can expect that at least every *infiltrating focus* of carcinoma will be found with high sensitivity. HARMS et al. (1994) reported that in 33% of their breast cancers, multifocal or multicentric disease was detected solely by MRI. In a study by HEYWANG-KÖBRUNNER (1993), in 18 out of 27 cases of multifocal carcinomas, only MRI was able to detect multifocality. GREENSTEIN OREL et al. (1995) reported that 20% of multifocal or diffuse carcinomas were unsuspected by conventional methods. OELLINGER et al. (1993) found eight multicentric carcinomas in a total of 25 breast cancers. The sensitivity of MRI in detecting multicentric carcinoma was 0.88, in comparison with 0.13 for mammography, although the sensitivities in the primary diagnosis of the lesions did not differ (0.96 for MRI and 1.0 for mammography).

Figure 14.22 depicts the right-sided mammogram and galactogram in a 61-year-old woman with bloody nipple discharge for 6 months. A multinodular structural disruption can be observed

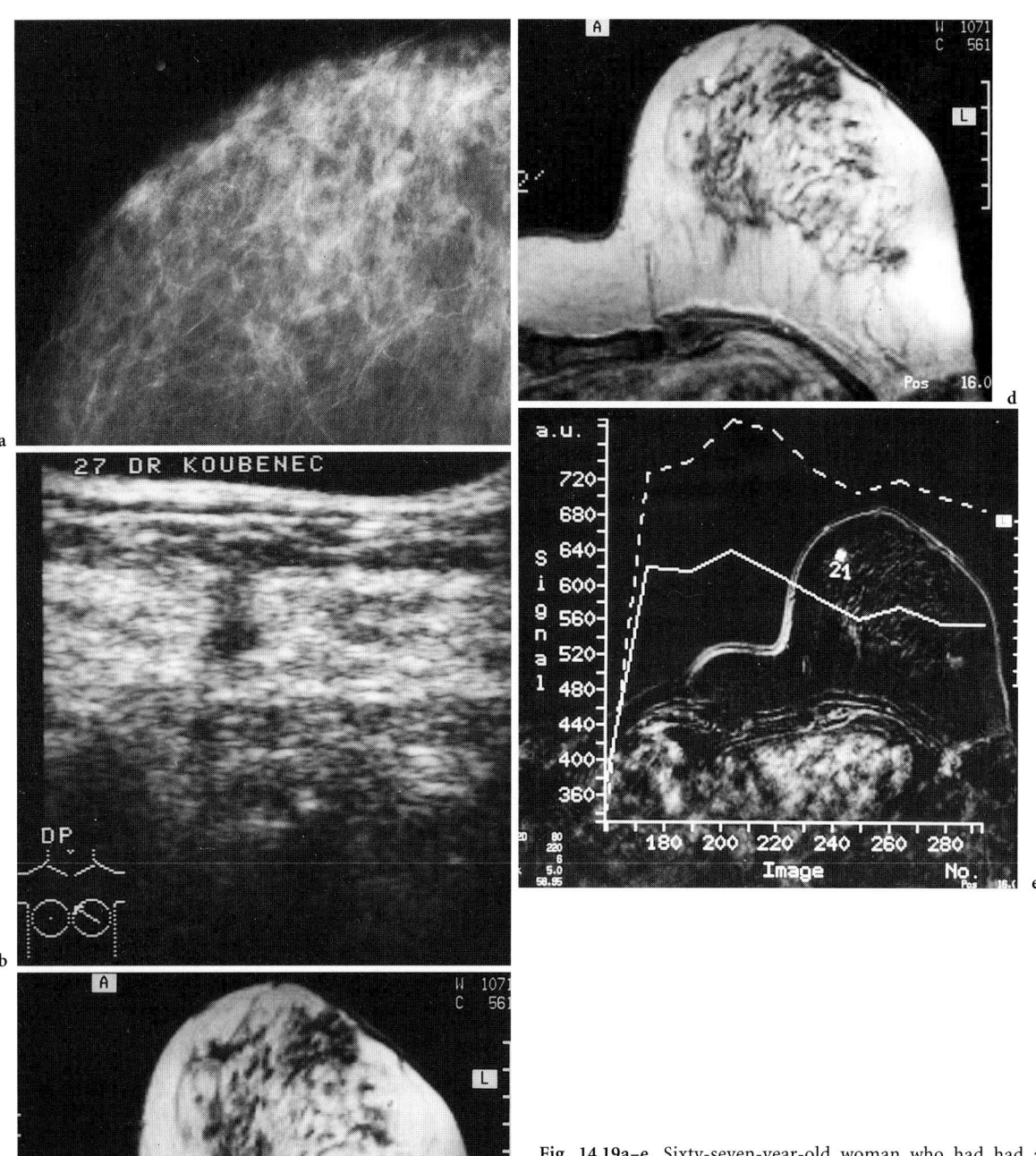

Fig. 14.19a–e. Sixty-seven-year-old woman who had had a right-sided mastectomy 6 years previously. **a** Unremarkable left craniocaudal mammogram. **b** Sonogram revealing a 7-mm hypoechoic lesion with faint shadowing. **c,d** Axial T1-weighted gradient-echo sequence (FLASH 2D, 80°/220/6 ms) before (**c**) and after (**d**) 0.1 mmol Gd-DTPA/kg, showing a small enhancing lesion with strong initial signal intensity increase. **e** Subtraction image (**d** minus **c**). Histological examination revealed an infiltrating intraductal carcinoma

Magnetic Resonance Imaging of the Breast 259

Fig. 14.20a–f. Slowly enhancing infiltrating carcinoma in a 52-year-old woman who presented with a nodule in the left outer breast region. **a** Craniocaudal mammogram showing a spiculated density in the left outer breast region. **b** Sonogram revealing a hypoechoic suspicious lesion. **c–f** Axial T1-weighted gradient-echo sequence (FLASH 2D, 80°/220/6 ms) before (**c**), 4 min (**d**) and 8 min (**e**) after 0.1 mmol Gd-DTPA/kg i.v. and subtraction image with time-intensity curve (**f**), showing slow, gradual contrast enhancement, not typical for a carcinoma. Histological examination revealed a moderately differentiated infiltrative ductal carcinoma pT1N0(0/14)G2

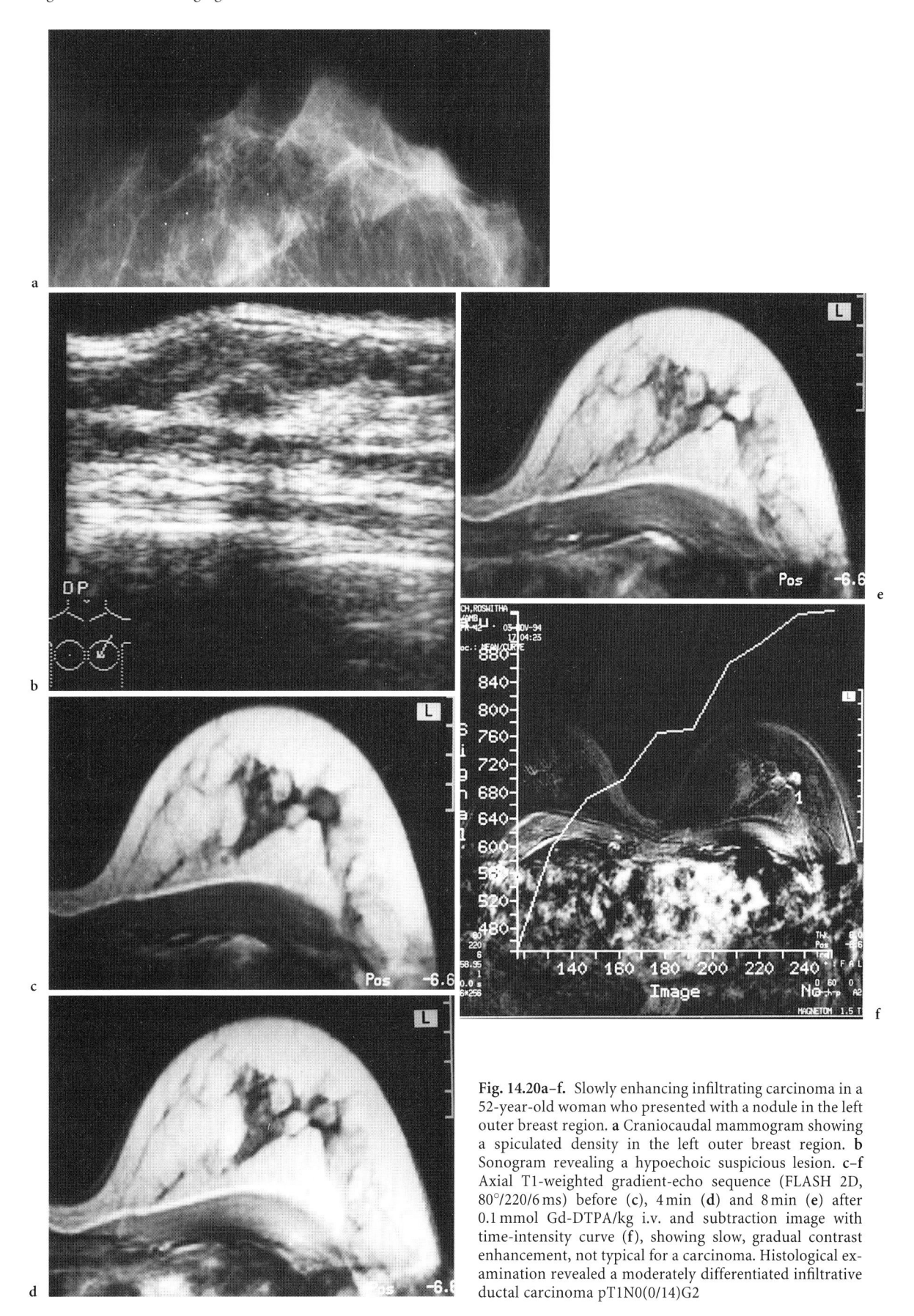

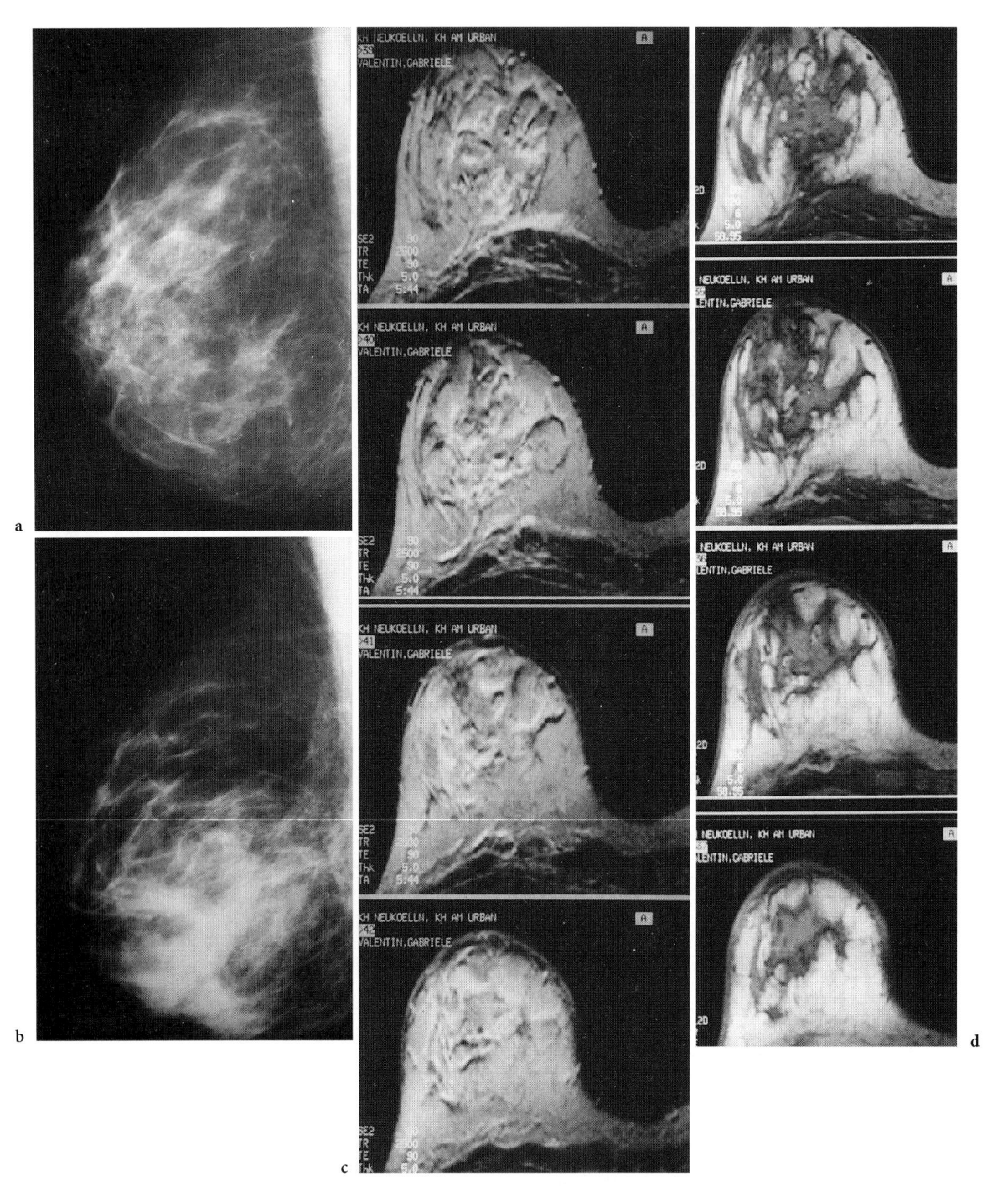

Fig. 14.21a–g. Forty-two-year-old woman with diffuse resistance and hyperthermia in the right lower breast half. **a** Right mediolateral premammogram 2 years previously and **b** current right mediolateral mammogram showing extensive density in the lower breast half with infiltration of the pectoral muscle. **c** Axial T2-weighted spin-echo sequence (SE 2500/90 ms), showing intense edema of the right breast reaching to the thoracic wall. **d,e** Axial T1-weighted gradient-echo sequence (FLASH 2D, 80°/220/6 ms) before (**d**) and after (**e**) i.v. administration of 0.1 mmol/kg body wt. Gd-DTPA with intense diffuse enhancement in the lower breast half. **f** Subtraction image after contrast enhancement. **g** Enhancement dynamic suggestive of a malignant lesion. Histological examination revealed an infiltrating ductal carcinoma with extensive lymphangiosis and infiltration of the pectoral muscle and interpectoral fat tissue and lymph nodes [pT2pN2(11/28)pMX]

Fig. 14.21e–g

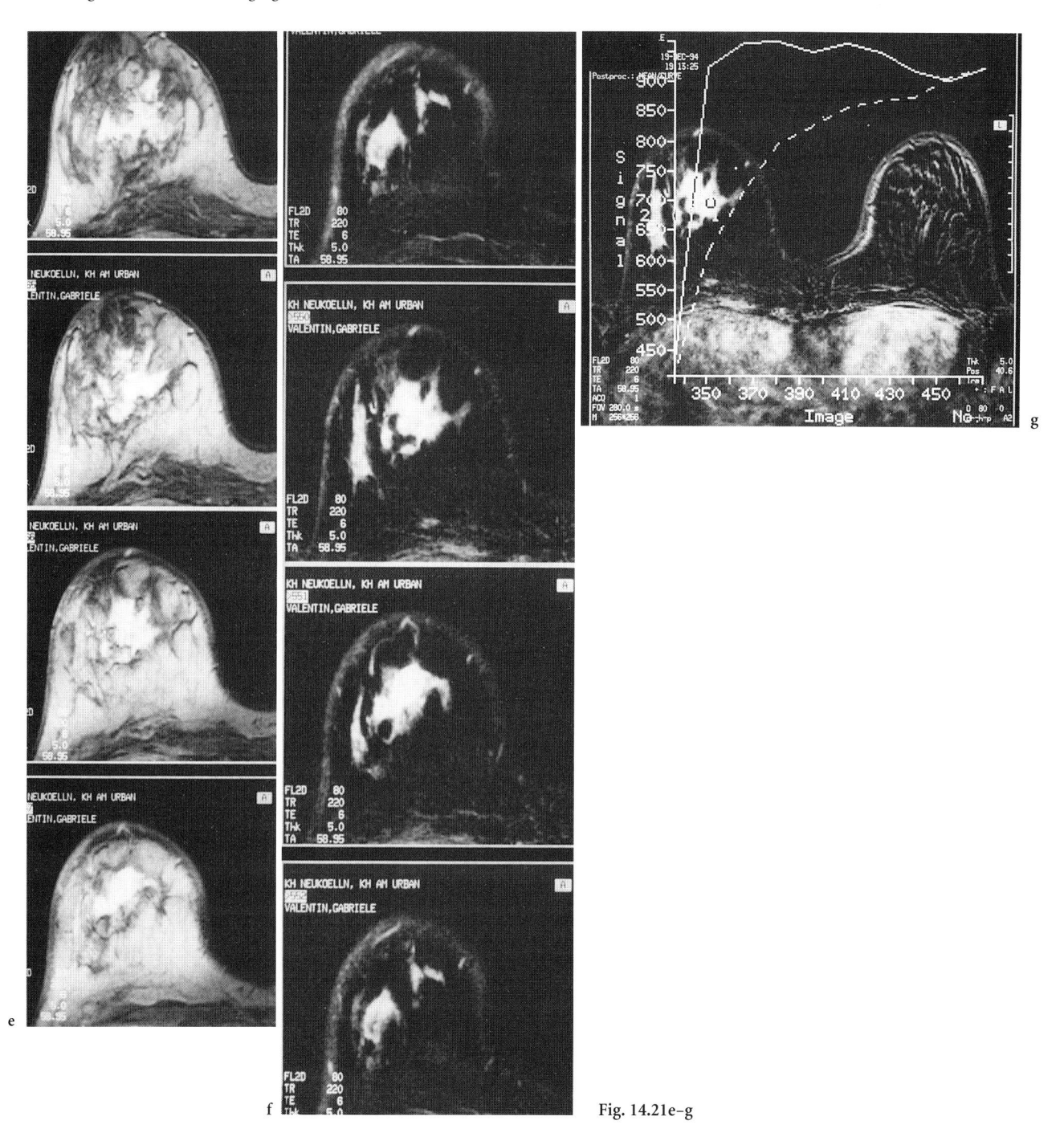

in the right upper breast with several spiculated densities (Fig. 14.22a,b). The galactogram shows diffuse irregularities in the milk ducts of the contrast-filled breast segment (Fig. 14.22c,d). Contrast-enhanced MRI clearly demonstrates the various individual foci of this multifocal infiltrating ductal carcinoma in the right breast (Fig. 14.22e,f).

14.4.2.3 Noninfiltrating (In Situ) Carcinoma

Whereas in early MRI publications no distinction was made between infiltrating and noninfiltrating (in situ) carcinoma, it soon became apparent that there are differences in the detection rates for these entities. Theoretically it may be questioned whether in

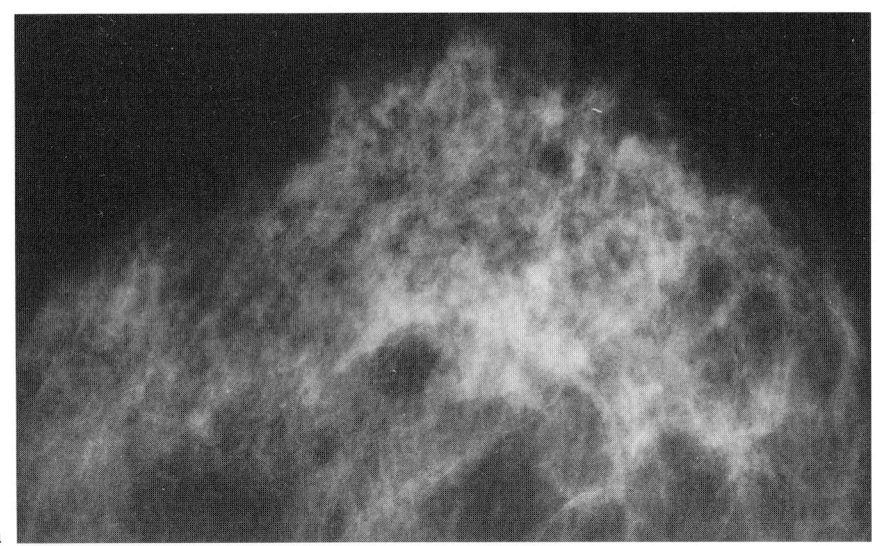

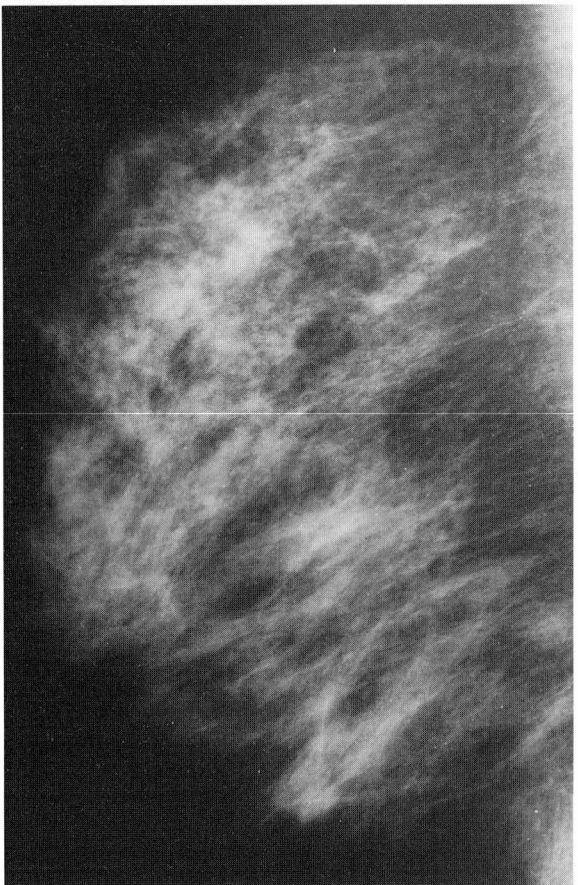

Fig. 14.22a–f. Multifocal intraductal infiltrative carcinoma of the right breast in a 61-year-old woman with bloody nipple discharge on the right side. **a,b** Craniocaudal and mediolateral mammograms demonstrate multiple nodular and several stellate densities in the upper breast region. **c,d** Craniocaudal and mediolateral galactograms show multiple irregular ducts. **e,f** Contrast-enhanced MRI: axial T1-weighted gradient-echo sequence (FLASH, 80°/220/6 ms) through the upper breast half depicts multiple foci of infiltrating ductal carcinoma in the right breast

Fig. 14.22c,d

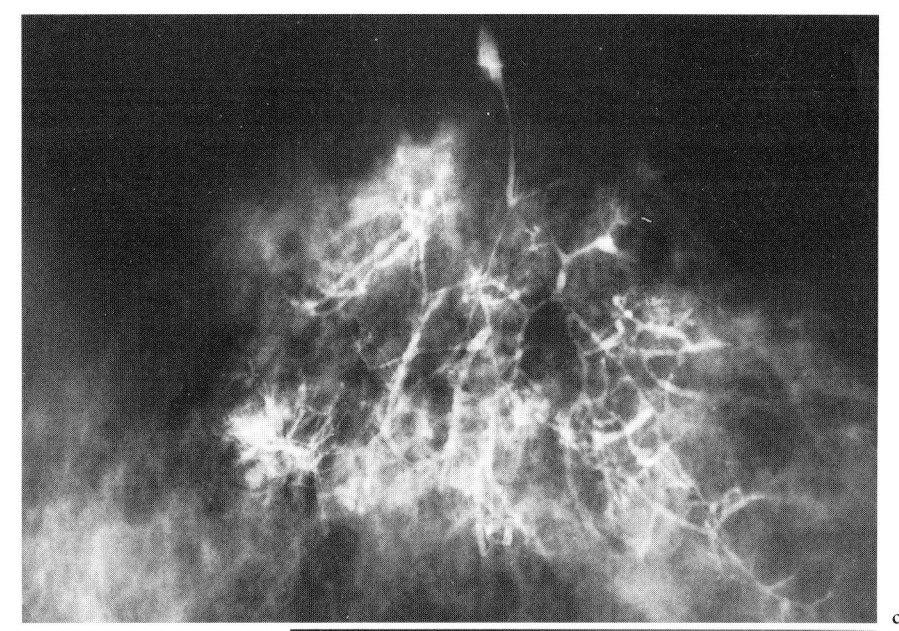

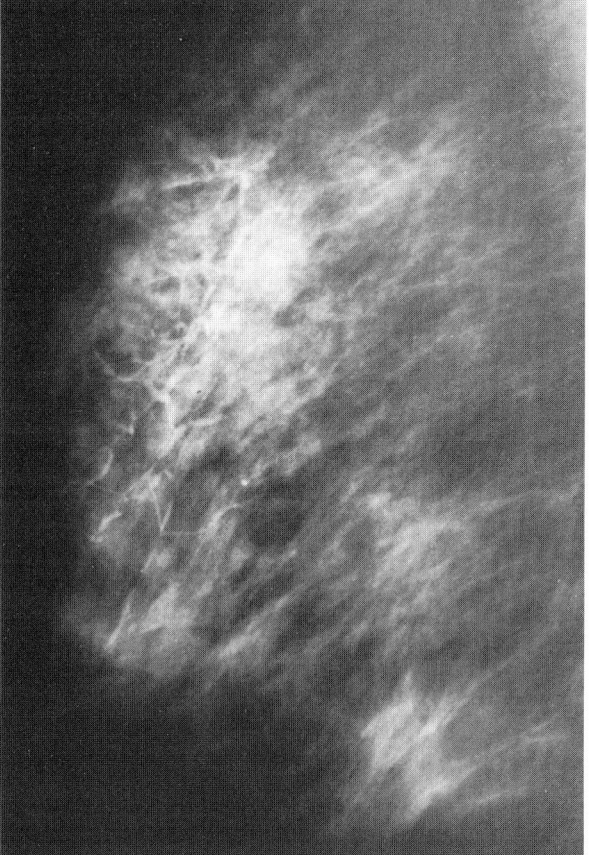

c

d

situ carcinoma can induce enough neovascularization so as to be detectable with contrast-enhanced MRI. This is also important with regard to the exact delineation of the tumor extent of infiltrating carcinoma, as many of these lesions have foci of in situ carcinoma in their vicinity which may remain undetected preoperatively.

Various groups have reported low sensitivities for the detection of in situ carcinoma with MRI. SITTEK et al. (1995b) reported a detection rate of infiltrating

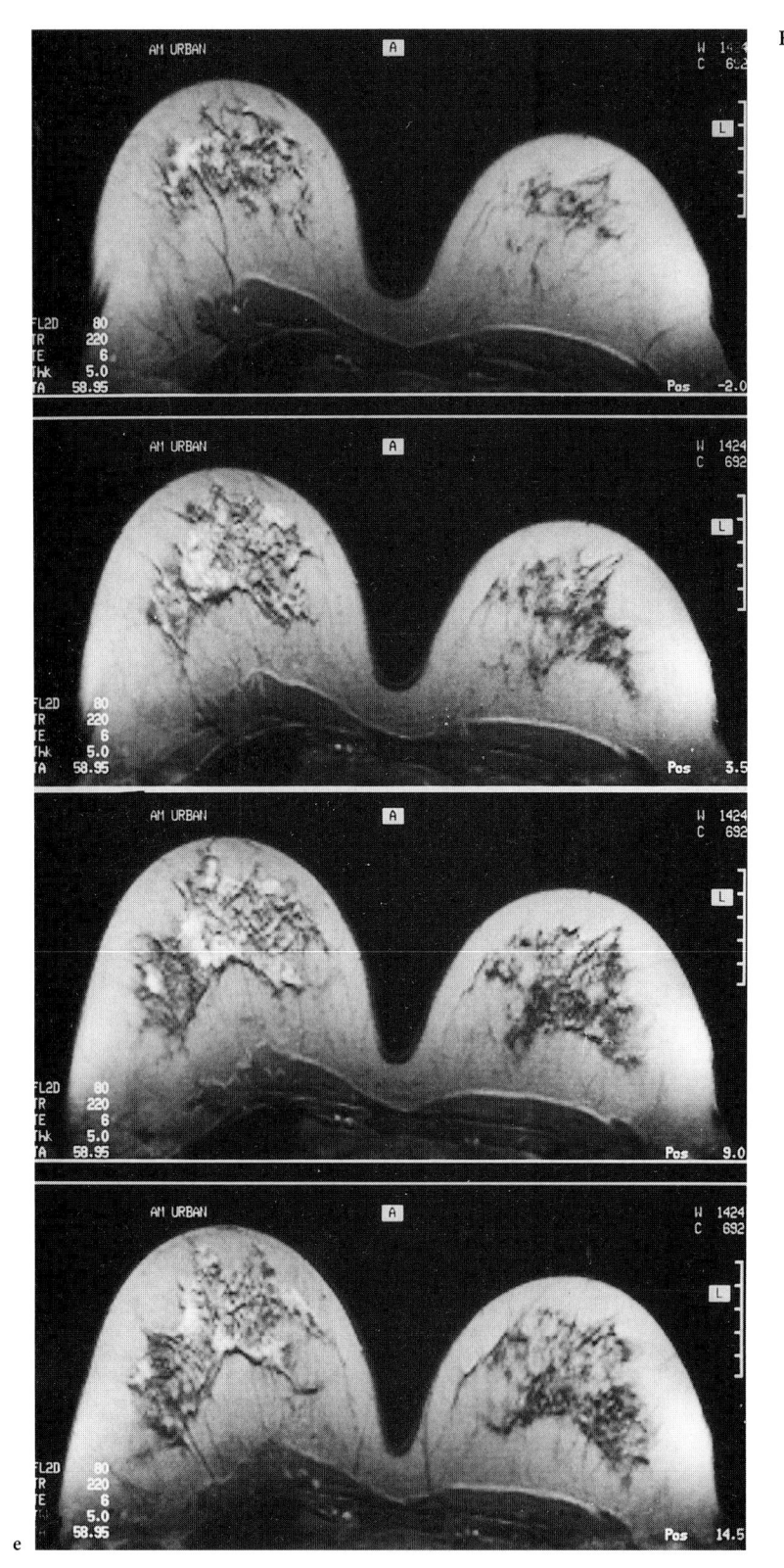

Fig. 14.22e

Magnetic Resonance Imaging of the Breast

Fig. 14.22f

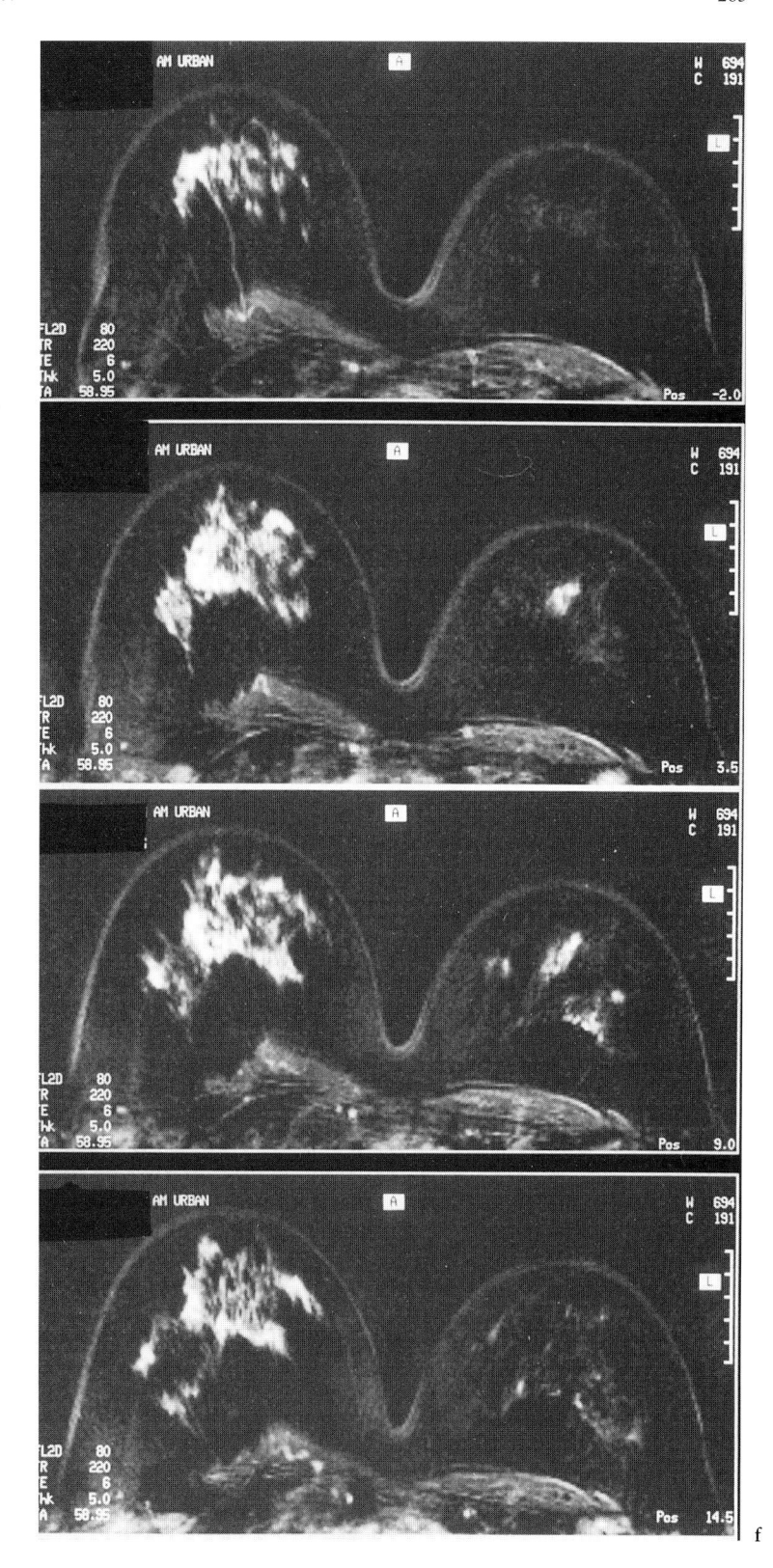

carcinoma of 87.9% with MRI compared to 85.2% with mammography, but only 38% with MRI compared to 88.4% with mammography for in situ carcinoma. FISCHER et al. (1995b) found contrast enhancement typical for carcinoma in only one-third of 37 in situ carcinomas. These were primarily comedo-type carcinomas. Twenty percent of the in situ carcinomas displayed no contrast uptake at all. GREENSTEIN OREL et al. (1995) found 9 of 15 in situ carcinomas with MRI.

BAUER et al. (1995) studied the detection rate of in situ foci surrounding infiltrating carcinomas. They found the following detection rates: within a distance of 2 cm from the infiltrating carcinoma ($n = 68$): MRI 17%, mammography 73%; more than 2 cm ($n = 39$): MRI 5%, mammography 72%. For satellite tumors within 4 cm ($n = 54$) they found a detection rate of 41% for MRI and 82% for mammography and ultrasonography. The detection rate of MRI (88%) was superior to that of mammography and ultrasonography (77%) only for satellite tumors further than 4 cm from the infiltrating focus. All 25 exclusively in situ carcinomas were detected only by mammography. BAUER et al. concluded that MRI is the preferred method for the detection of multicentric/-focal infiltrating carcinoma, but for the diagnosis of in situ carcinoma mammography remains the superior method.

14.4.3 Postoperative Status

14.4.3.1 Status After Breast Conservation Therapy

Early detection of an intramammary recurrence is the primary task of postoperative follow-up imaging of the breast after breast conservation therapy. Mammography is an accepted imaging method because it detects approximately half of all intramammary resurrences (STOMPER et al. 1987). Recurrences close to the chest wall are difficult to visualize, especially in operated and irradiated breasts, and are often missed by mammography. Scarring and postradiation fibrosis may obscure

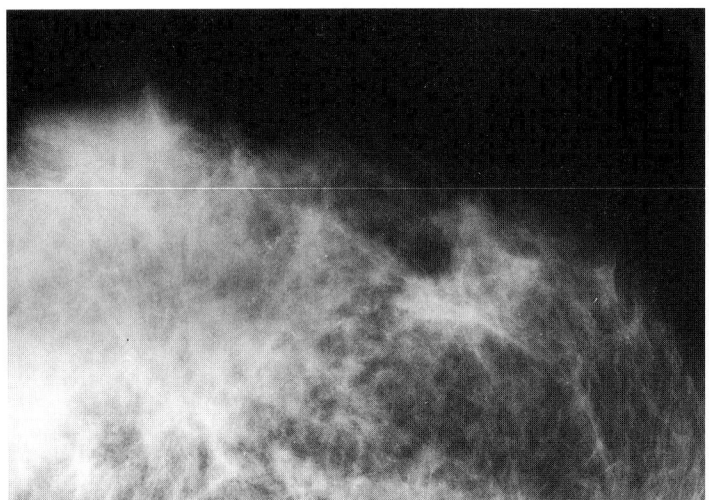

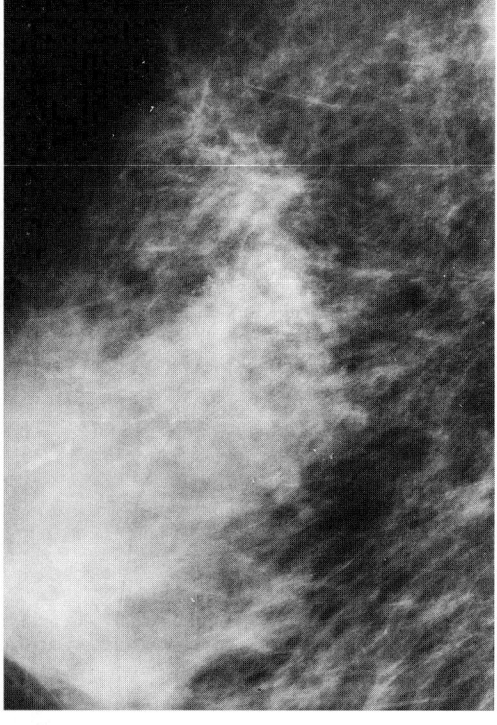

Fig. 14.23a–f. Sixty-one-year-old woman 3 years after local excision and postoperative radiation therapy of a 1.5-cm infiltrating ductal carcinoma in the upper right prepectoral region. **a,b** Craniocaudal and mediolateral mammograms; partial view showing multiple stellate coalescing densities in the upper prepectoral region and microcalcifications. **c** T2-weighted axial spin-echo image (SE 2500/90 ms) showing diffuse edema of the right retroareolar and central parenchyma. **d–f** Axial T1-weighted gradient-echo sequence (FLASH 2D, 80°/220/ 6 ms) before (**d**) and after (**e**) 0.1 mmol/kg Gd-DTPA and subtraction image (**f**) showing intense multifocal enhancement suggestive of multifocal recurrent carcinoma. Histological examination revealed a multifocal infiltrating intraductal recurrent carcinoma with beginning lymphangiosis

Fig. 14.23c–f

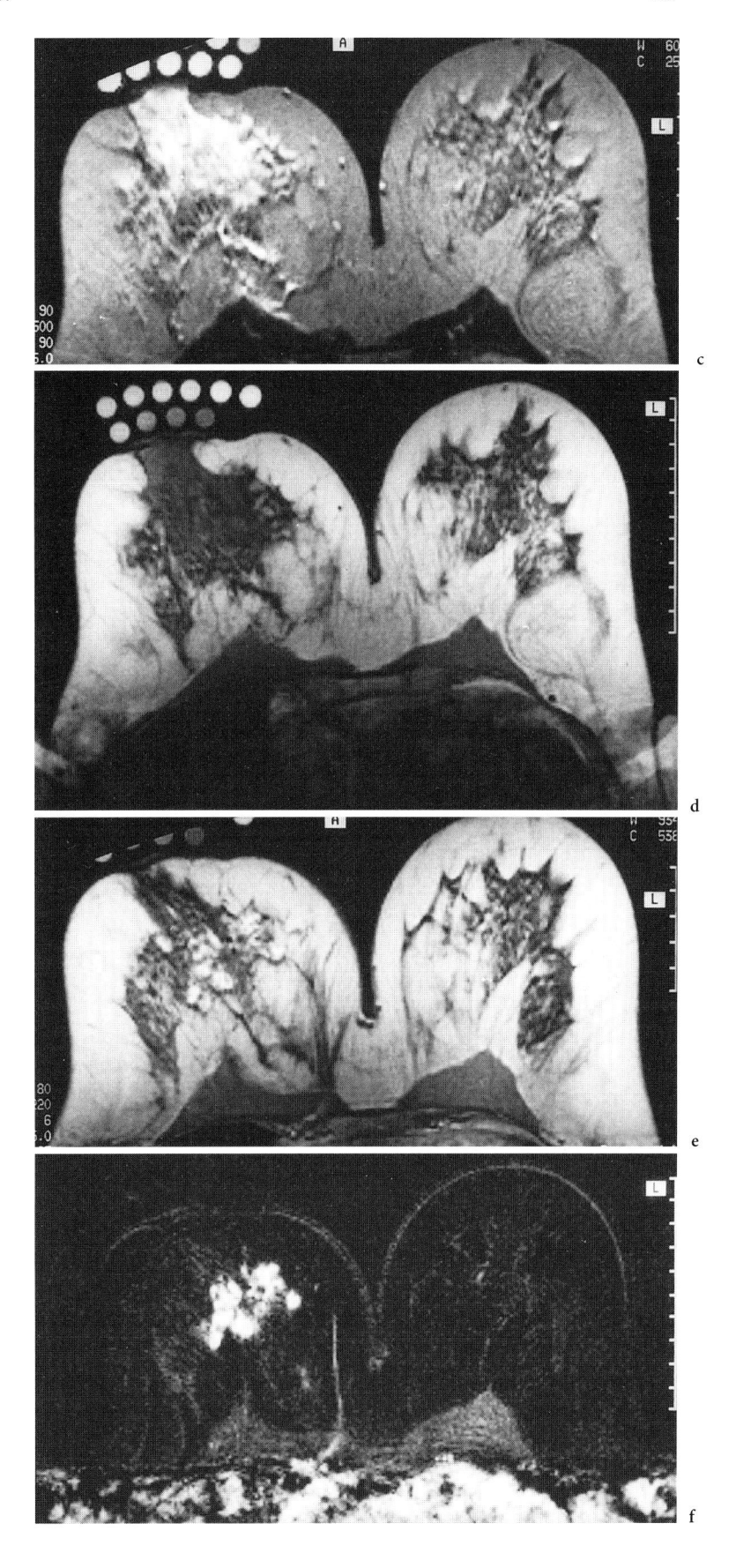

subtle changes in the radiographic image of the breast. MRI is therefore a welcome new imaging modality for this task. GILLES et al. (1993) and HEYWANG-KÖBRUNNER et al. (1993a,b) found contrast enhancement in all local recurrences. Of 11 local recurrences from the series of HEYWANG-KÖBRUNNER et al. (1993), four were detected exclusively by MRI. On the other hand, MRI produces equivocal results in one-third of the cases studied, because of nonspecific contrast uptake.

About half of all recurrences are detected using mammography by newly appearing microcalcifications (STOMPER et al. 1987). In Fig. 14.23 a compression view shows marked interstitial edema and diffuse scattered microcalcifications in the upper breast half of a woman who had undergone breast conservation therapy and radiation therapy 3 years previously because of infiltrating ductal carcinoma. She had noticed edema and firmness of her right breast. The T2-weighted MR image (Fig. 14.23c) demonstrates marked edema of the right breast, extending to the pectoralis muscle. Contrast-enhanced MRI (Fig. 14.23d–f) clearly shows numerous strongly enhancing foci of local recurrence in the right breast.

Figure 14.24 depicts the case of a 50-year-old woman who had had breast-conserving therapy and radiotherapy for an infiltrating ductal carcinoma 6 years previously. She presented for examination with a recently felt lump in the lower outer quadrant of her left breast. On the mammogram (Fig. 14.24a,b) the palpable nodule (with skin marker) can barely be recognized (cf. sonogram: Fig. 14.24c). MRI shows a lesion with pronounced ring enhancement suggestive of intramammary recurrence, which was confirmed at surgery.

14.4.3.2 Status After Silicone Implant (see also Chaps. 6 and 18)

Patients with silicone augmentation pose problems for mammographic examination because an estimated 22%–83% of the breast tissue is obscured by the radiodense silicone. In patients who have undergone mastectomy and silicone implant reconstruction it is especially difficult to visualize the remaining soft tissues and the prepectoral region on routine mammograms. With tangential views, targeted to the region of interest, one may successfully image a suspicious density, as in the case in Fig. 14.25a, which depicts a craniocaudal compression view of the right lateral margin of a silicone implant after subcutaneous mastectomy and radiation therapy 4 years previously. MRI confirmed the mammographic diagnosis of local recurrence, which was histologically confirmed (recurrent infiltrating ductal carcinoma).

Figure 14.26 shows the case of a 52-year-old woman who had had simple mastectomy of her left breast and implant reconstruction 3 years earlier. She had noticed a vague area of thickening behind her left nipple. On the mammogram a nonspecific oval density was recognized in the retroareolar region; ultrasonography showed a firm incompressible hypoechoic mass. MRI clearly demonstrated a strongly enhancing lesion behind the nipple which was proven to be recurrent carcinoma.

In a study by HEYWANG-KÖBRUNNER et al. (1993b) on 107 patients with silicone implants after mastectomy there was clear enhancement in all cancer recurrences (8); four out of the eight recurrences were detected solely by MRI. However, 14 patients had enhancing lesions found in the vicinity of silicone implants which corresponded to chronic fat granuloma and inflammatory processes, showing again that MRI is not specific for the diagnosis of cancer recurrence.

14.4.3.3 Extramammary Recurrence (Thoracic Wall/Mediastinum)

Local recurrence in the thoracic wall is often first noticed by the alert patient and is usually confirmed clinically by inspection and palpation. It can rarely be visualized by mammography. The experienced ultrasonographer, however, should be able to define the exact extent and in particular the infiltration of the thoracic wall. The retrosternal region is rather inaccessible for ultrasonography; up to now CT has been the procedure of choice to detect or exclude local recurrence in the thoracic wall or lymph node metastasis in the mediastinum. MRI can visualize both the thoracic wall and the retrosternal mediastinum.

Figure 14.26d–f depicts an axial section through the left thoracic wall of the same patient as in Fig. 14.26a–c, 2 years after explantation of the silicone implant and removal of a skin metastasis over the left thorax. Contrast-enhanced MRI clearly demonstrates a strongly enhancing local recurrence within the pectoralis minor muscle.

Figure 14.27 demonstrates the case of a 55-year-old woman who had partial mastectomy on the left side for infiltrating ductal carcinoma 3 months prior to examination. The MRI examination was carried

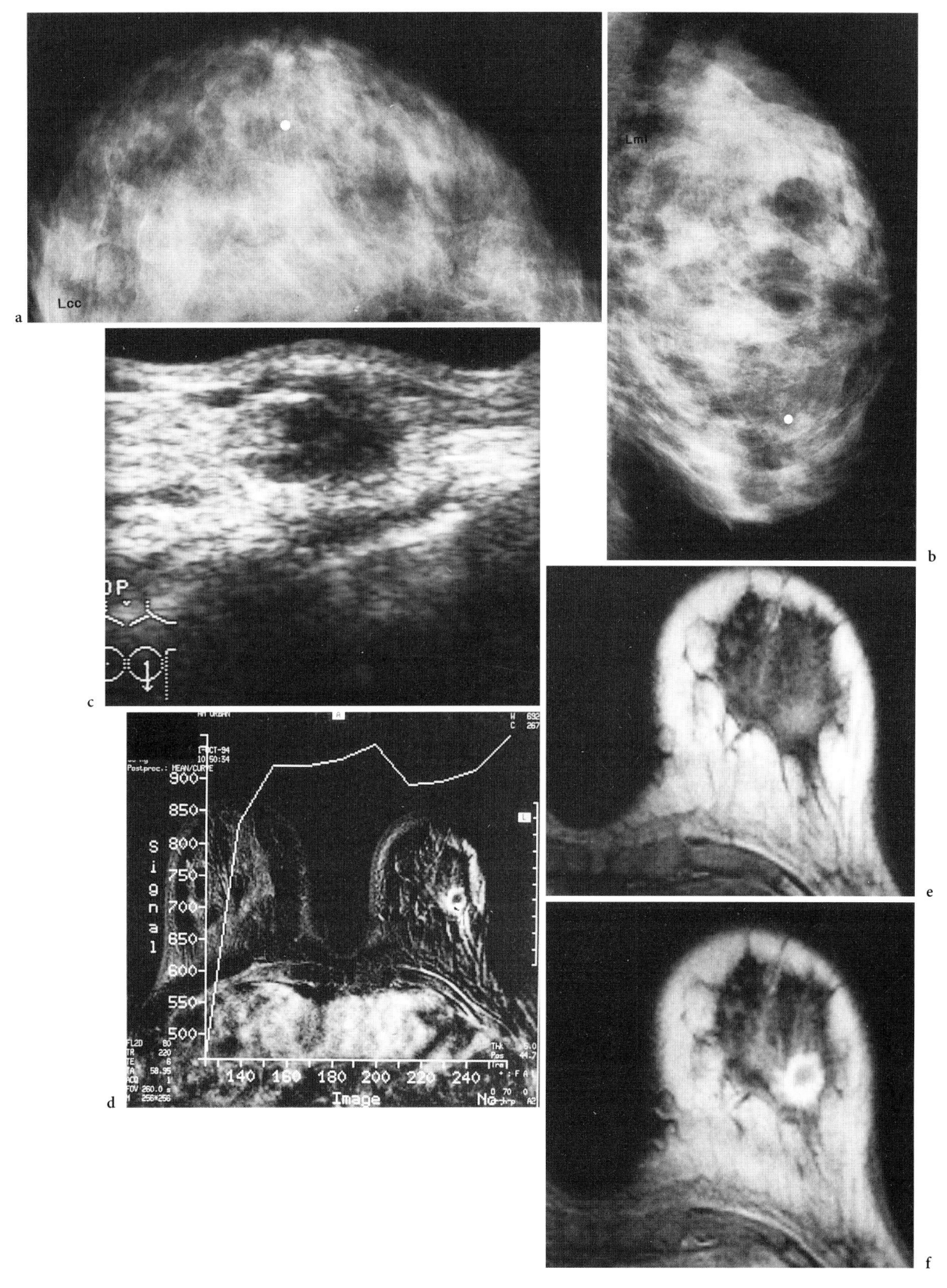

Fig. 14.24a–f. Fifty-year-old woman who had had breast-conserving surgery and radiotherapy of an infiltrating ductal carcinoma (pT2) 6 years previously. **a,b** Craniocaudal and mediolateral mammograms show an indistinct density in the middle of the breast only on the craniocaudal view. **c** Sonogram shows a highly suspicious solid lesion with jagged borders. **d–f** Axial T1-weighted gradient-echo sequence (FLASH 2D, 80°/220/6 ms) before (**d**) and 8 min after (**e**) 0.1 mmol Gd-DTPA/kg i.v., showing strong rim enhancement, and time-intensity profile showing a suspicious enhancement dynamic (**f**), also suggestive of a malignant tumor. Histological examination revealed an intraductal invasive carcinoma with central necrosis and hyalinosis

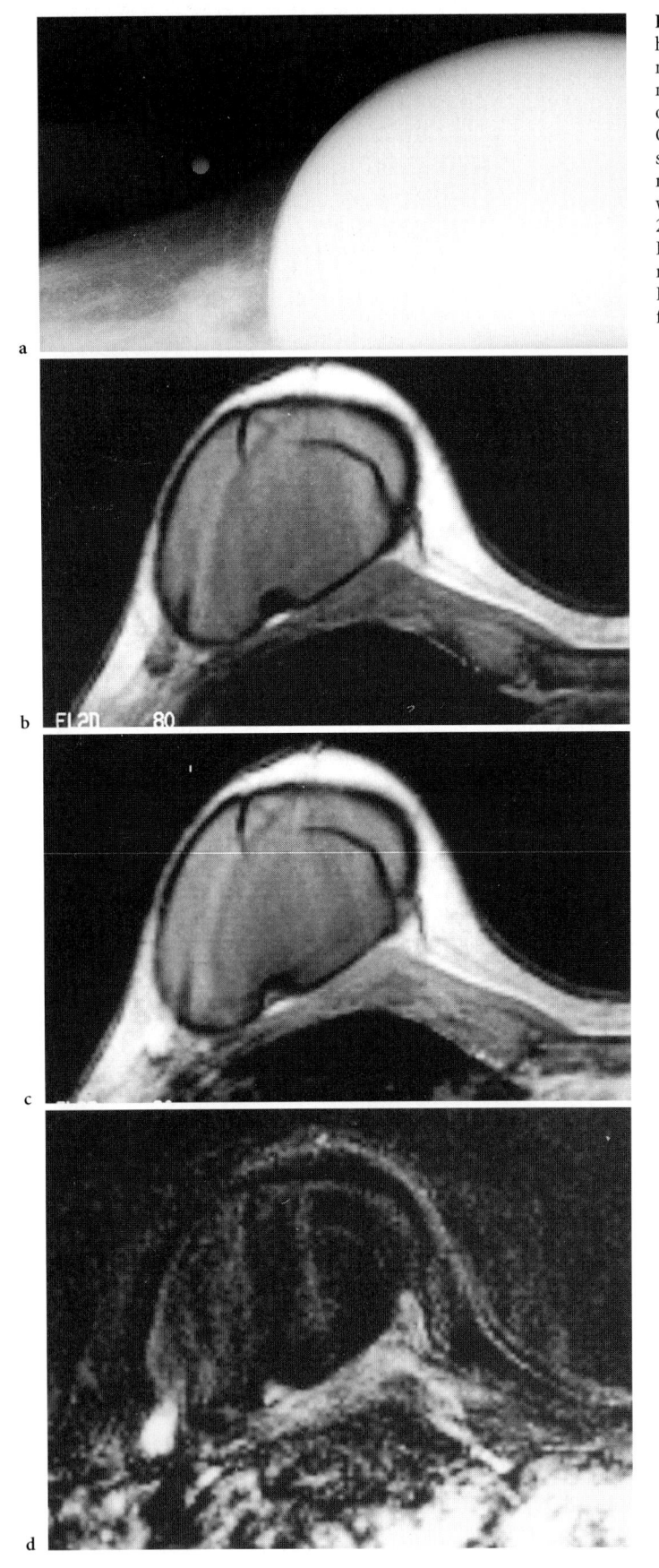

Fig. 14.25a–d. Forty-two-year-old woman who had undergone bilateral subcutaneous mastectomy because of right-sided breast carcinoma 4 years previously; no postoperative radio- or chemotherapy had been performed. **a** Craniocaudal mammogram shows a small spiculated density on the right lateral prepectoral margin of a silicone implant. **b, c** Axial T1-weighted gradient-echo sequence (FLASH 2D 80°/220/6 ms) before (**b**) and after (**c**) 0.1 mmol Gd-DTPA/kg shows a nodule with strong enhancement. **d** Subtraction image (**c** minus **b**). Histological examination revealed a recurrent infiltrating ductal carcinoma

Fig. 14.26a–c. Fifty-two-year-old woman with simple left-sided mastectomy in 1990 and implantation of an expander prothesis. **a–c** Axial T1-weighted gradient-echo sequence (FLASH 2D, 80°/220/6 ms) showing a recurrent carcinoma in left retroareolar region (1993). **d–f** Same region in 1995 after removal of the recurrent carcinoma and prosthesis, now with demonstration of recurrent carcinoma in the pectoralis minor muscle

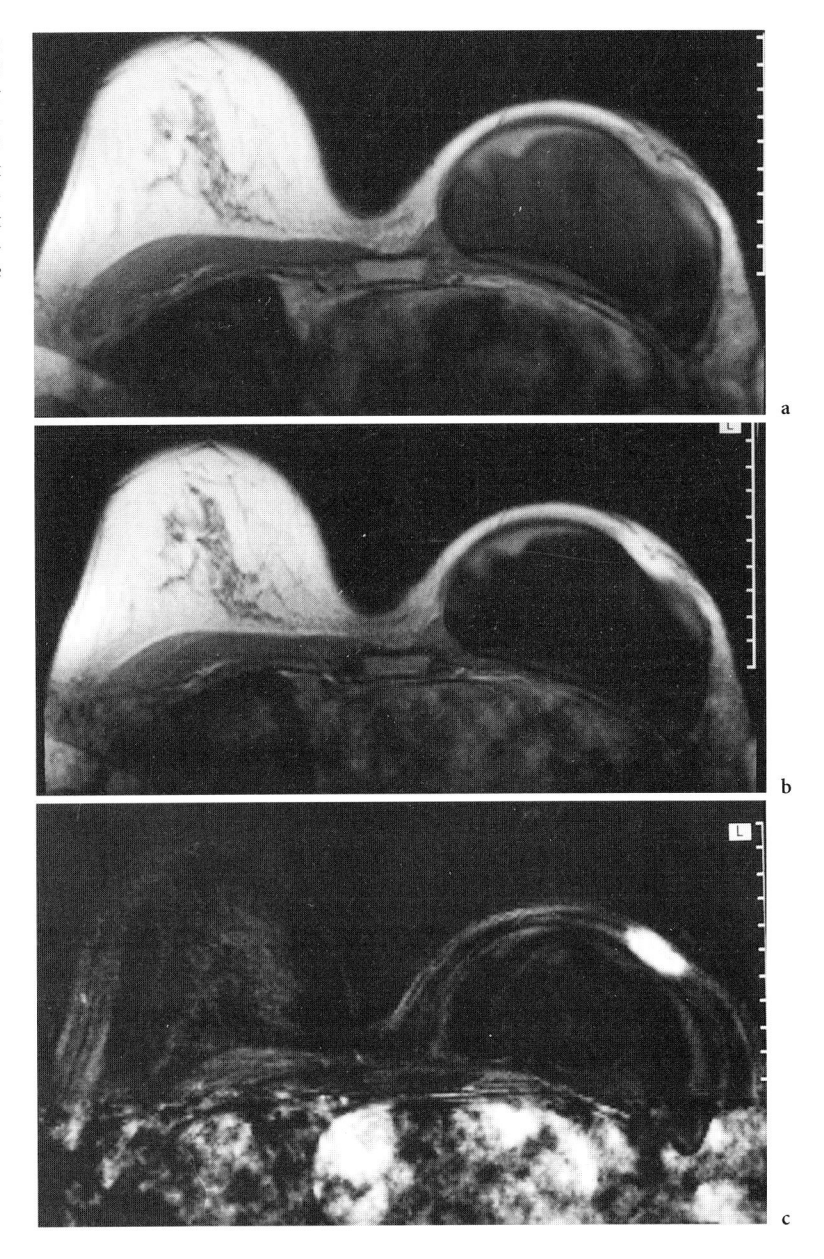

out to characterize a small subcutaneous nodule in the thoracic wall. In the left parasternal region a 1-cm strongly enhancing mass was detected which was proven to be a lymph node metastasis of the previously operated breast carcinoma by CT-guided core biopsy.

14.5 MR-Guided Biopsy

Contrast-enhanced MRI is a highly sensitive imaging modality which detects many lesions that would otherwise remain undetected by conventional methods. However, because of lack of specificity, it cannot ascertain a definite preoperative diagnosis. If MRI is integrated in clinical practice in order to improve *sensitivity*, many false-positive diagnoses and unnecessary operations will result. If, on the other hand, MRI is intended to improve *specificity*, that is to clarify equivocal cases with otherwise discrepant findings, it will nevertheless produce 10%–15% false-negative results at the expense of ~30% false-positives. Both approaches are, from a clinical point of view, unacceptable for preoperative patient management.

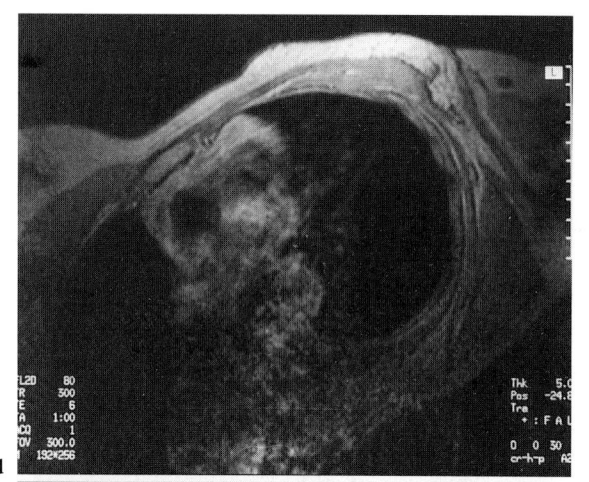

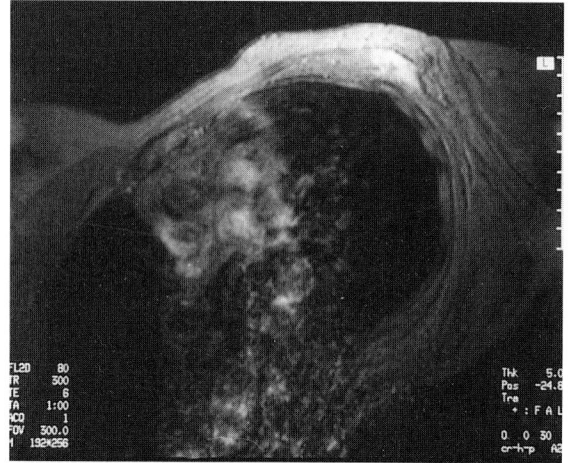

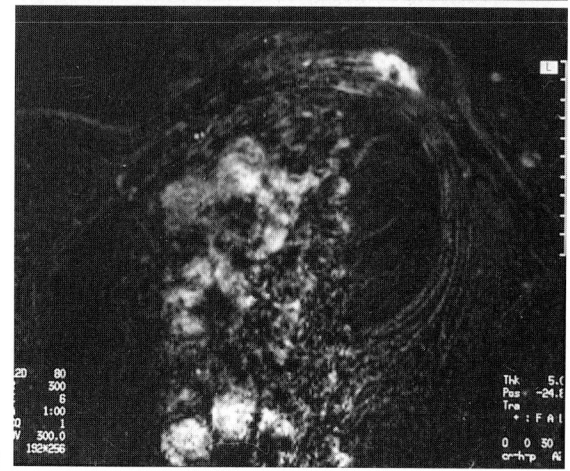

Fig. 14.26d-f

As *high sensitivity* is combined with *low specificity* in MRI, every positive result in MRI, especially when it is discrepant with the findings of conventional methods, must be verified by some kind of *biopsy*, which should be (a) *preoperative*, in order to avoid unnecessary surgery for falsely positive lesions and (b) *MRI-guided*, because many of the lesions found are seen only by MRI. Therefore the development of an *MRI-guided biopsy*, rather than a *localization technique*, is needed.

Pilot clinical results have been reported for various MRI-guided biopsy systems (FISCHER et al. 1995a; HEYWANG-KÖBRUNNER et al. 1995; HUSSMAN et al. 1993; KUHL et al. 1995b). Most systems use a perforated compression plate to immobilize the breast. The surface coil can be integrated into the compression plate. The exact localization of the slice position is achieved through contrast medium-filled markers in the stereotaxic device. After local anesthesia and a skin nick, a nonmagnetic coaxial needle is introduced through the appropriate hole of the compression plate and the correct position of the needle tip in relation to the target lesion is verified.

In Fig. 14.28a and b the mammogram of a 54-year-old woman with indeterminate complaints in her left breast is depicted. On the craniocaudal view (Fig. 14.28a) a spiculated density is demonstrated which could not be identified on the lateral view. As ultrasonography did not clearly delineate a lesion either, an MR examination was carried out which showed a slowly enhancing lesion at the corresponding site. In view of the still indeterminate diagnosis and the equivocal localization on the mammogram and sonogram, we decided to perform an MR-guided core biopsy with simultaneous charcoal marking of the lesion. Figure 14.28f-h demonstrates the breast positioned in the stereotaxic device before and after contrast administration and calculation of subtraction images. The prefire verification image (Fig. 14.28i) shows the coaxial system just in front of the enhancing lesion; the postfire image (Fig. 14.28j) shows the needle path through the lesion. After biopsy the lesion was marked by injection of 0.5 ml of a suspension of charcoal in Gd-DTPA solution. As an infiltrating ductal carcinoma was found at core biopsy and the lesion had already been marked during the procedure, definitive surgery could be performed without any further preoperative localization.

The ideal needle material for MR-guided interventional breast procedures is actively being sought. Special glass-fiber coaxial cannulas which produce no susceptibility artifacts in the image are being developed for core biopsy (FISCHER et al. 1995a). Fine-needle biopsy can be carried out with nonmagnetic titanium-iron fine needles (19G) (FISCHER et al. 1995). FISCHER et al. (1995) reported 19 of 23 MR-guided fine needle aspirations to have been successful, and 28 preoperative MR-guided lo-

Fig. 14.27a–c. Fifty-five-year-old woman who had had a mastectomy because of an infiltrating ductal carcinoma [pT1cpN0 (0/14)G3] 3 months previously. MRI examination to clarify a small subcutaneous nodule on the left thoracic wall. Axial T1-weighted gradient-echo sequence (FLASH 2D, 80°/220/6 ms) before/after 0.1 mmol Gd-DTPA/kg shows a nodule with strong enhancement in the left interior parasternal position, proven to be a lymph node metastasis by CT-guided core biopsy

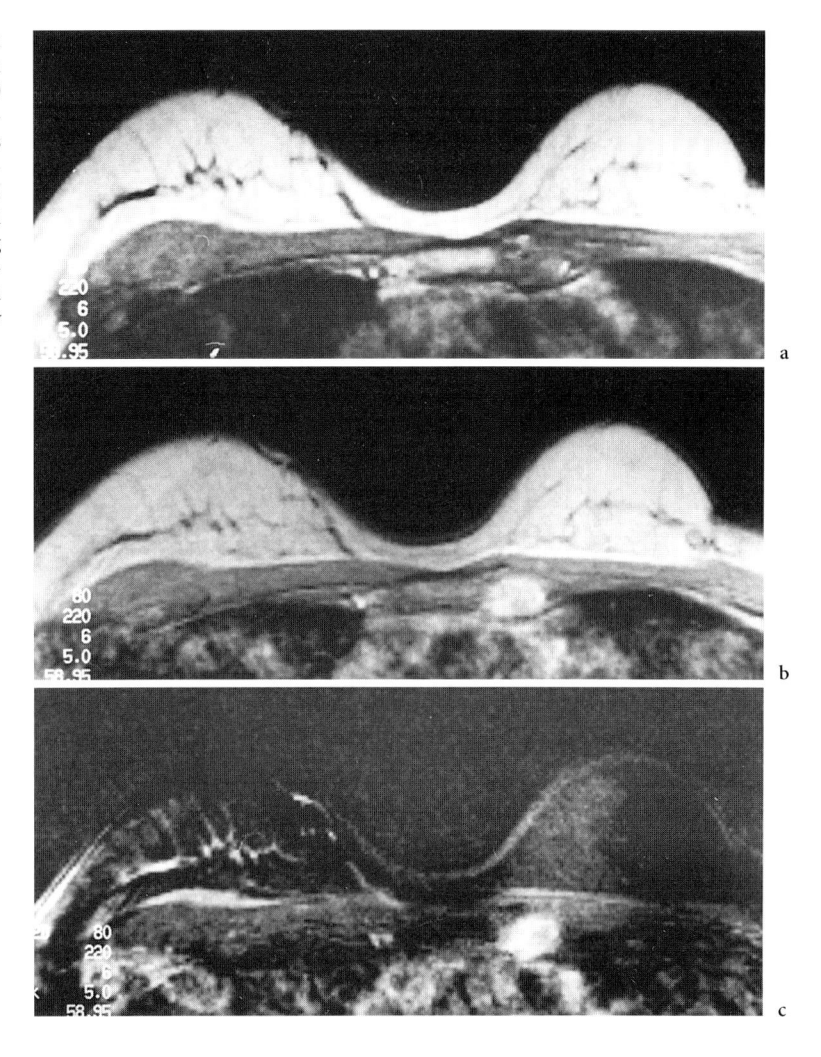

calizations. The future design of a stereotaxic device and needle material have to be further defined and a routine examination protocol for MR-guided breast biopsy needs to be implemented for most MR systems.

14.6 Diagnostic Value and Established Indications for MR of the Breast

Considering its principle of imaging (depicting vascularization and the extracellular space of a lesion), contrast-enhanced MRI of the breast can be expected to detect breast carcinomas which remain undetected by the conventional methods of mammography and ultrasonography. Although the published data show considerable variation, almost all authors report a *higher sensitivity* of MRI than conventional methods for the detection of infiltrating breast carcinoma (Table 14.1). However, with growing experience it has become apparent that, despite its high sensitivity, MRI has a definite rate of false-negatives in carcinoma detection (~10%). It has also become apparent that MRI fails to detect many of the in situ components of infiltrating carcinoma. There are, on the other hand, no reliable data about true-negative results of any method, as serial sectioning is rarely carried out on mastectomy specimens. Many diagnoses are established only on follow-up in patients in whom no histological examination has been carried out. Furthermore, a close correlation of MRI results with those of other imaging methods and pathology is not always provided, limiting the relevance of the data presented.

As often occurs with the advent of a new imaging modality, the diagnostic potential of MRI of the breast was greatly overestimated in the initial phase

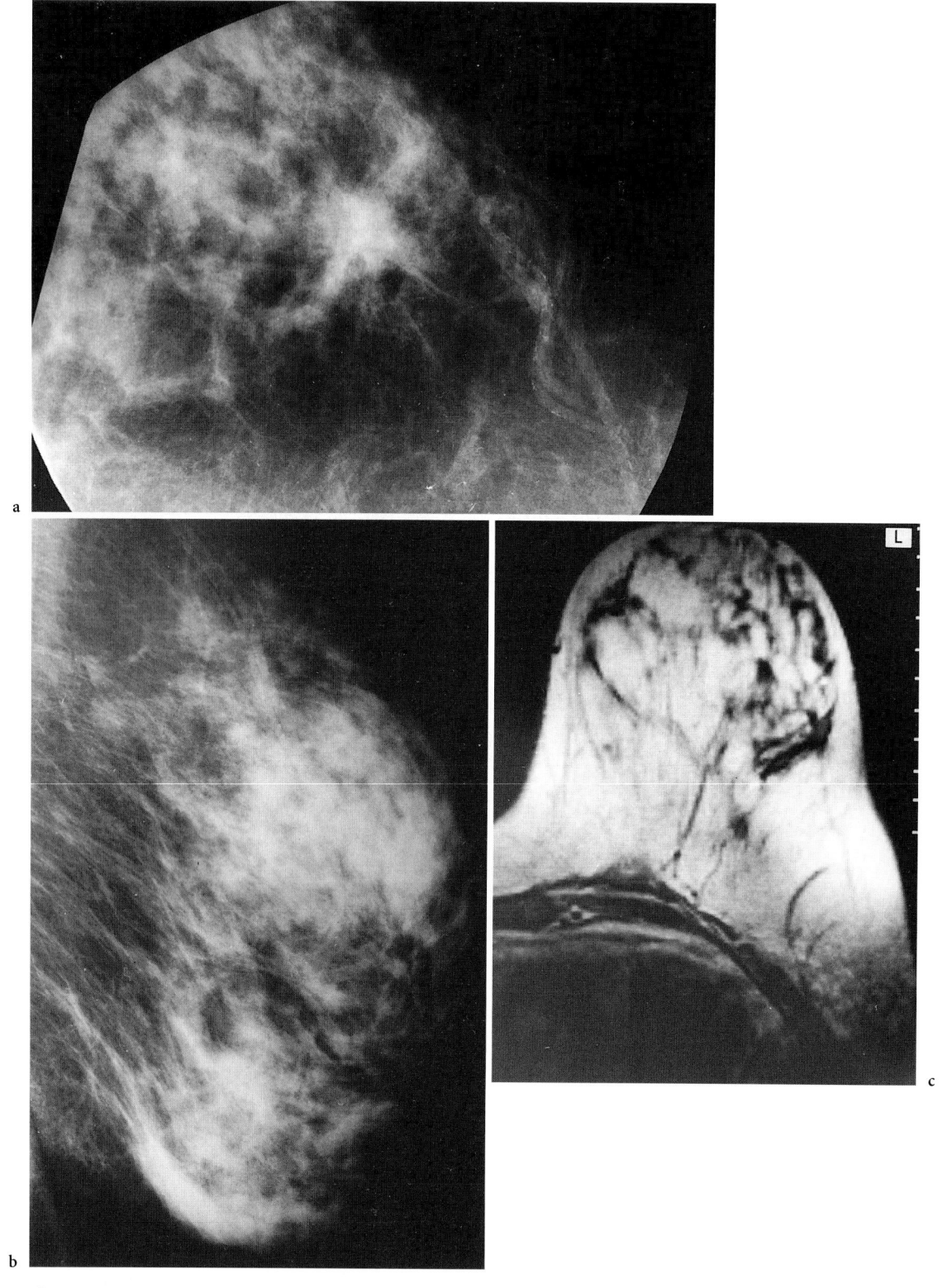

Fig. 14.28a–c

Magnetic Resonance Imaging of the Breast

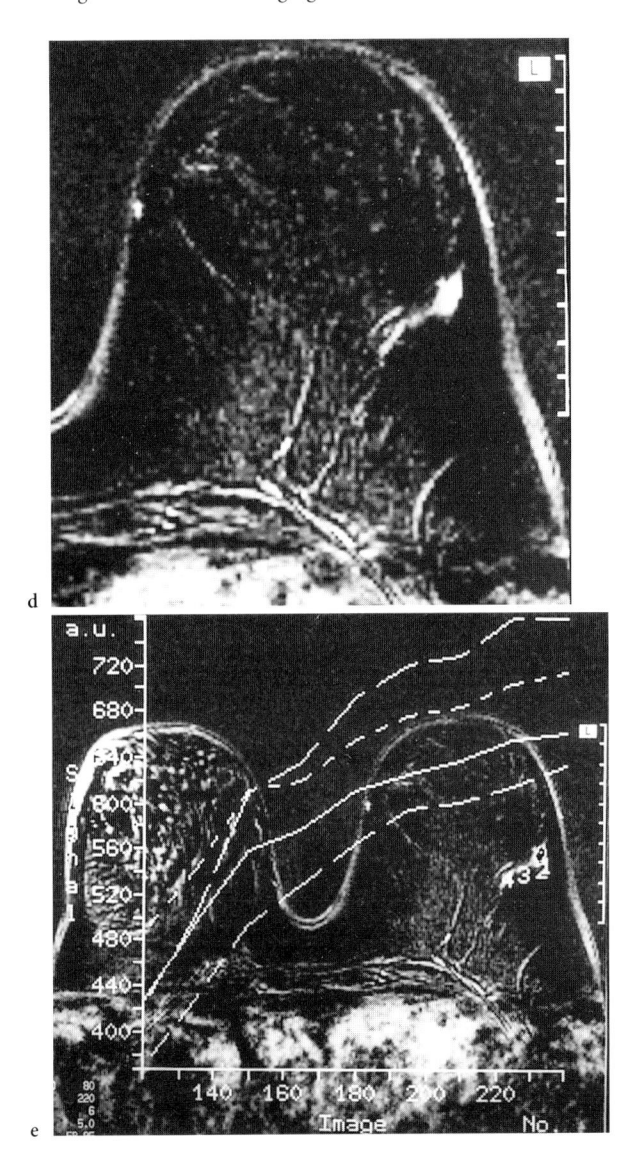

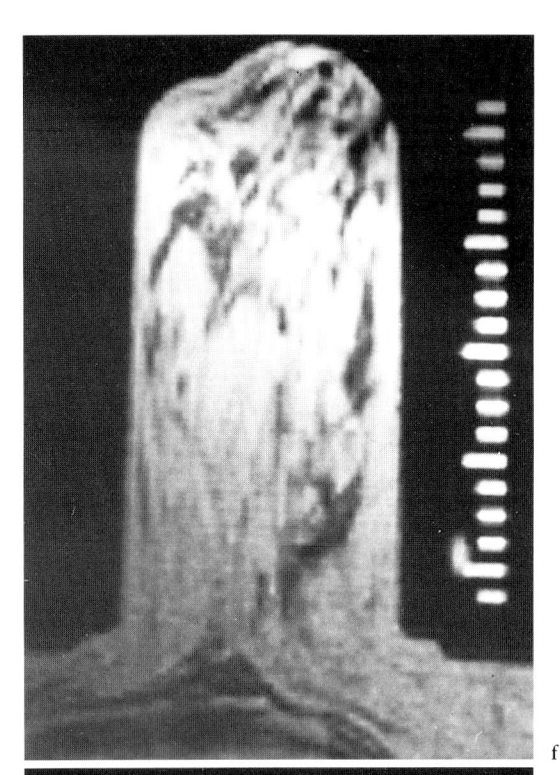

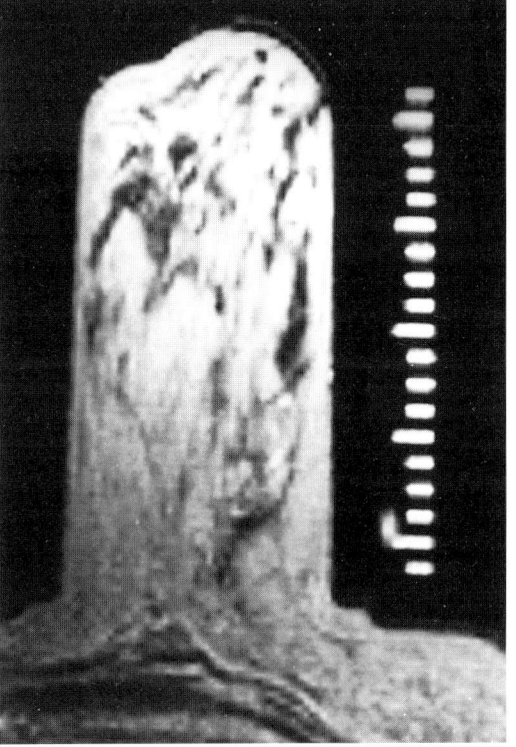

Fig. 14.28a–j. Fifty-four-year-old woman with indeterminate complaints between lateral quadrants of the left breast for the preceding 6 weeks; no palpable nodule was present. **a,b** Craniocaudal and mediolateral mammograms showing a stellate lesion in the cc projection, not easily identified on the mL projection. **c,d** Axial gradient-echo sequence (FLASH 2D, 80°/220/6 ms) after 0.1 mmol Gd-DTPA/kg i.v. and subtraction image showing a focal area of enhancement in the left lateral breast region. **e** Time-signal intensity curve shows a gradual signal increase without early signal maximum and no washout effect. **f–j** MR-guided core biopsy of an enhancing lesion. **f–h** Axial gradient-echo sequence (FLASH 2D, 80°/220/6 ms) after 0.1 mmol Gd-DTPA/kg i.v. and subtraction image after positioning of the breast in the stereotaxic localization device with a Gd-DTPA-filled localization plate. **i,j** Documentation of stereotaxic puncture procedure: **i** 16-G coaxial antimagnetic titanium needle in position, pointing to the enhancing lesion. **j** Postfire control scan after biopsy, demonstrating correct needle path through the lesion

Fig. 14.28h–j

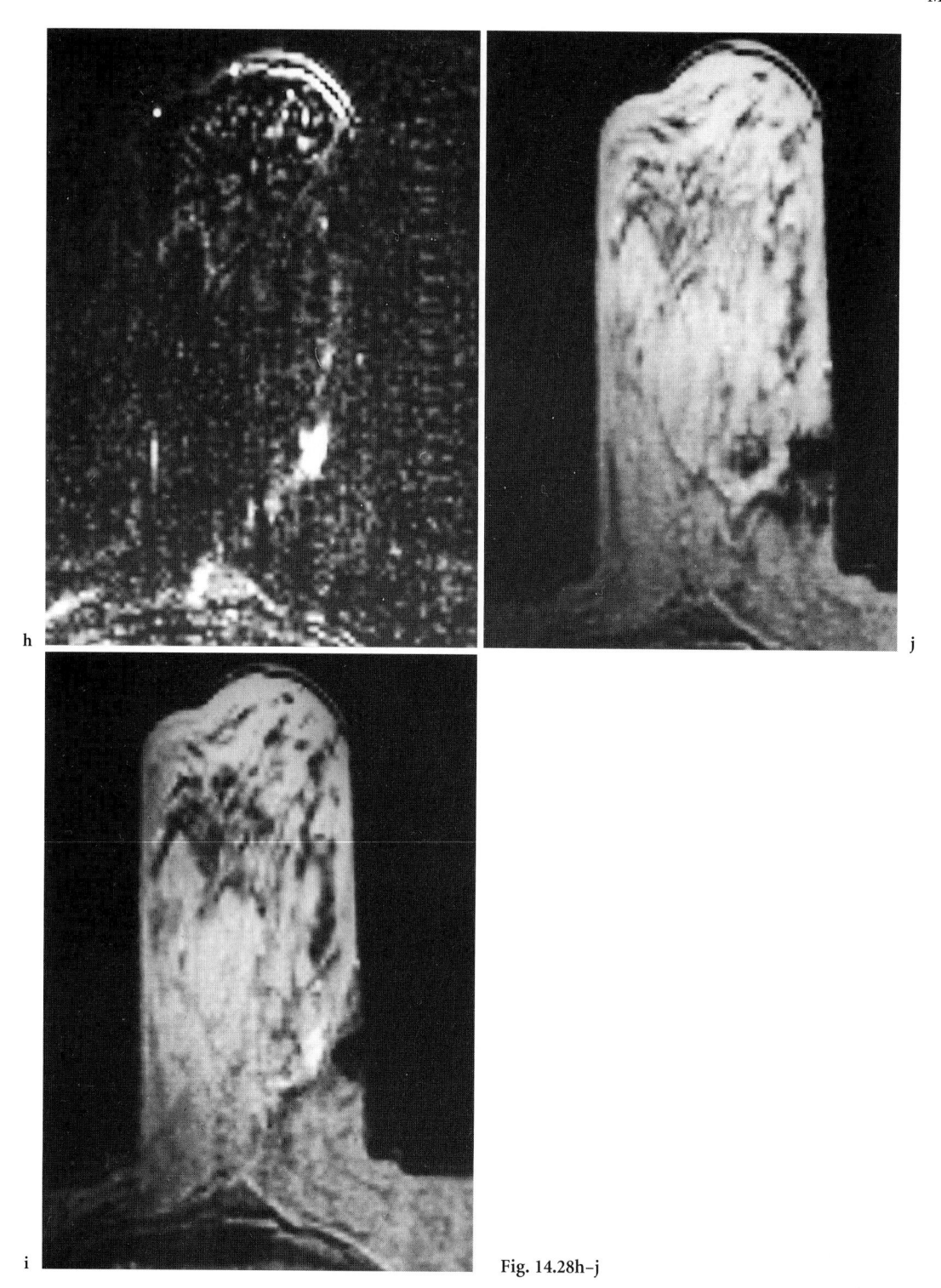

of experience (KAISER 1989, 1990, 1993). Some of these early studies were biased by methodological deficiencies insofar as conventional imaging methods were performed without careful attention to high standards of image quality. On the other hand, practical experience with MRI is too limited to allow a definitive validation of the new technology.

Table 14.1 gives some selected values of sensitivity, specificity, and positive and negative predictive values of various breast imaging methods. However,

Table 14.1. Published data on the sensitivity, specificity, and positive and negative predictive values of mammography, ultrasonography, and MRI

Reference	Mammography				US	MRI							
	5	6	7	8	5	1	2	3	4	5	6	7	8
Sensitivity (%)	85	82	55	89	76	85	89	98	95	91	99.5	94	93
Specificity (%)	92	16	89		88	57	29	97	89.5	79	28	37	
Pos. pred. value (%)	94	53			90	65		81	95.3	86	61		
Neg. pred. value (%)	81	47			72	80		99.8	89.5	86	98		

US, Ultrasonography; MRI, magnetic resonance imaging
1, KNOPP et al. (1995b); 2, ALLGAYER et al. (1993); 3, KAISER and HAHN (1995); 4, FISCHER et al. (1993); 5, MÜLLER-SCHIMPFLE et al. (1995b); 6, HEYWANG-KÖBRUNNER (1993); 7, HARMS et al. (1993); 8, SITTEK et al. (1995b)

Table 14.2. Results of our own clinical evaluation of mammography, ultrasonography, and contrast-enhanced MRI, alone and in combination, in 156 patients

	True +	True −	False +	False −
Mammography	73% (49/67)	67% (134/199)	31% (61/199)	19% (13/67)
Ultrasonography	78% (52/67)	75% (150/199)	21% (43/199)	16% (11/67)
Mammo. + US	94% (63/67)	77% (154/199)	22% (44/199)	7% (5/67)
MRI	93% (62/67)	78% (155/199)	22% (44/199)	7% (5/67)
Mammo. + US + MRI	97% (65/67)	90% (179/199)	10% (20/199)	3% (2/67)

comparability of the data is limited because the individual validation of each method by the authors differs too much and the study groups compared are too heterogeneous.

Table 14.2 summarizes the results of our own clinical evaluation of mammography, ultrasonography and contrast-enhanced MRI, independently of each other and in combination in 156 patients. As one can see, sensitivity of MRI for breast cancer detection was higher than that of mammography or ultrasonography separately. However, mammography and ultrasonography evaluated in combination yielded the same sensitivity as MRI alone. The lack of specificity of mammography (31% false-positives) could be improved by ultrasonography to 22% false-positives. Notwithstanding its high sensitivity, contrast-enhanced MRI missed 7% of carcinomas. On the other hand, the lack of specificity of MRI is documented by the 22% rate of false-positives in cancer detection. As would be expected, the combination of all three imaging modalities yielded the highest level of sensitivity and specificity.

These results cannot be regarded as a guideline for clinical practice because of cost constraints and limitation of patient compliance. Within this context, it should also be emphasized that the lack of specificity of mammography and ultrasonography can easily be overcome by image-guided fine-needle or core biopsy, at a fraction of the cost of an MRI examination.

Despite the ongoing evaluation of contrast enhanced MRI, the following statements about the current diagnostic value of this new modality can be made:

1. Contrast-enhanced MRI of the breast is probably the *most sensitive method* to detect breast pathology. MRI is a most valuable additional modality to improve the sensitivity of mammography and ultrasonography in selected patient groups in which conventional methods are known to be less sensitive (see indications).

2. Despite the superior sensitivity of MRI in breast cancer detection. 5%–12% of infiltrating carcinomas of the breast are not recognized as such with MRI, because they are not visualized with the morphological and dynamic MRI criteria established for carcinoma.

3. MRI is clearly inferior to mammography in detecting in situ carcinoma because a considerable number (according to the literature, 30%–70%) of noninfiltrating carcinomas are not visualized by MRI. The neovascularization induced through in situ carcinomas is often too faint to be detected by contrast-enhanced MRI. Thus MRI is unable to confidently exclude carcinoma.

4. MRI is a *nonspecific imaging modality* as far as distinction of benign and malignant lesions of the breast is concerned. It is of limited value for improving the specificity of mammography and ultrasonography, and is far inferior to image-guided fine-needle aspiration and core biopsy.

5. The numerous false-positive results of contrast-enhanced MRI encountered in the attempt to improve the sensitivity of mammography/ultrasonography must be counterbalanced by MRI-guided core biopsy before open surgery is considered.

The indications for MRI of the breast so far established may be defined as follows:

1. Patients with silicone implants with or without mastectomy
2. Patients whose breasts are difficult to evaluate by combined mammography and ultrasonography, who have:
   a) had breast conservation therapy
   b) axillary lymph node metastasis from an unknown primary tumor
   c) postoperative scarring
   d) proven carcinoma of one breast, MRI being performed to exclude multifocality/-centricity

Contrast-enhanced MRI of the breast is not indicated for:

1. Clustered or disseminated *microcalcifications* (because a positive result may represent proliferative mastopathy and a negative result cannot exclude in situ carcinoma)
2. Dense breasts
3. Circumscribed mammographic opacities proven to be solid by ultrasonography (probably benign lesions, requiring periodic mammographic surveillance alone)
4. Cancerophobic patients

In spite of the extensive literature on the subject, the exact value of contrast-enhanced MRI in breast cancer diagnosis needs to be defined more clearly through carefully designed studies comparing the various complementary imaging methods used independently and in combination.

References

Adam G, Spüntrup E, Mühler A et al. (1995) Vergleichende Untersuchungen benigner und maligner Mammatumoren mittels dynamischer MRT nach Gabe von Gadolinium-DTPA und einem neuen Blutpoolkontrastmittel 24-Gadolinium-Kaskaden-Polymer. 76th DRG Kongress, May 1995, Wiesbaden. Radiologe 35 (Suppl 1, issue 4)

Adler DD, Wahl RL (1994) New methods for imaging the breast: techniques, findings and potential. AJR 164:19–30

Allgayer B, Lukas P, Loos W, Kersting-Sommerhoff B (1993) MRT der Mamma mit 2D-Spinecho- und Gradientenechosequenzen in diagnostischen Problemfällen. Fortschr Röntgenstr 158:423–427

Bauer M, Schulz-Wendland R, Krämer S, Büttner A (1995) MR-mammography for evaluation of breast cancer and tumor-environment. ERC Congress, March 1995, Vienna. Eur Radiol 5 (Suppl)

Bradley Pierce WB, Harms SE, Flamig DP, Griffey RH, Evans WP, Hagans JE (1991) Three-dimensional gadolinium-enhanced MR imaging of the breast: pulse sequence with fat suppression and magnetization transfer contrast. Radiology 181:757–763

Buchberger W, Kapferer M, Stöger A, Chemelli A, Judmaier W, Felber S (1995) Dignitätsbeurteilung fokaler Mammaläsionen: Prospektiver Vergleich von Mammographie, Sonographie und dynamischer MRT. 76th DRG Kongress, May 1995, Wiesbaden. Radiologe 35 (Supple 1, issue 4)

Cooney BS, Orel SG, Schnall MD, Troupin RH (1993) Invasive lobular carcinoma in a patient with synchronous ductal carcinoma. In situ detection with MR imaging. AJR 162:1318–1320

Dao TH, Rahmouni A, Campana F, Laurent M, Asselain B, Fourquet A (1993) Tumor Recurrence versus fibrosis in the irradiated breast: differentiation with dynamic gadolinium-enhanced MR imaging. Radiology 187:751–755

Dash N, Lupetin AR, Daffner RH, Deeb ZL, Sefczek RJ, Shapiro RL (1986) Magnetic resonance imaging in the diagnosis of breast disease. AJR 146:119–125

Dilcher-Spies S, Venator M (1995) Diagnostische Wertigkeit der MR-Mammographie bei lobulärem Mamma-Carcinom – Retrospektive Analyse von 17 Patienten. 76th DRG Kongress, May 1995, Wiesbaden. Radiologe 35 (Suppl 1, issue 4)

Dresel V, Bühner M, Schulz-Wendland R, Bauer M (1995) Intraduktale Karzinome der Mamma – ist eine Diagnose in der Kernspintomographie (NMR) möglich? 76th DRG Kongress, May 1995, Wiesbaden. Radiologe 35 (Suppl 1, issue 4)

El Yousef SJ, Duchesneau RH, Alfidi RJ, Haaga JR, Bryan PJ, LiPuma JP (1984) Magnetic resonance imaging of the breast. Radiology 150:761–766

Fischer U, Heyden DV, Vosshenrich R, Vieweg I, Grabbe E (1993) Signalverhalten maligner und benigner Läsionen in der dynamischen 2D-MRT der Mamma. Fortschr Röntgenstr 158:287–292

Fischer U, Vosshenrich R, Döler W, Hamadeh A, Oestmann JW, Grabbe E (1995a) MR imaging-guided breast intervention: experience with two systems. Radiology 195:533–538

Fischer U, Westerhof JP, Vosshenrich R, von Heyden D, Oestmann JW, Grabbe E (1995b) Das präinvasive duktale Mammakarzinom in der MR-Mammographie. 76 DRG Kongress, May 1995, Wiesbaden. Radiologe 35 (Suppl 1, issue 4)

Fischer U, Brinck U, Schauer S, Grabbe E (1995c) Korrelation von Anreicherungsverhalten in der MR Mammographie mit immunhistochemischen Prognosefaktoren. 76 DRG Kongress, May 1995, Wiesbaden. Radiologe 35 (Suppl 1, issue 4)

Flickinger FW, Allison JD, Sherry R, Wright JC (1992) Differentiation of benign from malignant breast masses by dynamic time-intensity evaluation of contrast enhanced MRI

(abstract). Annual Meeting of the Society of Magnetic Resonance in Medicine, Berlin, 1992
Folkman J (1985) Tumor angiogenesis. Adv Cancer Res 43:175–199
Folkman J, Shing Y (1992) Angiogenesis. J Biol Chem 267:10931–10934
Friedmann BR, Jones JP, Chavez-Munoz G, Salmon AP, Merritt CR (1989) Principles of MRI. McGraw-Hill, New York
Friedrich M (1987) Kernspintomographie der Mamma. In: Frommhold W, Dihlmann W, Stender H-S, Thurn P (eds) Radiologische Diagnostik in Klinik und Praxis Allgemeine Grundlagen der radiologischen Diagnostik: Hals, Mediastinum, Zwerchfell, Mamma, kindlicher Thorax. Thieme, Stuttgart, pp 631–647
Friedrich M, Semmler W (1987) MR-Tomographie der Brust. Radiologe 27:165–177
Gilles R, Guinebretiere JM, Shapeero G et al. (1993) Assessment of breast cancer recurrence with contrast-enhanced subtraction MR imaging: preliminary results in 26 patients. Radiology 188:473–478
Gilles R, Guinebretière JM, Lucidarme O et al. (1994a) Nonpalpable breast tumors: diagnosis with contrast-enhanced subtraction dynamic MR imaging. Radiology 191:625–631
Gilles R, Guinebretière J-M, Toussaint C et al. (1994b) Locally advanced breast cancer: contrast-enhanced subtraction MR imaging of response to preoperative chemotherapy. Radiology 191:633–638
Greenstein Orel S, Schnall MD, LiVolsi VA, Troupin RH (1994) Suspicious breast lesions: MR imaging with radiologic-pathologic correlation. Radiology 190:485–493
Greenstein Orel S, Schnall MD, Powell CM et al. (1995) Staging of suspected breast cancer: effect of MR imaging and MR-guided biopsy. Radiology 196:115–122
Haase A, Frahm J, Matthaei D, Hänicke W, Merboldt KD (1986) FLASH-imaging: rapid NMR imaging using low flip angle pulses. J Magn Reson 67:258–266
Harms ST, Flamig DP, Hesley K et al. (1993) MR imaging of the breast with rotating delivery of excitation off resonance: clinical experience with pathologic correlation. Radiology 187:493–501
Harms ST, Flamig DP, Evans WP, Harries SA, Bown ST (1994) MR Imaging of the breast: current status and future potential. AJR: 1039–1047
Harms ST, Jensen RA, Meiches MD, Flamig DP, Evans WP (1995) Silicone-suppressed 3D MRI of the breast using rotating delivery of off-resonance excitation. J Comput Assist Tomogr 19:394–399
Hennig J, Nauerth A, Friedburg H, Ratzel D (1984) Ein neues Schnittbildverfahreu für die Kernspintomographie. Radiologe 24:579–588
Hess T, Knopp MV, Brix G, Hoffmann U, Junkermann H, Zabel H-J, van Kaick G (1993) Pharmacokinetic mapping of breast lesions by dynamic Gd-DTPA enhanced MRI. Proc Soc Magn Res Med, 12th Annual Meeting, 14–20 August 1993, New York
Heywang-Köbrunner SH (1993) Brustkrebsdiagnostik mit MR – Überblick nach 1250 Patientenuntersuchungen. Electromedica 61:43–52
Heywang-Köbrunner SH (1994) Contrast-enhanced magnetic resonance imaging of the breast. Invest Radiol 29:94–104
Heywang-Köbrunner SH, Hilbertz T, Pruss E, Wolf A, Permanetter W, Eiermann W, Lissner J (1988) Dynamische Kontrastmitteluntersuchungen mit FLASH bei der Kernspintomographie der Mamma. Digitale Bilddiagn 8:7–13
Heywang-Köbrunner SH, Wolf A, Pruss E, Hilbertz T, Eiermann W, Permanetter W (1989) MR imaging of the breast with Gd-DTPA: use and limitations. Radiology 171:95–103
Heywang-Köbrunner SH, Hilbertz T, Beck R, Bauer WM, Eiermann W, Permanetter W (1990) Gd-DTPA enhanced MR imaging of the breast in patients with postoperative scarring and silicone implants. J Comput Assist Tomogr 14:348–356
Heywang-Köbrunner SH, Schlegel A, Beck R et al. (1993a) Contrast-enhanced MRI of the breast after limited surgery and radiation therapy. J Comput Assist Tomogr 17:891–900
Heywang-Köbrunner SH, Beck R, Wendt T (1993b) Stellenwert der Kontrastmittel-Kernspintomographie bei der Diagnostik des Lokalrecidivs. In: Schmid L, Wilmanns W (eds) Praktische onkologie, vol III. Zuckschwerdt, München, pp 134–140
Heywang-Köbrunner SH, Haustein J, Pohl C, Beck R, Lommatzsch B, Untch M, Nathrath WBJ (1994) Contrast-enhanced MR Imaging of the breast: comparison of two different doses of gadopentetate dimeglumine. Radiology 191:639–646
Heywang-Köbrunner SH, Viehweg P, Kösling S, Spielmann RP (1995) Contrast-enhanced MRI of the breast: technical aspects and pitfalls. ERC Congress, March 1995, Vienna. Eur Radiol 5 (Suppl)
Hieschold V, Klengel ST, Neumann U, Köhler K (1995) Zur erforderlichen Zeitauflösung bei der dynamischen Kernspintomographie der Mamma. 76th DRG Kongress, May 1995, Wiesbaden. Radiologe 35 (Supple 1, issue 4)
Hittmair K, Turetschek K, Gomiscek G, Stiglbauer R, Schurawitzki H (1995) Field strength dependence of dynamic contrast-enhanced MRI of mammary tumors. ERC Congress, March 1995, Vienna. Eur Radiol 5 (Suppl)
Hussman K, Reuslo R, Philipps J, et al. (1993) MR mammographic localisation: work in progress. Radiology 189:915–917
Kaiser WA (1989) Magnetresonanztomographie der Mamma Erfahrungen nach 253 Untersuchungen. D Med Wochenschrift 114:1351–1357
Kaiser WA (1990) Dynamic magnetic resonance imaging using a double breast coil: an important routine examination of the breast. Front Eur Radiol 7:39–68
Kaiser WA (1992) MR-Mammographie bei Risikopatientinnen. Fortschr Röntgenstr 156:576–581
Kaiser WA (1993) MR-Mammography. Springer, Berlin Heidelberg New York
Kaiser WA, Deimling M (1990) Eine neue Multischicht-Maßsequenz für die komplette dynamische MR-Untersuchung an größeren Organen: Anwendung an der Brust. Fortschr Röntgenstr 152:577–582
Kaiser WA, Hahn D (1995) Technical pitfalls in dynamic MR-mammography. ERC Congress, March 1995, Vienna. Eur Radiol 5 (Suppl)
Kaiser WA, Kess H (1989) Prototyp-Doppelspule für die Mamma-MR-Messung. Fortschr Röntgenstr 151:103–105
Kaiser WA, Reiser MF (1992) MR mammography: experience with 650 examinations (abstract). SMRI Annual Meeting, New York
Kaiser WA, Zeitler E (1986a) Die Kernspintomographie der Mamma – Diagnose, Differentialdiagnose, Probleme und Lösungsmöglichkeiten Teil I: Untersuchungsverfahren. Fortschr Röntgenstr 144 4:459–465
Kaiser WA, Zeitler E (1986b) Kernspintomographie der Mamma: Diagnose, Differentialdiagnose, Probleme und

Lösungsmöglichkeiten. Teil II: Diagnostik. Fortschr Röntgenstr 144 5:572–579

Kaiser WA, Zeitler E (1989) MR imaging of the breast: fast imaging sequences with and without Gd-DTPA. Radiology 170:681–686

Kasumi F (1991) The diagnostic criteria of breast lesions of the Japan Society of Ultrasonics in Medicine and topical issues in the field of breast ultrasonography. In: Kasumi F, Ueno E (eds) Topics in breast ultrasound (in Japanese) Shinohara, Tokyo, pp 19–26

Kessler M, Sittek H, Milz P et al. (1995) Dynamic FLASH-3D-MRI of the breast: comparison with conventional X-ray-mammography and correlation with pathologic findings. Radiology (submitted for publication)

Knopp MV, Junkermann HJ, Sinn P, Dikic S, Hess T, Brix G, van Kaick G (1995a) MR-mammographic appearance of fibrodenomas: radiologic-histologic correlation. ERC Congress, March 1995, Vienna. Eur Radiol 5 (Suppl)

Knopp MV, Jundermann HJ, sinn P et al. (1995b) Assessment of MR-mammography in patients with screening detected lesions. ERC Congress, March 1995, Vienna. Eur Radiol 5 (Suppl)

Knopp MV, Hess T, Junkermann HJ et al. (1995c) Clinical evaluation of dynamic MR-mammography with automated processing. 76th DRG Kongress, May 1995, Wiesbaden. Radiologe 35 (Suppl 1, issue 4)

Knopp MV, Junkermann HJ, Hess T et al. (1995d) MR-Mammographie zum Monitoring von neoadjuvanter Therapie beim Mammacarcinom. 76th DRG Kongress, May 1995, Wiesbaden. Radiologe 35 (Suppl 1, issue 4)

Kuhl CK, Kreft BP, Hauswirth A, Gieseke J, Elevelt A, Reiser M, Schild HH (1995a) MR-Mammographie bei 0,5 Tesla, Teil II: Differenzierbarkeit maligner und benigner Läsionen in der MR-Mammographie bei 0,5 und 1,5 Tesla. Fortschr Röntgenstr 162:482–491

Kuhl CK, Elevelt A, Gieseke J, Schild HH (1995b) MR-mammographisch gesteuerte stereotaktische Markierung klinisch, mammographisch und sonographisch okkulter Läsionen durch eine Lokalisations- und Biopsiespule. 76th DRG Kongress, May 1995, Wiesbaden. Radiologe 35 (Suppl 1, issue 4)

Kuhl CK, Seibert C, Schild HH (1995c) Fokale und diffuse KM-anreichernde Läsionen in der MR-Mammographie bei gesunden Probandinnen: Bandbreite des Normalverhaltens und Zyklusphasenabhängigkeit. 76th DRG Kongress, May 1995, Wiesbaden. Radiologe 35 (Suppl 1, issue 4)

Kuhl CK, Deimling M, Bieling HB, Schild HH (1995d) Incrementalbilder in der dynamischen MR-Mammographie: Spielerei oder diagnostisch relevant? 76th DRG Kongress, May 1995, Wiesbaden. Radiologe 35 (Suppl 1, issue 4)

Lewis-Jones HG, Whitehouse GH, Leinster SJ (1991) The role of magnetic resonance imaging in the assessment of local recurrent breast cancer Clin Radiol 43:197–204

Liberman L, Dershaw D, Rosen PP, Abramson AF, Deutch BM, Hann LE (1994) Streotaxic 14-gauge breast biopsy: how many core biopsy specimens are needed? Radiology 192:793–795

Lufkin R, Teresi LM, Hanafee W (1987) New needle for MR-guided aspiration cytology of the head and neck. AJR 149:380–382

Müller-Schimpfle M, Rieber A, Kurz S, Stern W, Claussen CD (1995a) Dynamische 3-D-MR-Mammographie mit Hilfe einer schnellen Gradienten-Echo-Sequenz. Fortschr Röntgenstr 162:13–19

Müller-Schimpfle M, Stern W, Kurz S, Stoll P, Dammann F, Claussen CD (1995b) 3D-MR-Mammographie im Vergleich mit Mammographie und Sonographie – Ein Diskussionsbeitrag zur Mammadiagnostik heute. 76th DRG Kongress, May 1995, Wiesbaden. Radiologe 35 (Suppl 1, issue 4)

Oellinger H, Heins S, Sander B, Schoenegg W, Flesch U, Meissner R, Felix R (1993) Gd-DTPA enhanced MRI of breast: the most sensitive method for detecting multicentric carcinomas in female breast? Eur Radiol 3:223–226

Oppelt A, Graumann R, Barfuß H, Fischer H, Hartl W, Schajor W (1986) FISP – Eine neue schnelle Pulssequenz für die Kernspintomographie. Electromedica 54:15–18

Przetak C, Audretsch W, Schnabel T, Rezai M, Hartmann A, Hackländer T, Mödder U (1995) Therapiemonitoring des Mamma-Carcinoms durch Kernspintomographie bei neoadjuvanter Therapie. 76th DRG Kongress, May 1995, Wiesbaden. Radiologe 35 (Suppl 1, issue 14)

Reuther G (1993) Stellenwert der MR-Mammographie in der Problemfalldiagnostik unklarer Mammabefunde Fortschr Diagn 3:24–27

Revel D, Brasch RC, Paajanen H et al. (1986) Gd-DTPA contrast enhancement and tissue differentiation in MR imaging of experimental breast carcinoma. Radiology 158:319–323

Rubens D, Totterman S, Chacko AK et al. (1991) Gadopentate dimeglumine-enhanced chemical-shift MR imaging of the breast. AJR 157:267–270

Schnall MD, Orel S, Torosian M (1992) High resolution MRI of breast lesions in vivo. Soc Magn Reson Med, Berkeley, I, p 952

Schreiber W, Brix G, Knopp MV, Hess T, van Kaick G, Lorenz WJ (1995) Magnetization transfer weighted MR imaging of the breast: comparison with three-dimensional T1w FLASH imaging. ERC Congress, March 1995, Vienna. Eur Radiol 5 (Suppl)

Schwartz GF, Patchefsky AF, Feig SA et al. (1980) Multicentricity of nonpalpable breast cancer. Cancer 45:2913–2916

Schwickert HC, van Dijke CF, Roberts TPI et al. (1995) Einsatz der MRT mit makromolekularem Kontrastmittel zur Quantifizierung erhöhter Kapillarpermeabilität in bestrahlten Tumoren und zur Prädiktion einer gesteigerte Akkumulation von Chemotherapeutika. 76th DRG Kongress, May 1995, Wiesbaden. Radiologe 35 (Suppl 1, issue 4)

Sickles EA, Herzog KA (1980) Intramammary scar tissue: a mimic of the mammographic appearance of carcinoma. AJR 135:350–353

Sittek H, Kessler M, Bohmert H, Untch M, Lebeau A, Kohnert M, Reiser M (1995a) MR-mammography: differentiation of dysplasias. ERC Congress, March 1995, Vienna. Eur Radiol 5 (Suppl)

Sittek H, Kessler M, Bohmert H, Untch M, Lebeau A, Bredl T, Reiser M (1995b) Breast malignancies: comparison between MR-mammography and mammography. ERC Congress, March 1995, Vienna. Eur Radiol 5 (Suppl)

Stack JP, Redmond OM, Codd MB, Dervan PA, Ennis JT (1990) Breast disease: tissue characterization with Gd-DTPA enhancement profiles. Radiology 174:491–494

Stark DD, Bradley WG (1988) Magnetic resonance imaging. Mosby, St. Louis

Stelling CB, Wang PC, Lieber A, Mattingly SS, Griffen WO, Powell DE (1985) Prototype coil for magnetic resonance imaging of the female breast. Radiology 154:457–462

Stelling CB, Powell DE, Mattingly SS (1987) Fibroadenomas: histopathologic and MR imaging features. Radiology 162:399-407

Stelling CB, Runge VM, Davey DD et al. (1994) Dynamic enhancement of breast MRI at 30 seconds improves discrimination of sclerosing adenosis from invasive breast cancer. J Magn Reson Imaging 4(P):90

Stomper PC, Recht A, Berenberg AL, Jochelson MS, Harris JR (1987) Mammographic detection of recurrent cancer in the irradiated breast. AJR 148:39-43

Strohmaier A, Kotzan S, Barkow U, Lenk J, Friedrich M (1995) Evaluation of dynamic magnetic resonance mammography (MRM) with subtraction, parameter pictures and manual definition of the region of interest (ROI). ERC Congress, March 1995, Vienna. Eur Radiol 5 (Suppl)

Teubner J, Behrens U, Walz M et al. (1995) Dynamische Visualisierung der Kontrastmittelaufnahme bei der Mamma-MRT. 76th DRG Kongress, May 1995, Wiesbaden. Radiologe 35 (Supple 1, issue 4)

Tontsch P, Bauer M, Schulz-Wendtland R, Döinghaus K, Koch T, Lang N (1995) Dynamische MR-Mammographie bei 160 Hochrisikopatientinnen. 76th DRG Kongress, May 1995, Wiesbaden. Radiologe 35 (Suppl 1, issue 4)

Turner DA, Alcorn FS, Shorey WD et al. (1988) Carcinoma of the breast: detection with MR imaging versus xeromammography. Radiology 168:49-58

Turner DA, Wang JZ, Economou SG, Cobleigh M, Bloom KJ, Witt TR, Staren E (1993) Functional images from dynamic, contrast-enhanced 3DFT MR Images for the detection of breast cancer. Proc Soc Magn Reson Med. 12th Annual Meeting, August 14-20, 1993, New York

Utz JA, Herfkens MD, Glover G, Pelc N (1986) Three second initial NMR images using a gradient recall acquisition in a steady state mode (GRASS). Magn Reson Imaging 4:106

van Meulen P, Groon JP, Cuppen JJ (1985) Very fast MR imaging by field echoes and small angle excitation. Magn Reson Imaging 3:297-299

Weidner N, Semple J, Welch W, Folkman J (1991) Tumor angiogenesis and metastasis: correlation in invasive breast carcinoma. N Engl J Med 324:1-7

Weidner N, Folkman J, Pozza F et al. (1992) Tumor angiogenesis: a new significant and independent prognostic indicator in early-stage breast carcinoma. J Natl Cancer Inst 84:1875-1887

Wiener JI, Chako AC, Merten CW, Gross S, Coffey EL, Stein HL (1986) Breast and axillary tissue MR imaging: correlation of signal intensities and relaxation times with pathologic findings. Radiology 160:299-305

Wilhelm K, Grebe P, Teifke A, Halbsguth A, Mitze M, Thelen M (1992) Das lobuläre Mammakarzinom in der Kernspintomographie. Ein Fallbeispiel. Akt Radiol 2:373-375

Wolfmen NT, Moran R, Moran PR, Karstaedt N (1985) Simultaneous magnetic resonance imaging of both breasts using a dedicated receiver coil. Radiology 155:241-243

Zapf S, Halbsguth A, Brunier A, Mitze M, Klemencic J, Wilhelm K (1991) Möglichkeiten der Magnetresonanztomographie in der Diagnostik nicht palpabler Mammatumoren. Fortschr Röntgenstr 154:106-110

15 Prebiopsy Localization of Nonpalpable Breast Lesions

H. Junkermann and D. von Fournier

CONTENTS

15.1	Introduction	283
15.2	Methods of Localization	283
15.2.1	Geometric Localization	283
15.2.2	Grid Localization	283
15.2.3	Stereotactic Localization	284
15.2.4	Ultrasound Localization	285
15.3	Methods of Marking	286
15.3.1	Skin, Needle, and Dye Marking	286
15.3.2	Charcoal Marking	286
15.3.3	Guide Wire Marking	286
	References	289

15.1 Introduction

The increasing use of mammography for screening is leading to the detection of an increasing number of nonpalpable malignant and benign breast lesions. An excision for diagnostic or therapeutic reasons is necessary if further workup does not exclude malignancy. The ratio between benign and malignant results of biopsies on nonpalpable breast lesions is very variable. It depends not only on the expertise of the radiologist but also on the organization of the decision making (individual decision versus joint decision; Aitken et al. 1992) and especially on the availability of fine-needle or core biopsy (Svane et al. 1993). In the United States, malpractice-related concerns also may affect some decisions concerning biopsy.

The aim of the *diagnostic* excision is to achieve a definite pathological diagnosis without a disfiguring tissue defect. *Therapeutic* excision has the aim of complete excision of a malignant lesion, including an adequate margin. Prebiopsy localization in both cases guides the surgeon to the nonpalpable lesion.

H. Junkermann, MD, Universitäts-Kliniken, Abteilung Gynäkologische Radiologie, Voßstraße 9, 69115 Heidelberg, Germany
D. von Fournier, MD, Professor, Universitäts-Kliniken, Abteilung Gynäkologische Radiologie, Voßstraße 9, 69115 Heidelberg, Germany

Several methods of localization have been described, posing different demands on the technical equipment and personnel, with advantages and disadvantages depending on the situation in which they are used. Though simple and more refined methods have been used with similar results where the removal of the suspected lesion is concerned (Homer 1983b; Leinster et al. 1987; Tinnemans et al. 1987), a more precise localization allows the excision of smaller tissue pieces with less cosmetic distortion (Poole et al. 1986).

15.2 Methods of Localization

15.2.1 Geometric Localization

Localization of a lesion in relation to the nipple can be reconstructed from two orthogonal-projection mammograms. This method approaches the precision of needle-insertion procedures for small, firm breasts and superficially situated lesions. In large, pendulous breasts and with deeply situated lesions, however, this method is inaccurate. The different position of the breast at mammography (patient upright) and at operation (patient supine) adds to the inexactness of this method. The only advantage is that no additional tools are needed.

15.2.2 Grid Localization

Grids for the localization of breast lesions have been described (Brun del Re et al. 1977; Goldberg et al. 1983). A mammogram can be performed with the breast compressed by a plastic plate perforated with closely spaced holes. From the mammogram the hole closest to the lesion can be identified before needle insertion. Alternatively, the compression plate contains a single large hole marked at its edges by an alphanumeric grid that is both directly visible and seen on the mammogram, permitting the alphanumeric coordinates of the target lesion to be identified before needle insertion. Either approach allows very exact needle placement in the plane chosen. The depth of the lesion can be estimated only roughly from a pre-procedure mammogram taken in the perpendicular plane. It is advisable to insert the needle deeper than first anticipated and then to retract it, rather than having to push it in farther once breast compression is released. The depth of the needle can be adjusted after decompression and the taking of a second perpendicular view with the needle in situ.

15.2.3 Stereotactic Localization

This is the most sophisticated method of mammographic localization. With the breast compressed by a single-large-hole plate, two mammograms are taken at angles ±15° from perpendicular to the plane of compression (Figs. 15.1, 15.2). From the resultant parallax shift, the distance of the lesion from a marking on the supporting plate can be easily calculated. In modern units the depth calculation is automated and directly transformed into values for the manipulator. Theoretically, stereotaxis allows for a very exact localization with the needle placed within 1–2 mm of the lesion. The accuracy of the procedure is adversely influenced by factors such as movement of the patient's breast, the elasticity of the breast tissue, and the inability to locate exactly matching points on both stereoviews in diffuse lesions. Immobilization is easier to achieve with dedicated equipment, where the patient lies prone on a table, than with add-on units, where the patient sits upright. In

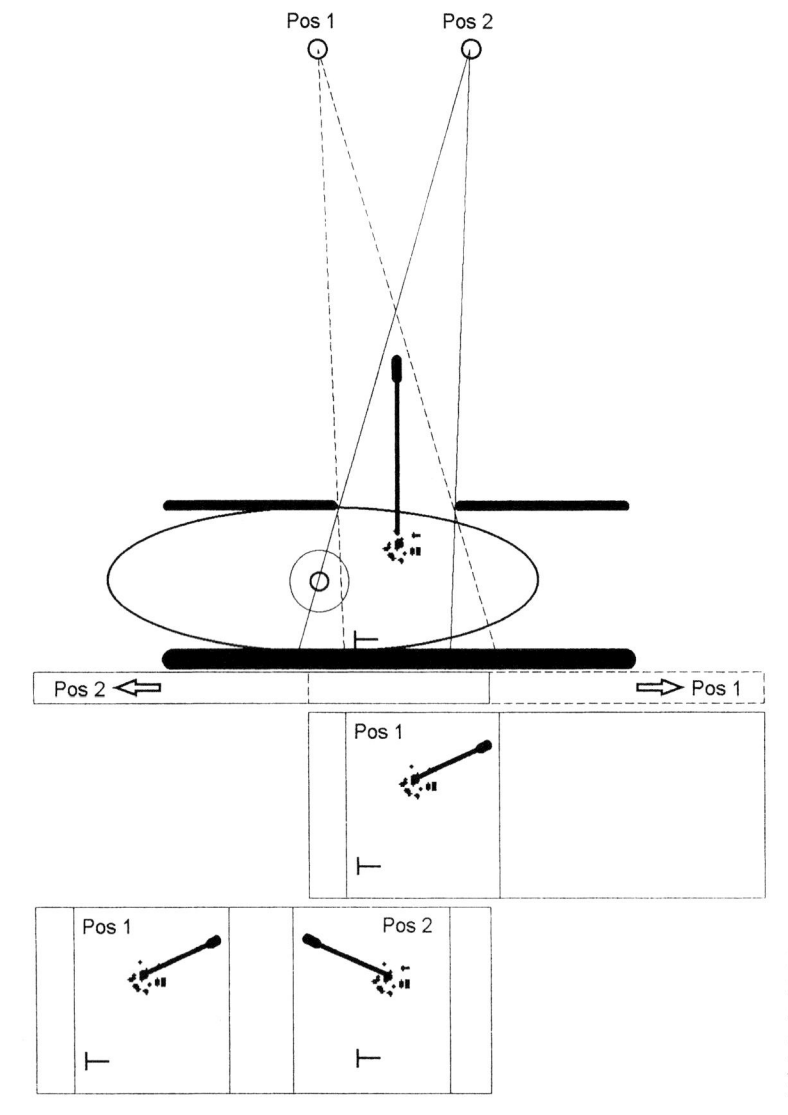

Fig. 15.1. Schematic representation of stereotactic localization of a group of microcalcifications. Two mammograms are taken at angles of ±15°. They are projected onto the same film. ⊢= fixed marking on the supporting plate

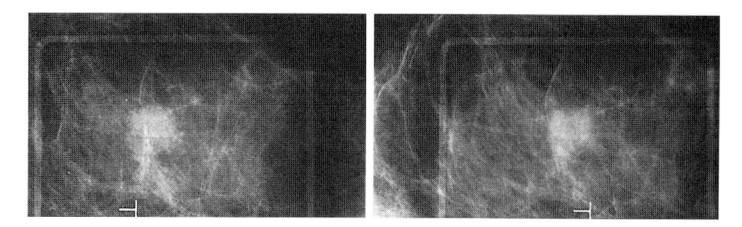

Fig. 15.2. Two stereotactic views on the same film. Depth is calculated from the displacement of the lesion in relation to the projection of the T-shaped marking

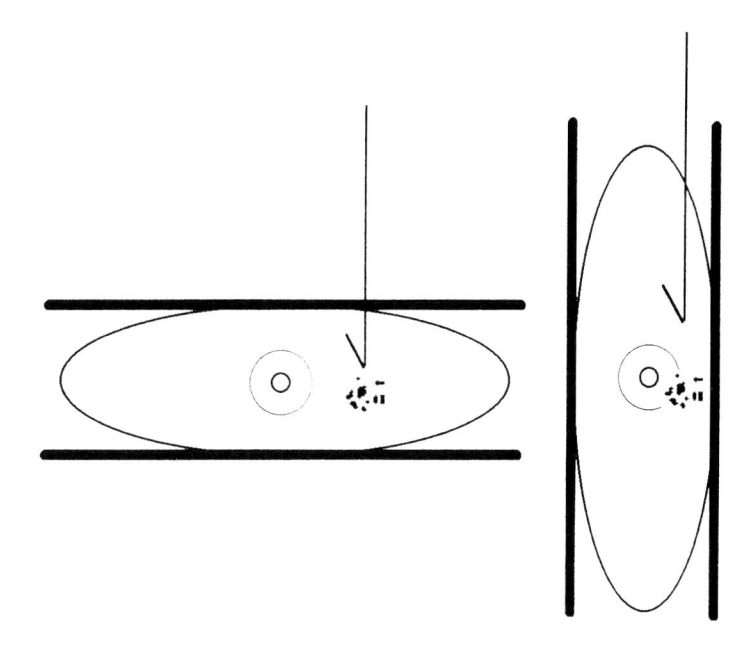

Fig. 15.3. Amplification of small placement error of hook wire (*left*) after compression in the perpendicular direction for confirmative mammography (*right*)

the latter case a comfortable chair, which supports the patient, is important. Digital equipment may speed up the acquisition of the image to a few seconds, as compared with the several minutes required for processing of conventional mammography film, thus shortening the overall time for the procedure and further minimizing the danger of patient movement. The elasticity of the breast tissue leads to amplification of small placement errors in the decompressed state (Fig. 15.3). This factor is responsible for deviations in the depth localization in vivo in comparison to in vitro. To account for the elasticity of the tissue it is advisable to insert the needle a few millimeters deeper than indicated on the manipulator. It is easier for the surgeon to locate the lesion if the marker passes the lesion than if the the lesion is not reached. Stereotactic localization is the most exact mammographic method of localization (GENT et al. 1986; BAUER and SCHULZ-WENDTLAND 1992).

15.2.4 Ultrasound Localization

In those cases where nonpalpable lesions can be detected with ultrasound, localization under ultrasonic guidance is faster and less cumbersome (KOPANS et al. 1984; MURAT et al. 1984). The needle can be easily seen in real time if it is advanced parallel to the transducer (Fig. 15.4). Thus a very precise placement is possible. Another advantage of the ultrasound method is that it is more flexible than the stereotactic method concerning the direction of access. The preferred ventrodorsal direction of access for the surgeon can be more easily used. SCHWARTZ et al. (1988) have described a method where the surgeon himself locates the lesion immediately before the operation. If necessary, ultrasound can be performed during the operation with a "gowned" transducer in the wound. With modern high-resolution transducers most masses identified at mammography can be localized by ultrasound. Microcalcifications, how-

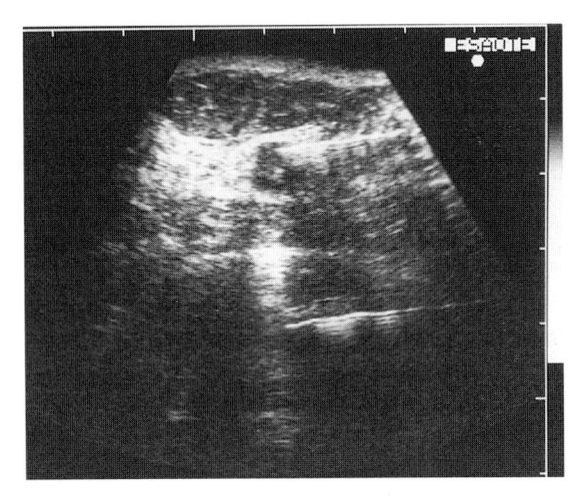

Fig. 15.4. Needle tip located within a 7-mm ductal invasive carcinoma. The needle (approaching from the right side) can be easily followed if kept parallel to the transducer

ever, can rarely be localized with ultrasound (WEBER et al. 1985; POTTERTON et al. 1994).

15.3 Methods of Marking

15.3.1 Skin, Needle, and Dye Marking

The geometric method of localization is the easiest way to mark the location of the lesion on the overlying skin. The accuracy of localization can be demonstrated with a small metal bead that is taped onto the skin before two orthogonal-projection mammograms are taken. The depth of the lesion can be estimated from a suitable tangential view of the breast. However, by inserting a needle instead of placing a metal bead one can more precisely take the depth of the lesion into account. Before removing the needle in the operating room, a dye like methylene blue can be injected to help the surgeon to find the suspected region intraoperatively. This method was used in our department for many years before we changed to wire marking (Fig. 15.5). A major disadvantage is the possible displacement of the needle on the way from the radiology department to the operating room or during preparation for surgery. Furthermore, if the dye is injected long before transport of the patient it may have diffused or resorbed by the time of the operation. The dye may be mixed with a radiopaque contrast agent to confirm the localization of the dye mammographically.

15.3.2 Charcoal Marking

A 4% charcoal solution in water is used to create a track between the lesion and the skin to guide the surgeon to the lesion. This method has been developed by SVANE (1983). Its main advantage is that the localization procedure can be done even several days in advance, for instance at the time of stereotactic fine-needle biopsy of a lesion that has to be removed irrespective of the result of cytology. Though this method is not widely used, it probably deserves further dissemination (POTCHEN et al. 1991; LANGLOIS and CARTER 1991). At the time of writing, charcoal injection has not been approved for use in the United States by the Food and Drug Administration.

15.3.3 Guide Wire Marking

The most widespread method of marking a nonpalpable lesion today is by guide wire (KOPANS and DELUCA 1980; MEYER and KOPANS 1982;

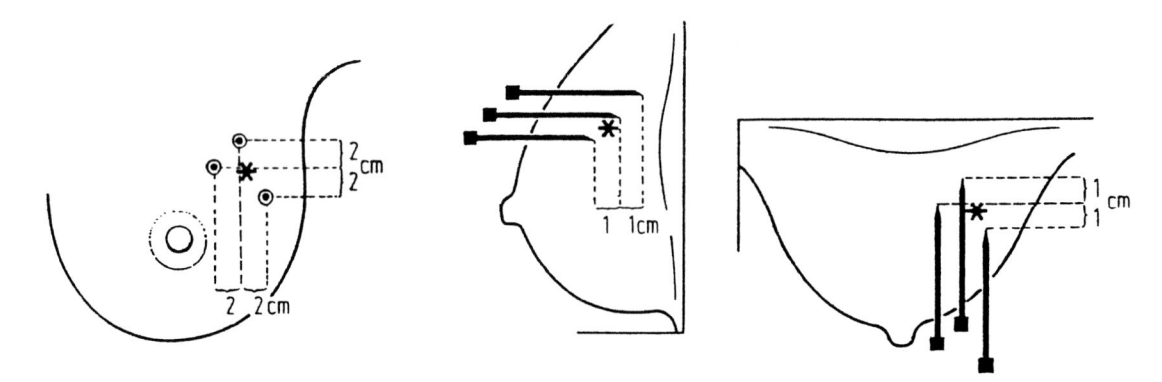

Fig. 15.5. Needle and dye marking of a lesion after geometric localization from two perpendicular mammograms. Three needles are introduced 2 cm apart at the estimated site of the lesion (*left*). The needle closest to the lesion is chosen from two perpendicular mammograms and dye is injected immediately preoperatively

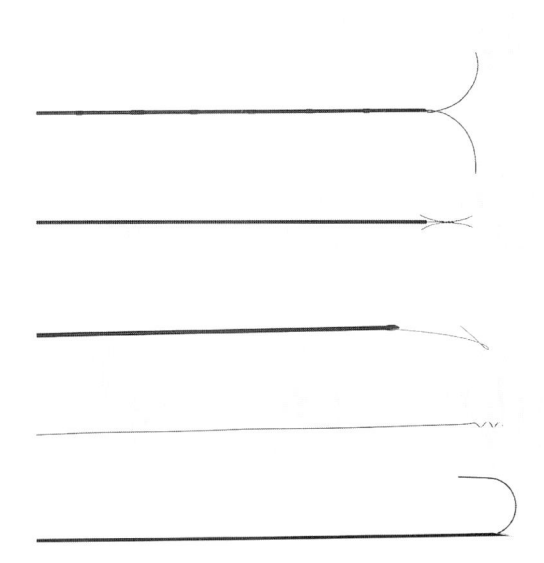

Prebiopsy Localization of Nonpalpable Breast Lesions

Fig. 15.6. A selection of localization wires. *From top to bottom:* BIP-Fixmarker, X-Reidy, Kopans type spring-hook wire, BIP-Twistmarker, Homer J-wire

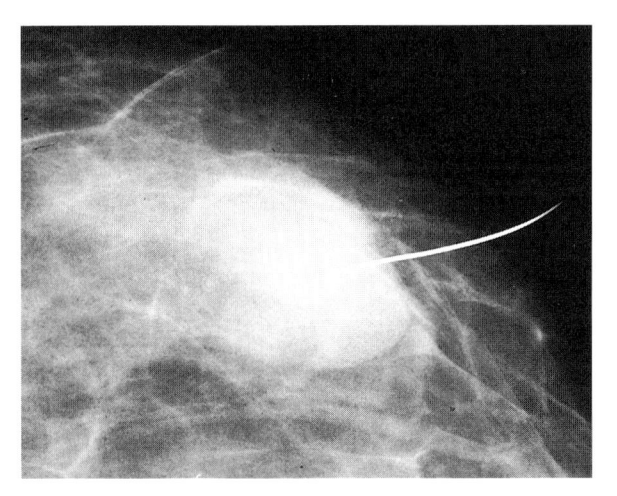

Fig. 15.7. A fibroadenoma localized with a BIP-Twistmarker using a 13-G coaxial system under ultrasonic guidance

(DAVIS et al. 1988). This complication seems to occur especially when a hook wire engages in muscular tissue. The wire should be resistant to cutting by scalpel or scissors. Thin wires may be cut without any remarkable effort of the surgeon (HOMER 1983a). It may then be difficult to find the small pieces of wire in the wound (Fig. 15.9). The hook

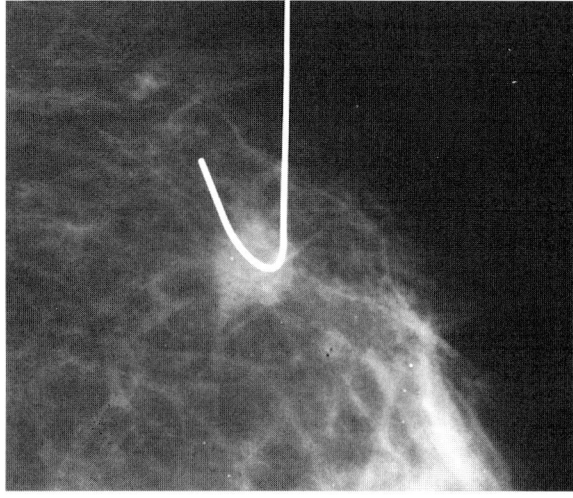

Fig. 15.8. A small invasive carcinoma localized using a Homer J-wire under stereotactic guidance

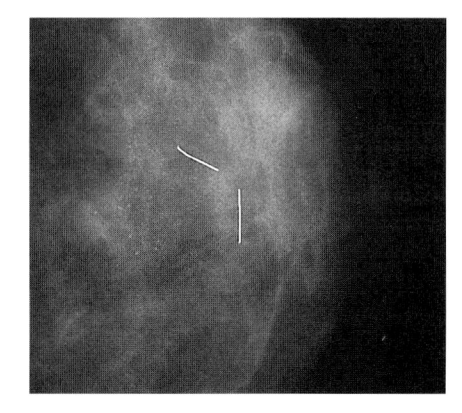

Fig. 15.9. Two pieces of localization wire that were left in the breast at localization biopsy

Table 15.1. Demands on a localization wire system

Resistance to inadvertent retraction in the breast irrespective of the breast texture (fatty or fibrous)
Resistance to forward dislocation of hook wires
Resistance to cutting of wire by scalpel or scissors
Resistance to inadvertent breaking of the hook wire tip
Stiffness for easy palpation of the wire during surgery
Flexibility for patient comfort if localization is done a considerable time before surgery

HOMER 1983b). This method has the advantage that the surgeon has a visible and palpable guide that leads him to the lesion. There are several kinds of localization wires on the market (Figs. 15.6–15.8), showing that it is difficult to meet all user demands, which are sometimes contradictory (Table 15.1): The wire tip should anchor firmly in the breast tissue irrespective of its fatty or fibrous texture, so that it is not inadvertently removed during transportation or during preoperative cleansing of the surgical site. It also should not move forward with a ratchet effect

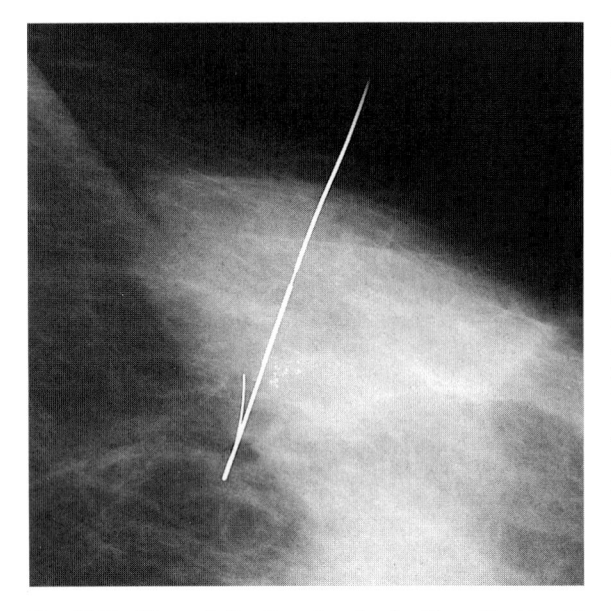

Fig. 15.10. Microcalcifications localized with a Hawkins II wire

should not break if the surgeon inadvertently pulls on the wire (BRONSTEIN et al. 1988). The wire should be stiff to ease palpation of the tip during surgery, especially if the lesion is not approached along the wire path (deeply and centrally located lesion). This can be accomplished by a stiffening cannula, which is slid over the wire before the operation (KWASNIK et al. 1987). If the interval between the localization and surgery is short, the same effect can be achieved by leaving in situ the guiding cannula used to introduce the wire (HOMER 1988).

We now use a hook wire with a flexible cable attached to it (URRUTIA et al. 1988; Fig. 15.10). This has been proven to hold fast in breast tissues of different texture (CZARNECKI et al. 1992). In order to prevent forward movement, the remaining end of the cable is taped firmly to the breast using a sterile foil. The woman is also asked to wear a bra during the night if the localization is done the day before surgery. The surgeon is given a sketch of the breast with an exact indication of the position of the wire and the lesion.

If the lesion is situated peripherally in the breast, the surgeon may easily follow the wire to its tip. If, however, the lesion is centrally located, it is more appropriate to make the incision over the presumed localization of the lesion and then to search for the wire tip within the breast.

It is important that the lesion has been adequately worked up before localization is scheduled. This helps to reduce the number of cancellations that occur because the presumed lesion shows a benign appearance during localization (MEYER et al. 1988). Equivocal lesions may be seen to be benign on the additional views that are taken as part of a complete breast imaging workup. Indeed, an apparent lesion may have been mimicked by superimposition of normal tissue structures.

For reasons of cost-efficiency, localization biopsy in the United States is usually performed on an outpatient basis using local anesthesia (HOMER et al. 1984; SMITH-BEHN and GHANI 1987; NORTON et al. 1988). This, however, should not affect the results negatively, as has been reported (RISSANEN 1993).

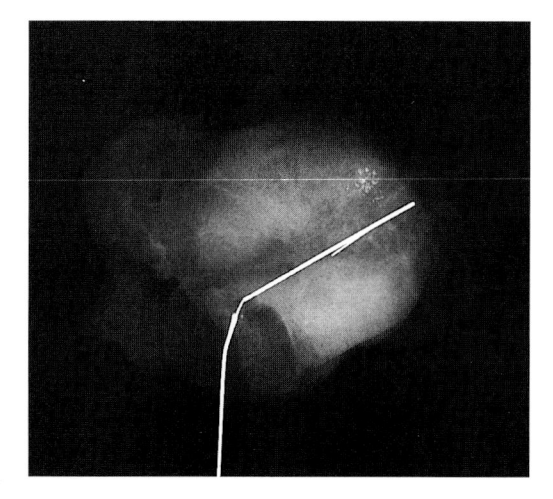

Fig. 15.11. Specimen radiography with the wire in situ. If the specimen is adequately marked with sutures or by other means, directed additional resection is possible if the lesion extends to the margin of resection

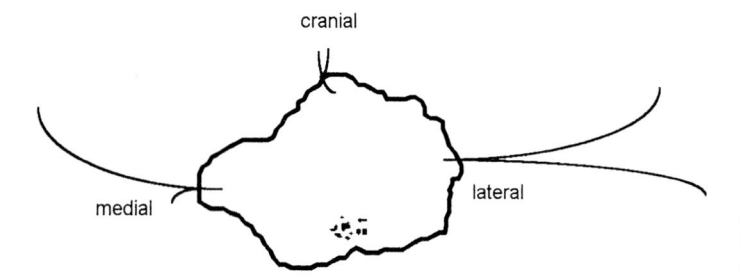

Fig. 15.12. Marking of a specimen with three sutures. This allows for reproducible orientation of the specimen at radiography

The surgeon may choose to approach the lesion from an incision directly above it, not necessarily following a guide wire that is introduced parallel to the chest wall. For confirmation of the removal of the lesion, a specimen x-ray should always be done (Figs. 15.11, 15.12), i.e., not only for calcified lesions. The great majority of noncalcified lesions may be identified on the specimen x-ray (STOMPER et al. 1988). If a specimen x-ray is not done, uncertainty will arise as to whether the lesion has actually been removed. Furthermore, on postoperative mammograms it may be difficult to decide whether a noncalcified lesion has actually been removed because of postsurgical sequelae such as edema, hematoma, or scar formation (KLUSEMANN et al. 1988).

References

Aitken RJ, Forrest AP, Chetty U, et al. (1992) Assessment of non-palpable mammographic abnormalities: comparison between screening and symptomatic clinics. Br J Surg 79:925–927

Bauer M, Schulz-Wendtland R (1992) Stereotaktische Lokalisation Mammaläsionen für Diagnostik und präoperative Markierung-Methodik, experimentelle Untersuchungen und klinische Ergebnisse bei 217 Patientinnen. RÖFO 156:286–290

Bronstein AD, Kilcoyne RF, Moe RE (1988) Complications of needle localization. Arch Surg 123:775–779

Brun del Re R, Stucki D, Herbst S, Almendral A (1977) Vorgehen bei mammographisch suspekten Veränderungen ohne lokalisierten palpablen Befund. Gynäkol Rundsch 17 (Suppl 1):85–87

Czarnecki DJ, Berridge DL, Splittgerber GF, Goell WS (1992) Comparison of the anchoring strengths of the Kopans and Hawkins II needle-hook-wire systems. Radiology 183:573–574

Davis PS, Wechsler RJ, Feig SA, March DE (1988) Migration of breast biopsy localization wire. AJR 150:787–788

Gent HJ, Sprenger E, Dowlatshahi K (1986) Stereotaxic needle localization and cytological diagnosis of occult breast lesions. Ann Surg 204:580–584

Goldberg RP, Hall FM, Simon M (1983) Preoperative localization of nonpalpable breast lesions using a wire marker and perforated mammographic grid. Radiology 146:833–835

Homer MJ (1983a) Transection of the localization hooked wire during breast biopsy. AJR 141:929–930

Homer MJ (1983b) Localization of nonpalpable breast lesions: technical aspects and analysis of 80 cases. AJR 140:807–811

Homer MJ (1988) Localization of nonpalpable breast lesions with the curved-end, retractable wire: leaving the needle in vivo. AJR 151:919–920

Homer MJ, Smith TJ, Marchant DJ (1984) Outpatient needle localization and biopsy for nonpalpable breast lesions. JAMA 252:2452–2454

Klusemann H, Link TM, Friedberg V, Thelen M (1988) Präoperative Lokalisation pathologischer Befunde in der Mammographie. RÖFO 149:636–641

Kopans DB, DeLuca SA (1980) A modified needle-hookwire technique to simplify preoperative localization of occult breast lesions. Radiology 134:781

Kopans DB, Meyer JE, Lindfors KK, Bucchianeri SS (1984) Breast sonography to guide cyst aspiration and wire localization of occult solid lesions. AJR 143:489–492

Kwasnik EM, Sadowsky NL, Vollmann RW (1987) An improved system for surgical excision of needle-localized nonpalpable breast lesions. Am J Surg 154:476–477

Langlois SL, Carter ML (1991) Carbon localization of impalpable mammographic abnormalities. Australas Radiol 35:237–241

Leinster SJ, Whitehouse GH, McDicken I (1987) The biopsy of impalpable lesions of the breast. Surg Gynecol Obstet 164:269–271

Meyer JE, Kopans DB (1982) Preoperative roentgenographically guided percutaneous localization of occult breast lesions. Arch Surg 117:65–68

Meyer JE, Sonnenfeld MR, Greenes RA, Stomper PC (1988) Cancellation of preoperative breast localization procedures; analysis of 53 cases. Radiology 169:629–630

Murat JL, Grumbach Y, Baratte B, Leflot P (1984) Estimation comparee des limites de la mammographie et de l'echographie en pratique senologique. Rev Fr Gynecol Obstet 79:807–819

Norton LW, Zeligman BE, Pearlman NW (1988) Accuracy and cost of needle localization breast biopsy. Arch Surg 123:947–950

Poole GV Jr, Choplin RH, Sterchi JM, Leinbach LB, Myers RT (1986) Occult lesions of the breast. Surg Gynecol Obstet 163:107–110

Potchen EJ, Sierra A, Mackenzie C, Osuch J (1991) Svane localization of non-palpable breast lesions. Lancet 338:816

Potterton AJ, Peakman DJ, Young JR (1994) Ultrasound demonstration of small breast cancers detected by mammographic screening. Clin Radiol 49:808–813

Rissanen TJ, Mäkäräinen HP, Mattila SI, Karttunen AI, Kiviniemi HO, kallioinen MJ, Kaarela OI (1993) Wire localized biopsy of breast lesions: a review of 425 cases found in screening or clinical mammography. Clin Radiol 47:14–22

Schwartz GF, Goldberg BB, Rifkin MD, D'Orazio SE (1988) Ultrasonography: an alternative to x-ray-guided needle localization of nonpalpable breast masses. Surgery 104:870–873

Smith-Behn J, Ghani A (1987) Non-palpable breast lesions: out-patient needle localization and biopsy. Postgrad Med J 63:17–18

Stomper PC, Davis SP, Sonnenfeld MR, Meyer JE, Greenes RA, Eberlein TJ (1988) Efficacy of specimen radiography of clinically occult noncalcified breast lesions. AJR 151:43–47

Svane G (1983) A stereotaxic technique for preoperative marking of non-palpable breast lesions. Acta Radiol 24:145–151

Svane G, Potchen EJ, Sierra A, Azavedo E (1993) Screening mammography: breast cancer diagnosis in asymptomatic women. Mosby, St. Louis

Tinnemans JG, Wobbes T, Hendriks JH, van der Sluis RF, Lubbers EJ, de Boer HH (1987) Localization and excision of nonpalpable breast lesions. A surgical evaluation of three methods. Arch Surg 122:802–806

Urrutia EJ, Hawkins MC, Steinbach BG, Meacham MA, Bland KI, Copeland EM, Hawkins IF (1988) Retractable-barb needle for breast lesion localization: use in 60 cases. Radiology 169:845–847

Weber WN, Sickles EA, Callen PW, Filly RA (1985) Nonpalpable breast lesion localization: limited efficacy of sonography. Radiology 155:783–784

16 Fine-Needle Aspiration and Core Biopsy

M. Bauer, P. Tontsch, and R. Schulz-Wendtland

CONTENTS

16.1 Introduction............................. 291
16.2 Methods of Localization and Targeting Aids..... 291
16.2.1 The Palpable Tumor....................... 291
16.2.2 Ultrasonography.......................... 291
16.2.3 Mammographic-Stereotaxic Guidance.......... 291
16.2.4 Guidance by Magnetic Resonance Imaging...... 293
16.2.5 Guidance by Computed Tomography.......... 293
16.3 Indications for Fine-Needle Aspiration and Core Biopsy............................ 294
16.3.1 Fine-Needle Aspiration..................... 294
16.3.2 Core Biopsy.............................. 295
16.4 Fine-Needle Aspiration or Core Biopsy?........ 297
References............................... 297

16.1 Introduction

Fine-needle aspiration cytology has been an established method in complementary breast diagnosis since the publications of Martin and Ellis in 1930. Core biopsy, however, has only recently found broader application with the introduction of automatic spring-acting puncture devices. Excellent results have been reported recently in the literature (Parker et al. 1994). The goal of both of the aforementioned interventional methods is to improve the specificity of breast diagnosis and thereby avoid unnecessary open breast biopsies with benign histology. The establishment of the diagnosis of invasive or noninvasive breast cancer preoperatively is of ever increasing importance for the individual tailoring of the operative treatment of breast carcinoma.

M. Bauer, MD, Professor, Münsterplatz 6, 79098 Freiburg i. Br., Germany
P. Tontsch, Münsterplatz 6, 79098 Freiburg i. Br., Germany
R. Schulz-Wendtland, MD, Universitätskliniken, Abteilung Gynäkologische Radiologie, Universitätsstraße 21, 91054 Erlangen, Germany

16.2 Methods of Localization and Targeting Aids

The precise localization of the target lesion plays a central role in cytologic puncture as well as in core biopsy. Basically, the methods of localization are identical for cytologic puncture and core biopsy. Results of palpation, ultrasonography, mammographic-stereotaxic methods as well as CT- or MR-imaging can serve as targeting aids.

16.2.1 The Palpable Tumor

While puncturing a palpable tumor, the target lesion is fixed between the forefinger and middle finger of one hand, while the other hand aims and guides the needle into the lesion (Fig. 16.1). An error rate of 30% due to false localization (not reaching the lesion) has been reported (Adam et al. 1989); furthermore, documentation of the needle position is not possible.

16.2.2 Ultrasonography

Ultrasonographically guided punctures are carried out tangentially to the transducer (Fig. 16.2). Even the smallest ultrasonographically detectable lesions of 3-4 mm can be aimed at safely with skilled hands. Correct positioning of the needle can be documented on a still-frame picture during the real-time ultrasonographic procedure (Fig. 16.3). The method is safe, fast, and inexpensive.

16.2.3 Mammographic-Stereotaxic Guidance

Lesions detected by mammography can be localized with dedicated breast stereotaxic equipment (e.g., TRC Equipment, Fischer Imaging, Lorad Stereoguide) as well as considerably cheaper stereotaxic add-on devices to standard mammographic units. Based on two stereo pictures the three-dimensional

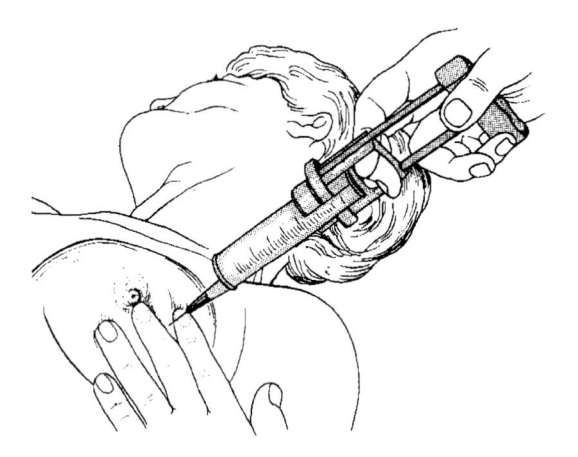

Fig. 16.1. Puncture method for palpable tumors (from BARTH 1979)

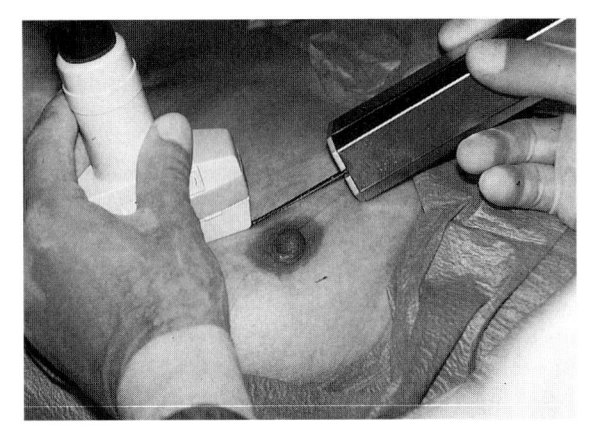

Fig. 16.2. US-guided core biopsy

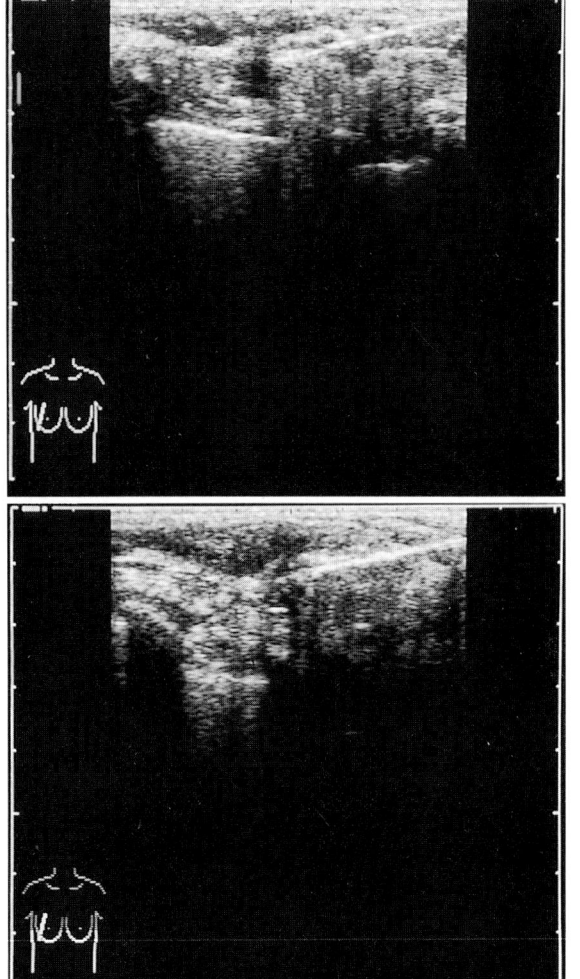

Fig. 16.3a,b. Documentation of US-guided core biopsy

coordinates of the lesion and a reference point are determined, for precise positioning of the puncturing device (Fig. 16.4). In most cases the puncture is done manually. Documentation of satisfactory needle position is highly precise in the x- and y-directions, whereas the z-axis (depth localization) has a higher failure rate due to the small stereo angle (e.g., ±15°) of the system and the considerable projective shortening of the depth distance. The precision of mammographic stereotaxis is 1 mm in the x- and y-axes. Under clinical conditions, several sources of error have to be considered (BAUER and SCHULZ-WENDTLAND 1992). In our own experience the needle deviation is less than 3 mm in over 90% of cases. Appropriate for localization are clearly defined lesions and clustered microcalcifications. One problem may arise when attempting to identify a subtle lesion (especially tiny microcalcifications) on stereo images, which are usually made without an antiscatter grid. One must be able to define the position of the lesion on both stereo pictures exactly. Input errors when identifying the lesion on the stereo pictures are extended disproportionately during calculation of the three-dimensional coordinates of the lesion, especially with regard to depth localization (z-axis).

The stereotaxic method enables localization of abnormalities visible primarily in one plane in mammography. Whereas stereotaxic localization with conventional film-screen technique may be rather time-consuming, newer digital equipment will enable control of the lesion position in a matter of seconds and noticeably reduce the time needed for the examination.

Fine-Needle Aspiration and Core Biopsy

Fig. 16.4. a Stereotaxically guided core biopsy. **b** Scheme of stereotaxic localization. The localization of the lesion is directly depicted in its x- and y-coordinates on the stereo images, whereas the depth localization (z-axis) is calculated from the lateral shift of the lesion in both stereotaxic images. The projection axis is tilted to either side by an angle of 15° (the stereo angle)

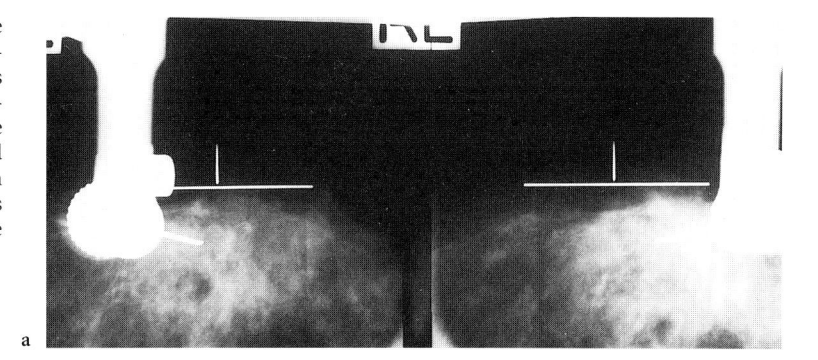

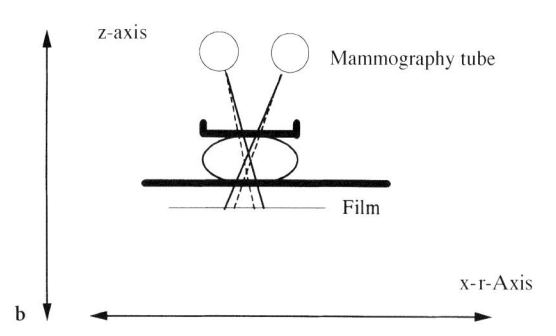

16.2.4 Guidance by Magnetic Resonance Imaging

Localization by MRI is now at the stage of clinical development and trial. This method is far more time-consuming and much more expensive than the other guidance systems. It is reserved for enhancing lesions recognizable only during dynamic MRI. Several prototype dedicated imaging coils are on trial for MRI-guided core biopsy, of which the method developed by HEYWANG-KÖBRUNNER et al. (1993) is more widespread. The breast to be examined is compressed between two evenly perforated sheets (Fig. 16.5). The perforated plates are at the same time a means of immobilization of the breast and an aid to guide the biopsy needle. During dynamic MRI examination the enhancing focus is localized and the needle is inserted. The coaxial needles are made either of a titanium alloy or of glassfiber in order to avoid susceptibility artifacts in the MR image. Control of the needle position relative to the lesion is achieved through thorough comparison of the slices intersecting the lesion and the needle tip. However, this slow and time-consuming control is not done in real-time and is not as interactive as with ultrasonography. On the other hand, documentation of the final needle position before and after firing of the biopsy gun is possible.

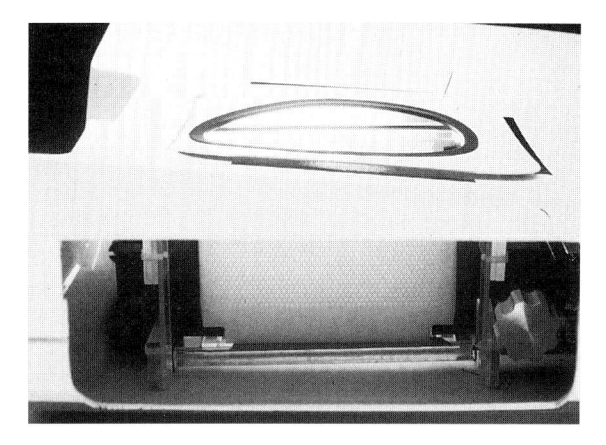

Fig. 16.5. MR coil for MR-guided core biopsy: prototype (by kind permission of Siemens)

16.2.5 Guidance by Computed Tomography

Using the same diagnostic principle as dynamic MRI (contrast enhancement of a lesion, clearly visualized after generating post- from precontrast subtraction images), CT also enables precise localization of a lesion with the patient is either the prone or the supine position. However, this procedure is currently time-consuming and only partially interactive. This may change with the future introduction of rapid spiral CT image acquisition techniques. In breast diagnosis this method has not achieved widespread use. It is of importance principally as an alternative to MRI localization and has the disadvantage of high radiation exposure.

16.3 Indications for Fine-Needle Aspiration and Core Biopsy

Fine-needle aspiration and core biopsy are carried out for the following indications:

1. Cytologic or histologic proof of the benign nature of a lesion in order to avoid unnecessary open biopsy
2. Preoperative cytologic and histologic proof of carcinoma:
   a) In order to plan the individual oncological operative approach
   b) Before neoadjuvant or primary chemotherapy of carcinoma
   c) Before primary radiation therapy of carcinoma
3. Histologic proof of recurrent breast carcinoma

16.3.1 Fine-Needle Aspiration

The goal of fine-needle aspiration is to gain enough representative material for cytologic analysis. This method also distinguishes cystic from solid lesions, except for cysts with thick, nonaspirable contents.

16.3.1.1 Technical Procedure

A hypodermic needle <2 mm (possibly thicker ones in more fibrous lesions) is put on a 20-ml syringe. A special holding device (Cameco fixture 12) allows the operator to produce negative pressure (suction) as well as safe handling. The puncture is done under sterile conditions. Local anesthesia is usually not needed. A palpable tumor is fixed between the forefinger and middle finger; for nonpalpable lesions the other aids for localization have been described in detail above. Under negative pressure the needle is moved back and forth with quick jerks in order to cut small pieces of tissue with the needle tip and suck them into the cannula. Before removing the needle the negative pressure is reduced to normal pressure so that the aspirated cells stay in the cannula. At an angle of about 35° the aspirate is carefully transferred onto a slide and smeared with a coverglass. The contents of cysts are centrifuged and the sediment transferred onto a slide. Besides cytologic examination, differential diagnosis of cysts can be accomplished by pneumocystography or ultrasonographic assessment of the inner cyst wall.

16.3.1.2 Results

Experienced cytodiagnosticians have lowered the rate of inadequate fine-needle aspiration specimens to less than 5%. In order to achieve this, at least three or four separate punctures of the lesion must be carried out. For less experienced examiners a rate of up to 30% has to be expected. Small palpable lesions are localized incorrectly in one-third of the cases. Here the method of choice is to correlate the clinical findings with real-time ultrasonographic guidance. The advantage of stereotaxic punctures is precise localization. However, due to the basic restrictions of needle aspiration, the sampling of the lesion is limited and the rate of nonusable specimens higher. In the literature this false-negative rate is reported to be between 9% and 20% (Bauer and Schulz-Wendtland 1992; Azavedo et al. 1989).

In each of two series of 1068 (Zajicek 1974) and 1745 (Zaidella et al. 1975) cases of clinically palpable tumors, more than 90% correct or correctly suspected malignant diagnoses were reported. There were 7.3% (Zajicek 1974) and 3.6% (Zaidella et al. 1975) false-negative results. Other authors reported a true-positive rate of about 90%, the rate of false-negatives varying between 8% and 14% (Prechtel and Rudzki 1973; Bothmann et al. 1974; Boquoi and Kreutzer 1974).

For 805 ultrasonographically guided punctures, Gordon et al. (1993) determined a very low (3%) rate of nonevaluable specimens. Among 225 cases of carcinomas confirmed by surgical histology and 580 benign lesions (of which 176 were confirmed histologically through surgery and 404 observed through follow-up) there were 5.3% false-negative and 7.7% false-positive results. Gordon et al. determined a sensitivity of 95% and a specificity of 92%; the positive predictive value was 15%, and the negative predictive value 98%.

Azavedo et al. (1989) reported their experience in 2594 mammographic-stereotaxic fine-needle aspirations between 1983 and 1987. In 2005 cases (77.3%) the combined mammographic and cytologic diagnosis was benign. During the subsequent observation period only one case turned out to be a carcinoma, i.e., one false-negative diagnosis in 2005 cases was found. A total of 589 (22.7%) cases were prospectively judged to need further assessment. In 22 cases (0.8%) surgical diagnosis and therapy were impossible in spite of suspected malignancy. In 567 (21.9%) women, diagnosis was histologically confirmed through surgery: In 60 (10.6%) cases pathologic though non-malignant changes were found. In 429 (75.7%) cases the suspicion of malignancy was histologically confirmed. i.e., in 86.3% surgical intervention was justified. In 49 (8.6%) cases the material obtained through stereotaxic fine-needle aspiration was not adequate; all of these women underwent surgery. The study by AZAVEDO et al. (1989) presents the most extensive experience worldwide with the mammographic-stereotaxic method and shows excellent results.

16.3.2 Core Biopsy

The goal of core biopsy is to obtain representative material for histologic examination of a lesion. This is possible due to modern high-speed biopsy devices and needles with a diameter greater than 1.2 mm. This method is suitable for diagnosis of noncystic clearly demarcated lesions.

16.3.2.1 Technical Procedure

Today, core biopsy is carried out mainly under ultrasonographic or mammographic-stereotaxic guidance. MRI-guided punctures are in clinical development.

Core biopsy uses special high-speed spring-activated biopsy guns, whose needle thrust can be adjusted between 1 and 2.5 cm. The needle diameter is between 1.2 and 2.1 mm. A cm scale on the needle surface is advantageous (see Fig. 16.1).

After disinfection of the puncture site the biopsy is carried out under aseptic conditions. The insertion site of the needle and the direction of the puncture should be chosen according to oncological considerations (e.g., location and direction of incision for breast-conserving therapy or masterctomy); during subsequent surgery, in the event that malignancy is found, it should be possible to excise the affected duct system. Under local anesthesia a skin nick is made with a scalpel and the needle is aimed at the lesion. The utilization of a coaxial cannula through which the biopsy needle is passed reduces tissue trauma and facilitates repeated tissue samplings.

Also, a marker wire can be inserted through the coaxial cannula, minimizing the risk of needle track seeding. After triggering, the core part of the needle is thrust into the lesion to the predetermined depth, using a high-speed spring-activated mechanism. The tissue volume which enters the sampling, notch of the biopsy needle is cut by the following outer cutting hollow needle (see Fig. 16.1). Between 2 and 12 tissue cylinders are usually obtained. When using ultrasonographic guidance, targeting and puncture itself are carried out tangentially to the linear 7.5-MHz transducer. The exact position of the needle within the lesion is documented before and after needle firing. Ultrasonographically, this can be done with high precision in two planes. Stereotaxic control is less exact in the depth localization (z-axis). When microcalcifications are biopsied, representative sampling of the lesion should be documented through specimen radiography.

After core biopsy, the incision is closed with steristips and the puncture site is compressed strongly. The tissue cylinders can be examined immediately by frozen section; with the technique of quick embedding the histologic diagnosis can be made on the same day.

16.3.2.2 Own Results

Since 1989 we have performed 1493 ultrasonographically guided high-speed core biopsies. i.e., 300–400 biopsies each year.

From May 1992 to April 1993 we performed 306 ultrasonographically guided core biopsies. The indication was the histologic verification of unclear or benign appearing ultrasonographically detected lesions as well as preoperative confirmation of suspected carcinoma. The average lesion size (ultrasonographically measured) was 1.68 cm (Table 16.1); five foci smaller than 5 mm and 41 foci smaller than 1 cm were specifically punctured. No infection was observed in this series. Local hematoma was seen in nine cases (2.9%). In ten cases (3.2%) there was not enough material for histologic examination.

Table 16.1. Distribution of target lesions according to size

≤5 mm	5 (1.7%)
6–9 mm	36 (12.1%)
10–15 mm	112 (37.6%)
16–19 mm	53 (17.8%)
20–29 mm	61 (20.5%)
≥30 mm	31 (10.4%)

Table 16.2. Histology of all 306 US-guided core biopsies

Histology	No. of patients
Invasive carcinoma	149 (48%)
In situ carcinoma	7 (2%)
Mastopathy (grade III)	2 (1%)
Simple mastopathy	20 (6%)
Fibroadenoma with noticeable proliferation	3 (1%)
Fibroadenoma with little proliferation	2 (1%)
Fibroadenoma without proliferation	86 (28%)
Papilloma	1 (0.5%)
Fibrosis	3 (1%)
Regular glandular parenchyma	10 (3%)
Fatty tissue/lipoid necrosis	9 (3%)
(Old) hematoma	1 (0.5%)
Lymph node	3 (1%)
Not enough material	10 (4%)

Table 16.3. Histology of the 119 benign core biopsies without operative confirmation

Histology	No. of patients
Simple mastopathy	13 (11%)
Fibroadenoma without proliferation	73 (61%)
Fibrosis	3 (3%)
Regular glandular parenchyma	10 (8%)
Fatty tissue/lipoid necrosis	9 (7%)
(Old) hematoma	1 (1%)
Lymph node	3 (3%)
Not enough material	7 (6%)

Table 16.4. Histologic results of surgery ($n = 187$)

Histology	No. of patients
Invasive carcinoma	151 (81%)
In situ carcinoma	8 (4%)
Mastopathy (grade III)	2 (1%)
Simple mastopathy	7 (4%)
Fibroadenoma with noticeable proliferation	3 (1%)
Fibroadenoma with little proliferation	2 (1%)
Fibroadenoma without proliferation	13 (7%)
Papilloma	1 (0.5%)

There was no correlation between lesion size and rate of inadequate tissue sampling (using a needle with a diameter of 2.1 mm). The diagnoses of all 306 core biopsies are listed in Table 16.2. In 119 cases (38.8%), operative verification of the lesion was not carried out on the grounds of the benign histologic result and the correlation with the other complementary breast diagnostic procedures (clinical examination, ultrasonography, mammography) (Table 16.3). Imaging follow-up at a 6-month interval and after an observation period of 18 months did not reveal any carcinoma.

A total of 187 patients (61.2%) underwent surgery in addition to core biopsy (Table 16.4). In 180 cases (96.3%) histologic diagnoses of core biopsy and surgery were identical, while in seven cases (3.7%) they were different. These cases are listed in detail in Table 16.5. There was no correlation between differing histologic diagnosis and lesion size. There were no false-positive results. However, we did produce three false-negative core biopsies (patients 1, 2, 3). These were two small carcinomas, 6 and 7 mm in size respectively, and one multicentric T2 tumor. In this latter case, there was already high suspicion of malignancy on the basis of the preceding imaging.

In summary, for the total of 306 ultrasonographically guided core biopsies we found a sensitivity of 98%, a specificity and positive predictive value of 100%, and a negative predictive value of 90%. If core biopsy diagnosis is combined with the results of complementary breast diagnostic procedures (mammography and ultrasonography) a sensitivity of 100% is achieved.

16.3.2.3 Results of Stereotaxic Core Biopsy Reported in the Literature

PARKER et al. (1994) reported on 6152 core biopsies of which 4744 were carried out stereotaxically and

Table 16.5. Seven discrepant histologic results of core biopsy and operative biopsy among 187 patients

No.	Cl/Ma/US	Operative biopsy	Core biopsy	Validation
1	Ca. T1, 6 mm	T1	Mastopathy	False-negative
2	Ca. T2 mult.	T2 mult.	Not enough material, fibrosis	False-negative
3	Ca. T1, 7 mm	T1	Not enough material, histology not possible	False-negative
4	DD Ca./fibrosis	DCIS	Ductal Ca.	True-positive
5	Ca. T1 mult.	T1 mult.	DCIS	True-positive
6	Extensive DCIS + 5 mm invasion	DCIS	Atypical growing cells, Ca. cannot be excluded	True-positive
7	Mastopathy	Mastopathy	Not enough material, no reliable diagnosis possible, open biopsy necessary	–

CL, Clinical examination; Ma, mammography; US, ultrasonography; mult., multicentric; DD, differential diagnosis; DCIS, ductal carcinoma in situ; Ca., breast cancer

1408 were ultrasonographically guided. A total of 3765 women underwent either surgical/histologic confirmation (1363 patients) or were followed by ultrasonography and mammography. The multicenter study revealed no false-positive but 15 false-negative diagnoses. Five of these false-negative results were confirmed histologically by surgery during follow-up. In 0.2% of patients, clinically significant complications were observed, which needed operative or medical treatment (three cases of hematoma requiring surgical drainage and three cases of infections).

When lesions with microcalcifications are core-biopsied, the mammographic documentation of microcalcifications in the core specimens is very important: Liberman et al. (1994a,b) showed that with microcalcifications included in the specimen the correct diagnosis was made in 81%, whereas this was possible in only 38% of cases when no microcalcifications were found.

In core biopsy a strong correlation between the rate of adequate tissue specimens and the number of tissue cylinders obtained was found. The rate of adequate tissue sampling rises from 81% taking two tissue cylinders up to 97% when six tissue samples are taken. Furthermore, adequate sampling is clearly higher in lesions appearing as circumscribed densities on the mammogram (99%) than with microcalcifications (87%) (Liberman et al. 1994a,b).

For carcinoma, Liberman et al. (1995a–c) found a positive predictive value of 98% (47 out of 48 carcinomas) with regard to the prediction of tumor invasion. The negative predictive value was 80% (12/15). When atypical ductal hyperplasia is found at core biopsy this must be considered an absolute indication for open biopsy because in about 50% of these cases carcinoma in situ is found in the neighboring tissue during open biopsy (Jackman et al. 1994).

16.4 Fine-Needle Aspiration or Core Biopsy?

For decades, fine-needle aspiration cytology has been an established method for the diagnostic assessment of clinical, ultrasonographic, and mammographic lesions. As with core biopsy, this tissue sampling method should be carried out under guidance using one of the modern imaging modalities. Within the scope of screening projects and in combination with mammographic diagnosis, this method has yielded excellent results when performed by experienced examiners (Azavedo et al. 1989). Furthermore, it is an efficient diagnostic procedure from an economic point of view (Lindfors and Rosenquist 1994). One remaining problem of this method is the relatively high rate of inadequate samples, especially in cases of the stereotaxic fine-needle aspiration cytology (Azavedo et al. 1989; Bauer et al. 1991). This can, however, be reduced considerably by taking at least four tissue samples.

Core biopsy has experienced a renaissance due to modern high-speed biopsy devices. Compared with aspiration cytology this method has a clearly lower rate of inadequate specimens. It offers the advantage of noninvasive histologic examination of a lesion. A disadvantage is the slightly higher degree of tissue trauma, which, however, can be reduced using coaxial cannulas. Today, ultrasonographically guided and mammographic-stereotaxic core biopsy has reached a stage of safe clinical application. The results published so far with this method, performed by experienced examiners, lead us to expect superior sensitivity, specificity, and positive/negative predictive values in comparison with fine-needle aspiration cytology. Through the widespread application of this method in the assessment of nonpalpable breast lesions, open biopsy can probably be avoided in the majority of cases.

References

Adam R, Falter F, Düll W, Reitzenstein M, Tulusan AH (1989) Erfahrungen mit der Drillbiopsie in der Diagnostik von Mammatumoren. Geburtshilfe Frauenheilkd 49:442

Azavedo E, Svane G, Auer G (1989) Stereotactic fine-needle biopsy in 2594 mammographically detected non-palpable lesions. Lancet 1033

Barth V (1979) Brustdrüse. Thieme, Stuttgart

Bauer M, Schulz-Wendtland R (1992) Stereotaktische Lokalisation kleinster Mammaläsionen für Diagnostik und präoperative Markierung-Methodik, experimentelle Untersuchungen und klinische Ergebnisse bei 271 Patientinnen. Fortschr Röntgenstr 156:286

Bauer M, Schulz-Wendtland R, Kommoss F, Prinz K, Richard F (1991) Small lesions in mammography: stereotactical localisation for cytological puncture and histological biopsy. Br J Radiol 64:91

Bauer M, Schulz-Wendtland R, Krämer S, Bühner M, Lang N, Tulusan AH (1994) Indikationen, Technik und Ergebnisse der sonographisch gezielten Stanzbiopsy in der Mammadiagnostik. Geburtshilfe Frauenheilkd 54:539–544

Boquoi E, Kreutzer G (1974) Punktionszytologie der Mamma. Dtsch Ärztebl 45:3229

Bothmann G, Rommel H, Kubli F (1974) Zur Stellung der Aspirationszytologie bei der Frühdiagnostik des Mammakarzinoms. Geburtshilfe Frauenheilkd 34:287

Burbank F (1994) Nine steps to a new breast biopsy paradigm. Diagn Imag May 1994: Supplement Stereotactic Core Breast Biopsy

Burbank F, Bellville J (1992) Core breast biopsy, research and what not to do. Radiology 185:639–644

Ciatto S, Catarzi S, Morrone D, Rosseli M (1993) Fine-needle aspiration cytology of nonpalpable breast lesions: US versus stereotaxic guidance. Radiology 188:195–198

D'Agincourt L (1994) Stereotactic breast biopsy invades surgical realm. Diagn Imag May 1994: Supplement Stereotactic Core Breast Biopsy

Dershaw DD, Fleischman RC, Liberman L, Deutch B, Abramson AF, Hann L (1993) Use of digital mammography in needle Localisation procedures. AJR 161:559–562

Dowlatshani K, Yaremko ML, Kluskens LF, Jokich PM (1991) Nonpalpable breast lesions: findings of stereotaxic needle core biopsy and fine needle aspiration cytology. Radiology 181:745–750

Elvecrog EL, Lechner MC, Nelson MT (1993) Nonpalpable breast lesions: correlation of stereotaxic large core needle biopsy and surgical biopsy results. Radiology 188:453–455

Evans WP, Cade SH (1989) Needle localisation and fine-needle aspiration biopsy of nonpalpable breast lesions with use of standard and stereotactic equipment. Radiology 173:53–56

Gisvold JJ, Goellner JR, Grant CS, et al. (1994) Breast biopsy: a comparative study of stereotaxically guided core and excisional techniques. AJR 162:815–820

Gordon PB, Goldenberg SL, Chan NHL (1993) Solid breast lesions: diagnosis with US-guided fine needle aspiration biopsy. Radiology 189:573–580

Harter LP, Curtis JS, Ponto G, Craig PH (1992) Malignant seeding of the needle track during stereotaxic core needle breast biopsy. Radiology 185:713–714

Helvie MA, Ikeda DM, Adler DD (1991) Localisation and needle aspiration of breast lesions: complications in 370 cases. AJR 157:711–714

Heywang-Köbrunner S, Schmidt F, Requardt H, Huynh A, Kloeppel R, Thiele J (1993) Prototype breast coil for MR imaging-guided needle localisation: first experiences. Radiology 189:138

Hopper KD, Abendroth CS, Sturtz KW, Mathews YL, Shirk SJ (1992) Fine needle aspiration biopsy for cytopathologic analysis: utility of syringe handles, automated guns, and the nonsuction mehod. Radiology 185:819–824

Jackman RJ, Nowels KW, Shepard MJ, Finkelstein SI, Marzoni FA (1994) Stereotaxic large-core needle biopsy of 450 nonpalpable breast lesions with surgical correlation in lesions with cancer or atypical hyperplasia. Radiology 193:91–95

Jackson VP, Reynolds HE (1991) Stereotaxic needle core biopsy and fine-needle aspiration cytologic evaluation of nonpalpable breast lesions. Radiology 181:633–634

Kopans DB (1993) Review of stereotaxic large-core needle biopsy and surgical biopsy results in nonpalpable breast lesions. Radiology 189:665–666

Kopans DB (1994) Caution on core. Radiology 193:325–328

Liberman L, Evans WP, Dershaw DD, Deutch BM, Abramson AF, Hann LE (1994a) Radiography of microcalcifications in stereotaxic mammary core biopsy specimens. Radiology 190:223–225

Liberman L, Dershaw DD, Rosen PP, Abramson AF, Deutch BM, Hann LE (1994b) Stereotaxic 14-gauge breast biopsy: how many core biopsy specimens are needed? Radiology 192:793–795

Liberman L, Cohen MA, Dershaw DD, Abramson AF, Hann LE, Rosen PP (1995a) Atypical ductal hyperplasia diagnosed at stereotaxic core biopsy of breast lesions: an indication for surgical biopsy. AJR 164:1111–1113

Liberman L, Dershaw DD, Rosen PP, Giess CS, Cohen MA, Abramson AF, Hann LE (1995b) Stereotaxic core biopsy of breast carcinoma: accuracy of predicting invasion. Radiology 194:379–381

Liberman L, Fahs MC, Dershaw DD, Bonnacio E, Cohen MA, Abramson AF, Hann LE (1995c) Impact of stereotaxic core breast biopsy on cost of diagnosis. Radiology 195:633–637

Lindfors KK, Rosenquist CJ (1994) Needle core biopsy guided with mammography: a study of cost-effectiveness. Radiology 190:217

Logan-Young WW (1994) Core biopsy would save $1 billion a year. Diagn Imag May 1994: Supplement Stereotactic Core Breast Biopsy

Logan-Young WW, Janus JA, Destounis SV, Hoffman NY (1994) Appropriate role of core breast biopsy in the management of probable benign lesions. Radiology 190:313–314

Lovin JD, Sinton EB, Burke BJ, Reddy VVB (1994) Stereotaxic core breast biopsy: value of providing tissue for flow cytometric analysis. AJR 162:609–612

Martin HE, Ellis EB (1930) Biopsy by needle puncture and aspiration. Ann Surg 92:169

Mittnick JS, Vasquez MF, Roses DF, Harris MN, Schechter S (1992) Recurrent breast cancer: stereotaxic localisation for fine-needle aspiration biopsy. Radiology 182:103–106

Morrow M (1995) When can stereotactic core biopsy replace excisional biopsy? A clinical perspective. Breast Cancer Res Treat 36:1–9

Parker SH, Lovin JD, Jobe WE, Luethke JM, Hopper KD, Yakes WF, Burke BJ (1990) Stereotactic breast biopsy with a biopsy gun. Radiology 176:741–747

Parker SH, Lovin JD, Jobe WE, Burke BJ, Hopper KD, Yakes WF (1991) Nonpalpable breast lesions: stereotactic automated large-core biopsies. Radiology 180:403–407

Parker SH, Jobe WE, Dennis MA, Stavros AT, Johnson KK, Yakes WF, Truell JE, Price JG, Kortz AB, Clark DG (1993) US-guided automated large-core breast biopsy. Radiology 187:507–511

Parker SH, Burbank F, Jackman RJ, et al. (1994) Percutaneous large-core breast biopsy: a multi-institutional study. Radiology 193:359–364

Prechtel K, Rudzki G (1973) Histomorphologisch nachweisbare Brustdrüsenveränderungen während des biphasischen Ovarzyklus. Geburtshilfe Frauenheilkd 33:370

Rubin E, Dempsey PJ, Pile NS, Bernreuter WK, Urist MM, Shumate CR, Maddox WA (1995) Needle-localisation biopsy of the breast: impact of a selective core needle biopsy program on yield. Radiology 195:627–631

Schulz-Wendtland R, Bauer M, Krämer S, Büttner A, Lang N (1994) Stereotaxie, eine Methode zur Punktion, Stanzbiopsie und Markierung kleinster mammographischer Herdbefunde. Gynäkol Prax 18:505–518

Sickles EA, Parker SH (1993) Appropriate role of core breast biopsy in the management of probably benign lesions. Radiology 188:315

Stephens T (1994) Digital mammographic guidance speeds breast biopsy. Diagn Imag May 1994: Supplement Stereotactic Core Breast Biopsy

Stomper PC, Cholewinski SP, Penetrante RB, Harlos JP, Tsangaris TN (1993) Atypical hyperplasia: frequency and mammographic and pathologic relationship in excisional biopsies guided with mammography and clinical examination. Radiology 189:667–671

Sullivan DC (1994) Needle core biopsy of mammographic lesions. AJR 162:601–608

Zaidella A, Ghosein NA, Pilleron JP, Ennuyer A (1975) The value of aspiration cytology in the diagnosis of breast cancer. Cancer 35:499

Zajicek J (1974) Monographs in clinical cytology, aspiration biopsy cytology. Part 1. Karger, Basel

17 Imaging the Breast After Radiation and Surgery

E.B. MENDELSON and C.E. TOBIN

CONTENTS

17.1	Introduction	299
17.2	Breast Conservation for Carcinoma	299
17.3	Breast Conservation: Imaging	301
17.3.1	Pre- and Perioperative Assessment	301
17.3.2	Posttreatment Follow-up Studies	301
17.3.3	Special Mammographic Views	310
17.3.4	Ultrasonography	311
17.3.5	Schedule for Follow-up Imaging After Breast Conservation Therapy	314
17.4	Imaging After Mastectomy	314
17.5	Advanced Cancer and Inflammatory Cancer	316
17.6	Conclusion	316
	References	317

17.1 Introduction

The breast is one of the most common sites of surgical procedures. About 183 000 new breast carcinomas will have been diagnosed during 1995 in the United States (WINGO et al. 1995). If this number represents 20%–40% of surgical breast biopsies, the total number of surgical procedures approximates 500 000 although the number of surgical procedures for biopsy may diminish with the rise in utilization of percutaneous core and fine-needle aspiration biopsy (FNAB) (LIBERMAN et al. 1995; RUBIN et al. 1995). It is important for radiologists to recognize postsurgical alterations and be aware that they may overlap with the radiographic features of malignancy.

Postoperative changes may be seen after benign biopsy as well as lumpectomy for carcinoma. Masses (fluid collections), architectural distortion and scarring, edema, skin thickening, and dystrophic calcifications occur after all surgical procedures (SICKLES and HERZOG 1981). Except for the development of dystrophic calcifications (Fig. 17.1), within the first year after benign biopsy these changes frequently resolve completely or with minor architectural distortion or scarring remaining. These alterations in the breast are accentuated and notably prolonged by radiation therapy. For analysis to be accurate, the mammograms must be placed in temporal context and correlated with the physical findings and procedures that have been performed. Errors will be avoided and the possibility of recurrent carcinoma can be suggested with greater confidence if mammograms are evaluated in sequence, always comparing with the earliest posttreatment study, not just the most recent examination. The preoperative study and specimen radiograph should also be reviewed along with the pathology report whenever available. When this is done, postsurgical and radiation changes are less likely to be misinterpreted as malignant, which is important in avoiding unnecessary biopsy of irradiated tissues in which the healing process may be disturbed.

17.2 Breast Conservation for Carcinoma

In the past two decades, breast cancer therapy has changed dramatically. For eligible women, equivalent survival rates have been demonstrated for breast conservation therapy (wide tumor excision and radiation therapy) and mastectomy (FISHER et al. 1985, 1993). Tumor recurrence varies from 6% to 10%, at rates reported as 1% to 2% or more per year after treatment (BARR et al. 1989; DUBOIS et al. 1990; FISHER et al. 1985; HAFFTY et al. 1989; STEHLIN et al. 1987; STOMPER and GELMAN 1989; STOMPER et al. 1987). In the first 7 years, the tumor generally recurs near the lumpectomy site, the mean time to recurrence being 3 years. Thereafter, tumor is found increasingly in other quadrants. The conservatively treated breast cancer patient with recurrent local tumor does not have the same poor prognosis as a patient with a mastectomy who has a chest wall recurrence. Salvage mastectomy to treat recurrence af-

---

E.B. MENDELSON, MD, Director, Mammography and Women's Imaging, Department of Radiology, The Western Pennsylvania Hospital, 4800 Friendship Avenue, Pittsburgh, PA 15224, USA
C.E. TOBIN, MD, Nassau Radiologic Group, P.C., 120 Mineola Blvd., Mineola, NY 11501, USA

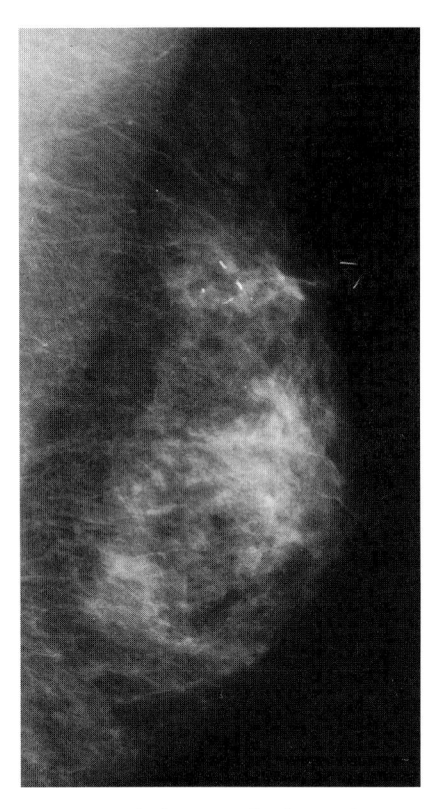

Fig. 17.1. Calcifications after benign biopsy. The biopsy site is marked with wire taped to the skin. One year after the procedure, coarse linear calcifications similar to secretory calcifications have developed

ter lumpectomy and radiation therapy does not jeopardize a patient's survival expectations. In some cases, the recurrent carcinoma has been reexcised without sacrificing the breast.

Careful selection and staging of patients for breast conservation therapy are important for optimal outcomes (RECHT et al. 1989; SUNDERLAND and MCGUIRE 1990). Although eligibility criteria may vary somewhat, candidates for lumpectomy and irradiation will have tumors less than 5 cm (T1 or T2), although most eligible tumors have been smaller than 4–4.5 cm (FISHER et al. 1985; NIH Consensus Conference 1991). Positive axillary lymph nodes are not a contraindication. An important selection criterion is that the tumor be removed with satisfactory cosmesis. Excision of a large tumor from a small breast may result in breast deformity and a poor cosmetic effect. No location in the breast is an absolute contraindication to breast conservation therapy. Retroareolar lesions require removal of the nipple-areolar complex, and for some patients, mastectomy may be preferable. Women with multicentric masses or diffuse, widespread malignant-appearing microcalcifications are not good candidates for lumpectomy and radiation therapy (NIH Consensus Conference 1991; SINGLETARY and MCNEESE 1988; SOLIN et al. 1990).

Breast conservation that requires radiation therapy is not an option for patients who are in the first and second trimesters of pregnancy. If lumpectomy is performed in the third trimester, the breast can be irradiated after delivery. Women who have collagen vascular disease are at risk of breast fibrosis after radiation therapy (HAFFTY et al. 1989; HARRIS et al. 1987; ROBERTSON et al. 1991). In patients who have previously had radiation therapy to an area that has included the breast, such as for Hodgkin's disease, irradiation for breast carcinoma results in an unacceptably high cumulative dose. Breast conservation therapy is not a good choice for debilitated patients for whom the long commitment to therapy would be a hardship. Those women who do not wish to undergo lumpectomy and radiation therapy should be offered other treatments.

Radiologists have primary responsibility for breast cancer patients in making the diagnoses of nonpalpable lesions, in assessing extent of disease radiographically to determine eligibility for breast conservation, in performing precise preoperative localizations, in careful interpretation of specimen radiographs correlated with mammograms, and in analyzing sequential follow-up studies after tumor removal and radiation therapy (MENDELSON 1992; PAULUS 1984; SADOWSKY et al. 1990). Radiologists are asked to make timely diagnoses of recurrent tumor, but are also obliged not to recommend unnecessary biopsies for postprocedural changes. For interpretation to be accurate, the radiographic findings must be correlated with the clinical history, the surgical procedures that have been performed, and the time intervals that have elapsed.

Although other procedures, such as segmentectomy, currently being reconsidered in the United States (JOHNSON et al. 1995), are performed in Europe, the *lumpectomy* or *wide excisional biopsy* is the most common operation used in the United States for breast conservation. Lumpectomy is ordinarily accomplished by means of a curvilinear incision made directly over the lesion, which is removed with a rim of tissue that is grossly free of tumor (Fig. 17.2) (WINCHESTER and COX 1992). If any skin is excised, it should be only a small ellipse.

In most lumpectomies, only the skin and subcuticular layers are sutured (WINCHESTER and COX 1992). The deeper layers of the surgical bed fill in gradually. Meticulous hemostasis decreases the

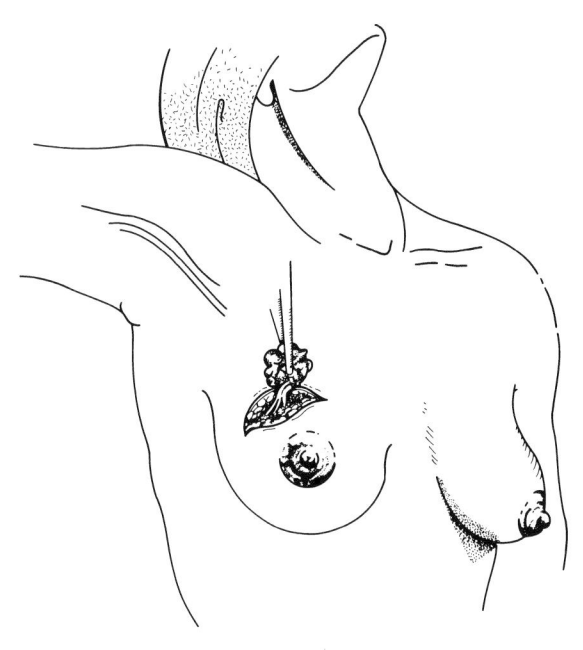

Fig. 17.2. Surgical technique for lumpectomy. A curvilinear incision is made directly over the tumor. The tumor bed is not drained, and the skin and subcuticular closure permits collection of fluid at the site, with slow resorption that helps preserve the breast contour. Axillary dissection is performed from a separate incision and a drain is placed

likelihood that large hematomas or seromas will form. Theoretically, a drain might result in formation of a crater-like cavity, and a drain is not placed in the lumpectomy site. The contour of the breast may be better preserved if fluid resorption and filling in of the surgical bed are gradual. Axillary dissection is often performed later through a separate incision into which a drain is placed.

Radiation therapy begins as soon as the surgical site has healed adequately, ordinarily 2–5 weeks after lumpectomy and axillary dissection. Between 40 and 50 Gy is delivered to the breast with an optional boost (ordinarily electron beam if available) to the lumpectomy site, bringing the total to 60–66 Gy. The axilla is not irradiated after axillary dissection.

17.3 Breast Conservation: Imaging

17.3.1 Pre- and Perioperative Assessment

To determine the appropriateness of lumpectomy and radiation therapy, mammography can be used to define the extent of the patient's disease, demonstrate multicentricity, and evaluate the contralateral breast. Mammographic analysis can further help to guide patient selection by suggesting the presence of certain prognostic indicators for tumor recurrence such as an extensive intraductal component (EIC) associated with an invasive carcinoma (HARRIS et al. 1987; RECHT et al. 1989; WINCHESTER and COX 1992). Pleomorphic microcalcifications seen within the tumor mass or stranding into the adjacent breast parenchyma are radiographic markers of EIC that should be evaluated with magnification radiography, which often shows many more calcifications and depicts morphology better than routine larger focal spot radiography.

Presurgical localization of nonpalpable masses and microcalcifications should be precise, with the tip of the hookwire or other marker usually no more than a few millimeters away from the target lesion. Specimen radiography is required to confirm removal of all presurgically localized nonpalpable and some palpable abnormalities. The specimen radiograph should be correlated with the mammogram, and an estimate made of the adequacy of the excision. Reliable assurance of a tumor-free margin cannot be obtained from specimen radiography, although if the mass or calcifications are seen at the margin of resection, in any view of the specimen, the surgeon should be advised to excise additional tissue. If the specimen is generous and the abnormality small, the radiologist can assist the pathologist further by needle-localizing the abnormality within the specimen using alphanumeric coordinates or another device. Full compression and magnification of the specimen can also increase visibility of the lesion. The specimen findings should immediately be communicated by the radiologist to the surgeon in the operating room and then reported formally (D'ORSI 1995).

17.3.2 Posttreatment Follow-up Studies

17.3.2.1 General Approach

For correlation with mammographic findings such as architectural distortion or new calcifications, scars are marked with thin wire cut to the length of the scar that are taped to the healed incision. The fine wires used for presurgical localization of nonpalpable lesions are suitable. These wires can be cut to the length of the scar and easily made to conform to its shape.

The scar may not always correspond to the area of tumor excision lying deeper within the breast (MACHTAY et al. 1994; MENDELSON 1992). It is im-

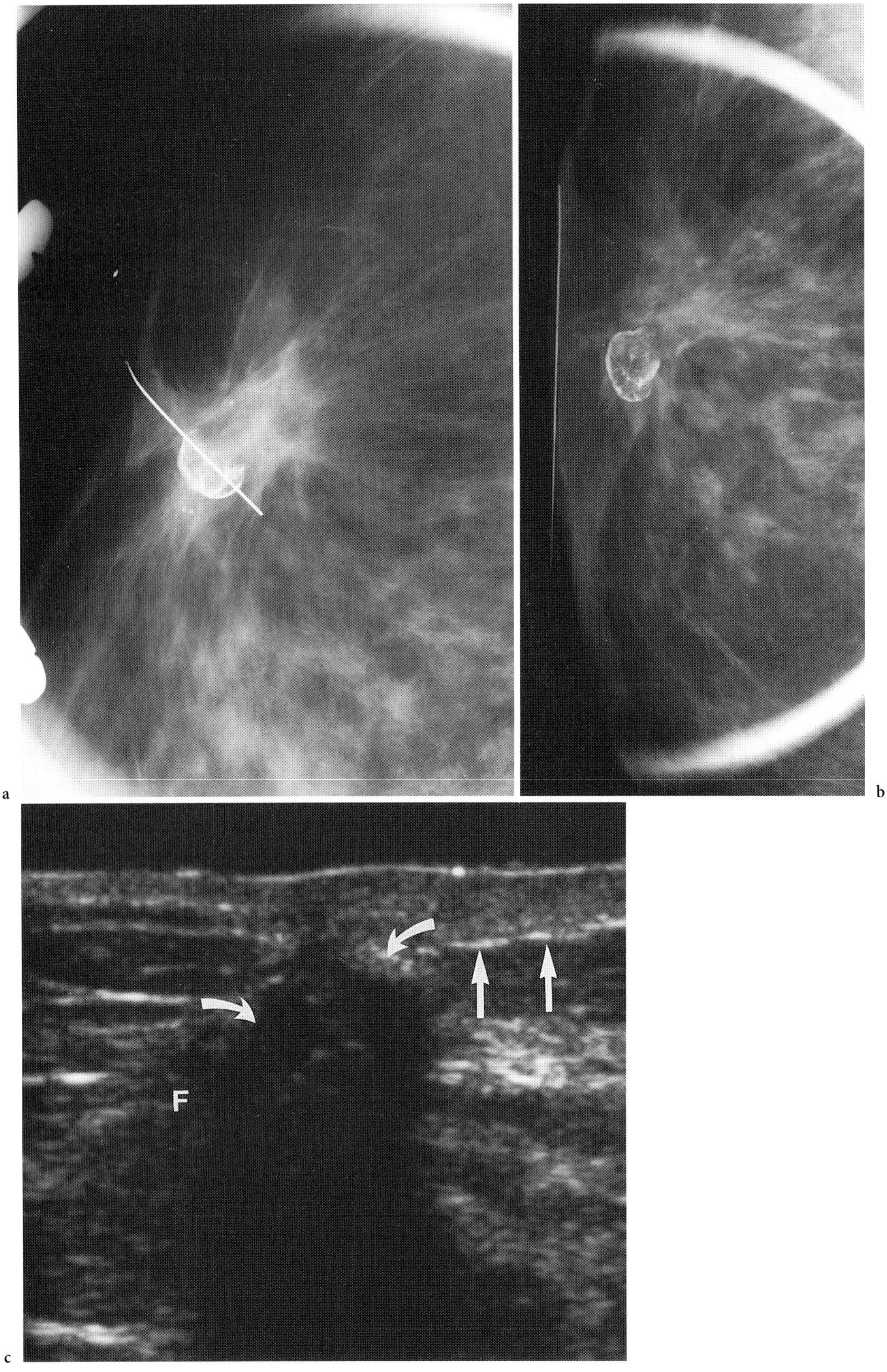
a
b
F
c

portant to identify and focus on the tumor bed because more than 65% of recurrences are at or within a few centimeters of this site (HARRIS and RECHT 1991; HARRIS et al. 1987; FOWBLE et al. 1990; MENDELSON 1992; STOMPER et al. 1987). A mammographic view tangential to the skin incision site will permit differentiation of thickened skin from the tumor bed deeper in the breast (Fig. 17.3).

Ultrasonography can be used as well to distinguish the cutaneous incision from the lumpectomy site. With ultrasonography, the surgical bed is a distinct hypoechoic oval area showing posterior acoustic enhancement if fluid is present or an irregularly shaped hypoechoic area with posterior acoustic shadowing after fibrosis has developed (Fig. 17.3).

A third method of identifying the tumor bed, helpful for radiation therapy planning and for subsequent follow-up imaging studies, involves placement of surgical clips at the margins of the tumor bed at the time of lumpectomy (MACHTAY et al. 1994). Neither clips in the breast nor wires on the skin should compromise mammographic visualization of the breast tissue. The wires also do not interfere with gadolinium-enhanced magnetic resonance, a technique under study for its applicability in differentiating mature scar tissue from recurrent tumor after lumpectomy and radiation therapy (HEYWANG et al. 1990). The wires or clips may cause only small signal-void artifacts.

17.3.2.2 Findings Expected After Breast Conservation

17.3.2.2.1 Fluid Collections. During the first year after breast conservation therapy, at the lumpectomy site, the mammogram often shows an oval mass that is fairly dense and well marginated but usually with a few spiculations or irregularities. The mammographic appearance and timing are suggestive of a postoperative fluid collection; it is unlikely that a carcinoma will regrow to larger than its preoperative dimensions within the first year, particularly if the margins of resection have been free of tumor. If there is doubt, ultrasonography can be used to identify the mass as fluid filled (Fig. 17.4).

17.3.2.2.2 Scars. As the tumor bed is imaged on follow-up mammograms during the first 6–18 months, the discrete, dense fluid collection will be replaced by architectural distortion or a spiculated soft tissue density representing an evolving scar. Areas of radiolucency representing entrapped fat are interspersed with the soft tissue density. The scar may elongate and develop jagged borders.

Because both scarring and carcinoma appear as spiculated, poorly marginated soft tissue densities on mammograms, to distinguish them, the clinical history, physical examination, and comparison with previous studies are necessary. On physical examination, scarring uncomplicated by fat necrosis is perceived as induration rather than a mass. Radiolucencies within the central area of soft tissue density suggest scarring.

Another finding observed in intramammary scars is a changing appearance in different projections. In one view, the spiculated soft tissue densities are mass-like, but they elongate in other projections.

A more reliable sign of scarring that is helpful in follow-up of the conservatively treated breast is contraction and shrinkage of the evolving scar as it matures in the first year or two. The size of the resection, volume of the postsurgical fluid collection, and whether it was drained postsurgically may affect the rate of scar formation (Fig. 17.5). After two successive studies have shown no change, recurrent tumor should be suspected if the scar increases in size or becomes more nodular (Fig. 17.6) (MENDELSON

Fig. 17.3a–c. Importance of tangential views. **a** Nontangential view of lumpectomy site 3 years after tumor removal and irradiation shows soft tissue density from the skin incision site projecting over the tumor bed. Changes, such as true increased density, size, or new nodularity, may be difficult to appreciate in this view, making exclusion of recurrence problematic. Wire taped to the skin, a calcifying oil cyst, and a few benign dystrophic calcifications are seen. **b** The lumpectomy site is seen to better advantage in the tangential spot compression view. Here the skin incision site marked by the wire taped to the skin is clearly separate from the tumor bed, which shows only fibrotic strands with some entrapped fatty tissue and the calcifying oil cyst indicative of fat necrosis. Recurrence can be excluded more confidently. The lumpectomy site should be scrutinized as the area where recurrent tumor will develop within 2.5–7 years following breast conservation therapy on average. **c** Sonogram of lumpectomy site, for correlation with mammogram, shows, in the tumor bed, the thickened skin (*arrows*) and a poorly marginated rounded hypoechoic area with posterior acoustic shadowing, the oil cyst, with calcifications in its rim and within it (*curred arrows*). The surrounding fatty tissue shows architectural distortion representing the fibrosis (*F*) seen mammographically. In addition to tangential views, ultrasonography can separate the skin incision from the tumor bed, which is easily identified

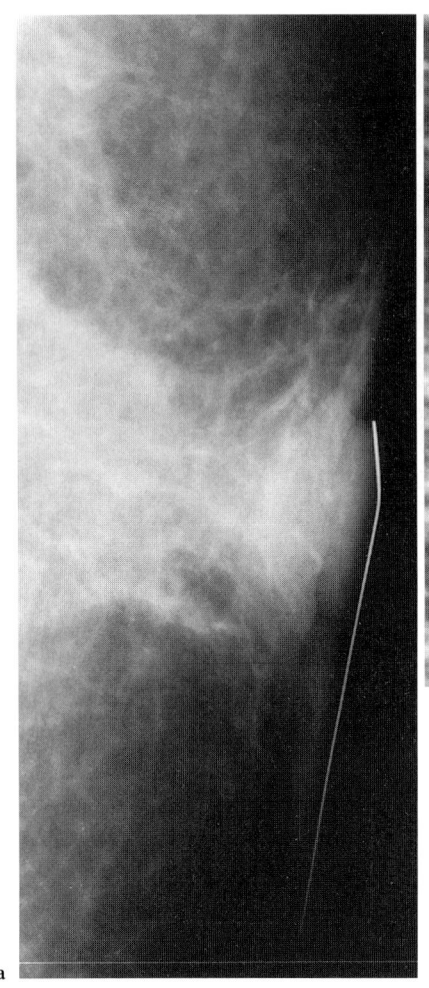

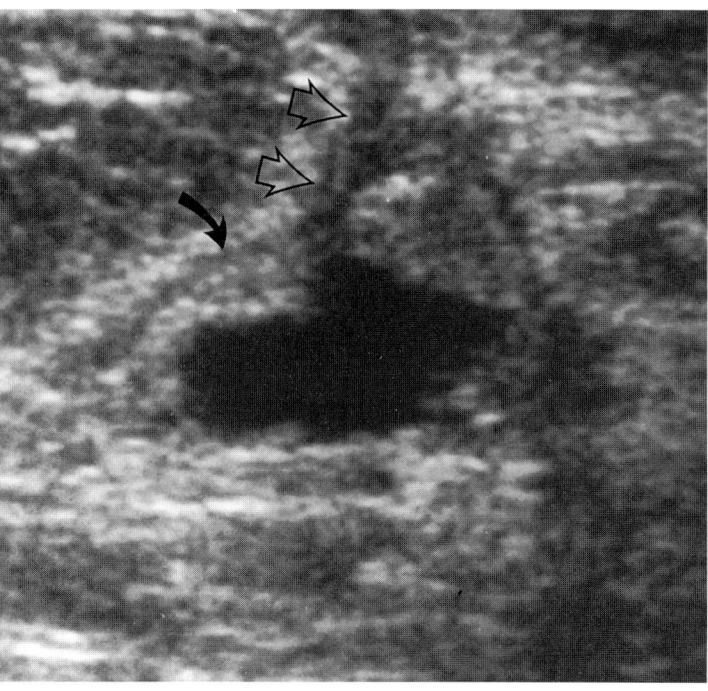

Fig. 17.4a,b. Fluid collection after lumpectomy and radiation therapy. **a** Magnification lateral tangential view of the lumpectomy site posterior to the nipple shows soft tissue density and mild breast edema. A wire is taped to the incision site. **b** Fluid collection seen in tumor bed on sonogram. A track from the incision site (*arrows*) leads to the fluid collection. Breast edema can be recognized with ultrasonography as hypoechoic angular lines (*curved arrow*) and increased echogenicity of the surrounding tissues and subcutaneous fat. The fluid resorbs during the first year to 18 months and is replaced by the scar which then develops

1992). Core biopsy or surgical excision may confirm recurrent tumor as the cause of increasing soft tissue density. Large-needle core biopsy may be preferable to fine-needle aspiration cytology because radiation therapy itself may cause cytologic atypia difficult to distinguish from neoplastic changes.

17.3.2.2.3 Edema. Nearly all patients who have had axillary dissection or radiation therapy have breast edema (Fig. 17.7). Increased breast density and thickened, stringy linear parenchymal trabeculations are seen when edema is moderately severe. The breast enlarges and adequate mammographic compression is impeded by the edema involving the parenchyma, subcutaneous tissues, and skin. These changes are most evident in the periareolar and dependent areas of the breast.

Breast edema gradually diminishes and resolves in many patients within 2 years (LIBSHITZ et al. 1978). Mild edema remains in a small percentage of patients. After breast density has stabilized, recurrent edema is a cause for concern.

17.3.2.2.4 Skin Thickening. Skin thickening and breast edema are companion findings that have similar time courses for maximal change and resolution after lumpectomy and breast irradiation. The skin's thickness may reach 1 cm or even greater in the periareolar region and dependent portion of the breast. By 2 years after breast conservation therapy, the skin has returned to near-normal thickness although mild thickening persists in approximately 20% of patients (LIBSHITZ et al. 1978; MENDELSON 1992). If the skin again thickens and the breast becomes edematous after return to the new baseline, recurrent tumor should be considered although inflammatory carcinoma is the least common form of recurrence (Fig. 17.8).

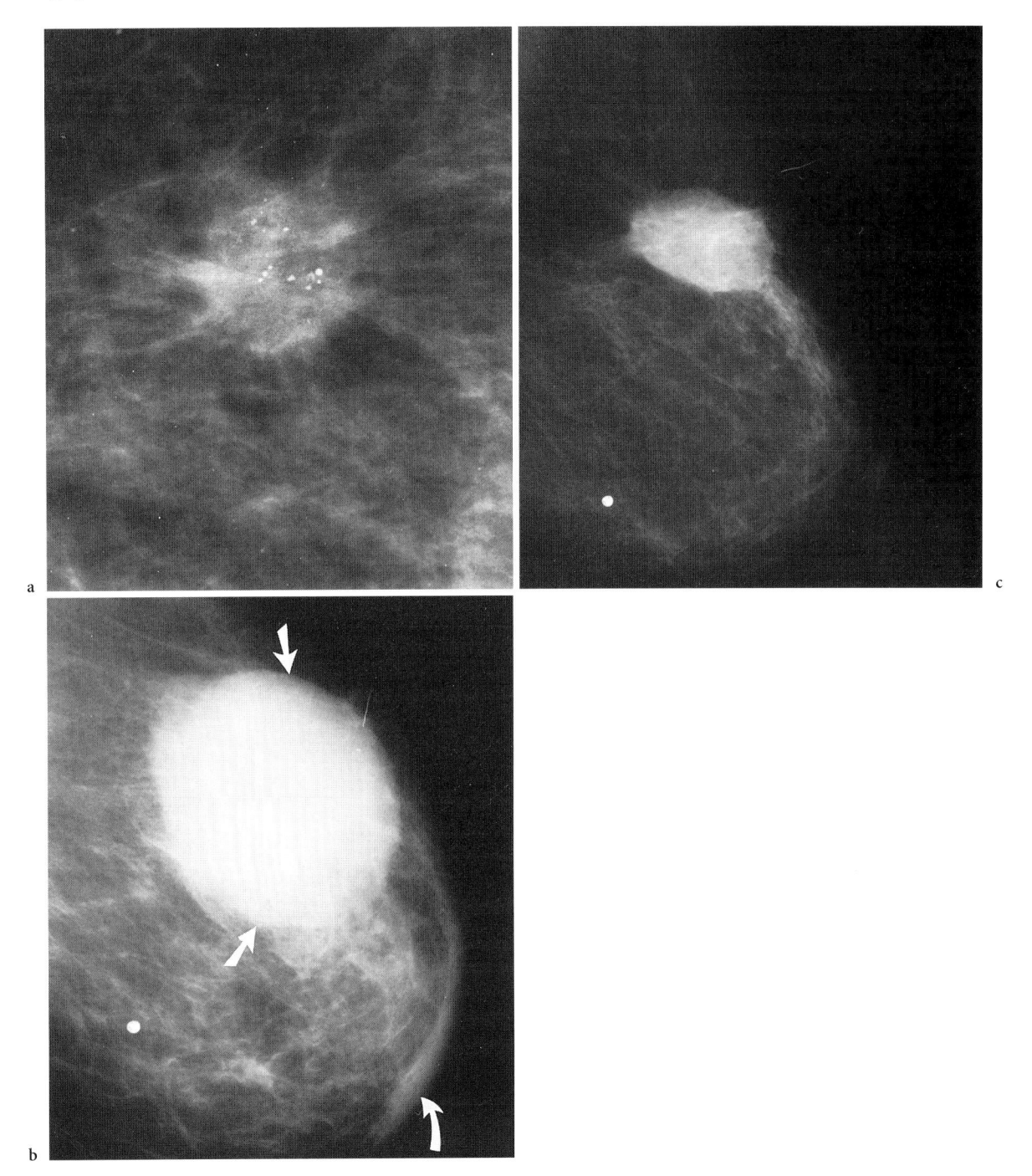

Fig. 17.5a–c. Resolving fluid collection and evolving scar. a Specimen radiograph (magnification with spot compression) shows 1-cm spiculated infiltrating ductal carcinoma containing microcalcifications representing an extensive intraductal component. b Six months after excision and following radiation therapy, there is a 5 × 6 cm oval fluid collection (*arrows*) at the lumpectomy site, marked by wire, skin thickening (*curved arrow*), and mild edema. These are typical findings at 6 months, with variability in size of the fluid collection and degree of edema. c Eighteen months after breast conservation, the fluid collection has decreased in size and density, with areas of low density probably representing oily material of oil cysts/fat necrosis. Marginal spiculation signifies development of scarring and is to be expected

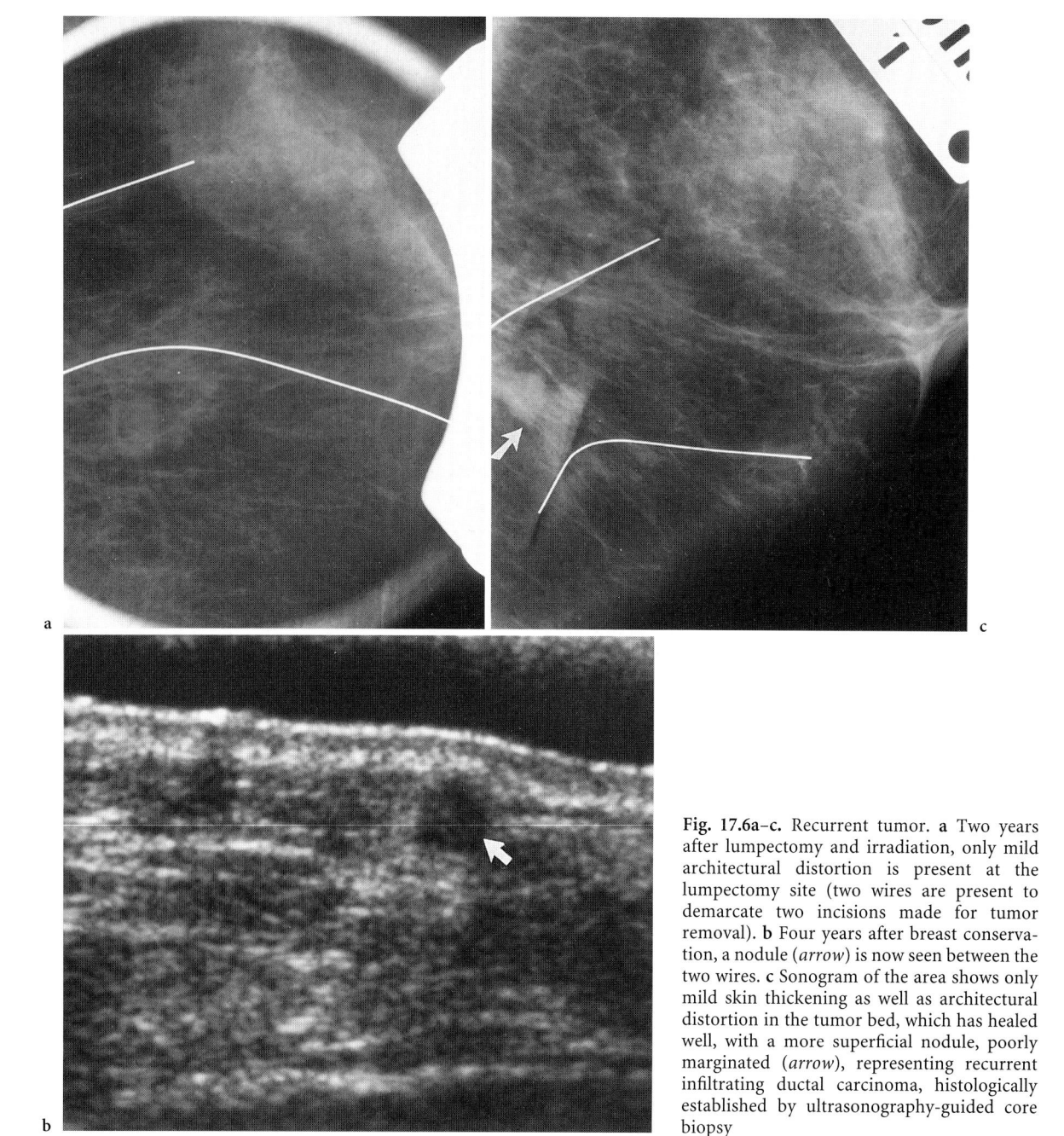

Fig. 17.6a-c. Recurrent tumor. a Two years after lumpectomy and irradiation, only mild architectural distortion is present at the lumpectomy site (two wires are present to demarcate two incisions made for tumor removal). b Four years after breast conservation, a nodule (*arrow*) is now seen between the two wires. c Sonogram of the area shows only mild skin thickening as well as architectural distortion in the tumor bed, which has healed well, with a more superficial nodule, poorly marginated (*arrow*), representing recurrent infiltrating ductal carcinoma, histologically established by ultrasonography-guided core biopsy

17.3.2.2.5 Calcifications. Calcifications are a most important marker of new or recurrent breast carcinoma. The same morphologic and distributional features used preoperatively to classify calcifications are applicable to the treated breast. Postoperative, preradiation magnification radiography should be performed to detect residual calcifications at the tumor excision site. Commonly, the surgical bed will be reexcised if microcalcifications remain (Fig. 17.9).

New calcifications occur frequently at the site of tumor excision. Several types of benign calcifications are found at the lumpectomy site. Although they will coarsen later, calcifications may be quite fine, faint, and difficult to characterize as they begin to precipitate in scars, fibrotic tissue, or areas of fat necrosis. Once residual calcifications have been excluded, calcifications that occur soon (6-18 months) after surgery and radiation therapy are most often benign.

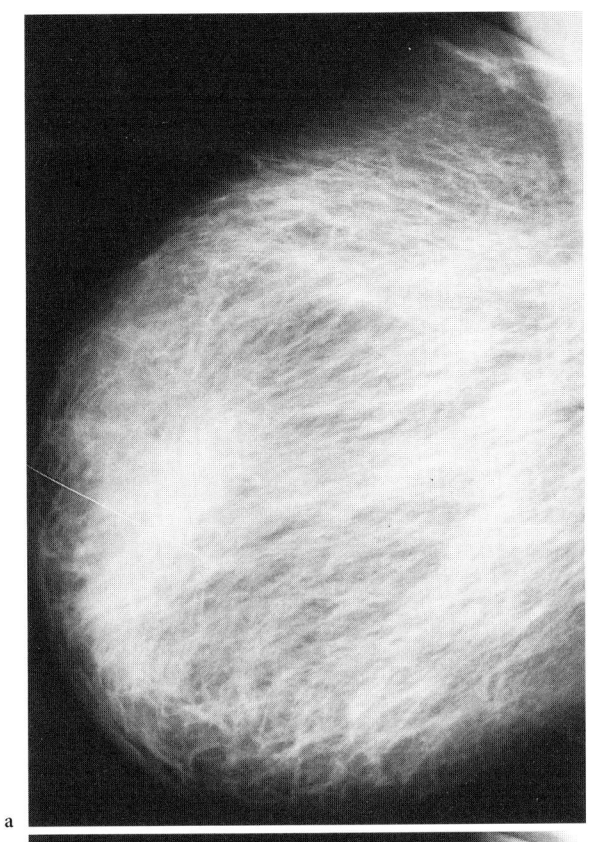

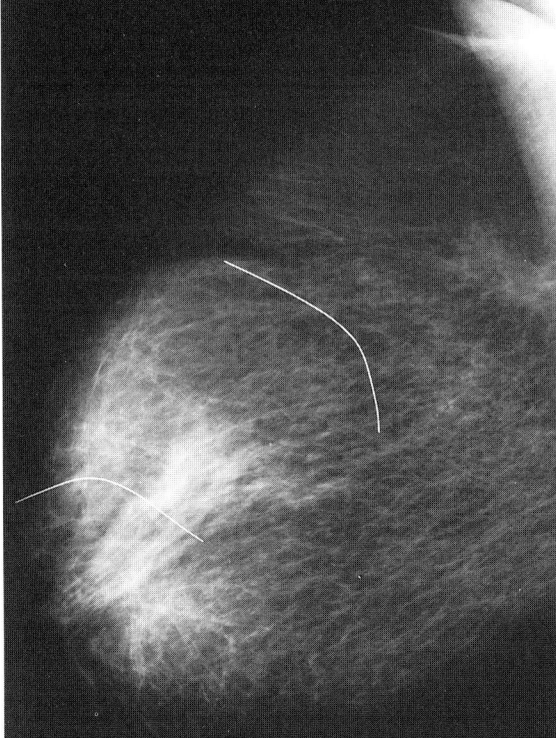

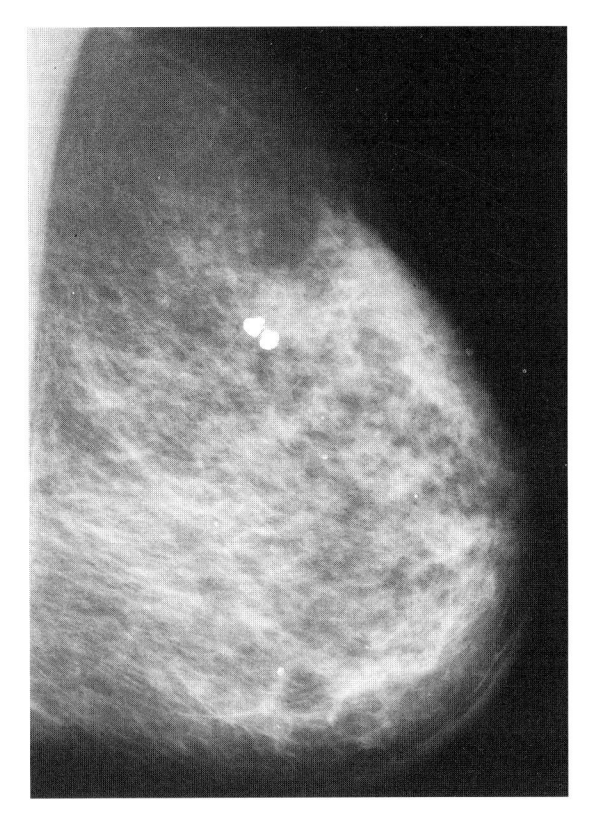

Imaging the Breast After Radiation and Surgery

Fig. 17.8. Recurrence as inflammatory carcinoma. Four years earlier, lumpectomy and radiation therapy had been performed for contralateral infiltrating ductal carcinoma with an extensive intraductal component (comedocarcinoma). After 2½ years, the tumor recurred at the lumpectomy site and salvage mastectomy was performed. One year later, shown here, the skin of the remaining breast is thickened. Mild edema was also present. Inflammatory carcinoma was diagnosed on biopsy.

Fig. 17.7a,b. Breast edema. **a** Breast edema is most marked 6 months after lumpectomy and radiation therapy. The florid edema masks the site of tumor excision, marked by a wire. The anterior and dependent skin is thickened. **b** Eighteen months later, edema has regressed, leaving a mild residuum. The anterior wire marks the lumpectomy site; the more superior and posterior wire was the site of a benign biopsy in the past. The lumpectomy site is better seen, with stranding and fibrotic change

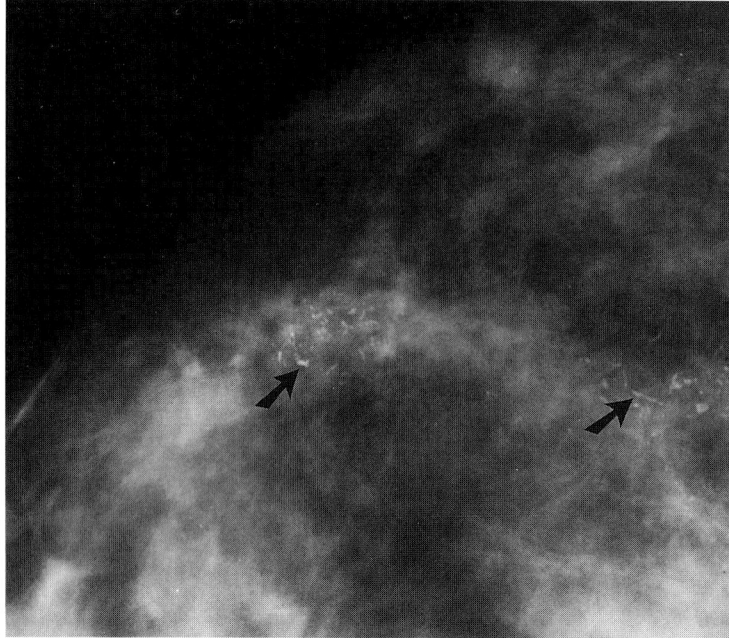

Fig. 17.9a,b. Residual microcalcifications after lumpectomy. **a** Preoperative spot compression view with magnification shows malignant microcalcifications (*arrows*) that were demarcated with two hook wires to delineate the area of involvement and then excised surgically. **b** Postsurgical preradiation view of the tumor bed shows fluid collection and scarring (*arrowhead*). A wire taped to the skin denotes the incision site. Residual microcalcifications of comedocarcinoma (*arrows*) are present anterior to the lumpectomy site. They were localized and removed prior to radiation therapy

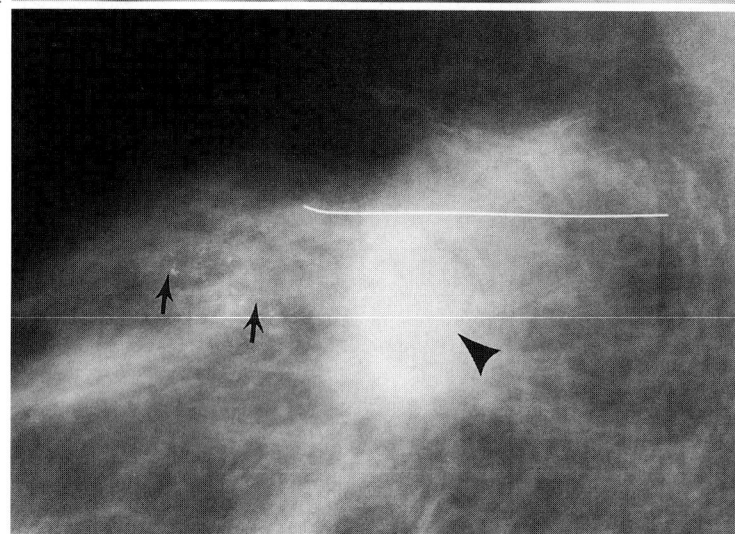

Fat necrosis is associated with all types of surgical procedures in the breast. In vague, patchy soft tissue densities, calcifications may be needle-like, of varied shapes, bizarre, disorganized appearing, and alarming. These dystrophic calcifications will become thick, calcified plaques. Thin arcs of calcification may form complete circles to define the rims of rounded, radiolucent oil cysts (Figs. 17.3, 17.10).

After tumor excision and radiation therapy, small, round, and smooth dystrophic calcifications are common at the lumpectomy site. They resemble the calcifications of secretory disease or ductal ectasia and may have a similar origin, forming in areas of necrotic tissue, sloughed cells, and cellular detritus.

Also benign appearing and somewhat less common are more coarse, plaque-like, angular calcifications. These larger calcifications are also dystrophic, developing in scars and in disturbed subcutaneous tissue.

Calcified remnants of suture material at the lumpectomy site have distinctive shapes, often containing knots (Fig. 17.11). Branching linear calcifications and double tracking may suggest malignancy, but these linear sutural calcifications can be several millimeters long and quite wide. They resemble the thick straight calcifications of ductal ectasia or secretory disease (Fig. 17.12).

Imaging the Breast After Radiation and Surgery

Fig. 17.10. Calcifications of fat necrosis. Four years after lumpectomy and radiation therapy, coarse calcifications are encircling and filling in oil cysts of fat necrosis. The central portion of the spiculated scar is fat filled, and dystrophic, benign calcifications (*arrows*) are also seen. These are typical postsurgical changes with no sign of recurrence present

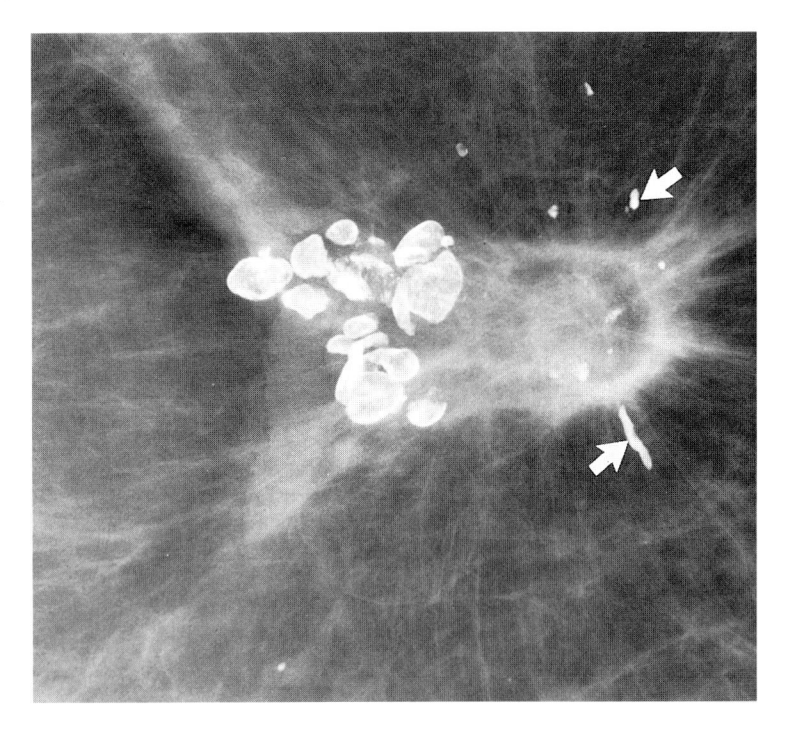

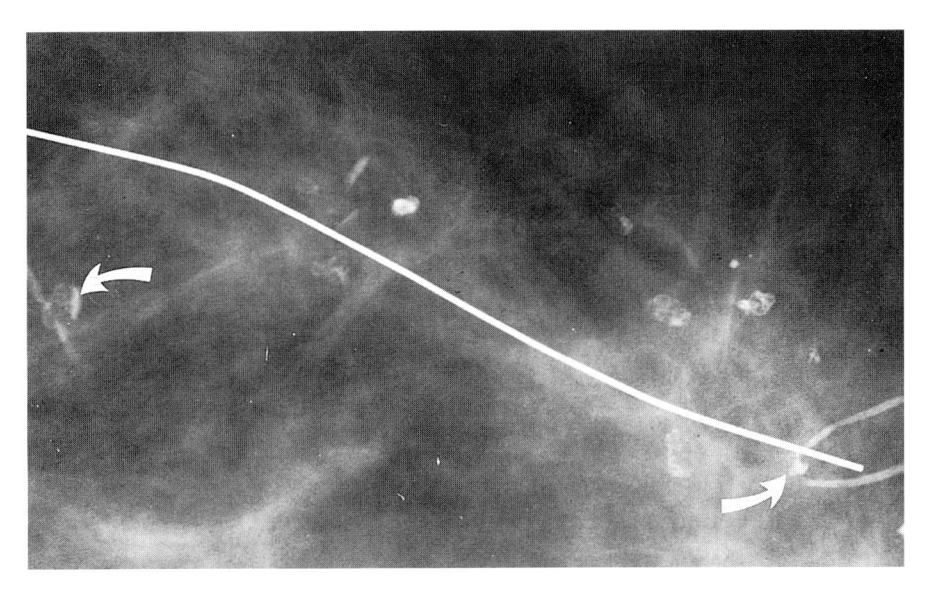

Fig. 17.11. Sutural calcifications. Calcified remnants of suture at the lumpectomy site are thick, can be long, and often contain knots (*arrows*). These linear calcifications resemble secretory calcifications and should not be mistaken for linear microcalcifications of ductal carcinoma in situ

Microcalcifications, a common radiographic sign of recurrent tumor, account for a substantial percentage of mammographically detected recurrences (REBNER et al. 1989). An active search with magnification radiography should be made for new indeterminate or malignant-appearing calcifications at the lumpectomy site.

Unexcised calcifications may or may not disappear following radiation therapy, and their persistence does not necessarily indicate viable tumor. The expectation of recurrence will be higher after excision of invasive carcinoma with EIC or with large areas of the comedocarcinoma variant of ductal carcinoma in situ (JOHNSON et al. 1995; LAGIOS 1990).

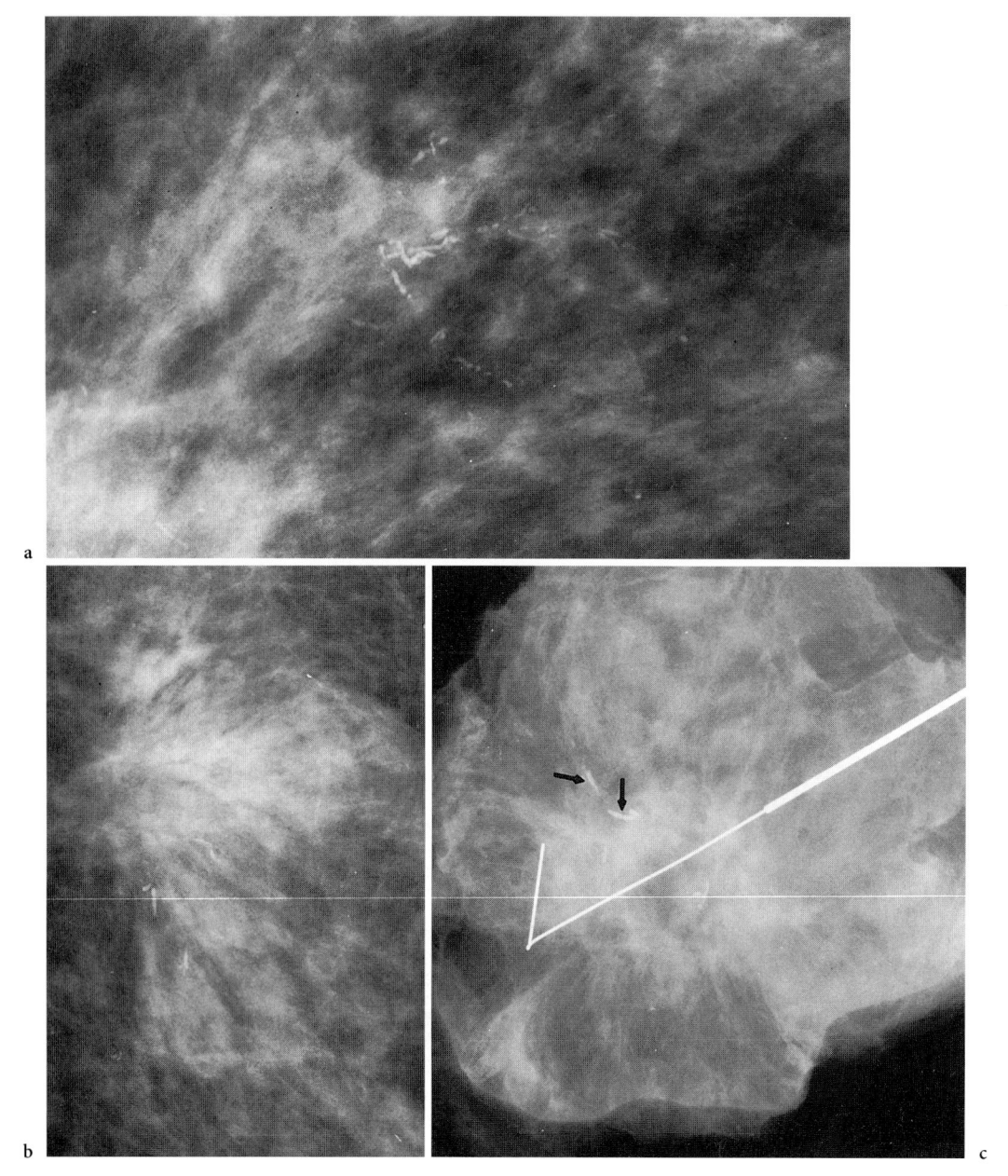

Fig. 17.12a–c. Recurrence versus sutural calcifications. **a** Preoperative spot compression view with magnification shows linear, broadening, malignant-appearing pleomorphic microcalcifications of comedocarcinoma. **b** One year later, magnification view of tumor bed obtained as part of a follow-up study shows linear calcifications considered as a possible recurrence, not ordinarily seen this soon if the margins of resection are free of tumor. **c** Specimen radiograph shows soft tissue density representing scarring. The thick linear calcifications (*arrows*) were sutural; no recurrence was present

17.3.3 Special Mammographic Views (Table 17.1)

The standard mediolateral oblique and craniocaudal views require supplementation with additional mammographic projections directed to visualization of the lumpectomy site. The scar should be marked with wire or another radiopaque marker that does not obscure the breast tissue. The area of excision should be imaged fully in two projections. A view with the x-ray beam tangential to the marker will show the skin incision in profile, separate from the deeper area of tumor excision (Fig. 17.3). This tangential view is of great value in analyzing changes at the operative site and should be standard in the follow-up of breast conservation patients. Spot compression and magnification radiography of the

Imaging the Breast After Radiation and Surgery

Table 17.1. Mammographic evaluation after breast conservation

Mark scars: wires taped to scar for correlation with
    architectural distortion
Routine views: mediolateral oblique and craniocaudal
Additional views nearly always of value:
    Tangential views to separate skin incision site from deeper
        tumor bed
    Spot compression: better compression in inaccessible
        areas
        For posterior lesions, retroareolar area
        With magnification for calcifications
Particular view depends on location of lesion (place film
    closest to lesion): e.g., mediolateral or lateromedial,
    exaggerated axillary, or medially rotated craniocaudal
    views

tumor bed should also be performed in the projection in which the surgical site is seen most completely. If the tumor has presented as microcalcifications, magnification views in two projections force the interpreter to scrutinize the surgical bed for new microcalcifications. Particularly if the surgical site is near the posterior edge of the compression plate, a small spot compression device will be useful both in fixing the area and in spreading apart the tissue elements (Fig. 17.13).

17.3.4 Ultrasonography

In the postoperative breast, ultrasonography can be used to characterize a mammographic or palpable mass as fluid-filled or solid (Fig. 17.14). Ultrasonography is an alternative method of imaging sequential changes such as skin thickening and decreasing scar size. Ultrasonography is also useful as a supplement to mammography in confirming resolution of fluid collections and evaluating the tumor bed for new, hypoechoic masses that might represent tumor recurrence.

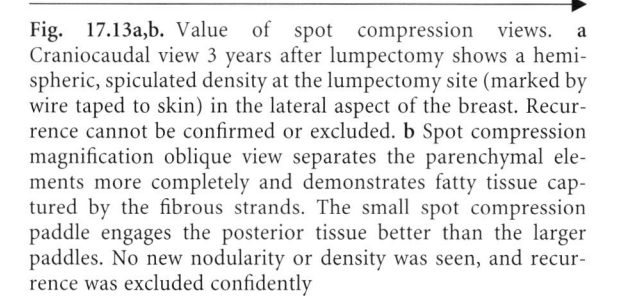

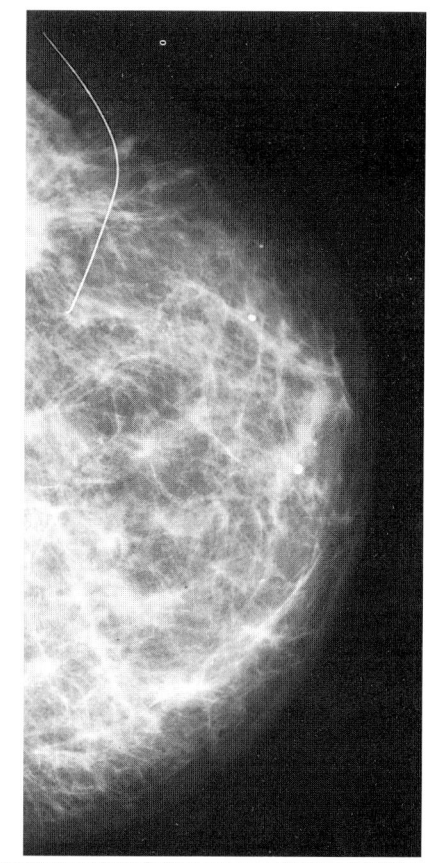

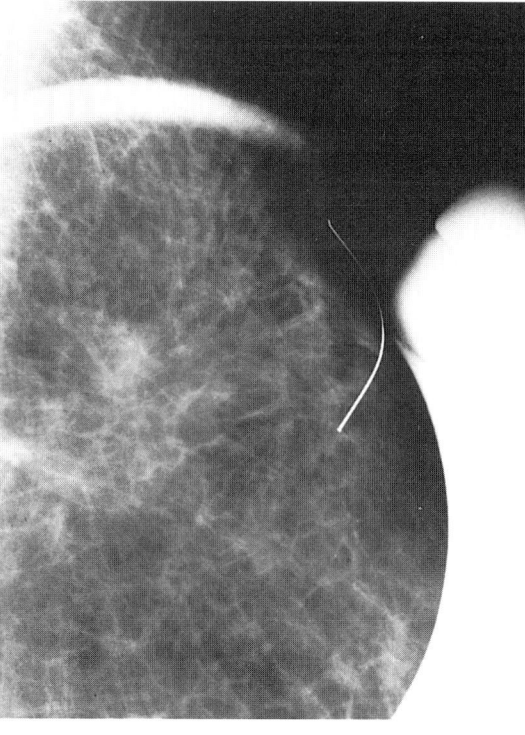

Fig. 17.13a,b. Value of spot compression views. a Craniocaudal view 3 years after lumpectomy shows a hemispheric, spiculated density at the lumpectomy site (marked by wire taped to skin) in the lateral aspect of the breast. Recurrence cannot be confirmed or excluded. b Spot compression magnification oblique view separates the parenchymal elements more completely and demonstrates fatty tissue captured by the fibrous strands. The small spot compression paddle engages the posterior tissue better than the larger paddles. No new nodularity or density was seen, and recurrence was excluded confidently

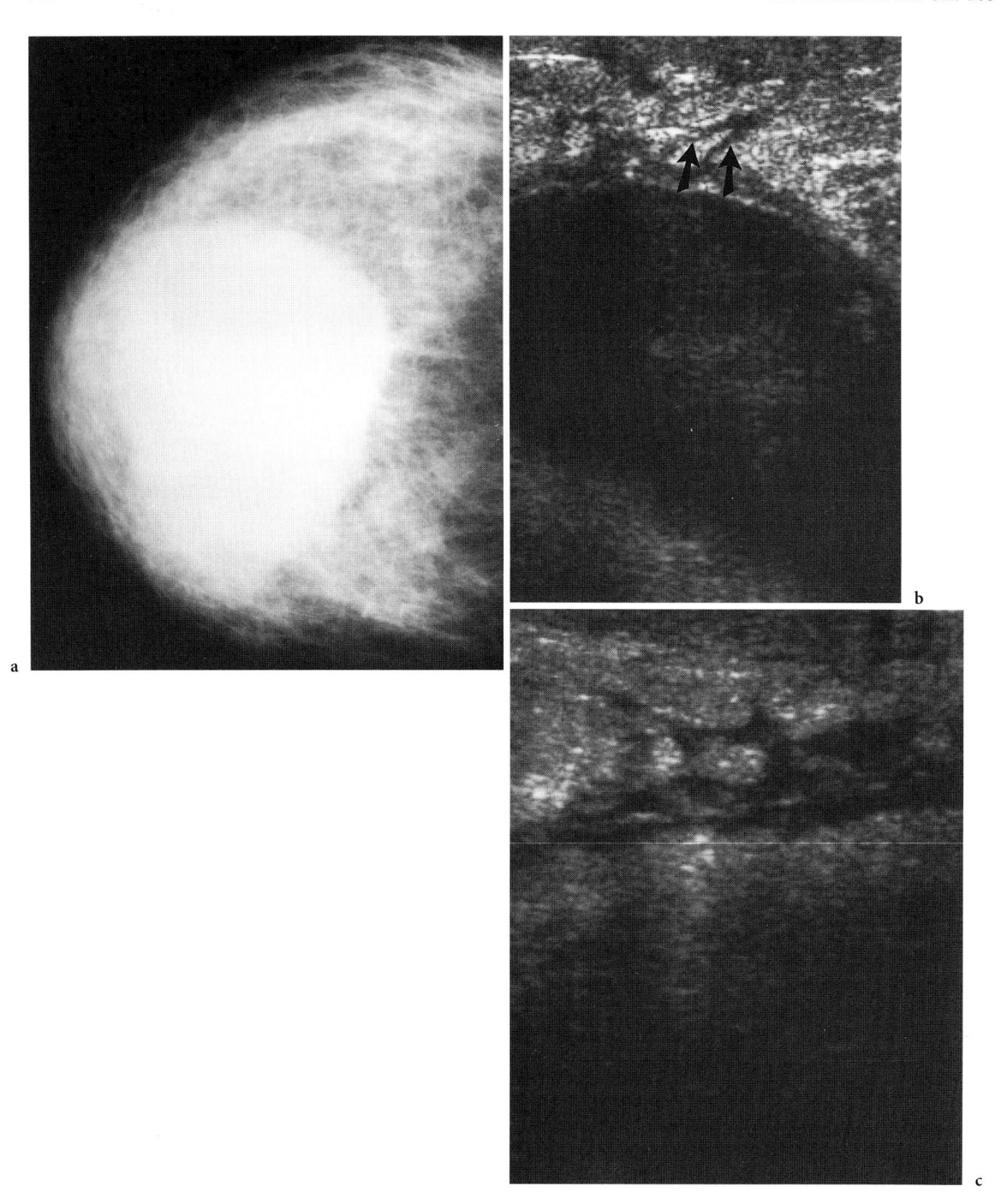

Fig. 17.14a–c. Abscess. **a** At the completion of radiation therapy, a large fluid collection is seen at the lumpectomy site. There is marked edema and skin thickening. The patient was febrile and had leukocytosis. As a complication of irradiation, the skin had become quite erythematous, and a small area of ulceration developed at the site of incision. **b** The oncologic team proposed percutaneous drainage of the 13-cm abscess visualized in part on the sonogram. Edema is signified by the increased echogenicity and hypoechoic tubular structures (*arrows*) around the purulent collection. **c** Only edema remains after the collection was evacuated using ultrasonographic guidance for a 16 gauge needle. The patient, who received antibiotics intravenously, defervesced. The collection refilled, as expected, and was redrained 3 times. When clear, a residual 5-cm fluid collection was left to resorb gradually, as is ordinarily done

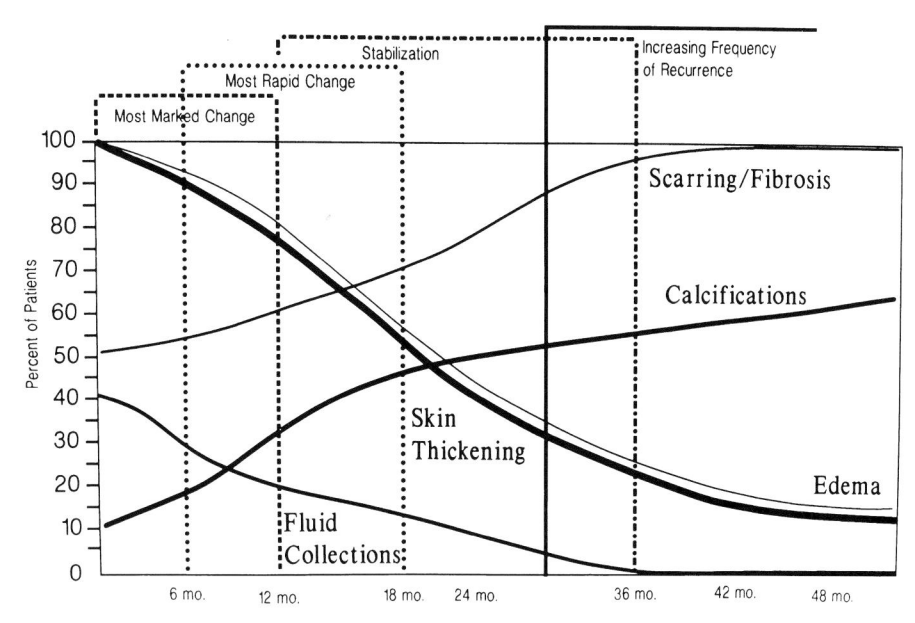

Fig. 17.15. Changing appearance of the conservatively treated breast. At each visit, evolving or resolving changes must be anticipated and tracked horizontally as well as vertically (temporal changes) to detect tumor recurrence early and to avert misidentification of posttreatment changes as recurrent tumor, which might result in an unnecessary surgical or percutaneous interventional procedure

Table 17.2. Imaging after breast conservation therapy

Timing of the study	Rationale
Treated breast	
Perioperative specimen radiography	To assure excision of the abnormality and grossly assess the need for additional tissue removal.
Postoperative preradiation (2–5 weeks lumpectomy)	Detection of residual carcinoma – important for microcalcifications (Fig. 17.9).
6 months	Baseline study: Peak of postprocedural changes: masses, skin thickening, edema. Early calcifications form.
12 months	Assess changes listed above; begin to look for mammographic stability (no change on two successive studies).
18 months	End of time of most rapid change; confirm stability.
24 months	Expect stabilization for most patients. More confident recognition of benign postprocedural changes.
30 months	Mammogram should be stable for nearly all patients.
36 months	Stable mammogram: Suspect recurrence if direction of change is unexpected.
Annual studies can be resumed after stabilization (usually by 18–36 months)	Detect recurrence: For patients at increased risk of recurrence (EIC and young patients), consider intervals of 6 months.
Contralateral breast	
Annually	Screening; increased risk of breast carcinoma.

17.3.5 Schedule for Follow-up Imaging After Breast Conservation Therapy

There is considerable geographic variation within the United States in the treatment of breast cancer. On the east and west coasts, the majority of breast cancer patients are treated with wide excision and irradiation, but in some other areas up to two-thirds of women eligible for breast conservation are not being offered this option. Somewhat dependent on the prevailing surgical practices, there is also wide variation in experience with the radiologic follow-up of these patients. Currently, beyond the first year after therapy, no guidelines have been adopted for intervals between follow-up studies, although many recommendations have appeared in the literature.

Two major objectives of imaging after breast conservation therapy are (a) early diagnosis of recurrence, prior to development of metastases, and (b) minimization of misinterpretations of postprocedural change as tumor recurrence to avoid unnecessary biopsy of radiation-treated tissue that may be slower to heal. The key to achieving these objectives is familiarity with the time course of postoperative and irradiation changes (Fig. 17.15). The period of greatest change occupies the first 18 months, with the most marked changes occurring around 6 months. In general, if the margins of resection have been free of tumor, recurrence will not be anticipated at the lumpectomy site until 2–3 years have elapsed.

Perhaps most important is recognition of stability of the breast, which we have defined as lack of change on two successive mammograms. Subsequently, a change counter to the direction of resolution would suggest recurrent tumor.

There is agreement that mammography at 6 and 12 months after tumor excision will record the greatest changes in the postprocedural breast. Beyond the 1-year study (HASSELL et al. 1990; OREL et al. 1993), various schedules have been proposed for follow-up mammograms. Most authors have supported studies every 6 months after the first year for some period of time (HASSELL et al. 1990; MENDELSON et al. 1989; SADOWSKY and SEMINE 1990; SADOWSKY et al. 1990; SICKLES 1991). We request a postoperative preradiation mammogram of the lumpectomy site, useful for exclusion of residual microcalcifications (Fig. 17.9). Studies are then performed every 6 months until the breast is stable, generally a period of 1–3 years, as much to avoid unnecessary biopsies of postprocedural benign changes as to diagnose recurrent tumor. The achievement of stability coincides with the time that recurrences begin to appear, which is 2–3 years after conservation therapy. After the breast appears stable mammographically, we advise annual studies of both the treated and the contralateral breast (Table 17.2).

Mammographic interpretation and follow-up imaging of the conservatively treated breast cancer patient can challenge the radiologist. Only with an understanding of the time course of changes can imaging evaluation of the postoperative breast be accurate.

17.4 Imaging After Mastectomy

When mastectomy is performed, the most common surgical procedure is modified radical mastectomy (KINNE 1991), with removal of the breast tissue and

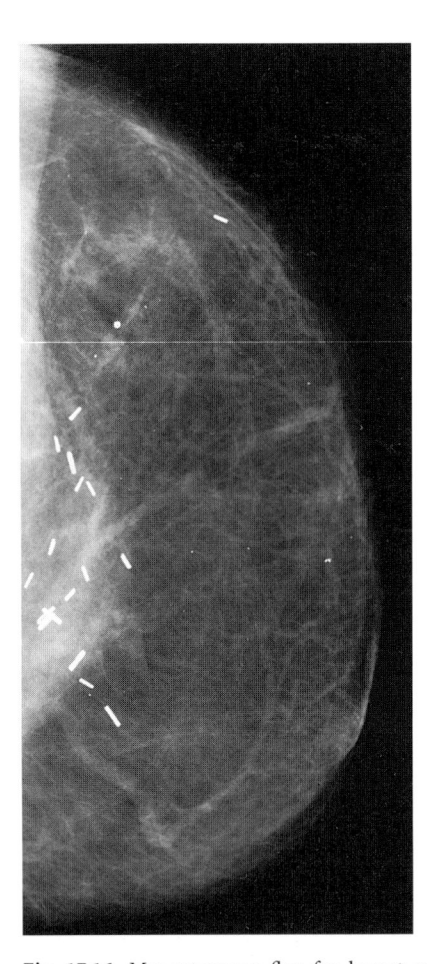

Fig. 17.16. Myocutaneous flap for breast reconstruction. A transverse rectus abdominis (TRAM) flap is seen in place. Surgical clips are present near the muscular pedicle. Only vascular, fatty, and connective tissue elements are seen. No radially oriented ducts are present

pectoralis major muscle and a generous ellipse of skin overlying the tumor. In contrast to lumpectomies, where the axillary lumphadenectomy is performed from an incision separate from that used to excise the tumor, the mastectomy incision extends to the axilla for nodal dissection or sampling. With mastectomy, as much of the breast tissue is removed as possible, although shreds may remain at the chest wall or at the incision site, the locations of local/regional recurrent carcinoma in more than 50% of cases (RECHT and HAYES 1991).

In modified radical mastectomies, with preservation of the pectoralis minor (the pectoralis major is removed in radical mastectomies), redundant tissue, frequently fatty, may be present at the mastectomy site. For reassurance of an anxious patient, to evaluate a mass palpated on clinical examination, or in a patient whose lymph nodes remain in the axilla, the mastectomy site can be imaged.

Mediolateral oblique, craniocaudal, and spot compression views with a narrow paddle, the x-ray beam being directed tangential to the area of concern, can be performed (EKLUND and CARDENOSA 1992; FAJARDO et al. 1993). The routine use of these views has not been established as cost-effective, most recurrences being evident on physical examination or manifested by chest wall pain, with skeletal metastases suggested by radionuclide bone scans (FAJARDO et al. 1993). Mammography and ultrasonography are reserved for palpable masses or suspected recurrences (RISSANEN et al. 1993). The consensus of these studies is that annual or other routine surveillance of the tissue remaining at the mastectomy site is unnecessary.

Another view of the mastectomy site is the uncompressed axillary view performed with higher kilovoltage technique (31–42 kV) using an aluminum filter. This view will show skeletal structures of the shoulder and portions of the ribs as well as soft tissues of the axilla. Having found only one case of bone metastases, which was already known, we abandoned this view approximately 6 years ago (MENDELSON 1992). More recently, other authors have reported similar findings and concluded that routine axillary views are not useful in women after mastectomy (PROPECK and SCANLAN 1993).

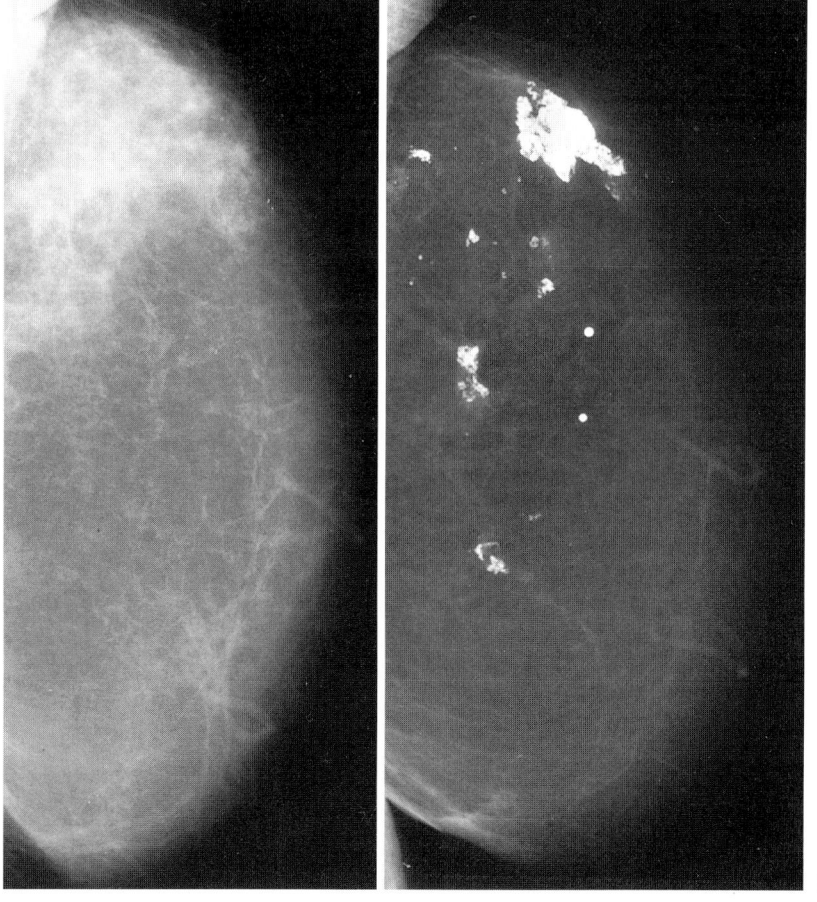

Fig. 17.17a,b. Fat necrosis in a TRAM flap. **a** One year after reconstruction, a bubbly area of density is seen in the superior flap, representing developing oil cysts. **b** Seven years later, the patient returned with palpable masses (areas of radiopaque markers) caused by a benign coalescence of calcifications in the area of fat necrosis. Mammography in the intervening years had shown formation of calcifications around the oil cysts that gradually became coarser and heavier, ultimately conglomerating. No recurrent tumor is present. Recognition of fat necrosis is important to avoid unnecessary interventions

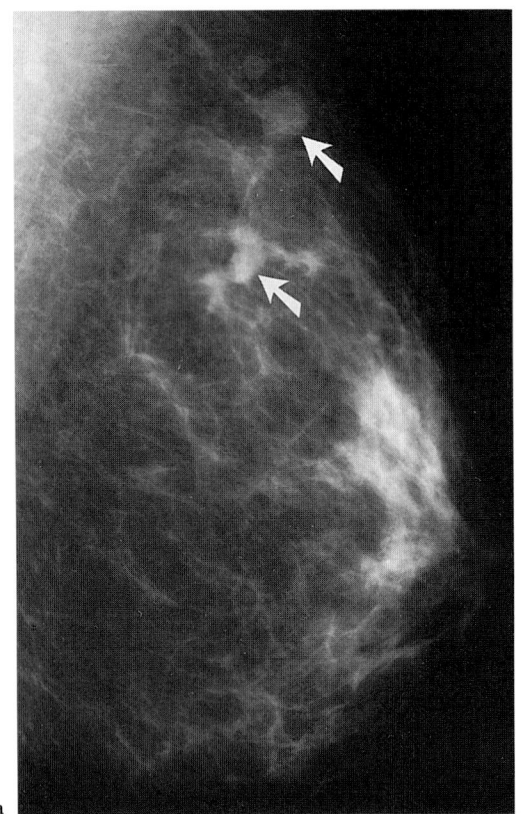

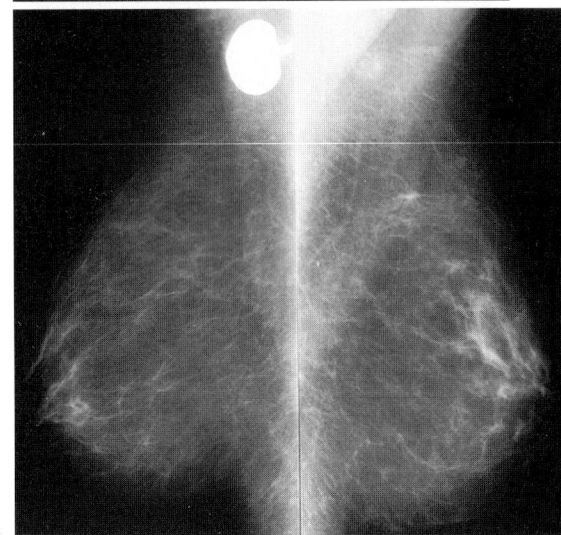

Fig. 17.18a,b. Response to chemotherapy. **a** Multicentric carcinoma in a 38-year-old woman with nodules (*arrows*) in the upper outer and upper inner left breast. A large metastatic axillary node was also present. **b** Five months later, with the infusion port seen in the right axilla, there has been a dramatic response to the chemotherapeutic regimen. The nodules have disappeared, and there has been some fatty replacement of fibroglandular tissue

The necessity to image the reconstructed breast has not been established. The mastectomy patient with and without a simulated breast would share the same risk of tumor recurrence. Although film-screen compression mammography can be performed on a reconstructed breast either with an implant or with a myocutaneous flap, in asymptomatic patients with myocutaneous flap reconstruction (as in the unreconstructed mastectomy patient) we no longer perform routine follow-up studies because of the low yield of significant radiographic findings. If findings on physical examination or breast self-examination suggest an abnormality, however, mammography will be performed.

With myocutaneous flap reconstruction, no radial ductal organization is seen. Behind the created nipple, no ducts are present. The simulated breast is fatty with vascular and connective tissue elements scattered randomly. Clips may be seen near the muscular pedicle (Fig. 17.16). The skin at the sites of suturing may be thickened. When physical findings, such as a mass are present, mammography can frequently confirm fat necrosis and exclude carcinoma. Because of the frequency of occurrence of fat necrosis, a baseline study of an autologous reconstruction may not be unreasonable (Fig. 17.17).

17.5 Advanced Cancer and Inflammatory Cancer

Little has been written about the need for imaging studies, the specific modalities, and the intervals that might be appropriate in the follow-up of patients who received chemotherapy or radiation therapy prior to any surgical treatment. These are areas for future study. Empirically, we have followed up patients who have received chemotherapy within a month after completion of the initial course of chemotherapy and all the subsequent courses (Fig. 17.18). At those times, we have followed up mammographically with magnification views if microcalcifications were involved and with ultrasonography to provide three dimensions for volumetric calculation of decrease in tumor size.

17.6 Conclusion

For accurate interpretation of mammograms of the breast that has undergone surgical alterations, it is important to be aware of the nature of the surgical procedure, the period that has elapsed since the procedure was performed, and other clinical changes that may have occurred. For greatest accuracy and interpretive confidence, preoperative studies, specimen radiographs, and pathology reports should be reviewed and all of the breast imaging studies should be looked at in chronological sequence along with the current examination.

References

Barr LC, Brunt AM, Goodman AG et al. (1989) Uncontrolled local recurrence after treatment of breast cancer with breast conservation. Cancer 64:1203-1207

D'Orsi CJ (1995) Management of the breast specimen. Radiology 194:297-302

Dubois JB, Saumon-Reme M, Gary-Bobo J et al. (1990) Tumorectomy and radiation therapy in early breast cancer: a report on 392 patients. Radiology 175:867-871

Eklund GW, Cardenosa G (1992) The art of mammographic positioning. RCNA 30:21-53

Fajardo LL, Roberts CC, Hunt KR (1993) Mammographic surveillance of breast cancer patients: should the mastectomy site be imaged? AJR 161:953-955

Fisher B, Bauer M, Margolese R et al. (1985) Five year results of a randomized clinical trial comparing total mastectomy and segmental mastectomy with and without radiation in the treatment of breast cancer. N Engl J Med 312:665-673

Fisher B, Costantino J, Redmond C et al. (1993) Lumpectomy compared with lumpectomy and radiation therapy for the treatment of intraductal breast cancer. N Engl J Med 328:1581-1586

Fowble B, Solin LJ, Schultz DJ et al. (1990) Breast recurrence following conservative surgery and radiation: patterns of failure, prognosis, and pathologic findings from mastectomy specimens with implications for treatment. Int J Radiat Oncol Biol Phys 19:833-841

Haffty BG, Goldberg NB, Rose M et al. (1989) Conservative surgery with radiation therapy in clinical stage I and II breast cancer. Arch Surg 124:1266-1270

Harris JR, Recht A (1991) Conservative surgery and radiotherapy. In: Harris JR, Hellina S, Henderson IC, Kinne DW (eds) Breast disease. Lippincott, Philadelphia, p 395

Harris JR, Schnitt SJ, Connolly JL (1987) Conservative surgery and radiation therapy for early breast cancer. Arch Surg 122:754-755

Hassell PR, Olivotto IA, Mueller HA et al. (1990) Early breast cancer: detection of recurrence after conservative surgery and radiation therapy. Radiology 176:731-735

Heywang SH, Hilbertz T, Beck R (1990) Gd-DTPA enhances MR imaging of the breast in patients with postoperative scarring in silicon implants. J Comput Assist Tomogr 14:348

Johnson JE, Page DL, Winfield AC, Reynolds VH, Sawyers JL (1995) Recurrent mammary carcinoma after local excision. Cancer 75:1612-1618

Kinne DW (1991) Primary treatment of breast cancer: surgery. In: Harris JR, Hellman S, Henderson IC et al. (eds) Breast diseases. Lippincott, Philadelphia, pp 347-373

Lagios MD (1990) Duct carcinoma in situ: pathology and treatment. Surg Clin North Am 70:853-871

Liberman L, Fahs C, Dershaw DD, Bonaccio E, Abramson AF, Cohen MA, Hann LE (1995) Impact of stereotaxic core breast biopsy on cost of diagnosis. Radiology 195:633-637

Libshitz HI, Montague ED, Paulus DD (1978) Skin thickness in the therapeutically irradiated breast. AJR 130:345-347

Machtay M, Lanciano R, Hoffman J, Hanks GE (1994) Inaccuracies in using the lumpectomy scar for planning electron boosts in primary breast carcinoma. Int J Radiat Oncol Biol Phys 30:43-48

Mendelson EB (1992) Evaluation of the postoperative breast. Radiol Clin North Am 30:107-138

Mendelson EB, Harris KM, Doshi N, Tobon H (1989) Infiltrating lobular carcinoma: mammographic patterns with pathologic correlation. AJR 153:265-271

NIH Consensus Conference (1991) Treatment of early stage breast cancer. JAMA 265:391-395

Orel SG, Fowble BL, Solin LJ, Schultz DJ, Conant EF, Troupin RH (1993) Breast cancer recurrence after lumpectomy and radiation therapy for early-stage disease: prognostic significance of detection method. Radiology 188:189-194

Paulus D (1984) Conservative treatment of breast cancer: mammography in patient selection and follow-up. AJR 143:483-487

Propeck PA, Scanlan KA (1993) Utility of axillary views in postmastectomy patients. Radiology 187:769-771

Rebner M, Pennes DR, Adler DD et al. (1989) Breast microcalcifications after lumpectomy and radiation therapy. Radiology 170:691-693

Recht A, Hayes DF (1991) Local recurrence following mastectomy. In: Harris JR, Hellman S, Henderson IC et al. (eds) Breast diseases. Lippincott, Philadelphia, p 529

Recht A, Connolly JL, Schnitt SJ et al. (1989) Therapy of in situ cancer. Hematol Oncol Clin North Am 3:691-708

Rissanen TJ, Makarainen HP, Mattila SI, Lindholm EL, Heikkinen MI, Kiviniemi HO (1993) Breast cancer recurrence after mastectomy: diagnosis with mammography and US. Radiology 188:463-467

Robertson JM, Clarke DH, Pavzner MM et al. (1991) Breast conservation therapy in severe breast fibrosis after radiation therapy in patients with collagen vascular disease. Cancer 68:502-508

Rubin E, Dempsey PJ, Pile NS, Bernreuter WK, Urist MM, Shumate CR, Maddox WA (1995) Needle-localization biopsy of the breast: impact of a selective core needle biopsy program on yield. Radiology 195:627-631

Sadowsky NL, Semine A (1990) Good mammography finds postop cancer recurrence. Diagn Imaging, pp 100-106

Sadowsky NL, Semine A, Harris JR (1990) Breast imaging: a critical aspect of breast conserving treatment. Cancer 65:2113-2118

Sickles EA (1991) Periodic mammographic follow-up of probably benign lesions: results in 3,184 consecutive cases. Radiology 179:463-468

Sickles EA, Herzog KA (1981) Mammography of the postsurgical breast. AJR 136:585-588

Singletary SE, McNeese M (1988) Segmental mastectomy and irradiation in the treatment of breast cancer. Am J Clin Oncol 11:679-683

Solin LJ, Fowble BL, Schultz DJ et al. (1990) Definitive irradiation for intraductal carcinoma of the breast. Int J Radiat Oncol Biol Phys 19:843-850

Stehlin JS, deIpolyi PD, Greeff PJ et al. (1987) A ten year study of partial mastectomy for carcinoma of the breast. Surg Gynecol Obstet 165:191–198

Stomper PC, Gelman RS (1989) Mammography in symptomatic and asymptomatic patients. Hematol Oncol Clin North Am 3:611–640

Stomper PC, Recht A, Berenberg AL et al. (1987) Mammographic detection of recurrent cancer in the irradiated breast. AJR 148:39–43

Sunderland MC, McGuire WL (1990) Prognostic indicators in invasive breast cancer. Surg Clin North Am 70:989–1003

Winchester DP, Cox JD (1992) Standards for breast-conservation treatment. CA Cancer J Clin 42:135–162

Wingo PA, Tong T, Bolden S (1995) Cancer statistics 1995. CA Cancer J Clin 45:8–30

18 Imaging After Breast Implants

N.D. DeBruhl, D.P. Gorczyca, and L.W. Bassett

CONTENTS

18.1	Introduction 319
18.1.1	Injectable Materials 319
18.1.2	Implantable Prostheses 319
18.2	Silicone Breast Implants 320
18.2.1	Encapsulation of Silicon-Gel Implants......... 321
18.2.2	Rupture................................ 321
18.2.3	Gel Bleed............................... 321
18.3	Mammography.......................... 321
18.3.1	Mammographic Findings 322
18.3.2	Mammography for Evaluation of Implant Rupture 323
18.4	Ultrasonography......................... 323
18.4.1	Normal Sonographic Findings 323
18.4.2	Sonographic Signs of Implant Rupture 325
18.4.3	Intracapsular Ruptures 325
18.4.4	Extracapsular Ruptures 325
18.4.5	Limitations in the Sonographic Evaluation of Implants............................. 326
18.5	Magnetic Resonance Imaging 326
18.5.	Technical Factors 326
18.5.2	Imaging Protocols 327
18.5.3	Appearance of Normal Implants 328
18.5.4	Intracapsular Rupture 329
18.5.5	Extracapsular Rupture 330
18.5.6	Gel Bleed............................... 331
18.6	Comparison of Different Imaging Modalities 331
	References 331

18.1 Introduction

During the past century, many different methods have been tried to augment or reconstruct the breast. Unfortunately, the majority of the approaches have proved disappointing, with many associated complications (Bridges and Vasey 1993; Letterman and Schurter 1989; Steinbach et al. 1993). Methods

---

N.D. DeBruhl, MD, Iris Cantor Center for Breast Imaging, 165-43 Department of Radiological Sciences, 200 UCLA Medical Plaza, Los Angeles, CA 90095-6952, USA
D.P. Gorczyca, MD, Iris Cantor Center for Breast Imaging, 165-43 Department of Radiological Sciences, 200 UCLA Medical Plaza, Los Angeles, CA 90095-6952, USA
L.W. Bassett, MD, Iris Cantor Center for Breast Imaging, 165-43 Department of Radiological Sciences, 200 UCLA Medical Plaza, Los Angeles, CA 90095-6952, USA

used to augment or reconstruct the breast can be placed into one of three categories: autogenous tissue transplantation, injectable materials, and implantable prostheses.

18.1.1 Injectable Materials

During the last century, many different materials have been injected into the breast for augmentation. One of the first materials injected was paraffin. Several other materials were also injected but most resulted in a poor cosmetic outcome and secondary complicatons. Complications ranged from granulomatous and inflammatory reactions to necrosis, pulmonary embolism, and death. Direct silicone injections were first used in the 1950s, and eventually had complications similar to those identified with paraffin injections (Letterman and Schurter 1989; Steinbach et al. 1993). Silicone injections in the breast can result in palpable masses that mimic carcinoma. Silicone injections may also obscure the breast parenchyma, greatly compromising the accuracy of mammography (Fig. 18.1).

18.1.2 Implantable Prostheses

In the 1950s, synthetic implantable sponge prostheses, composed of polyvinyl alcohol or Ivalon, were first used for breast augmentation. Initial reports were promising; however, scar tissue quickly made these implanted prostheses hard and caused them to shrink. Other synthetic materials were used such as etheron, polyether polyurethane, polypropylene, and even polytef (Teflon), all resulting in poor cosmetic results and other complications.

In 1963 Cronin and Gerow first described their use of a silicone-gel prosthesis (Cronin and Gerow 1964). Today the majority of the estimated 2 million American women with breast implants have the silicone-gel type, placed either for augmentation or reconstrucion. A large number of different types of

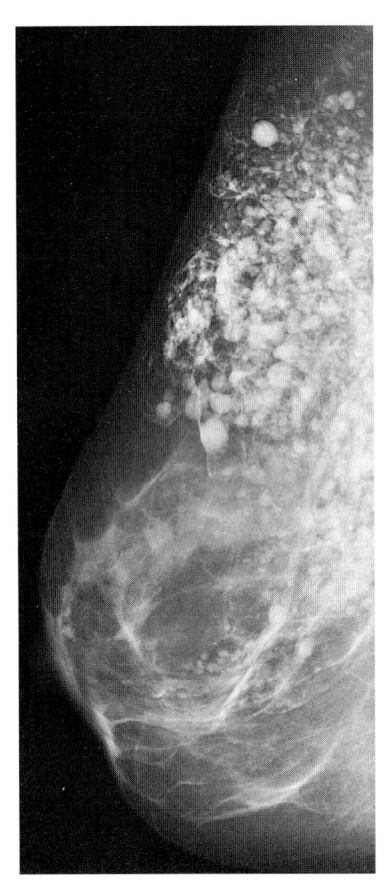

Fig. 18.1. Mediolateral mammogram demonstrating silicone injections. The dense silicone granulomas have migrated to the superior aspect of the breast and were also present in the axilla and upper arm. Due to the density of the silicone, the granulomas limit the mammographic examination

silicone-gel implant have been manufactured. The types of implant fit into four major categories, the two most common of which are the single-lumen implant and the double-lumen implant (Fig. 18.2a). The single-lumen implant has a smooth or textured outer silicone membrane coating which contains the silicone gel. The double-lumen type has a saline outer chamber surroundign the inner silicone-gel implant. For augmentation mammoplasty the implants are placed either anterior (subglandular) or posterior (subpectoral) to the pectoralis major muscle (Fig. 18.3). Although subpectoral implants are technically more difficult to place, they offer the advantages of improved mammography, decrease in capsular contracture, and less obvious surgical scar.

18.2 Silicone Breast Implants

Silicone breast implants have been manufactured for more than 30 years. However, despite initial enthusi-asm, complications with silicone implants have not been uncommon. These complications have included rupture and leakage, fibrous or calcific contracture, localized pain, paresthesias, and possi-

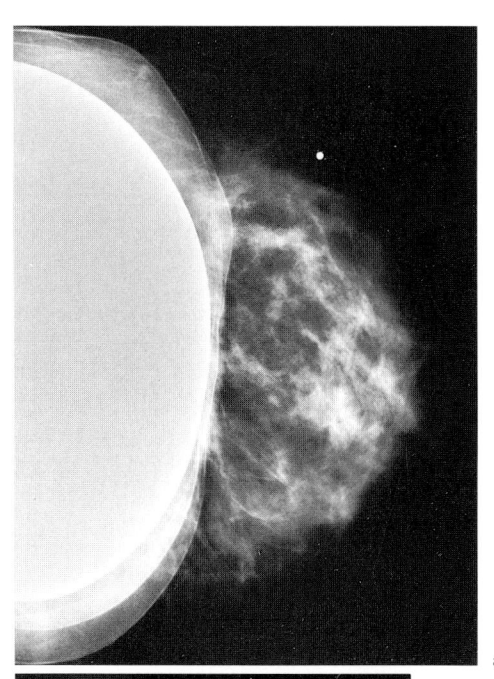

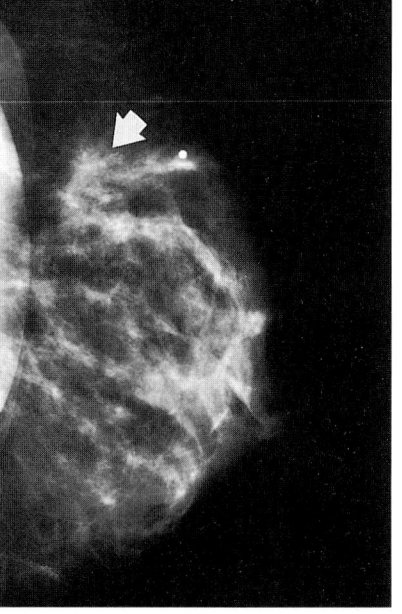

Fig. 18.2a,b. Implant-included and implant-displaced views. The woman complained of a palpable mass, which the technologist localized by placing a BB directly over it. **a** Mediolateral oblique (MLO), implant-included view. The implant is subglandular and of the double-lumen type, with a silicone inner chamber surrounded by saline. **b** 90° lateral, implant-displaced view. Displacement of the implant combined with improved compression of the anterior tissue discloses a spiculated mass (*arrow*) at the site of the palpable abnormality

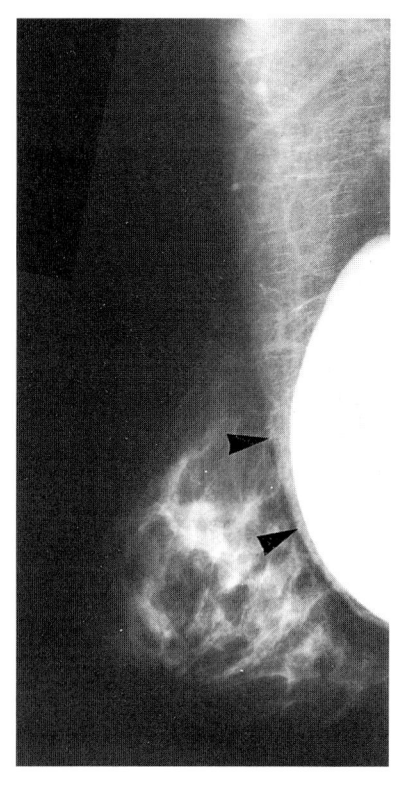

Fig. 18.3. Subpectoral implant. MLO view shows the border of the overlying pectoral muscle (*arrowheads*)

bly even generalized autoimmune disorders (MARIK et al. 1990; SPIERA 1988; WEINER 1991). In 1992, the U.S. Food and Drug Administration (FDA) held hearings about potential complications resulting from the use of silicone-gel implants. As a result, the FDA banned the use of silicone-gel implants, except under specific conditions (KESSLER 1992).

The majority of silicone implants are composed of an outer silicone membrane and inner silicone gel. The composition of the silicone membrane is an elastic polymer of silicone. The purpose of the soft membrane is to contain the silicone gel and provide a natural feeling and contour to the augmented breast.

18.2.1 Encapsulation of Silicone-Gel Implants

A fibrous capsule always forms around a breast implant (McINNIS 1990). The capsule that forms may be soft and impalpable, or hard and resistant. When a hard capsule forms, the breast may have an undesirable contour and feel. Closed capsulotomy, a procedure by which the surgeon uses vigorous manual compression to disrupt a hard fibrous capsule, was once used as a method to restore a more natural feeling to the breast (BAKER et al. 1976). However, this procedure has been discontinued because of its association with significant herniation and rupture of the breast implant (GRUBER and JONES 1981).

18.2.2 Rupture

Implant ruptures can be divided into two major categories, intracapsular and extracapsular rupture (AHN et al. 1993). *Intra*capsular implant rupture, the most common type, is defined as rupture of the implant membrane (elastomer envelope) allowing the release of silicone gel which does not extend beyond the intact fibrous capsule. *Extra*capsular rupture is defined as rupture of both the implant membrane and the fibrous capsule, with silicone leakage extending into surrounding tissues.

18.2.3 Gel Bleed

Gel bleed is microscopic silicone leakage through an intact implant membrane (BRODY 1977). Most if not all implants will eventually have gel bleed, but it is usually not extensive enough to be detected.

18.3 Mammography

Women with silicone breast implants are not at increased risk for developing breast cancer, and therefore regular mammographic screening is recommended at intervals appropriate for the woman's age (BERKEL et al. 1992). However, implants usually limit the amount of tissue visualized on mammograms. It is important to emphasize that the positioning of the breasts of women with silicone-gel implants requires special expertise by radiologic technologists. In general, more tissue can be visualized in the mammograms of women with subpectoral than in the mammograms of women with subglandular implants. Special views, called implant displaced views, have been developed to better visualize the native breast tissue anterior to silicone breast implants (EKLUND et al. 1988).

Both implant-included and implant-displaced views should be performed whenever possible (American College of Radiology 1992; BASSETT et al. 1994). Implant-included views are performed first, utilizing only moderate compression. Implant-displaced views are done next. The displacement of the implant posteriorly allows for taut compression of the anterior native tissues, and may show more of these tissues (Fig. 18.2) (DESTOUET et al. 1992). A hard, fixed capsule can prevent the performance of implant-displaced views due to immobility of the implant.

Due to the more complex nature of the examination, even a screening examination of a woman with implants should be reviewed for technical quality before she leaves the mammography facility. Women with implants are often more anxious about mammography and may have questions about the examination or the results. Therefore, for scheduling purposes, we assign asymptomatic women with implants to have diagnostic examinations, which are performed with a radiologist on site. We do not currently recommend that women with silicone implants have their mammograms performed in either mobile or fixed site screenig facilities where a radiologist is not on site.

There are no documented cases of implant rupture due to mammography compression. However, we are aware of several unsubstantiated cases of rupture attributed to mammography. While new, nonimplanted silicone-gel bags can withstand considerable mammographic compression, it is suspected that over time implanted silicone-gel bags may be subject to fatigue and trauma, making them vulnerable to rupture. Therefore, radiologists should at least be aware of the potential for implant rupture during mammography and should have a protocol within their facilities to deal with any complicatiosn that may arise. Clinical signs of implant rupture include palpable silicone nodules, decreased breat size, asymmetry, tenderness, and a change in texture of the implant. Breakage of the fibrous capsule around the implant may occur with compression, and may be accompanied by an audible "pop." Thus, mammographic compression can potentially convert an intracapsular rupture to an extracapsular rupture.

The possibility of implant rupture from mammography compression has led some professional liability carriers to suggest that a signed consent form be obtained prior to the performance of mammography on women with breast implants. Radiologists have voiced concern over the need of such informed consents in the absence of any documented evidence of a relationship between mammography and implant rupture. Radiologists are also concerned that informed consents might alarm women and prevent them from having mammograms done (BASSETT and BRENNER 1992). The American College of Radiology does not recommend that routine consent forms be obtained for mammography of women with breast implants, but educational information for these women is encouraged.

18.3.1 Mammographic Findings

Mammographic features that are specific to breast implants include a measurable periprosthetic dense band or rim of tissue that correlates with a fibrous capsule around the implant, periprosthetic calcification, asymmetry of implant size or shape, focal herniation of the implant, and implant rupture with deflation of the envelope and extravasation of silicone outside the membrane (Figs. 18.4, 18.5) (DESTOUET et al. 1992; DERSHAW and CHAGLASSIAN 1989; LEIBMAN and KRUSE 1990; YOUNG et al. 1989). Free silicone in the breast may be manifested by dense masses, linear streaks, or lymph node opacification (Fig. 18.6).

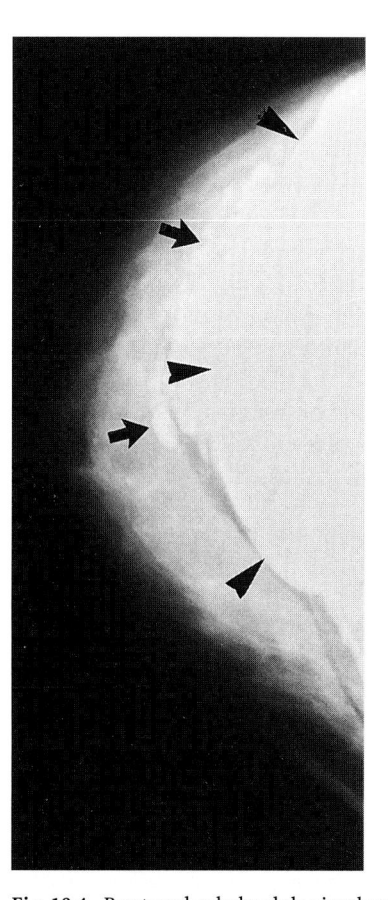

Fig. 18.4. Ruptured subglandular implant. Craniocaudal view with mild compression shows coalescence of free silicone granulomas (*arrows*) anterior to the implant (*arrowheads*)

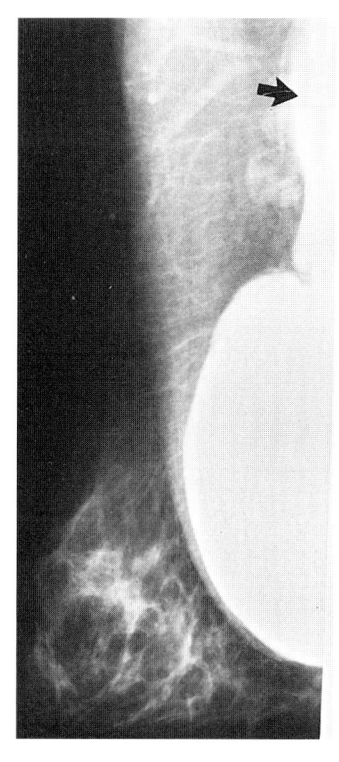

Fig. 18.5. Ruptured subpectoral implants. The extruded free silicone gel (*arrow*) is seen extending into the axilla

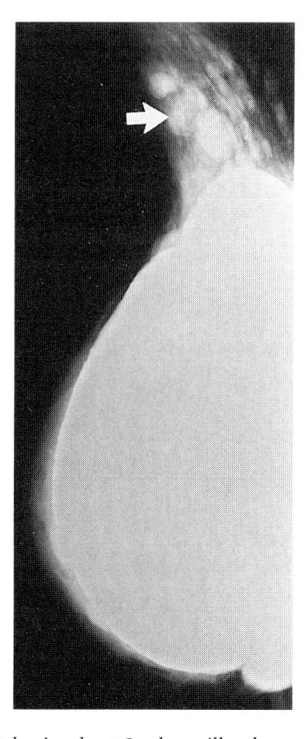

Fig. 18.6. Ruptured subglandular implant. In the axilla, there are several dense silicone granulomas (*arrow*) anterior to lymphatic channels with streaky opacification from uptake of silicone gel

18.3.2 Mammography for Evaluation of Implant Rupture

Since clinical examination may fail to disclose an implant rupture and its extent, radiologists are often requested to evaluate the integrity of breast prostheses. In our experience, mammography has not been useful in the detection intracapsular implant ruptures. While mammography can identify free silicone after a silicone implant rupture, the silicone may be obscured by an overlying implant.

Due to the limitations of clinical breast examinaion and mammography in the evaluation of breast implants, ultrasonography and magnetic resonance (MR) imaging have been investigated as adjunctive methods.

18.4 Ultrasonography

There are conflicting reports on the usefulness of ultrasonography for detecting implant ruptures (GANNOTT et al. 1992; HARRIS et al. 1993; ROSCULET et al. 1992). The varying results in the literature may reflect the experience of the operators and technical factors. Ultrasonography is operator dependent and requires on-site evaluation to accomplish the best results. A high-resolution transducer (7.5–10 MHz) is necessary to evaluate the integrity of a silicone implant. However, a 5-MHz transducer may be required to depict the posterior aspects of the implant or to better visualize a subpectoral implant. The implant should be exmined systematically, to ensure evaluation of all areas of the implant, surrounding breast, and axila. Clockwise scanning of the breast is used in our practice to be sure that the examination is complete. Selected hard copy images are obtained for documentation.

18.4.1 Normal Sonographic Findings

Table 18.1 reports the common sonographic findings in 57 surgically proven normal and ruptured breast implants (DEBRUHL et al. 1993). The most reliable sign of an intact implant is an anechoic interior (Fig. 18.7). However, reverberation artifacts are commonly encountered in the anterior aspect of the implant and should not be confused with abnormalities (Fig. 18.8). The reverberation artifact is usually no thicker than the breast tissue anterior to the implant. The implant membrane, sometimes visualized as a thin echogenic line at the parenchymal tis-

Table 18.1. US signs in 57 surgically removed implants (from DeBruhl et al. 1993)

Surgical findings	Anechoic interior	Anterior reverberations	Stepladder sign	Heterogeneous aggregates
Ruptured (20)	0	15	14	5
Intracapsular (16)	0	12	10	4
Extracapsular (4)	0	3	4	1
Intact (37)	8	25	3	1

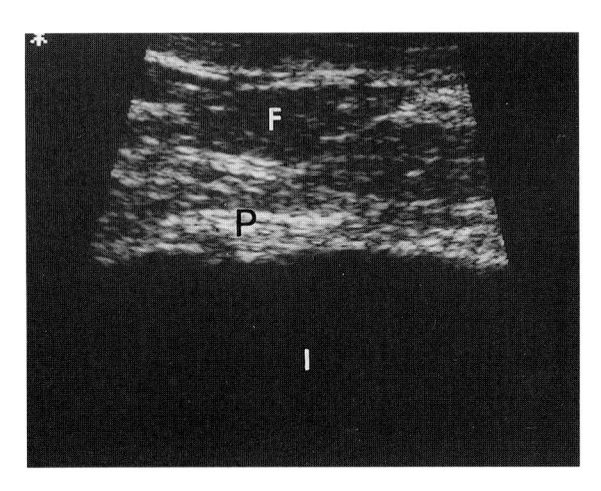

Fig. 18.7. Normal subglandular silicone implant has anechoic interior. *I*, implant interior; *F*, subcutaneous fat: *P*, parenchyma

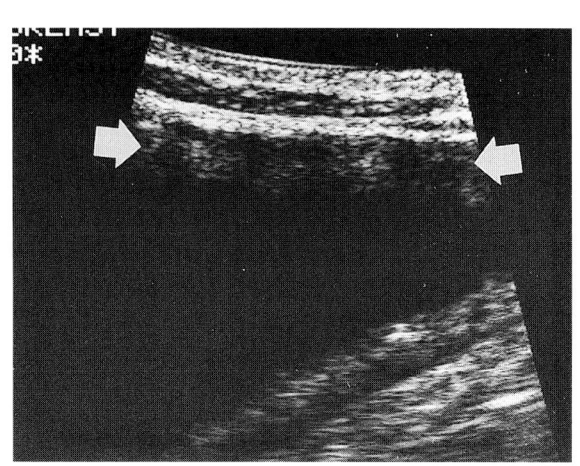

Fig. 18.8. Normal silicone implant. Artifactual echoes (*arrows*) due to reverberation are commonly seen and should not be mistaken for ruptured implant. Posterior to this the interior prosthesis is anechoic

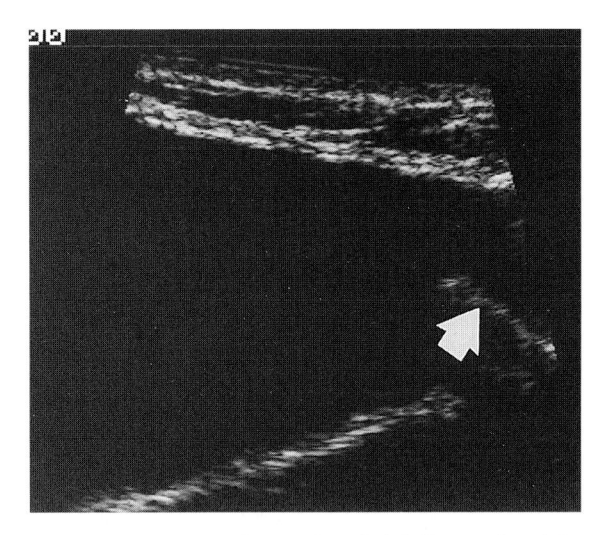

Fig. 18.9. Silicone implant with radial fold, manifested by single echogenic line (*arrow*) which extends from the periphery of the implant

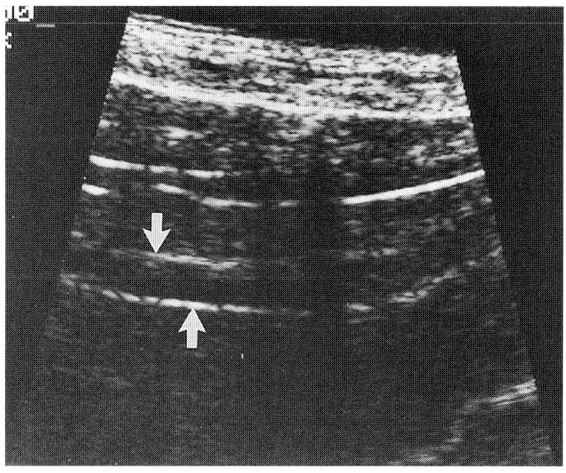

Fig. 18.10. Intracapsular rupture. The "stepladder sign" is manifested by multiple horizontal echogenic lines (*arrows*) which are roughly parallel to each other. These lines represent the collapsed implant membrane

sue–implant interface, should be continuous and intact.

Radial folds present as echogenic lines that extend from the periphery to the interior of the implant (Fig. 18.9). These folds are normal infoldings of the implant membrane into the silicone gel. Radial folds are commonly found in normal implants but are more frequently seen and may be more prominent in the presence of capsular contracture.

18.4.2 Sonographic Signs of Implant Rupture

The reported signs of implant rupture include hyperechoic or hypoechoic masses, dispersion of the sonographic beam ("snowstorm" or "echogenic noise"), discontinuity of the implant membrane, multiple parallel echogenic lines within the implant interior (stepladder sign), and aggregates of medium- to low-level echoes within the interior of the implant (DeBruhl et al. 1993; Levine and Collins 1991; Rosculet et al. 1992).

18.4.3 Intracapsular Ruptures

In our experience, the stepladder sign if the most reliable sonographic evidence of an intracapsular rupture (Table 18.1) (DeBruhl et al. 1993). The stepladder sign is a series of horizontal echogenic straight or curviliner lines, somewhat parallel, traversing the interior of the implant (Fig. 18.10). This sign represents the collapsed implant membrane floating within the silicone gel, and is analogous to the "linguine sign" seen on MR imaging (see below). The contnuity of these echogenic lines is usually not obvious on ultrasonography because of the narrow field of view.

In our experience, the presence of aggregates of low- to medium-level echoes within the implant is not a reliable sign of intracapsular rupture because it can also be seen with gel bleed. The etiology of these aggregates of echoes is uncertain, but it has been hypothesized that they are related to chemical and physical changes of the silicone gel secondary to its exposure to tissue fluids.

18.4.4 Extracapsular Ruptures

The most reliable sign of an extracapsular rupture is the presence of hyperechoic or hypoechoic nodules, which are often surrounded by hyperechoic parenchyma (Fig. 18.11). The nodules represent silicone granulomas, composed of free silicone and surroundign fibrous tissue reaction, lying outside the confines of the fibrous capsule (Levine and Colins 1991). These granulomas have been associated with loss of sonographic information distally, a phenomenon termed "echodense noise" (Rosculet et al. 1992) (Fig. 18.11). Sometimes this noise is present without any recognizable nodules (Harris et al. 1993) (Fig. 18.12). The granulomas are differentiated from breast tumors through correlation of clinical, mammographic, and sonographic findings. Occasionally, extracapsular rupture is associated with discontinuity of the breast–implant fibrous capsule interface (Fig. 18.13). This latter finding may represent the extrusion of silicone through the ruptured fibrous capsule and into the anterior breast tissue.

As would be anticipated, sonographic signs of intracapsular rupture can be expected to accompany extracapsular rupture (Fig. 18.13). Therefore, when sonographic signs of intracapsular rupture are present, a careful search for extracapsular rupture should made, including a search for silicone nodules in the axilla.

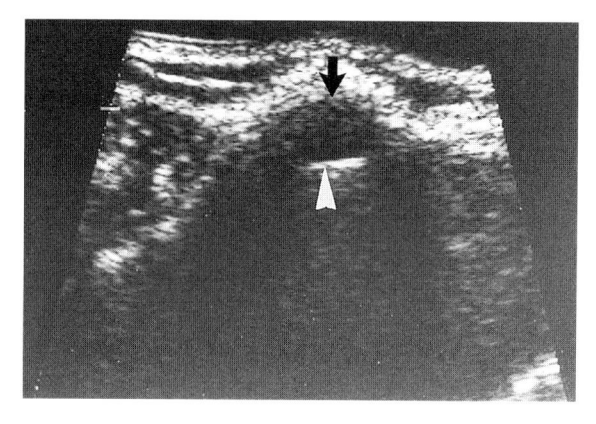

Fig. 18.11. Extracapsular rupture. A hypoechoic silicone granuloma (*arrow*) is identified in the tissue anterior to the implant. There is a hyperechoic interface (*arrowhead*) directly posterior to the granuloma, and behind this an area of "echogenic noise" in which all sonographic information is lost

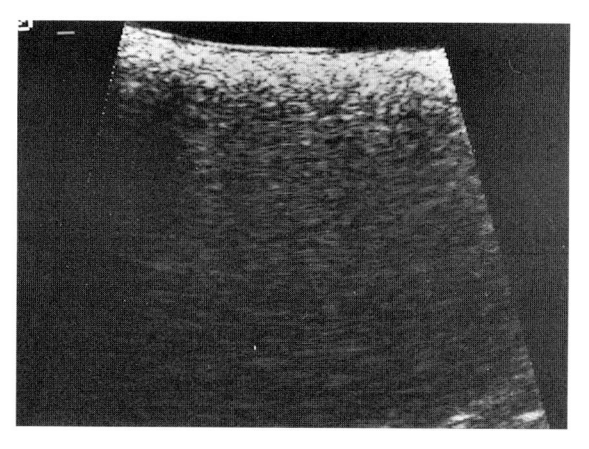

Fig. 18.12. Dispersion of the ultrasound beam by free silicone is referred to as a "snowstorm" appearance

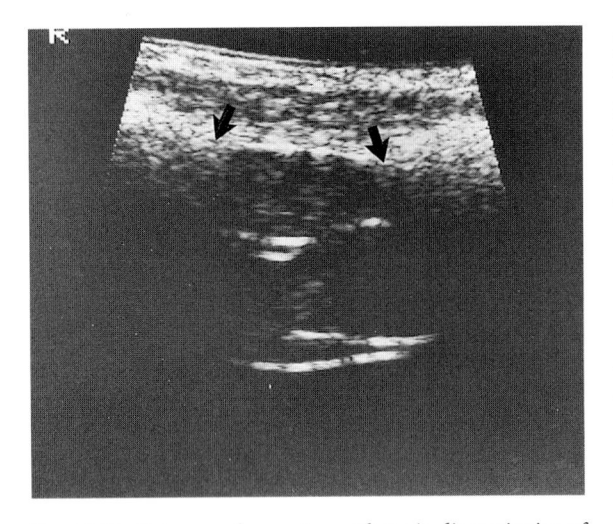

Fig. 18.13. Extracapsular rupture. There is discontinuity of the parenchyma–implant fibrous capsule interface. This finding is believed to be due to the extravasation of silicone through the ruptured membrane and fibrous capsule. Note the echogenic lines within the implant representing the collapsed implant membrane

18.4.5 Limitations in the Sonographic Evaluation of Implants

We have encountered some important limitations in the sonographic evaluation of implants. Due to marked attenuation of the ultrasound beam by silicone, ultrasonography is limited in the evaluation of the back wall of an implant and the tissue posterior to it. Prominent reverberation artifact can be confused with abnormalities of the implant. Previous silicone injections make it impossible to rule out extracapsular rupture in patients who have subsequent placement of silicone prostheses. In addition, extensive silicone injections can make it extremely difficult to evaluate the interior of a subsequently placed silicone implant, due to attenuation of the ultrasound beam by the injected silicone and granulom formation. In the same way, residual silicone granulomas from extracapsular rupture of explanted silicone implants compromise the evaluation of a new implant.

18.5 Magnetic Resonance Imaging

Magnetic resonance imaging has proved to be the most accurate method for the detection of breast implant ruptures. An understanding of the MR characteristics of silicone will be helpful to understand the different MR sequences that can be used to differentiate silicone from surrounding breast parenchyma. The chemical composition of most medical-grade silicones is dimethyl polysiloxane with varying degrees of polymerization (Habal 1984). The MR signal is derived from the protons of the methyl groups. The implant membrane is also composed of silicone but differs from the gel because of the many additional cross-linkages between the methyl groups that result in an elastic solid. Although the implant membrane is composed of silicone, only minimal MR signal is produced from the silicone membrane because of the cross-linkages between the methyl groups (Gorczyca et al. 1994b).

18.5.1 Technical Factors

The selection of MR pulse sequences used to image breast implants is determined by the relative a Larmor precessional frequencies, as well as the T1 and T2 properties of the tissues (fat, muscle, and silicone). The relative resonance frequency of silicone is approximately 100 Hz lower than that of fat

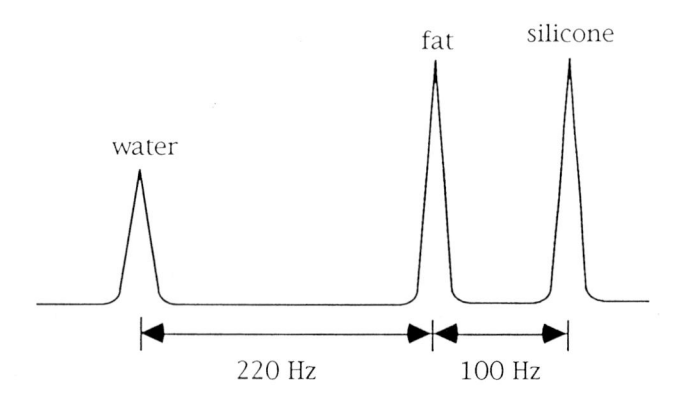

Fig. 18.14. Relative resonance frequency differences between water, fat, and silicone at 1.5 T. The resonance frequency of silicone is approximately 320 Hz lower than that of water and 100 Hz lower than that of fat

Table 18.2. Signal intensities of silicone, fat, and water with different MR pulse sequences

MR sequence	Silicone	Fat	Water
FSE T2-weighted (TR/TE 5000/200)	High	Medium	Very high
FSE with water suppression	High	Medium	Low
Inversion recovery FSE (IRFSE) (TR/TE 5000/90, TI = 150)	High	Low	Very high
IRFSE with water suppression	High	Low	Low
Three-point Dixon (3PD) silicone only	High	None	None

and 320 Hz lower than that of water at 1.5 T (Fig. 18.14). Since the resonance frequency of silicone is close to fat, when chemical suppresion techniques (chemical fat or water suppression) are used, the MR signal from silicone behaves similar to the signal from fat. As a result, the silicone signal is high when chemical water suppression is used and the silicone signal is low when chemical fat suppression is used (Table 18.2).

The relative relaxation times of silicone, fat, and water can also be used to obtain MR sequences which selectively emphasize the signal from silicone. The relaxation time of fat is shorter than that of silicone. Therefore, one can use the relaxation time properties of silicone and fat to suppress the fat while maintaining a strong signal from silicone. The use of inversion recovery with a short T1 (STIR) will suppress the signal from fat while maintaining signal from silicone (MUKUNDAN et al. 1993; MUND et al. 1993). To obtain a more selective silicone image, a chemical water suppression pulse can be used in conjunction with a STIR sequence to produce a silicone selective sequence.

Chemical shift imaging (CSI) is another way to selectively image silicone (GARRIDO et al. 1993; GORCZYCA et al. 1994c; SCHNEIDER and CHAN 1993). This method uses the differences between the Larmor frequencies of silicone, fat, and water to separate the MR signal of silicone from the signals of fat and water. An example of a CSI MR sequence is the modified three-point Dixon technique (GORCZYCA et al. 1994c; SCHNEIDER and CHAN 1993). This sequence produces a silicone-only sequence and a simultaneous fat/water image with a single MR sequence.

18.5.2 Imaging Protocols

In our practice, MR imaging is performed using a dedicated breast coil with the patient prone (SINHA et al. 1993). A 1.5-T superconducting magnet is used to acquire an axial scout image, fast gradient-recalled acquisition in the steady state (GRASS), followed by a sagittal T2-weighted fast-spin-echo (FSE) and axial T2-weighted FSE with water suppression sequences. A 192 × 256 matrix, 2 NEX with slice thickness between 3 and 5 mm to cover the entire implant is used to image the patients. Heavily T2-weighted FSE images, with TE approximately 200, are used to decrease the signal from the breast adipose tissue while keeping the signal from the silicone fairly high. This

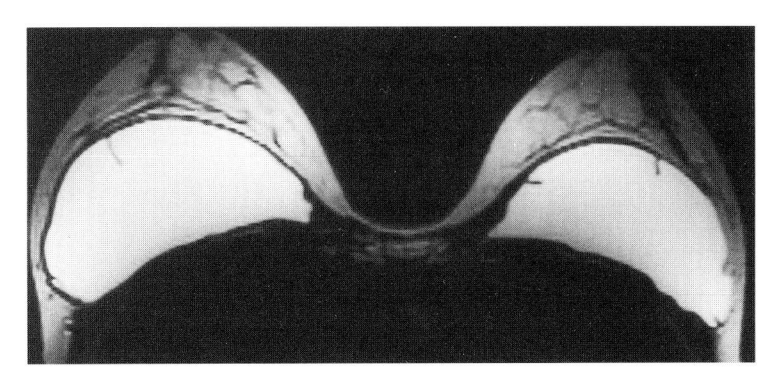

Fig. 18.15. Axial T2-weighted MR image without water suppression of normal single-lumen implant

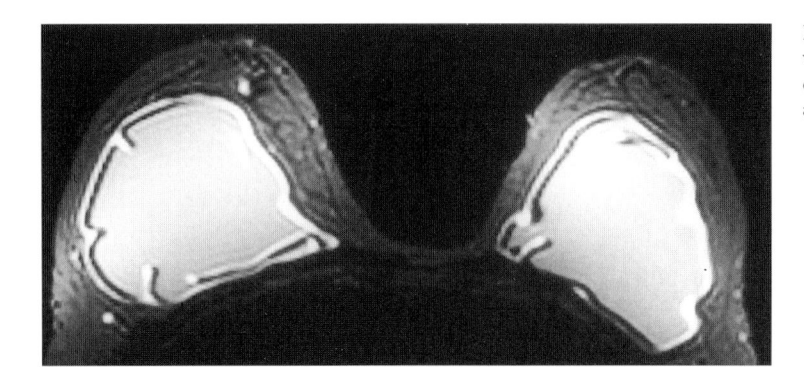

Fig. 18.16. Axial T2-weighted MR image without water suppression of normal double-lumen implant (outer saline lumen around inner silicone lumen)

examination requires between 20 and 30 min to complete. The relative signal intensities of silicone, fat, and water with various pulse sequences are summarized in Table 18.2.

18.5.3 Appearance of Normal Implants

On MR imaging, a normal single-lumen silicone implant has an outer Silastic membrane containing

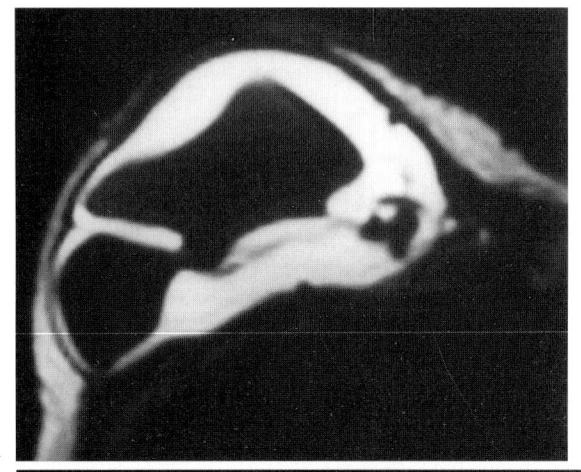

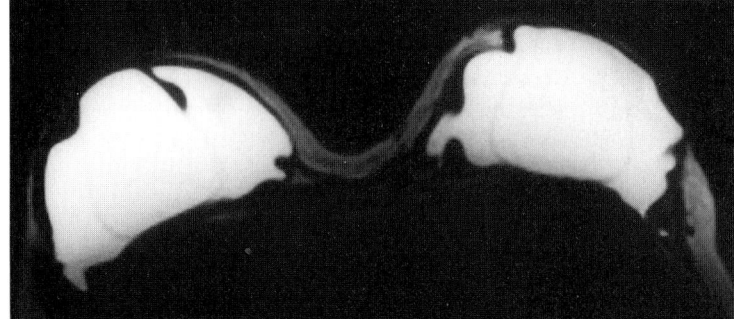

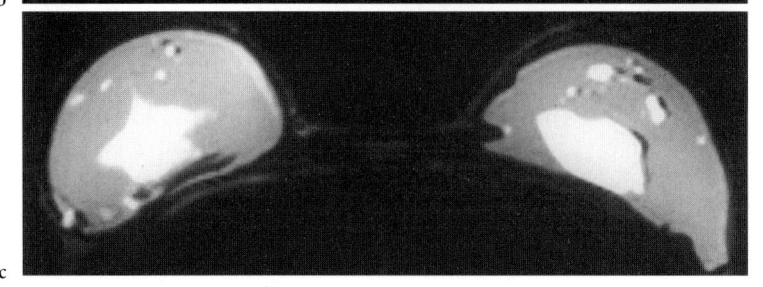

Fig. 18.17a–c. Three different type of breast implant as seen on MR imaging. **a** Reversed double-lumen: silicone-filled outer lumen surrounding inner saline-filled lumen (saline suppressed by chemical water suppression). Axial T2-weighted FSE images with water suppression. **b** Multicompartmental implant composed of an outermost saline-filled lumen (saline suppressed by chemical water suppression) surrounding two inner silicone-filled compartments. Axial T2-weighted FSE images with water suppression. **c** Single-lumen silicone implant with saline injected into the silicone at the time of surgery to increase the volume of the prostheses. T2-weighted STIR without water suppression

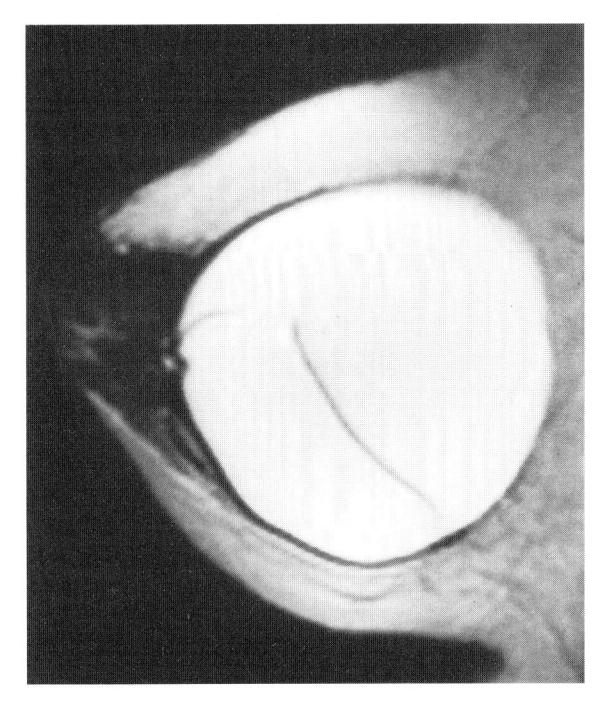

Fig. 18.18. Radial folds. Sagittal T2-weighted FSE image with water suppression shows prominent radial folds in a single-lumen implant. Radial folds extend to the periphery of the implant and are usually few in number. These folds are not indicative of rupture or leak

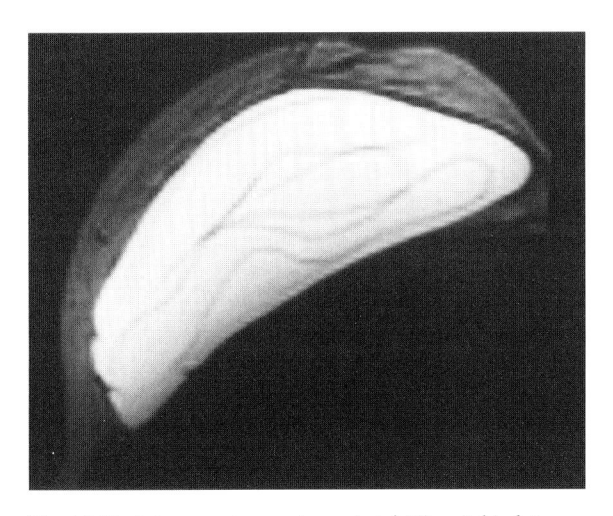

Fig. 18.19. Intracapsular rupture. Axial T2-weighted image shows multiple curvilinear low-signal-intensity lines within the implant, the "linguine" sign

on the pulse sequence (Table 18.2, Fig. 18.16). A variety of other types of implantable prostheses are occasionally encountered, which alter the MR appearance. These other varieties include expander implants (reverse double lumens: saline in the inner lumen, silicone in the outer lumen), multicompartmental implants, foam implants, and single-lumen silicone implants with saline directly injected into the silicone at the time of surgery (Fig. 18.17). Occasionally, two or even more implants are placed in one breast, a configuration commonly known as "stacked implants." Some implants have a coating of polyurethane covering the surface of the silicone envelope. These implants typically have a moderate to large amount of reactive fluid surrounding the implant. Saline implants have become more popular since the FDA limited the use of silicone-gel limplants in 1992.

One of the most commonly encountered variations seen in normal implants is the presence of prominent radial folds, normal infoldings of the silastic elastomer membrane (Fig. 18.18). These folds may be prominent enough to suggest an appearance of implant rupture. However, radial folds, even when prominent, can be recognized because they should extend to the periphery of the implant and are relatively few in number.

18.5.4 Intracapsular Rupture

The most reliable sign of intracapsular rupture on MR maging is the presence of multiple curvilinear low-signal-intensity lines within the high-signal-intensity silicone gel, the so-called linguine sign (Fig. 18.19) (Gorczyca et al. 1992). These curvilinear lines represent the collapsed implant membrane floating within the silicone gel (Gorczyca et al. 1994b). In early stages, the curvilinear lines may be located near the periphery of the implant.

The "teardrop" sign is sometimes the only indication of implant rupture. This sign represents silicone that has leaked out of the ruptured silicone implant and entered one of the radial folds on the exterior of the implant (Fig. 18.20). This finding is not definitive for a rupture in the implant membrane, because it has also been attributed to extensive gel bleed (see below).

Rarely, intracapsular rupture is associated with multiple hyperintense foci within the implant lumen on T2-weighted images, or multiple hypointense foci on water-suppression images. When only a few (less than six) of these water droplets are seen within a

homogeneous high-signal-intensity silicone (Fig. 18.15). A double-lumen silicone implant typically has an inner lumen of high-signal-intensity silicone surrounded by a smaller outer lumen which contains saline and has different signal intensities depending

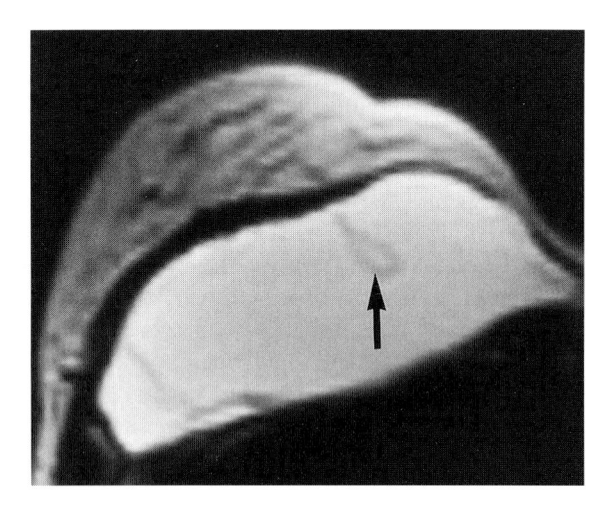

Fig. 18.20. Teardrop sign. Axial T2-weighted image shows a radial fold which contains silicone within it (*arrow*) ("teardrop" sign). Even after close inspection, at surgery no rupture could be found in the implant. The silicone outside the membrane was determined to be due to extensive gel bleed

silicone implant we do not diagnose a ruptured implant unless there is other supporting evidence of rupture. We have seen numerous cases in which these small water droplets have been present in intact implants.

Bulges and other contour deformities are not reliable signs of implant rupture (Fig. 18.21). In addition, fluid may be seen around the periphery of the implant and this should not be considered a sign of rupture. This fluid may represent saline in the outer component of a double-lumen implant or possibly reactive fluid.

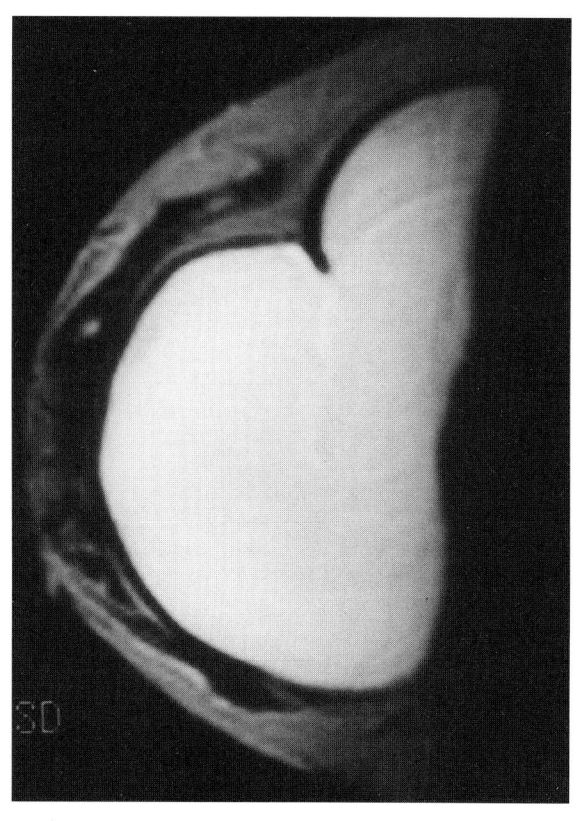

Fig. 18.21. Contour irregularity. Sagittal T2-weighted image of a normal single-lumen silicone implant with bulging of the contour of the implant

18.5.5 Extracapsular Rupture

The definitive sign of extracapsular rupture is the presence of free silicone in the breast parenchyma. On MR imaging free silicone presents as focal areas of high signal intensity outside the confines of the implant (Fig. 18.22) (MUND et al. 1993). The multiplanar capabilities of MR imaging allow precise localization of free silicone. Other causes of silicone in the parenchyma are previous silicone injections or silicone remaining from previous rupture of a silicone implant that has been removed.

Since extracapsular rupture is an extension of intracapsular rupture, all of the signs of intracapsular rupture can be present as well. For example, the linguine sign, the most reliable sign of intracapsular rupture, is almost always seen in cases of extracapsular rupture.

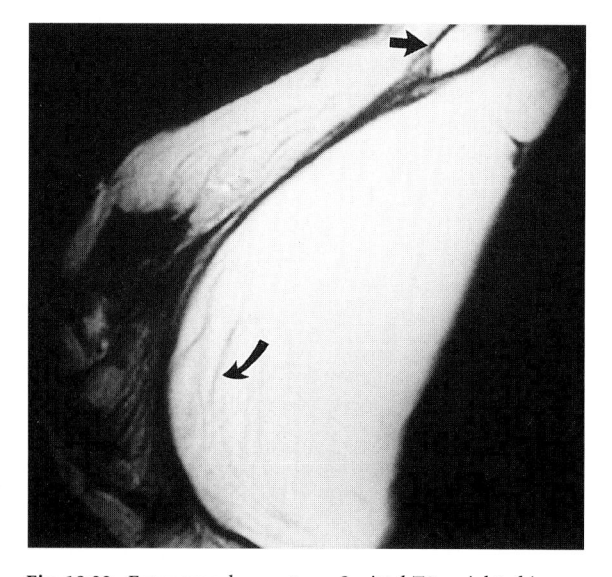

Fig. 18.22. Extracapsular rupture. Sagittal T2-weighted image demonstrates extracapsular silicone (*arrow*) and collapse of the silicone membrane indicated by the linguine sign (*curved arrow*)

18.5.6 Gel Bleed

Gel bleed is microscopic leakage of silicone through an intact implant membrane (BRODY 1977). Most if not all implants will eventually have gel bleed; however, the majority of gel bleeds are so small that they cannot be detected by MR imaging. Only when gel bleed is extensive can silicone gel be detected outside the silicone membrane, presenting with a teardrop sign when the silicone enters a radial fold. A focal or early intracapsular rupture can have a similar appearance to an extensive gel bleed and it can be difficult, if not impossible, to differentiate these two entities on MR images (Fig. 18.20) (GORCZYCA et al. 1992).

18.6 Comparison of Different Imaging Modalities

Mammography, ultrasonography (US), MR imaging, and computed tomography (CT) have all been used to evaluate the integrity of silicone breast implants (BERG et al. 1993; EVERSON et al. 1994; MUND et al. 1993). We conducted an investigation to compare these imaging modalities in an animal model (GORCZYCA et al. 1994a). We found that MR imaging and CT are more accurate than US and mammography for detection of intracapsular silicone implant ruptures when only the images were available for review.

Overall, MR imaging appears to be the most accurate method for evaluating the integrity of breast implants, with a reported sensitivity of 94% and specificity of 97% when two orthogonal sequences are used to evaluate the implant (GORCZYCA et al. 1994c).

Computed tomography is also accurate in detecting intracapsular ruptures, and is capable of depicting the linguine sign (GORCZYCA et al. 1994a; SCOTT et al. 1988). The ability of CT to detect extracapsular ruptures is still under investigation. Although CT probably should not be the modality of choice for imaging a young patient with implants because of the radiation exposure, it is useful for radiologists to be familiar with the CT findings of implant rupture because silicone implants may be imaged during CT examination of the chest and upper abdomen.

As indicated earlier, mammography is limited in its ability to detect silicone rupture and leakage, particularly intracapsular ruptures (DESTOUET et al. 1992). US is capable of detecting both intracapsular and extracapsular rupture with a reported sensitivity of 70% and specificity of 92% (DEBRUHL et al. 1993). However, US is very operator dependent and a steep learning curve is needed to be proficient in the US evaluation of implants. US only approaches the sensitivity of MR imaging when the US examination is performed by an experienced operator who also interprets the examination at the time it is performed.

References

Ahn CY, Shaw WW, Narayanan K, Gorczyca DP, Sinha S, DeBruhl ND, Bassett LW (1993) Definitive diagnosis of breast implant rupture using magnetic resonance imaging. Plast Reconstr Surg 94:681–691

American College of Radiology (1992) ACR committee on quality assurance in mammography. Patient positioning. In: Mammography quality control. American College of Radiology, Reston, VA, pp 57–99

Baker JL, Bartels RJ, Douglas WM (1976) Closed compression technique for rupturing a contracted capsule around a breast implant. Plast Reconstr Surg 58:137–141

Bassett LW, Brenner RJ (1992) Considerations when imaging women with breast implants. AJR 159:979–981

Bassett LW, Hendrick RE, Bassford TL, et al. (1994) Quality determinants of mammography. Clinical Practice Guideline, N. 13. AHCPR Publication no. 95-0632. Agency for Health Care Policy and Research, Public Health Service. U.S. Department of Health and Human Services, Rockville, Md, pp 1–170

Berg WA, Caskey CI, Hamper UM, et al. (1993) Diagnosing breast implant rupture with MR imaging, US, and mammography. Radiographics 13:1323–1336

Berkel H, Birdsell DC, Jenkins H (1992) Breast augmentation: A risk factor for breast cancer? N Engl J Med 326:1649–1653

Bridges AJ, Vasey FB (1993) Silicone breast implants: history, safety, and potential complications. Arch Intern Med 153:2638–2644

Brody GS (1977) Fact and fiction about breast implant "bleed." Plast Reconstr Surg 60:615–616

Cronin TD, Gerow F (1964) Augmentation mammaplasty: a new "natural feel" prosthesis. In: Transactions of the third international congress of plastic surgeons. Excerpta Medica, Amsterdam, pp 41–49

DeBruhl ND, Gorczyca DP, Ahn CY, Shaw WW, Bassett LW (1993) Silicone breast implants: US evaluation. Radiology 189:95–98

Dershaw DD, Chaglassian TA (1989) Mammography after prosthesis placement for augmentation or reconstructive mammoplasty. Radiology 170:69–74

Destouet JM, Monsees BS, Oser RF, Nemecek JR, Young VL, Pilgram TK (1992) Screening mammography in 350 women with breast implants: prevalence and findings of implant complications. AJR 159:973–978

Eklund GW, Busby RC, Miller SH, et al. (1988) Improved imaging of the augmented breast. AJR 151:469–473

Everson LI, Parantainen H, Detlie T, et al. (1994) Diagnosis of breast implant rupture: imaging findings and relative efficacies of imaging techniques. AJR 163:57–60

Ganott MA, Harris KM, Ilkhanipour ZS, Costa-Creco MA (1992) Augmentation mammoplasty: normal and abnormal findings with mammography and US. Radiographics 12:281–295

Garrido L, Kwong KK, Pfleiderer B, Crawley AP, Hulka CA, Whitman GL, Kopans DB (1993) Echo-planar chemical shift imaging of silicone gel prostheses. Magn Reson Imaging 11:625–634

Gorczyca DP, Sinha S, Ahn CY, et al. (1992) Silicone breast implants in vivo: MR imaging. Radiology 185:407–410

Gorczyca DP, DeBruhl ND, Ahn CY, et al. (1994a) Silicone breast implant ruptures in an animal model: comparison of mammography, MR imaging, US, and CT. Radiology 190:227–232

Gorczyca DP, DeBruhl ND, Mund DF, Bassett LW (1994b) Linguine sign at MR imaging: does it represent the collapsed silicone implant shell? Radiology 191:576–577

Gorczyca DP, Schneider E, DeBruhl ND, et al. (1994c) Silicone breast implant rupture: comparison between three-point Dixon and fast spin-echo MR imaging. AJR 162:305–310

Gruber RP, Jones HW (1981) Review of closed capsulotomy complications. Ann Plast Surg 6:271–275

Habal MB (1984) The biologic basis for the clinical application of the silicones. Arch Surg 119:843–848

Harris KM, Ganott MA, Shestak KC, Losken HW, Tobon H (1993) Silicone implant rupture: detection with US. Radiology 187:761–768

Kessler DA (1992) The basis of the FDA's decision on breast implants. N Engl J Med 326:1713–1715

Leibman AJ, Kruse B (1990) Breast cancer: mammographic and sonographic findings after augmentation mammoplasty. Radiology 174:195–198

Letterman G, Schurter M (1989) History of aesthetic breast surgery. In: Lewis JR (ed) The art of aesthetic plastic surgery, vol I. Little, Brown & Co, Boston, pp 21–27

Levine RA, Collins TL (1991) Definitive diagnosis of breast implant rupture by ultrasonography. Plast Reconstr Surg 87:1126–1128

Marik PE, Kark AL, Zambakides A (1990) Scleroderma after silicone augmentation mammoplasty: a report of two cases. S Afr Med J 77:212–213

McInnis WD (1990) Plastic surgery of the breast. In: Mitchell GW, Bassett LW (eds) The female breast and its disorders. Williams & Wilkins, Baltimore, pp 203–210

Mukundan S, Dixon WT, Kruse BD, Monticciolo DL, Nelson RC (1993) MR imaging of silicone gel-filled breast implants in vivo with a method that visualizes silicone selectively. J Magn Reson Imaging 3:713–717

Mund DF, Farria DM, Gorczyca DP, DeBruhl ND, Ahn CY, Shaw WW, Bassett LW (1993) MR imaging of the breast in patients with silicone-gel implants: spectrum of findings. AJR 161:773–778

Rosculet KA, Ikeda DM, Forrest ME, ONeal RM, Rubin JM, Jeffries DO, Helvie MA (1992) Ruptured gel-filled silicone breast implants: sonographic findings in 19 cases. AJR 159:711–716

Schneider E, Chan TW (1993) Selective MR imaging of silicone with the 3-piont Dixon technique. Radiology 187:89–93

Scott IR, Muller NL, Fitzpatrick DG, et al. (1988) Ruptured breast implant: computed tomographic and mammographic findings. Can Assoc Radiol J 39:152–154

Sinha S, Gorczyca DP, DeBruhl ND, Shellock FG, Gausche VR, Bassett LW (1993) MR imaging of silicone breast implants: comparison of different coil arrays. Radiology 187:284–286

Spiera H (1988) Scleroderma after silicone augmentation mammoplasty. JAMA 260:236–238

Steinbach BG, Hardt NS, Abbitt PL, Lanier L, Caffee HH (1993) Breast implants, common complications, and concurrent breast disease. Radiographics 13:95–118

Weiner SR (1991) Silicone augmentation mammoplasty and rheumatic disease. In: Stratmeyer ME (ed) Silicone in medical devices: proceedings of a conference held in Baltimore, MD, Feb 1–2, 1991. Department of Health and Human Services (Publication FDA 92-4249), Bethesda, MD, pp 81–102

Young VL, Bartell T, Destouet JM, Monsees B, Logan SE (1989) Calcification of breast implant capsule. South Med J 82:1171–1173

19 Breast Cancer Screening Projects: Results

I. Schreer and H.-J. Frischbier

CONTENTS

19.1	Introduction	333
19.2	Deficiencies in Analyzing Screening Results	333
19.3	Randomized Studies	335
19.3.1	Health Insurance Plan	335
19.3.2	Swedish Trial Results	335
19.3.3	The Edinburgh Trial	337
19.3.4	The Canadian National Breast Screening Study	337
19.4	Case-Control Studies	338
19.4.1	The Florence Study	338
19.4.2	The DOM Project	338
19.4.3	The Nijmegen Screening Program	338
19.5	Further Screening Studies	339
19.5.1	The Breast Cancer Detection Demonstration Project (BCDDP)	339
19.5.2	United Kingdom Trial of Early Detection of Breast Cancer (TEDBC)	340
19.5.3	National Health Service Breast Screening Program, United Kingdom	340
19.5.4	The German Mammography Study	341
19.6	Screening Mammography in Women Aged 40–49 years	342
	References	345

19.1 Introduction

The most effective means of reducing mortality in patients with breast cancer is early detection. Furthermore, the detection of cancer at an earlier stage allows treatment with breast conservation and hence a better quality of life.

Several controlled or randomized clinical studies carried out in North America and in European countries have shown that screening by periodic mammography can significantly reduce mortality from breast cancer. The follow-up of the populations studied is now long enough to allow firm conclusions regarding the efficacy of the early detection of breast cancer by screening mammography. Due to its sensitivity and high specificity, mammography is the most valid diagnostic test. An overview of the results of screening projects indicates an approximately 30% reduction in mortality in randomized trials and a greater than 50% reduction in case-control studies. Overall both sets of results are statistically significant, indicating that the reductions in mortality are very unlikely to have arisen by chance; indeed, the evidence from the randomized studies, which by their design avoid bias, suffices to demonstrate that breast cancer screening is effective in reducing mortality from breast cancer. On the other hand, when analyzing the epidemiologic effects of mass breast cancer screening by mammography, it is argued that the benefits and adverse effects of a screening program must be measured in terms of absolute risk. According to this measure the mortality reduction achieved by a mass screening program is only one death per ca. 15 000 woman-years. Many thousands of mammograms are thus needed to prevent one cancer death, and the criticism has been made that breast cancer screening has not been shown to produce a statistically significant reduction in total mortality: Breast cancer screening can be expected to reduce mortality from all causes of death by only 1%. Moreover, it could be possible that adverse effects of breast cancer screening contribute to mortality from other causes.

19.2 Deficiencies in Analyzing Screening Results

The possibility of detecting an early, clinically occult breast cancer is dependent on image quality and personal experience. However, image quality has been documented in none of the published screening studies. Sickles and Kopans (1993) pointed out that mammographic images from the randomized controlled studies are not all comparable with state-of-the-art mammography. They stated that "there should be no doubt that relatively poor quality mammography in all the randomized controlled

---

I. Schreer, MD, Universitäts-Frauenklinik, Strahlenabteilung, Martinistraße 52, 20246 Hamburg, Germany
H.-J. Frischbier, MD, Professor, Universitäts-Frauenklinik, Strahlenabteilung, Martinistraße 52, 20246 Hamburg, Germany

trials has reduced the ability of mammography to demonstrate the benefits achievable at current levels of performance." We agree that the improved technique of modern mammography results in a higher diagnostic benefit, especially in younger women aged 40-49 years. Therefore the conclusion originally drawn from randomized screening programs, that screening mammography in this age group consistently demonstrates no benefit in the first 5-7 years after study entry and only uncertain, at best marginal, benefit at 10-12 years (FLETCHER et al. 1993), is not relevant to the mammography now available.

The difference between the results from the two types of study – randomized versus case-control – is at least partly due to the fact that randomized trials have been analyzed on an "intention to treat" bias, that is, according to the groups to which the women were allocated regardless of whether they were actually screened. Such a procedure will yield a lower estimate of effect that would be obtained if all women offered screening were to accept the offer. The case-control studies indicate the possible extent of reduction in mortality from breast cancer among women who actually attend for a screening examination compared with women who do not, bearing in mind that some of this difference is likely to be due to women at high risk of dying from breast cancer being less likely to be screened than others; for example, those with a breast lump may have seen their doctors directly without formally entering a screening program. Nevertheless, randomized clinical trials are the preferred setting for the evaluation of the effects of mammography on reduction of mortality due to breast cancer. Comparisons between the different randomized clinical trials have to be assessed carefully (HOLMBERG 1993), however, because there are important differences in the trial designs in respect of: (a) compliance among invited women, (b) violation by also using clinically indicated mammography in the uninvited group, (c) use of mammography alone or in combination with physical examination, (d) age groups included, (e) use of mammography in one or two views, and (f) screening interval time (Table 19.1). On the other hand case-control studies are threatened by an additional factor: the self-selection of women to the screening group. HOLMBERG (1993) pointed out that this bias is "unpredictable and can work as a healthy screen effect or the reverse."

Table 19.1. Selected characteristics of the design and conduct of eight randomized controlled trials of breast cancer screening (from FLETCHER et al. 1993)

Study (year begun)	Age at entry (yr)	Screening modality	Periodicity (mo)	Randomization	Sample size Study	Sample size Control	% screened at 1st examination
HIP (1963)	40-64	2-view MM + CBE	12	Individual	30 239	30 756	67
Sweden Two-County (1977)	40-74	1-view MM	24 (age <50 yr) 33 (age ≥50 yr)	Cluster: geographic	78 085	56 782	89
Malmö (1976)	45-69	2-view MM	18-24	Cluster: birth cohort	21 088	21 195	74
Stockholm (1981)	40-64	1-view MM	28	Cluster: birth cohort	39 164	19 943	81
Göteborg (1982)	40-59	2-view MM	18	Individual (age 40-49 yr) Cluster (age 50-59 yr)	20 724	28 809	84
Edinburgh (1976)	45-64	2-view MM + CBE initially (later. usually 1-view MM)	12 24	Cluster: physician	23 226	21 904	61
Canada NBSS 1 (1980)	40-49	2-view MM + CBE	12	Individual: volunteers	25 214	25 216	−100[a]
Canada NBSS 2 (1980)	50-59	2-view MM + CBE versus CBE only	12	Individual: volunteers	19 711	19 694	−100[a]

CBE, Clinical breast examination; MM, mammography
[a] Study design included randomization of volunteers after clinical breast examination; accordingly, virtually 100% had their first screening examination

Currently available data are adequate to judge the effectiveness of screening mammography in reducing mortality in patients with breast cancer. In evaluating results of the different screening tests, it is also useful to compare the following additional measures: sensitivity, specificity, biopsy rate, positive predictive value, prevalence ratio, ratio of in situ to invasive cancers, size of detected cancers, and frequency of axillary lymph node metastases. However, most publications reporting screening results are incomplete in these respects. Further studies to determine age-specific onset, optimal screening intervals, and quality control should be undertaken.

19.3 Randomized Studies

19.3.1 Health Insurance Plan

The Health Insurance Plan (HIP) study is the oldest randomized trial. From 1963 to 1970 the HIP of New York offered about 31 000 women aged 40–64 years initial mammography and three additional examinations at annual intervals combined with physical examinations (STRAX et al. 1973). A control population of the same size received the normal care offered by the HIP which did not include screening. One-third of breast cancers diagnosed in this study would not have been detected without mammography. In patients over 50 years of age, 38% of cancers were found only by mammography alone, while in those below age 50 the figure was 20%. The rate of interval cancers between annual screening was 34%. Breast cancer in the study group had a lower rate of axillary node involvement (43% vs 54% in the control group). Of the cases detected through screening, 71% had no histologic evidence of node involvement. After 10 years the reduction of breast cancer mortality was 29% compared with the control group (SHAPIRO 1988). During the early follow-up period there was no reduced mortality among women in the 40- to 49-year age group. In the ≥50-year age group the percent difference in breast cancer deaths diminished to 23% at 18 years of follow-up.

Diagrams of cumulative deaths from breast cancer diagnosed within 5 years of entry for the study and control groups, stratified according to age, demonstrated that in women under 50 years old a significant difference appeared after more than 6 years (SHAPIRO 1988). However, analysis of the cumulative number of breast cancer deaths in the HIP study and control groups by 18 years of follow-up according to age at entrance showed that the differences among the young women were based on a small numbers of deaths and were not significant (RUTQVIST et al. 1990). Accordingly, not all investigators are convinced of the significance of the HIP data for women between 40 and 49 years of age, especially given that some of their cancers were diagnosed after the age of 50. It should be noted, however, that the technical standard of mammography during the period of the HIP study, i.e., 1963–1970, was much lower than that of present-day mammography, and that its ability to detect early cancers in the denser breasts of younger women was very limited.

19.3.2 Swedish Trial Results

After pilot studies by LUNDGREN in the early 1970s, the Swedish National Board of Health and Welfare initiated a large controlled study in two counties (Two-County Study) Kopparsberg (W) and Östergötland (E), in 1977. Further studies had already started in three cities: Malmö, Stockholm, and Gothenburg. All these studies were randomized trials and population based, i.e., they included all women of a selected age group within a defined geographic area. Invited women constituted the study group, and uninvited women, the control group. Randomization, age at entry, and study design differed between these five trials (Table 19.2).

In 1993 NYSTRÖM et al. gave an overview of the results of these trials. This revealed a significant, 24% [95% confidence interval (CI) 13%–34%] reduction in breast cancer mortality among women invited to mammography compared to the control group. The largest reduction was obtained in the 50- to 69-year age group (29%). Among women aged 40–49 years the reduction was 13%. During the first 8 years of follow-up in the latter age group the cumulative breast cancer mortality was similar in the study (invited) and the control group; however, after 8 years a difference was observed in favor of the study group. In the group of patients aged 70–74 years screening mammography "seems to have had only a marginal impact" (NYSTRÖM et al. 1993).

To assess uniformly the results of screening by a blind review of all deaths due to breast cancer in the five Swedish studies, an independent "end-point committee" (EPC) was founded. Based on Swedish cancer and cause of death registries, this committee divided the dead women into those with "breast cancer as the underlying cause of death" and those with "breast cancer present at death". The results are summarized in Table 19.3. We can conclude that the

Table 19.2. Basic characteristics of the five randomized trials in Sweden (from Nyström et al. 1993)

Characteristics	Screening center				
	Malmö	Kopparberg (W)	Östergötland (E)	Stockholm	Gothenburg
Study area	Municipality	Province	Province	Southern part of the province	Municipality
Randomization	Individual	Cluster	Cluster	Cluster	Individual (40–49 yr) Cluster (50–59 yr)
Cluster		Municipality, parish, tax district	Parish, municipality	Day of birth	Day of birth
Age at randomization	45–70	40–74	40–74	40–65	40–59
Year and month of randomization for invited members of control group first round:					
Start for invited group	Oct 76–Aug 78	July 77–Feb 80	May 78–March 81	March 81–May 83	Dec 82–April 84
End for control group		Sept 82–Dec 86	April 86–Feb 88	Oct 85–Dec 86	Nov 87–June 91
No. of invited women 40–74 years:					
Invited group[a]	20 695	38 562	38 405	38 525	20 724
Control goup[a]	20 783	18 478	37 145	20 651	28 809
Study design:					
Number of views	Two[b]	One	One	One	Two
Screening interval	18–24	24, 33[c]	24, 33[c]	28	18
Attendance rate, 1st round	74%	89%	89%	82%	84%

[a] Women with breast cancer diagnosed before date of randomization excluded
[b] From round 3, one or two views were used according to the parenchymal pattern
[c] Averages for the 40–49 and 50–74 age groups respectively

Table 19.3. Number of person-years of follow-up and events by invited (IG) and control group (CG) for "breast cancer as underlying cause of death" and for "breast cancer present at death" according to the End-Point Committee by screening center and age at entry. "Follow-up" model. Relative risks and 95% confidence intervals (CI) are shown (from Nyström et al. 1993)

Screening center	Age at entry (yr)	Person-years of follow-up ×1000		"Breast cancer as under-lying cause of death"				"Breast cancer present at death"			
				Events		Relative risk	95% CI	Events		Relative risk	95% CI
		IG	CG	IG	CG			IG	CG		
Malmö	45–70	239	240	87	108	0.81	0.62–1.07	99	116	0.85	0.65–1.12
Kopparberg (W)	40–74	403	192	132	91	0.68	0.52–0.89	141	91	0.73	0.56–0.95
Östergötland (E)	40–74	372	362	119	139	0.82	0.64–1.05	118	146	0.78	0.61–0.99
Stockholm	40–65	287	164	53	40	0.80	0.53–1.22	55	41	0.81	0.53–1.23
Gothenburg	40–58	129	181	27	47	0.86	0.54–1.37	27	48	0.84	0.52–1.35
All	40–74	1430	1139	418	425	0.77	0.67–0.88	440	442	0.78	0.68–0.89

reduction of mortality was similar for these two different end-points. For analysis of the study results the authors used two models: a "follow-up" and an "evaluation" model. The follow-up model included all breast cancer deaths among women with a primary diagnosis after the date of randomization and before a common fixed study end-point of 31 December 1989. The evaluation model ignored breast cancer deaths among women whose primary tumor, according to the cancer register, was diagnosed after completion of the screening of the controls. In Table 19.4 the number of person-years of follow-up and events by study and control group according to these two models are summarized. The overall relative risk in the follow-up model was 0.77 (95% CI 0.67–0.88) and in the evaluation model, 0.76 (95% CI 0.66–0.87).

Besides reduction in breast cancer mortality, another factor was studied in the Swedish trials: the

Table 19.4. Number of person-years of follow-up and events by invited (IG) and control group (CG) for "breast cancer as underlying cause of death" according to the End-Point Committee by screening center, age at entry, and model of analysis ("follow-up" and "evaluation" models). Relative risks and 95% confidence intervals (CI) are shown (from Nyström et al. 1993)

Screening center	Age at entry	Person-years of follow-up ×1000 IG	Person-years of follow-up ×1000 CG	"Follow-up" model Events IG	"Follow-up" model Events CG	"Follow-up" model Relative risk	"Follow-up" model 95% CI	"Evaluation" model Events IG	"Evaluation" model Events CG	"Evaluation" model Relative risk	"Evaluation" model 95% CI
Malmö	45–70	239	240	87	108	0.81	0.62–1.07	87	108	0.81	0.62–1.07
Kopparberg (W)	40–74	403	192	132	91	0.68	0.52–0.89	114	79	0.68	0.51–0.90
Östergötland (E)	40–74	372	362	119	139	0.82	0.64–1.05	113	129	0.84	0.65–1.08
Stockholm	40–65	287	164	53	40	0.80	0.53–1.22	40	32	0.72	0.45–1.16
Gothenburg	40–59	129	181	27	47	0.86	0.54–1.37	25	44	0.84	0.51–1.39
All centers	40–49	427	350	84	75	0.90	0.65–1.24	73	68	0.87	0.63–1.20
	50–59	540	454	151	174	0.72	0.58–0.90	137	162	0.71	0.57–0.89
	60–69	372	271	130	138	0.69	0.54–0.88	121	126	0.71	0.56–0.91
	70–74	91	64	53	38	0.98	0.63–1.53	48	36	0.94	0.60–1.46
	40–74	1430	1139	418	425	0.77	0.67–0.88	379	392	0.76	0.66–0.87

screening interval. As demonstrated in Table 19.2, the screening interval varied in these studies from 18 to 33 months. No study included a randomization of different intervals. Tabar et al. (1987) analyzed the results of the Two-County Study. They reported that although the average interval in that study was 33 months for women aged 50 years or more, the optimum interval between screening examinations in this age group is 24 months at most. Moreover, Tabar et al. concluded that women below 50 years of age should be screened at shorter intervals to ensure a high probability of detecting rapidly growing tumors while they are still small. Their results indicate that to achieve a high reduction in breast cancer mortality, 50% of screen-detected invasive cancers should be less than 15 mm in diameter and 70% should not have lymph node metastases.

19.3.3 The Edinburgh Trial

The Edinburgh Trial of screening for breast cancer involved approximately 45 000 women aged 45–64 years between 1979 and 1981. The women who attended underwent two-view mammography and physical examination at their prevalence screen. The incidence screen involved physical examinations alone in years 2, 4, and 6 and physical examination combined with oblique-view mammography in years 3, 5, and 7.

The cancer detection rate was 6.2 per 1000 women attending at the first visit and around 3 per 1000 women in the following visits when both mammography and physical examination were performed (Roberts et al. 1990). The detection rate was around 1 per 1000 at the intervening visits with physical examinations alone. At the first screen 96% of the cancers were detected by mammography and 74% by physical examination. Only 61% of the invited women attended the screening examination and the percentage decreased year by year. Therefore a large proportion (53%) of the study population was never screened.

After 7 years of follow-up the mortality reduction was 17% (95% CI 0.58–1.18), which was statistically not significant. In women aged over 50 years the mortality reduction was 20%.

19.3.4 The Canadian National Breast Screening Study

The Canadian trials, performed between 1980 and 1988, comprised two parts: The first trial (NBSS 1) compared (a) combined screening by mammography and physical examination repeated three or four times and (b) a single physical examination in women aged 40–49 years, while the second trial appraised the same examination procedure in women aged 50–59 years (NBSS 2). All women were instructed in breast self-examination. In the 40- to 49-year age group there was an excess of advanced cancers in the group undergoing mammography plus physical examination at the first and the following courses up to 5 years (Mettlin and Smart 1993). Seven years after starting this trial the breast cancer death rates in the 40- to 49-year age group were 14.7 in the screened group and 10.4 per 10 000 person-years for those who received only physical examination. The death rates in the 50- to 59-year age group were 18.5 compared to 19.0. The authors concluded that, "The differences in death rates were not statistically significant in either the younger or older women."

The Canadian trials are affected by more contaminations than other studies. In the study group 7% and in the control group 26% of women had mammograms outside of the trial. In each of the study arms 10%–15% of women failed to have their scheduled mammograms. A criticized point in this study was that deaths in the control group of women may have been ascertained less completely than those in the study group. But the most important argument against the value of the trials was the use of volunteers who selected themselves to participate.

Because the quality of mammograms in the trials had been questioned by some experts, a retrospective review was undertaken by three experts. They stated that between 1980 and 1985 only 49%–75% of mammograms received satisfactory scores for contrast, density, and image quality. In 1986 and 1987, a significant improvement in technical quality occurred, with a satisfactory score of 85%–89% (Baines et al. 1990). All of these factors may have led to contamination and affected the results.

19.4 Case-Control Studies

19.4.1 The Florence Study

In 1970 a population-based screening program for breast cancer was started in Florence (Italy). Women between 40 and 70 years old were offered mammography at an interval of 2.5 years. Physical examination was performed only in selected cases. Between 1970 and 1981 approximately 25 000 women were invited to attend for screening. The average compliance upon the first invitation was 60% (Palli et al. 1986). For the evaluation of the efficacy of this screening program a case-control study design was used: the screening histories of all women who died from breast cancer between 1977 and 1984 were compared with those of a matched group of living controls. The authors found a relative risk of 0.57 (95% CI 0.35–0.92) and of 0.32 (95% CI 0.20–0.52) for women screened only once or at least twice. No significant protective effect was shown for women below the age of 50 years. In 1990 Paci et al. examined the early indicators of efficacy of the Florence program. They studied the observed number of interval cancers and compared them with the expected incident cancers, examining their ratio at different time intervals. The prevalence/incidence (P/I) ratio can be calculated as an early indicator of efficacy. For the 40- to 49-year age group, the P/I ratio was 1.09; for the 50- to 59-year age group it was 3.14, and for the the 60- to 69-year age group, 4.82.

19.4.2 The DOM Project

In Utrecht (The Netherlands) the so-called DOM project was started in 1974 to evaluate screening for breast cancer. Nearly 15 000 women aged 50–64 years at entry to the study were examined by physical examination and xeromammography at intervals of 12, 18, 24, and 48 months.

A matched case-control study was performed to evaluate the risk of mortality from breast cancer (Collette et al. 1984). The relative risk in the group of screened women compared to women never screened was 0.30 (95% CI 0.13–0.70). From the data no conclusions can be drawn about the ideal screening interval. Lengthening of the interval from 1 to 2 years did not seem to worsen the staging of screen-detected cancers (Day et al. 1986).

19.4.3 The Nijmegen Screening Program

In 1975 a population-based screening program with mammography was introduced in the city of Nijmegen, The Netherlands. At 2-year intervals up to 1986 six screening rounds were performed, with mammography as the only screening procedure, in women aged over 35 years. Peeters et al. (1989) examined rates of attendance, referral, biopsy, and detection. Positive predictive values for biopsy were 30% on average for women aged under 50 years and 60%–70% for elderly women. In the younger age group the ratio between screen-detected and interval cancers was about 1:1 and in patients over the age of 50 years, 2:1.

Van Dijck et al. (1993) performed a review of the mammograms of the eighth screening round of the Nijmegen program. They compared the mammograms of 40 patients with interval cancers to those of 44 screen-detected cancers. All patients had been examined by mammography in the seventh round between 1987 and 1988. The interval cancers were classified in 13% of cases as "screening error," in 38% as "minimal sign present," in 43% as "radiographically occult," and in 6% as "radiographically occult at diagnosis." They concluded that annual instead of biennial screening may detect most "screening error" cases and some of the "minimal sign present" and "radiographically occult" cases at an earlier stage. Prevention of screening errors can be achieved "by thorough training of the radiologists and mammography radiographers, by ensuring a high technical quality of the mammographic films, and by applying double reading."

KOPANS (1993) pointed out that many of the cancers that were not detectable on the index screen in the Nijmegen program could have been diagnosed earlier if the screening interval had been shortened to 1 year. He mentioned the observation of MOSKOWITZ (1986), who reported that in women under the age of 50 a 2-year interval would be too long, as during that time cancers could grow to clinically detectable sizes.

19.5 Further Screening Studies

19.5.1 The Breast Cancer Detection Demonstration Project (BCDDP)

In 1973 the American Cancer Society and National Cancer Institute initiated a national screening program. In 29 widely distributed locations throughout the United States, more than 280000 women between the ages of 35 and 74 years were examined annually by physical examination and two-view mammography. Almost half of the women were under the age of 50 years; 51.7% completed all five screening courses, and 86.7% had two or more examinations.

In 1982 BAKER analyzed the cancer detection rates and compared the rates of biopsy performance, minimal cancer detection, and interval cancers for the years 1–5 (Table 19.5). The total nonmalignant to malignant biopsy ratio was 5.4; in the 35- to 39-year age group it was 16.4, and in the 70- to 74-year age group, 2.7. The age-specific interval cancer rates between years 1 and 5 ranged between 5.3 (in the 35- to 39-year age group) and 10.1 (in the 60- to 64-year age group). In the 40- to 49-year age group 35.4% of the cancers were diagnosed by mammography alone.

SEIDMANN et al. (1987) evaluated the efficacy of screening in the BCDDP by survival. In patients with screen-detected cancers survival adjusted for lead time was constantly 1 year longer compared to analyses in the study by the HIP.

In 1988 MORRISON et al. analyzed breast cancer incidence and mortality in the BCDDP and reported a 9-year cumulative mortality from breast cancer of only 79.6% of that expected in women who did not have breast cancer diagnosed by the screening procedure. In those aged 35–49 years at entry the ratio was 0.89, in those aged 50–59 years 0.76, and in those aged 60–74 years, 0.74. In a 14-year follow-up study of women participating in the BCDDP, SMART et al. (1993) evaluated the data from 64185 women who had been selected for inclusion in the long-term follow-up program. This group included 4275 patients with breast cancer diagnosed during the screening project. Distribution of breast cancer cases according to both stage and histology and 14-year adjusted survival rates were analyzed by three age groups (Tables 19.6, 19.7). The differences in 14-year survival rates for these age groups were small: 90.2% in women aged 40–49 years, 86.2% in those aged 50–59 years, and 87.6% in those aged 60–69 years. This analysis indicates that both for stage distribution and for survival rates there are no significant differences between women under and women over 50 years of age.

The benefit of screening for women in the 40- to 49-year age group observed in the HIP study after 18 years of follow-up was confirmed by the BCDDP. It must be emphasized that BCDDP screening was performed as an annual procedure with two-view

Table 19.5. Five-year results of BCDDP: comparison of crude detection rates, biopsy performance rates, minimal cancer detection rates, minimal cancer detection rates, and interval cancer rates for years 1–5 (from BAKER 1982)

	Year								
	1	1.5	2	2.5	3	3.5	4	4.5	5
Biopsy performance rates	358.1		187.6		173.4		145.9		117.8
Cancer detection rates	55.8		26.5		25.2		25.4		23.6
Minimal cancer detection rates	18.4		8.5		8.6		8.0		7.0
Interval cancer rates		8.0		7.7		8.0		7.5	

Rates are per 10000 annual screenings
Minimal cancers are defined as noninfiltrating cancers, or infiltrating tumors <1 cm in diameter

Table 19.6. Distribution of breast cancer cases by age for histology and lymph node status, size, and stage (from SMART et al. 1993)

Characteristic	No.				%			
	Total	40–49 yr	50–59 yr	60–69 yr	Total	40–49 yr	50–59 yr	60–69 yr
Histology								
In situ	528	166	232	130	15	17	15	13
Invasive	2683	742	1180	761	75	74	76	76
−LNS	2009	544	866	599	56	54	56	60
+LNS	674	198	314	162	19	20	20	16
Unknown	354	96	148	110	10	10	9	11
Total	3565	1004	1560	1001	100	100	100	100
Size of lesion								
In situ	528	166	232	130	22	25	22	19
Size <1 cm	301	78	117	106	13	12	11	16
Size 1–1.9 cm	842	211	362	269	35	32	35	40
Size 2–4.9 cm	611	181	286	144	26	27	27	21
Size >5 cm	101	27	49	25	4	4	5	4
Total	2383	663	1046	674	100	100	100	100
Stage at diagnosis								
0	524	165	229	130	15	16	15	13
1a + 1b	259	65	99	95	7	6	6	9
1c	644	157	278	209	18	16	18	21
2	459	139	205	115	13	14	13	11
3	498	136	235	127	14	14	15	13
Unknown	1181	342	514	325	33	34	33	32
Total	3565	1004	1560	1001	100	100	100	100
Mode of detection[a]								
MM alone	780	170	311	245	40	40	44	52
MM and PE	847	207	349	201	41	49	50	43
PE alone	105	40	35	22	9	10	5	5
Neither	17	3	9	4	10	1	1	1
Total	1749	420	704	472	100	100	100	100

LNS, lymph node status; MM, two-view mammographic screenings; PE, physical examinations
[a] Recommended for biopsy before May 1977

mammography and in combination with physical examination. Screening studies with intervals of 2 years or longer, with only one-view mammography, and without physical examination are inadequate to evaluate screening efficacy in women under the age of 50 years. Therefore it is not surprising that the randomized studies with an inadequate study design failed to find significant evidence of benefit in women aged 40–49 years.

19.5.2 United Kingdom Trial of Early Detection of Breast Cancer (TEDBC)

In 1979 a first screening round in the TEDBC was carried out in Guildford. This trial is a comparative population study for women aged 45–64 years registered with a general practioner. For 7 years an annual clinical examination was combined with mammography at the first, third, fifth, and seventh rounds. During this trial the detection rate increased "by some 40%" (THOMAS 1989). At the seventh round (12575 women) screen sensitivity was 95%, clinical sensitivity 34%, mammographic sensitivity 93%, and predictive value 65%.

19.5.3 National Health Service Breast Screening Program, United Kingdom

In 1991 the U.K. National Health Service introduced a screening program for women aged 50–64 years. All women who are registered with general practitioners are invited to attend for screening mammography at 3-year intervals. CHAMBERLAIN et al. (1993) reported the results of this program for 1991–1992. Of 1.4 million women who were invited for screening, 71.3% accepted the invitation. In the first round 6.3 breast cancers were detected per 1000 women screened. In the second round 3 years later, 3.4 breast cancers per 1000 were diagnosed. On the basis of the experience of two screening clinics in

Table 19.7. Fourteen-year adjusted survival rates from breast cancer cases by age for histology and lymph node status, size, and stage (from SMART et al. 1993)

Characteristic	Overall	Age-specific survival		
		40–49 yr	50–59 yr	60–69 yr
Histology				
In situ	98.8	99.4	99.0	97.7
Invasive	80.3	81.8	79.1	81.1
Invasive (−LNS)	86.4	86.0	85.1	89.0
Invasive (+LNS)	61.6	70.3	61.6	51.6
Unknown	78.8	81.0	78.6	79.6
Size of lesions				
In situ	98.8	99.4	99.0	97.7
Size <1 cm	90.1	91.9	99.0	97.7
Size 1–1.9 cm	84.0	85.6	83.8	82.1
Size 2–4.9 cm	73.7	74.1	73.6	74.9
Size >5 cm	63.3	[a]	[a]	[a]
Stage at diagnosis				
0	98.8	99.4	99.2	97.7
1a + 1b	92.7	96.4	85.1	97.7
1c	91.3	90.2	91.6	92.1
2	82.2	80.3	83.6	82.5
3	59.5	67.7	59.6	50.6
Unknown	79.6	81.0	78.6	79.6
Mode of detection				
MM alone	87.5	90.2	86.2	87.6
MM and PE	80.0	82.9	79.9	77.4
PE alone	85.3	84.6	83.8	[a]
Neither	75.6	77.8	73.3	[a]

Values are percentages. MM, two-view mammography screening; PE, physical examination
[a] Too few cases to calculate rate

Edinburgh and Guildford (THOMAS 1989) a number of target performance indicators were suggested: an acceptance rate of 70%, a referral rate of 10% or less, a biopsy rate of 3% or less with a malignant to benign ratio greater than 0.5, a cancer detection rate in the first round of at least 5 per 1000, and a detection rate of invasive cancers less than 10 mm of at least 1.5 per 1000. Only 6 out of 17 regions and 32% of individual programs reached the target of 1.5 breast cancers less than 10 mm per 1000 screened women. It is the aim of this national program to reduce breast cancer mortality by 25% by the year 2000.

19.5.4 The German Mammography Study

In 1971 a prospective screening study was started at the University Hospital in Hamburg. Up to 1986 a total of 14000 women aged over 35 years without clinically suspicious findings were examined by two-view mammography and physical examination at 2-year intervals. In parallel with the screening study a prospective study was carried out in which all patients with clinically manifest breast cancers treated in Department of Gynecology of the University Hospital were followed up. Thus it was possible to compare the results of two studies performed over the same period and with identical histologic assessment, staging, therapy, and follow-up.

Figure 19.1 shows the survival rate of patients with breast cancer who participated in the screening program ($n = 176$) as compared with that of patients with clinically manifest tumors ($n = 338$). Of the screen-detected cases, 22 were interval cancers, and in 28 patients the screen interval was longer than 3 years. Fifty-three cancer patients (32.5%) were under the age of 50 years. In Fig. 19.2 the survival rate of these patients is compared with that of older patients. There was no significant difference ($P = 0.4452$) in the survival rate between the two age groups. Of the screen-detected cancers, 22% were noninvasive and 58% were less than 2 cm in diameter; in 15% axillary lymph node metastases were found histologically.

Based on these results in 1989 a pilot study was set up (German Mammography Study) to develop and test quality assurance measurement under the special conditions of the decentralized German health care system and to work out recommendations for establishing mammographic screening as a nationwide activity. All women in two study regions of northern Germany attending a regular cancer screening examination were eligible if they were at least 40 years old, had no suspicious findings on

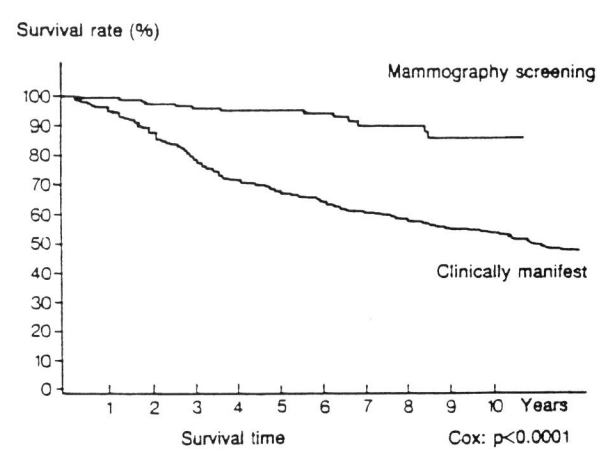

Fig. 19.1. Survival rate of patients who participated in the Hamburg Mammography Screening Study compared to that of patients with clinically manifest breast cancers, treated in the Gynecological Department of the University Hospital, Hamburg

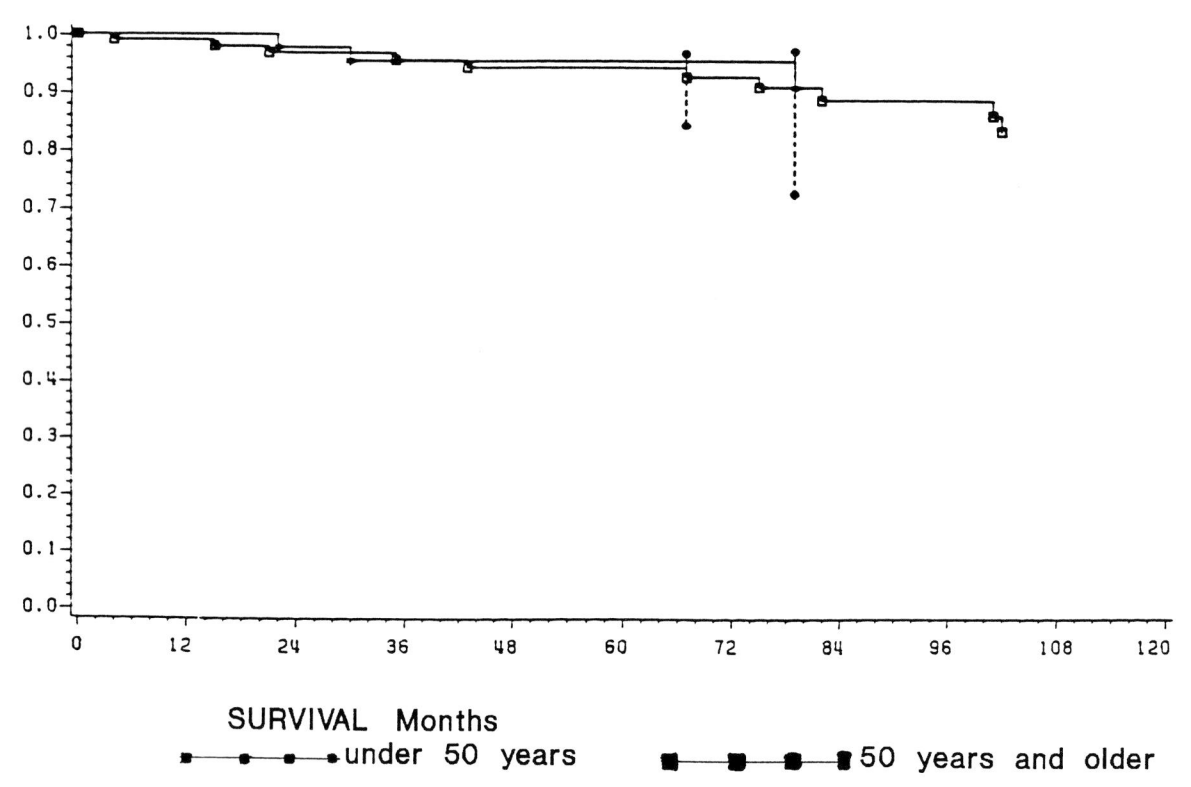

Fig. 19.2. Survival rate of patients with breast cancer detected by mammography in the Hamburg Mammography Screening Study. Comparison between patients aged under 50 ($n = 53$) and over 50 ($n = 110$) years (Cox: $P = 0.4452$)

physical examination, and had not undergone mammography during the preceding year. The rescreening interval was 1 year. In 170 patients a breast cancer was detected by mammography. In the first round 110 cancers were diagnosed: 14% ductal cancer in situ (DCIS), 20% invasive cancers <1 cm, and only 10% axillary lymph node metastases. This study demonstrated that office-based physicians in a decentralized fee for service health system will cooperate effectively in a quality assurance program which results in measurable improvements of operation (FRISCHBIER et al. 1994).

19.6 Screening Mammography in Women Aged 40–49 Years

In the United States among women between 40 and 49 years of age, breast cancer is the most common malignant tumor and the leading cause of death from cancer. Approximately 30%–40% of the years of life lost to breast cancer are due to malignant disease found in women aged 40–49 years. In 1993, 28 900 women developed breast cancer in the 40- to 49-year age group compared with 31 500 in the 50- to 59-year age group. Thus early detection in the younger age group is a major challenge.

We have significant scientific proof of a 20%–40% reduction in mortality in randomized controlled trials of women starting at age 40, but all these studies are flawed by low statistical power, especially when subgroup analyses for women 40–49 years of age are performed. None of the trials had been designed or performed properly to evaluate this subsegment of the population. Only the Canadian National Breast Screening Study (CNBSS) has been designed prospectively to assess the specific age period of 40–49. The screen modality consisted of two-view mammography in conjunction with physical examination at 1-year intervals. After 7 years of follow-up the published results demonstrated no evidence that screening for breast cancer was effective among young women. It seemed that mammography did not offer any additional advantage over skilled physical examination in women aged 50–59. Major concern exists about this study with regard to image quality, skill of the radiologists, the lack of blinded randomization, cross-over between the study population and the control group, and insufficient length of follow-up, so that no conclusions regarding breast cancer screening in younger women should be drawn from the study at this time.

The HIP study demonstrated a 24% mortality reduction becoming evident after 9 years of follow-up, but is also considered to have too low a statistical power.

To date we are unable to establish proven mortality benefit in the younger age group due to too few patients and too few "events." Therefore no further meta-analyses are considered helpful. A large study population is needed with a long follow-up. The UICC Meeting in Geneva stipulated an enrollment of 1 500 000 women from the United States and Europe with results not to be expected for another 10–15 years. Instead of waiting, and because additional information is urgently needed, surrogate measures (FEIG 1994) and surrogate end-points have been used to assess screening efficacy. These data can provide results years before mortality reduction rates become available. These surrogate measures include tumor size, rate of DCIS and small invasive cancers, lymph node involvement and grading, prevalence/incidence ratio, interval cancer rates, stages, and survival. They have been analyzed from a number of observational studies.

The largest study in the world, The BCDDP, demonstrated identical percentages of "minimal cancers" in the various age groups. No difference was found between the 40- to 49-year and 50- to 59-year age groups concerning lymph node status, but the number of lymph nodes involved was higher in the 60- to 69-year age group, resulting in a somewhat poorer survival rate than among women in the two younger groups.

Comparable results were reported from smaller studies. The population-based Uppsala Screening Program, started in 1988, was divided into two age subgroups, women aged 40–54 years and women aged 55–59 years. In the first round the younger age group was examined with mediolateral oblique and craniocaudal views without a grid. The intended screening interval was 18 months for the younger age group and 24 months for the older age group. The average screening interval turned out to be 23.4 months. In the first screening round the participation rate was 44.6% for women aged 40–49. The proportion of minimal cancers in the 40- to 49-year group was the same or greater than for the older women and greater than the proportion surfacing between screenings.

In an observational study comparing women under 50 years of age with mammographically detected cancer or cancer detected by clinical examination, STACEY-CLEAR et al. (1992) reported the rate of DCIS to be 40% in the former group but only 9% in the latter group. Fifty percent of the mammographically detected cancers were stage I, as opposed to just 30% in the women with palpable cancers. Excluding DCIS, the survival rates were 91% for women with mammographically detected infiltrating cancers and 72% for women with palpable tumors.

Subsequent screening mammography permits detection of tumors at an earlier stage, resulting in a reduced breast cancer mortality (FRANKEL et al. 1995). Therefore reduction in stage could be a reliable, intermediate outcome indicator of decreased mortality.

A recently published screening study (CURPEN et al. 1995) running from 1985 to 1994 also demonstrated no statistically significant differences between women aged 40–49 and women aged 50–64 years old in terms of tumor size, lymph node status, or stage of breast cancer detected. The median size of breast cancers was 10 mm for women aged 40–49 versus 11 mm for women aged 50–64. In both age groups 88% of the patients showed no evidence of metastases to axillary lymph nodes. The rate of advanced breast cancer was even lower (19%) than in the older group (26%). Comparable results concerning tumor size and stage have been published by TABAR et al. (1993). They reported a nonsignificant 26% reduction in mortality in the 40- to 49-year age group in the Kopparberg part of the Swedish Two-County Trial. The data consisted of 115 tumors in the 40- to 49-year age group in Kopparberg county, 94 consecutive cases diagnosed in Kopparberg county between 1989 and 1992, and 88 cases from the Screening Mammography Program of British Columbia. Whilst the older series was done without a grid over 2-year intervals, both of the later series used two-view mammography with a grid. Tumor size was found to be similar among the different age groups. Only a slightly better prognosis was found for the node-positive women in the group 40–49 years of age.

Poorly differentiated tumors are likely to grow more quickly than well-differentiated ones. In the Swedish Two-County Trial, cancers diagnosed in refusers had not only an unfavorable size and nodal status but also an adverse grade. This suggested the hypothesis that for some tumors the grade deteriorates as the tumor grows. Comparing the tumors from the PSP (passive study population) with the interval and incidence of screen-detected tumors and refusers' tumors from the ASP (active study population), more grade 3 tumors were found in the control group. If controlled for size, however, the difference was no longer significant, suggesting that the effect of earlier detection on grade can be predicted by the effect of earlier detection on size. Four important conclusions were drawn:

1. Tumor size is very strongly related to detection status (control, prevalence screen, subsequent screen, interval, refuser) and to grade and node status.
2. Grade and size are significantly and independently associated with each other and with detection status.
3. The earlier detection of tumors by screening is associated with more prognostically favorable categories of all the tumor characteristics.
4. It is likely that for some cancers early detection actually confers a more favorable malignancy grade, but there are still considerable numbers of grade 3 screen-detected tumors.

Screening should be detecting grade 3 tumors, and as many as possible before their size exceeds 15 mm. To assume possible differences in tumor biology in women aged 40–49 could be shown to be incorrect. On the contrary, "the prognosis for women in their forties is, if anything, better than for older women" (TABAR et al. 1993). Regardless of age, it is the prognostic factors tumor size, nodal status, and tumor grade that influence subsequent survival. In consequence the effectiveness and success of a screening program can be predicted by analyzing these tumor characteristics.

Difficulty in demonstrating a significant reduction in mortality therefore may be considered a reflection of the adequacy or otherwise of the screening process itself.

Further insight into the specific problems of screening younger age groups can be gained when taking into account the interval cancers and advanced cancers detected during the screening process. The incidence of interval cancers depends on both the frequency of screening and the sensitivity of the screening modality. Studies of interval cancers have revealed that mammographic sensitivity is lower in young women and the cancer growth rate is faster (TABAR et al. 1987). Data from the Nijmegen study group showed the median volume doubling time of breast cancer diagnosed in women aged 50–70 years to be 157 days (95% CI 121–204 days), while for women younger than 50 years it was 80 days (95% CI 44–147 days) (TABAR et al. 1992). The authors concluded that more frequent screening is needed for women younger than 50 years. The "so journ time" (i.e., the time spent in the preclinical detectable state) was estimated to be 1.25 years for women aged 40–49 compared with 3.8 years for women aged 50 and over.

Fifty-eight percent of the interval cancers in the Two-County Trial were stage II or worse. Women whose cancers were diagnosed during the first or second year after screening correspondingly had the same unsatisfactory survival rates as the control group. This was also confirmed by the HIP study.

In the 40- to 49-year age group in the Two-County Trial, interval cancers were found to contribute more than half of the total breast cancer deaths (TABAR et al. 1987). In these younger women one-view mammography detected only about 60% of the cancers that would have surfaced in the succeeding 12 months and 30% of those that would have appeared in the second year. Comparable data resulted from the Florence screening program (PACI et al. 1990). Clearly, the lower the proportion of interval cancers, the greater will be the reduction of breast cancer mortality.

It was also found in the Two-County Trial that 38% of the cancers in the young age group were stage II whereas the figures were 25% for women 50–59 years old and 17% for those 60–69 years old (TABAR et al. 1987). The authors concluded that "for women aged 40–49 years single-view mammography every two years is not a sufficiently effective screening policy."

The sensitivity of mammography is considered to be lower in younger women. Poorer efficiency in early studies was due to poor technical quality compared to today's high-quality equipment. Comparisons are possible between the HIP study and the BCDDP. In the HIP study only 38.8% of cancers in the age group 40–49 were detected with mammography, as compared to 85.4% in the BCDDP.

Higher sensitivity and specificity are achievable with two views (BASSET et al. 1987; IKEDA and SICKLES 1988; THURFJELL 1990; SICKLES et al. 1990). An improvement in image quality of 34% since 1985 has been determined in the United States (CONWAY et al. 1994).

Further results reflecting the influence of modern high-quality mammographic technique are as follows (SICKLES and KOPANS 1993):

1. The lower rate of T2 tumors in modern series in which women 40–49 years old are screened (12%–13% of cases vs 22%–30% in randomized controlled trials).

2. A lowering of the rate of lymph node-positive cancers (12%–13% vs 23%–43%)
3. A reduced number of stage 2 or higher cancers (15%–19% vs 24%–58%)

The high costs of a screening program for younger women are the source of controversy. These costs arise from the lower prevalence or incidence, the lower positive predictive value, the fact that more biopsies are needed per detected cancer, and the further procedures required to evaluate abnormal examinations (KERLIKOWSKE et al. 1993). Economic problems in Europe and North American countries have led to restrictions on public health care. Nevertheless, we should try to distinguish strictly between financial aspects and scientific evidence. There is every reason to believe that screening 40- to 49-year-old women will be effective and of benefit. This can only be achieved if quality assessment and control are strictly implemented and continuously improved. It is equally vital to evaluate all prognostically important data.

References

Baines CJ, Miller AB, Kopans DB, Moskowitz M, Sanders DE, Sickles EA, To T, Wall C (1990) Canadian National Breast Screening Study: assessment of technical quality by external review. AJR 155:743–747
Baker LH (1982) Breast Cancer Detection Demonstration Project: five-year summary report. CA Cancer J Clin 32:194–225
Bassett LW, Bunnell DH, Jahanshahi R (1987) Breast cancer detection: one versus two views. Radiology 165:95–97
Cardenosa G, Eklund GW (1995) Screening mammography in women 40–49 years old. AJR 164:1104–1106
Chamberlain J, Coleman D, Ellmann R et al. (1993) First results in mortality reduction in the UK trial of early detection of breast cancer. Lancet 2:411.
Collette HJA, Day NE, Rombach JJ, De Ward F (1984) Evaluation of screening for breast cancer in a non-randomized study (The Dom Project) by means of a case-control study. Lancet 1224–1226
Conway BJ, Suleiman OH, Rueter FG, Antonsen RG, Slayton RJ (1994) National survey of mammographic facilities in 1985, 1988, and 1992. Radiology 191:323–330
Curpen BN, Sickles EA, Sollitto RA, Ominsky SH, Galvin HB, Frankel SD (1995) The comparative value of mammographic screening for women 40–49 years old versus women 50–64 years old. AJR 164:1099–1103
Day NE, Baines CJ, Chamberlain J, Hakama M, Miller AB, Prorok P (1986) UICC project on screening for cancer: report of the workshop on screening for breast cancer. Int J Cancer: 38:303–308
Dodd GD (1988) Screening for the early detection of breast cancer. Cancer 62:1781–1783
Feig SA (1994) Determination of mammographic screening intervals with surrogate measures for women aged 40–49 years. Radiology 193:311–314
Fletcher SW, Black W, Harris R, Rimer BK, Shapiro S (1993) Report of the International Workshop on Screening for Breast Cancer
Frankel SD, Sickles EA, Curpen BN, Sollitto RA, Ominsky SH, Galvin HB (1995) Initial versus subsequent screening mammography: comparison of findings and their prognostic significance. AJR 164:1107–1109
Frischbier HJ (1994) Beitrag zur kontroversen Einschätzung des Mammographie-Screenings bei asymptomatischen Frauen zwischen dem 40. und 50. Lebensjahr. Geburtsh u Frauenheilk. 54:1–11
Frischbier HJ, Hoeffken W, Robra BP (1994) Mammographie in der Früherkennung, Qualitätssicherung und Akzeptanz. Ergebnisse der Deutschen Mammographie-Studie. Ferdinand Enke Verlag, Stuttgart, Germany
Holmberg L (1993) Evaluation of breast cancer screening programs. Cancer 72:1433–1436
Ikeda DM, Sickles EA (1988) Second-screening with mammography: one versus two views per breast. Radiology 168:651–656
Kerlikowske K, Grady D, Barclay J, Sickles EA, Eaton A, Ernster V (1993) Positive predictive value of screening mammography by age and family history of breast cancer. JAMA 270:2444-2450
Kopans DB (1993) Mammography screening for breast cancer. Cancer 72:1809–1812
Mettlin CJ, Smart CR (1993) The Canadian National Breast Screening Study. An appraisal and implications for early detection policy. Cancer 72:1461–1465
Morrison AS, Brisson J, Khalid N (1988) Breast cancer incidence and mortality in the Breast Cancer Detection Demonstration Project. J Natl Cancer Inst 80:1540–1547
Moskowitz M (1986) Breast cancer: age-specific growth rates and screening strategies. Radiology 161:37–41
Nyström L, Rutqvist LE, Wall S, et al. (1993) Breast cancer screening with mammography: an overview of the Swedish randomized trials. Lancet 341:974
Paci E, Ciatto S, Buiatti E, Cecchini S, Palli D, Rosselli Del Turco M (1990) Early indicators of efficacy of breast cancer screening programmes. Results of the Florence District Programme. Int J Cancer 46:198–202
Palli D, Roselli Del Turco M, Buiatti E, Carli S, Ciatto S, Toscani L, Maltoni G (1986) A case-control study of the efficacy of a non-randomized breast cancer screening program in Florence (Italy). Int J Cancer 38:501–504
Peer PGM, Van Dijck JAAM, Hendriks JHCL, Holland R, Verbeek ALM (1993) Age-dependent growth rate of primary breast cancer. Cancer 71:3547–51
Peeters PHM, Verbeek ALM, Straatman H, et al. (1989) Evaluation of overdiagnosis of Nijmegen Programme. Int J Epidemiol 18:295–299
Roberts MM, Alexander FE, Anderson TJ, et al. (1990) Edinburgh trial of screening for breast cancer; mortality at seven years. Lancet 335:241
Rutqvist LE, Miller AB, Anderson I, et al. (1990) Reduced breast-cancer mortality with mammography screening: an assessment of currently available data. Int J Cancer Suppl 5:76–84
Schreer I, Frischbier HJ (1991) Predictive value of mammography in early detection of breast cancer: analysis of histological findings in breast biopsies indicated only by mammography. Eur J Radiol 1:165–168
Seidmann H, Gelb SK, Silverberg E, La Verda N, Lubera JA (1987) Survival experience in the Breast Cancer Detection Demonstration Project. CA Cancer J Clin 37:258–290
Shapiro S (1988) Final results of the breast cancer screening randomized trial: The Health Insurance Plan (HIP) of

greater New York study. In: Day NE, Miller AB (eds) Screening for breast cancer. Sam Huber, Toronto

Sickles EA, Kopans DB (1993) Deficiencies in the analysis of breast cancer screening data. J Natl Cancer Inst 85:1621–1624

Sickles EA, Ominsky SH, Sollitto RA, Galvin HB, Monticciolo DL (1990) Medical audit of a rapid-throughput mammography screening practice: methodology and results of 27 114 examinations. Radiology 175:323–327

Smart CR, Hartmann WH, Beahrs OH, Carfinkiel L (1993) Insights into breast cancer screening of younger women: evidence from the 14-year follow-up of the Breast Cancer Detection Demonstration Project. Cancer 72:1449–1456

Stacey-Clear A, McCarthy KA, Hall DA, et al. (1992) Breast cancer survival among women under age 50: is mammography detrimental? Lancet 340:991–994

Strax P, Venet L, Shapiro S (1973) Value of mammography in reduction of mortality from breast cancer in mass screening. AJR 117:686–689

Tabar L, Faberberg G, Day NE, Holmberg L (1987) What is the optimum interval between mammographic screening examinations? An analysis based on the latest results of the Swedish two-county breast cancer screening trial. Br J Cancer 55:547–551

Tabar L, Fagerberg G, Duffy SW, Day NE, Gad A, Grontoft O (1992) Update of the Swedish two-county program of mammographic screening for breast cancer. Radiol Clin North Am 30:187–210

Tabar L, Duffy SW, Warren Burhenne L (1993) New Swedish breast cancer detection results for women aged 40–49. Cancer 72:1437–1448

Thomas BA (1989) The place of clinical examination in breast cancer screening. In: Ziant G (ed) practical modalities of an efficient screening for breast cancer in the European Community. Proceedings of an International Symposium of the Association Against Cancer, Brussels, Belgium, January 20–21, 1989. Excerpta Medica, Amsterdam

Thurfjell E (1990) One versus two view mammography screenings: a prospective trial. Svenska Läkaresälskapets Handlingar Hygiea 99:220

Van Dijck JAAM, Verbeek ALM, Hendriks JHCL, Holland R (1993) The current detectability of breast cancer in a mammographic screening program: a review of the previous mammograms of interval and screen-detected cancers. Cancer 72:1933–1938

20 Breast Cancer Screening: General Guidelines, Program Design, and Organization

L.J. Warren Burhenne

CONTENTS

20.1	Introduction	347
20.2	General Guidelines	348
20.2.1	Introduction	348
20.2.2	Age Group Selection	348
20.2.3	Screening Modalities	349
20.2.4	Eligibility Requirements	349
20.2.5	Mechanisms for Investigation of Screen-Detected Abnormalities	349
20.2.6	Goals	350
20.3	Administrative Design	350
20.3.1	Administrative Structure	350
20.3.2	Committee Functions	350
20.3.3	Financial Organization	351
20.4	Organization and Methods	351
20.4.1	Screening Center Models and Geographic Coverage	351
20.4.2	Promotion	352
20.4.3	Compliance with Rescreening	353
20.4.4	Screening Center Operation	353
20.4.5	Selection of Facilities and Screening Radiologists	354
20.4.6	Report Format	354
20.4.7	Report Generation	354
20.4.8	Diagnostic Investigation	355
20.4.9	Data Collection, Analysis, and Quality Control	355
20.4.10	External Review	356
20.4.11	Pathology Review	356
20.5	Results	356
20.5.1	Demographics	357
20.5.2	Mammography Results	357
20.5.3	Cost Analysis	358
20.5.4	Cost-effectiveness	360
20.6	Summary	361
20.6.1	Planning and Organization	361
20.6.2	Service and Administration	362
20.6.3	Quality Control and Continuous Quality Improvement	362
	Appendix. SMPBC Quality of Image Audit	363
	References	364

L.J. Warren Burhenne, MD, Executive Director, Screening Mammography Program of British Columbia, Suite #414, 750 West Broadway, Vancouver, BC V5Z 1H3, Canada

20.1 Introduction

Screening for cancer has been and remains the subject of worldwide study, analysis, and scrutiny. The philosophy – which is based upon early detection, diagnosis, and treatment – of interrupting the spread of disease before it becomes advanced carries with it broad implications for society. For diseases such as cervical and breast cancer, primary prevention cannot be applied, since the causes are not known, and, in the case of breast cancer, it is very likely that there are multiple causes. For these malignancies, screening tests are applied to improve survival and achieve mortality reduction. Breast cancer is considered suitable for screening because of (a) the potential for serious morbidity and high mortality, (b) the fact that there is a detectable preclinical phase, (c) the established effectiveness of early treatment, and (d) the high prevalence among the screened population. From a practical point of view, however, breast cancer screening requires the examination of large numbers of healthy women in order to designate for more thorough assessment the small proportion that will likely be diagnosed with breast cancer Richert-Boe and Humphrey 1992). It is understandable, therefore, because of the economic consequences of such wide-scale screening and the physical implications of the screening and diagnostic tests, that there should be intensive scrutiny both of the test itself and of its effect on the population.

Mammography has undergone more scrutiny than most diagnostic tests in radiology. It has been assessed for the required attributes of an effective screening test, such as high sensitivity and specificity, acceptance by those screened and by the personnel providing the screening procedures, and acceptably low risk and cost.

Various randomized and nonrandomized controlled trials, cohort and case-controlled studies, and demonstration projects have been performed over the past several decades and have established the effectiveness of screening mammography, either alone or with clinical breast examination, in reducing mortality from breast cancer (STRAX et al. 1973; SHAPIRO 1977; BEAHRS et al. 1979; BAKER 1982; SHAPIRO et al. 1982, 1988; VERBEEK et al. 1984; COLLETTE et al. 1984; TABAR et al. 1985a,b, 1992; PALLI et al. 1986; SEIDMAN et al. 1987; UK Trial 1988, 1993; ROBERTS et al. 1990; BJURSTAM and BJORNELD 1994). The recent trend toward reduced mortality from breast cancer has been acknowledged by the National Cancer Institutes of Canada and the American Cancer Society to be related to earlier detection (Canadian Cancer Statistics 1993; GARFINKEL 1994). Ten-year survival rates of >95% for in situ and small invasive breast cancers are contrasted with expected 10-year survival of <55% for women with axillary lymph node involvement (LETTON and MASON 1989).

The success of the scientific studies having reported mortality reductions ranging to 32% has been dependent upon adequate compliance; it is generally considered that 70% compliance of the population at risk is needed to achieve such success. However, despite the fact that mammography screening is successful in reducing mortality from breast cancer, increasingly it will be funding agencies which will decide whether or not mass screening is practical, based upon analysis of the unit cost of the procedure.

20.2 General Guidelines

20.2.1 Introduction

Whether or not mass screening is to be conducted as part of a publicly funded program, as in Sweden (COLLETTE et al. 1984; VERBEEK et al. 1984; PEETERS et al. 1989; National Board of Health and Welfare 1990; PAMILO et al. 1990; HAKAMA et al. 1991; KLEMI et al. 1992; TABAR et al. 1992; THURFJELL and LINDGREN 1994), the Netherlands (COLLETTE et al. 1984; VERBEEK et al. 1984; National Board of Health and Welfare 1990), Finland, the United Kingdom (AUSTOKER 1991), and five Canadian provinces and one territory (Canadian Cancer Statistics 1993), or through institutions or private facilities, as in most states of the United States (BIRD and MCLELLAND 1986; SICKLES et al. 1986; SICKLES 1988; BIRD 1989; KRON et al. 1989; RUBIN et al. 1990; DEBRUHL et al. 1994), various critical decisions must be made before the program is established. These include considerations as to the age groups that will be recruited and other eligibility requirements, whether or not mammography will be offered alone or in combination with clinical breast examination, whether diag-

nostic investigations will be performed in specialized review or assessment facilities, whether preexisting facilities and equipment will be used or new facilities will be required, and finally, what goals will be set for the screening process.

20.2.2 Age Group Selection

The eight randomized controlled studies conducted since 1963 in the United States, Sweden, and the United Kingdom, when considered together, comprised women aged 40-74 (TABAR and DEAN 1989; FLETCHER et al. 1993; WALD et al. 1993). A reduction in mortality for women aged 50-69 of approximately one-third is accepted by all authorities, and all screening programs currently in operation include women in this age group. Although randomized controlled trials have proven mortality reduction for women aged 40-74 (SICKLES and KOPANS 1993; FEIG 1994; KOPANS 1994; KOPANS et al. 1994), proof is more difficult to show for women aged 40-49 and women aged 70 and older, when attempts are made to stratify overall results retrospectively. However, a recent report from Gothenburg, Sweden and a recent combined analysis have shown statistically significant mortality reduction for women aged 40-49 (SMART et al. 1995). While it is generally accepted that more information is required for this younger age group, the International Union Against Cancer (UICC), has determined that "available data can support a range of guidelines including recommendations to begin screening at age 40 or to begin at age 50" (ECKHARDT et al. 1995). Similarly, there is variation in recommended screening intervals, with recommendations for screening women aged 50 and over at intervals of from 1 to 3 years and for screening women aged 40-49 at intervals of from 1 to 2 years (ECKHARDT et al. 1995; METTLIN and SMART 1994). Such decisions will influence critically the costs involved, in view of the lower prior probability of breast cancer in younger women. Similarly, the acknowledged increase in interval cancers in the second year of a screening interval must be balanced against the increased costs of annual screening (FRISELL et al. 1987). In addition to the actual costs of screening, costs related to diagnosis and various social costs must be considered. Cost-effectiveness analyses can be performed, once the program is in operation, using actual program data to permit comparison of the standard unit of gain – cost per woman-year of life saved – among various breast screening programs and among other medical interventions. Such analyses assist funding agencies in determining allocations among the various interventions and in designing efficient screening programs.

20.2.3 Screening Modalities

The accepted screening modalities include mammography, clinical breast examination, and breast self-examination. Evidence for benefit with both mammography alone and mammography combined with physical examination is strong. However, since no studies have been performed to study the effect of clinical breast examination alone, it is accepted as complementary to mammography. Similarly, as with clinical examination, although studies of breast self-examination indicate that the more frequent use of this technique is associated with more favourable clinical staging, evidence of mortality reduction has not been established. Also, there is a suggestion that there may be fundamental differences between women who practice and women who do not practice breast self-examination, which affect breast cancer prognosis (RICHERT-BOE and HUMPHREY 1992).

The choice of complementing mammography with clinical breast examination in mass screening is influenced directly by the added costs involved.

20.2.4 Eligibility Requirements

As the goal of screening is to detect breast cancer early enough to impact upon its natural history, women who have clinical signs or symptoms of the disease should be excluded (RICHERT-BOE and HUMPHREY 1992). Women with symptoms require problem-solving breast imaging directed at the symptomatic site to supplement the survey imaging of both breasts in search of occult malignancy. In addition, women with breast prostheses often are excluded from screening and advised to be investigated at diagnostic facilities because specialized imaging techniques are needed to fully evaluate both native breast tissue and prostheses.

Since women may be encouraged to seek screening by various means, including invitation letters, physician's advice, and media promotion, it is quite common for women to initiate their own screening referrals. For programs which do not require that screenees name a referring physician, the role of the screening radiologist is rendered nontraditional. Under these circumstances, the radiologist effectively takes on the role of the primary physician with its attendant medical/legal liabilities. For the Screening Mammography Program of British Columbis (SMPBC), women are permitted to refer themselves. However, if they do not have family physicians to whom reports can be sent and who would be willing to supervise any diagnosis or treatment required, women are referred to a list of family physicians who are prepared to accept new patients under such circumstances (WARREN BURHENNE et al. 1992a; BURHENNE 1993).

20.2.5 Mechanisms for Investigation of Screen-Detected Abnormalities

Screening mammography can be equated with detection of abnormalities which confer an increased risk for breast cancer. By contrast, diagnostic imaging workup of screen-detected abnormalities, as for the imaging evaluation of clinical signs and symptoms suggestive of breast cancer, is much more complex than a standard screening examination. Such studies are tailored for the patient and may include additional standard or nonstandard projections and magnification views. Ordinarily, a breast physical examination is performed and a breast history taken. Both the technologist and the radiologist monitor the images, and ancillary tests (such as breast ultrasonography, with or without needle aspiration biopsy) are often included. The complexity of the process carries with it increased time commitment for all personnel and, therefore, higher costs (SICKLES et al. 1986; KOPANS et al. 1994).

Where review or assessment clinics are provided and administered by screening programs, such facilities tend to be fewer in number, as in the Universal Screening Programs in operation in Sweden, the Netherlands (COLLETTE et al. 1984; VERBEEK et al. 1984; AUSTOKER 1991; TABAR et al. 1992), the United Kingdom (The Essendon Breast x-ray Program Collaborative Group 1992; UK Trial 1992; CHAMBERLAIN et al. 1993; RICHARDS 1994), and Australia. In North America, diagnostic workup is typically performed by radiologists in community facilities by referral from the family physician (BIRD and MCLELLAND 1986; SICKLES et al. 1986; SICKLES 1988; BIRD 1989; PEETERS et al. 1989; WARREN BURHENNE et al. 1992a,b; BURHENNE 1993; ELWOOD et al. 1993). Wherever the diagnostic tests are conducted, efficient, high-volume screening is best performed separate from diagnostic mammography.

20.2.6 Goals

The implicit goal of breast cancer screening is to reduce mortality from the disease in the population examined. An important requirement for success, however, is to ensure compliance sufficient to achieve this end. In planning screening programs, one may set additional specific goals directly related to program results, such as cancer detection rates, abnormal call rates, and interval cancer rates. Additional general goals may be stated such as ensuring that diagnostic workup and treatment proceed promptly (SICKLES et al. 1990; WARREN BURHENNE et al. 1992; WALD et al. 1993; FEIG 1994), avoiding harm to those not in need of treatment, and working together with other members of the health care team to provide the service. Whatever the case, quality assurance will relate directly to frequent and regular appraisal of results.

20.3 Administrative Design

The SMPBC, established in 1988, is the largest multiple center breast cancer demonstration project in North America (WARREN BURHENNE et al. 1992). This program will be used as the model for purposes of discussion of design and organization, with comparisons to and contrasts with other programs where pertinent.

20.3.1 Administrative Structure

In the province of British Columbia (BC), 99% of residents are insured with the Medical Services Plan of BC, which funds all required medical services. The Ministry of Health provides special grant funds for the Program, through the BC Cancer Agency, which is administered by a Board of Trustees.

The SMPBC Steering Committee establishes Missions, Goals, and Objectives and general policies for the Program. The physician Executive Director and Program Administrator oversee and administer the functions of the Central Office, its staff, and the original (model) center. Various services including Human Resources, Finance, SMPBC Pathologist, SMPBC Physicist, and acquisition of goods and equipment are purchased through a contract with the BC Cancer Agency. Only the model center is managed by the Central Office. All other regional centers have contracted management with either publicly funded institutions or private radiologists. Each of the regional centers is staffed by a Chief Technologist as well as technical and clerical staff.

The Central Office staff comprises the Program Administrator, Program Evaluator, Office Systems Coordinator, and Registry Staff, as well as the Administrative Executive Secretary. The Program Evaluator, a statistician, is responsible for the overall quality management program, and the Mammography Registry – a Central Office function of data collection including coding and classification, analysis, and presentation of data – and for the development and implementation of central computerization. One facet of central computerization is linkage to the BC Cancer Registry, to track interval cancers.

The Central Office provides program-wide financial management, data collection, quality control, public relations, promotion, planning, and execution of educational activities, the Mammography Registry service, and central scheduling of appointments. In addition, it provides administration of the model center, develops all program policies, and coordinates the establishment of new centers. All subcommittees are coordinated through the Central Office. The individual centers operate within overall program guidelines and with annual budgets which are determined by annual screening quotas, in consultation with the program administration. Day-to-day management of the regional centers is the responsibility of either the locally appointed radiologist administrator or, as in the case of public institutions, the radiology department manager.

This system of administration bears some similarities to that of the National Health Service Breast Screening Program in the United Kingdom, which also commenced in 1988. In the United Kingdom, the Department of Health, which accepts advice from the Breast Screening Advisory Committee, oversees the screening operations managed by the various regional health authorities or health boards throughout the country (AUSTOKER 1991).

20.3.2 Committee Functions

The SMPBC Steering Committee comprises representatives from the BC Cancer Agency, BC Medical Association, BC Radiological Society, University of BC, the Canadian Cancer Society, and the Health Ministry. In addition, there are lay appointees from the BC Cancer Agency Board of Trustees and from the community, as well as BC Cancer Agency and SMPBC administrative staff. This representation ensures that not only health care providers and those responsible for funding, but also consumers are involved with policy making. The interdisciplinary Committee physicians include diagnostic radiologists, radiation oncologists, breast surgeons, pathologists, epidemiologists, and family practitioners (WARREN BURHENNE et al. 1992a).

The Administrative Committee reviews the operations of the program and advises the Steering Committee, recommending policies for approval.

The Academic Committee, which comprises physicians chosen from the Steering Committee and administrative staff, reviews and recommends approval of research projects and evaluates their impact upon the program, provides a central resource of information on the Program, sets standards for candidate screeners and for their continuing medical education, and organizes and coordinates the visiting professor program and the External Review program.

The Quality Management Committee maintains quality assurance standards and monitors reporting and compliance with the standards, recommending changes as required.

The Screeners' Advisory Committee, comprising chief radiologists from all of the screening centers, assists the Academic Committee in establishing the acceptance standards for program screeners and in establishing and maintaining standards for a review process to monitor program outcome.

20.3.3 Financial Organization

A global budget is derived for all centers, including the Central Office. Individual budgetary items for operating expenses such as salaries, benefits, radiologist fees, and supplies are projected for each of the centers.

Privately managed centers receive an additional amount for capital equipment amortization and leasehold improvements based upon the projected number of annual examinations.

One of the goals of the original model center project was to determine the annual unit cost. The unit cost and cost per cancer detected will be dependent upon not only the total cost and number of screens performed, but also the number of cancers detected. This latter figure will be directly related to the proportion of returning women, as compared with first screened women.

20.4 Organization and Methods

20.4.1 Screening Center Models and Geographic Coverage

Whether or not centralized mass mammography screening is conducted from a few centers, as in Sweden and the Netherlands (COLLETTE et al. 1984; VERBEEK et al. 1984; TABAR et al. 1985a, 1992; PEETERS et al. 1989), or in multiple, logistically separated centers, as in the United Kingdom, Australia, and British Columbia (AUSTOKER 1991; The Essendon Breast X ray Progiam Collaborative Group 1992; UK Trial 1992; CHAMBERLAIN et al. 1993; RICHARDS 1994; WARREN BURHENNE 1994), consideration must be given to placement of facilities to provide convenient access for women to screening.

In British Columbia, screening is provided in facilities based on various models. The model is chosen based upon the unique needs of the communities (WARREN BURHENNE 1994).

The fixed center model, including free-standing centers in shopping malls and medical centers as well as centers based in hospitals, is more suitable for large communities in which screening can be expected to attract up to 15 000 eligible women. Mobile centers are more suitable for smaller communities without sufficient population to support a full-time operation. A unique variation on the fixed center theme – the ancillary center – refers to part-time screening centers set-up in hospitals in smaller communities in which the mammography equipment is chronically underutilized. In these hospitals, screening is performed on a part-time basis according to program specifications, usually by dedicating selected half-days exclusively to screening.

Where screening is conducted in a facility which is government-funded, screening program budget funding is not provided for rental of the premises, leasehold improvements, or equipment amortization, since these costs are funded by the global budget of the facility. These costs are, however, reimbursed where private radiologists manage facilities. Ancillary facilities, which are always located in hospitals, are funded in the same way as full-time institutional centers.

The multiple model concept was developed based upon the particular geographic conditions in British Columbia and the population distribution. British Columbia is 365 900 square miles in area with a population of 3 082 388. The majority of the population (63%) live within 100 miles of the United States border; about half of the provincial population reside in the Vancouver area and the remainder are concentrated on Vancouver Island and scattered in numerous smaller communities throughout the province.

The difficulty in providing a screening mammography service to women in remote communities with a population density much less than the provincial average of 8/square mile has been a challenge to the evolution of the current models. A variation of the ancillary center model suggested to provide service to women from very remote communities is the provision of a dedicated charter bus, rented at various intervals, to transport women from the remote communities to the nearest ancillary center.

Our experience has shown that as long as screening program standards are applied equally to all of the centers, the quality of mammographic imaging can be maintained. In addition, the use of otherwise underutilized equipment can result in overall cost savings.

20.4.3 Promotion

There are numerous established barriers to the success of widespread mammography screening. Some are attributed to prospective screenees, including concern about discomfort, perceived risks of radiation, fear as to diagnosis, lack of awareness of the advantages of screening, absence of a general positive attitude towards health, and limited access to screening facilities. Other factors, such as knowledge of current guidelines, concerns as to effectiveness, false-positive and false-negative results, and incorrect assumptions as to radiation effects, remain prevalent and are ascribed primarily to physician attitudes. However, there is general agreement that all so-called barriers can be classified into two categories: awareness and access. These concepts and their possible effects upon compliance require consideration during the process of planning a screening program, to ensure that screening centers are sited in appropriate locations and that both physicians and consumers are well informed ahead of time.

Adequate preparation of community physicians is of particular importance, especially when screening involves mammography alone and the responsibility for performance of clinical breast examination and for the initiation and supervision of diagnostic workup rests with the referring physicians. One important mechanism to ensure that community physicians have appropriate current information about breast cancer screening and the screening program, is to include family practitioners, diagnostic radiologists, breast surgeons, radiation and clinical oncologists, and pathologists in the planning process and, ideally, on a steering committee. A helpful policy is to send a detailed letter with information about the philosophy of the program, the eligibility requirements for screenees, the reporting mechanism, and current statistics to all physicians in the community, to prepare these physicians for the opening of a screening center. It is particularly important to prepare and consult with community diagnostic radiologists, who may feel that dedicated screening centers will impact upon their practices. It has been shown that if there is a reduction in the number of screening examinations performed in the community facilities, this is typically offset by increased numbers of diagnostic workup cases generated from screening (SICKLES 1988).

In addition, it is helpful to provide active education to family physicians. We have designed a family doctor awareness program which involves sending teams of specially trained radiologists and family physicians to visit various hospitals and community facilities to give a prepared presentation to community physician groups. This can be conveniently performed where physicians meet for hospital rounds and other similar planned gatherings. The personal contact between the program and community physicians provides a forum for questions and answers and an opportunity for valuable education. Program brochures and information on making appointments and screening center locations are provided to physicians before screening centers open. Family physicians also receive regular documentation of the clinical outcomes of their patients who have attended the screening program. An annual scientific meeting, at which program results are presented and challenging cases are discussed, is held for all program radiologists as well as for community diagnostic radiologists and breast surgeons.

Promotional strategies for screenees fall into two main categories: general publicity and personal invitation letters. Direct advertising in newspapers and on local cable television is one of the most effective means of attracting women to screening. However, it is important and advisable to have an ongoing organization to provide presentations to special groups – for example, a multicultural outreach program directed toward specific ethnic groups, supplemented by regular distribution of program brochures and updated results to community groups and various seniors centers and health offices. A program-produced educational videotape presentation aired regularly on local cable television stations has proved very effective in attracting potential screenees who would not otherwise respond to written material. We have found it helpful to work together with the Canadian Cancer Society and other volunteer organizations with such productions, to ensure that the public receives a consistent message as to the value of mammography, clinical breast examination, and self-examination.

Direct letters of invitation, whether generated from family practitioner lists or election rolls, as in Australia, or from public insurance registration lists, will improve attendance (Austoker 1991; The Essendon Breast X-ray Program Collaborative Group 1992).

20.4.3 Compliance with Rescreening

In order to achieve the goal of mortality reduction through screening, it is critical to ensure that women return for serial studies after an initial screen.

The Widespread use of computerization facilitates the generation of annual reminder letters when women are due for repeat screening. A standard reminder letter can be conveniently mailed directly to the screenee and/or to the physician (who will then forward it to the patient or arrange a telephone reminder). Current cumulative data from the SMPBC show that 63% of women have returned for rescreening by 18 months, 70% by 24 months, and 80% by 36 months, based upon a reminder for annual screening.

With only 25% of women actually returning by 12 months, these data imply that it would be inappropriate to increase the recommended screening interval to 2 years (or to 3 years, as in the United Kingdom), since it has been demonstrated in Sweden and the Netherlands that the interval cancer rate would increase to unacceptable levels (Frisell et al. 1987; vanDijck et al. 1993).

20.4.4 Screening Center Operation

20.4.4.1 Hours of Operation and Appointments

The hours of operation are determined by the demand for service. For example, 50–60 examinations can be conveniently performed in a standard 8-h shift. Since evening and weekend hours are convenient for some patients, extended hours into the evening and/or weekend hours are available in many centers. In addition, one of the mobile van facilities provides screening on a 7 day/week basis. Because of the need for high-volume throughput on an ongoing basis, examinations must be spaced evenly throughout the workday and appointments are required. In addition to screening-center-specific telephone numbers, we provide a toll-free long-distance appointment service for women who wish to attend the mobile van and remote ancillary facilities.

20.4.4.2 Eligibility and Registration

Eligibility is determined through the previously described telephone interview. Upon arrival, women complete a brief registration form and background data questionnaire including questions on reproductive history, hormonal therapy, and general activities determining health consciousness. The background data questionnaire is available in English, Chinese, Hindi, Punjabi, and German.

20.4.4.3 The Mammography Examination

After registration, women are provided with a disposable gown and when ready, are taken to the mammography room. Our current promotional videotape plays continuously in the prescreening waiting area. The technologist performing a screening examination interviews each screenee briefly to determine whether and where a previous mammography examination has been performed, whether or not the screenee is currently taking estrogen therapy, and whether or not there has been previous breast surgery, documentation the sites of scars, if any, as well as obvious skin lesions or nipple inversion on the reporting form. Although women with any breast complaints are deemed to be ineligible at the time they contact the screening centers to make appointments, very rarely a screenee will report a breast symptom or sign after she has been registered. The examinations for these women are completed, however, with a notation made on the reporting form for the radiologist, who will contact the family physician directly and emphasize the need for a prompt clinical breast examination.

Bilateral, craniocaudal, and mediolateral oblique mammographic views are performed. Depending upon the time available, the technologist either will develop the images immediately or will batch develop them at some later time. The technologist will repeat a projection only if it is quite clear that the entire breast cannot be included with one exposure or in the very unlikely event that the screenee has been observed to move during the exposure.

The technologists mount all cases on a specialized alternating illuminator and arrange the reporting forms for the screening radiologists. If there are previous films in the screening center, they are mounted for comparison; previous films from outside the screening center are obtained for comparison before reporting only under special circumstances, such as in the mobile van system and in other facilities where the previous examinations are available promptly from a nearby diagnostic facility, and when an undue delay in reporting would not occur because of a comparison.

Screenees are told that they will receive a letter advising them of the results within 5–7 days and that their physicians will receive an official report. In addition, technologist ordinarily reminds all screenees of the recommendation to return in 1 year for follow-up screening.

Since screening is provided by government funding, no payment is required. However, women are requested to show their insurance cards at the time of registration to confirm eligibility.

20.4.4.4 Equipment

A dedicated mammography unit with a molybdenum target tube, molybdenum filter, and beryllium window, and a dedicated processor with extended-cycle processing are Program requirements. High-voltage power supply, automatic exposure control, movable grids in two sizes, and an actual focal spot size of 0.3 or 0.4 mm are also required. However, there is no specific requirement as to mammography film, screen, cassettes, or processing chemistry. Rather, a random selection of clinical images is reviewed by a team of experienced screening radiologists and the overall image quality is judged as acceptable or not, based upon Program audit standards (Appendix) On-board processing, for example, has proved to be acceptable for the mobile van facilities. All equipment and phantom and clinical images undergo both objective and subjective tests both before acceptance, at 6 months, and thereafter at yearly intervals.

20.4.5 Selection of Facilities and Screening Radiologists

The Screening Program Steering Committee annually determines the locations in greatest need of service. The Program then solicits all radiologists performing mammography in these communities, inviting proposals to administer a screening center. When the best proposal is chosen, the radiologists in the facilities are invited to nominate candidates to become Screening Program radiologists. These candidates must possess certain acceptance criteria, including two formal mammography training courses that involve a screening mammography component (at least one within the past 3 years), documented interpretation of at least 2500 mammograms, and an acceptable curriculum vitae.

In addition, the Program has designed a standardized interpretation test and requires satisfactory performance on the test before a screening radiologist can be accepted. Those whose performance is not within the Program standards must take additional training. All screeners undergo a day of orientation at the Central Office and model center. Chief radiologists have a 2-day orientation. In addition, each radiologist screener is required to attend an annual conference with mammography content for which funding is provided by the Screening Program. As described above, the Program holds an annual scientific meeting for its screening radiologists and other Program physicians.

20.4.6 Report Format

Screening radiologists initial the reporting form, and, using a check-off system, designate the breast density category (< or ⩾50% dense tissue), whether or not there is a significant abnormality, and whether or not the abnormality requires further study. A degree of suspicion (A, B, or C) is chosen for the abnormalities requiring further study. The radiologists also indicate the location of the abnormality. Furthermore, for those cases in which additional study is required, the screening radiologist writes a brief handwritten note on the form describing the imaging features of the abnormality.

All data entered on the reporting form are coded directly into the Program computer by the Registry staff.

20.4.7 Report Generation

A brief letter is sent to all screenees indicating either that the examination does not reveal any sign of breast cancer or that further assessment is required. In either case, these screenees are reminded to see their family physicians for an annual breast physical examination and instruction in breast self-examination. The coded information is also used to generate specialized reports to physicians. These reports state either that the examination is negative, or that there is a specific abnormality for which recommendation for diagnostic study is being made. The radiologist's written comment is reproduced as directly as possible. These procedures have been refined over the years and have proven to be acceptable to both women and their physicians. In particular, the practice of notifying both screenee and physician renders it very unlikely that diagnostic investigations are not performed due to loss of reports or letters. Central mailing of screenee reports is delayed until at least 3 days after the mailing of the physician reports, in order to ensure that the physician receives the information first and is prepared, should the screenee contact him for an appointment and advice as to additional investigation.

20.4.8 Diagnostic Investigation

Family physicians have accepted the responsibility for initiating and coordinating all diagnostic studies. The first diagnostic study ordinarily performed is the clinical breast examination. However, it is very common for family physicians who receive a report of an abnormal screening mammography examination to directly contact a diagnostic radiologist who then takes over coordination of the various diagnostic tests. Specifically, available previous films are solicited and a comparison is made. If required, additional studies such as diagnostic mammography or diagnostic ultrasonography with or without needle aspiration biopsy or core biopsy are performed. If an open biopsy is required, the diagnostic radiologist informs the family physician, who then makes arrangements for the appropriate surgical referral. Similarly, for lesions considered "probably benign" after diagnostic evaluation, the radiologist would make the appropriate recommendation for serial follow-up. Although a formal review clinic or facility is not part of the Program, the physicians involved tend to organize themselves into multidisciplinary teams which work together cohesively for the most efficient and most economical diagnostic process.

20.4.9 Data Collection, Analysis, and Quality Control

20.4.9.1 Data Collection

20.4.9.1.1 Abnormal Screening Examinations. Information on the results of diagnostic workups is solicited directly from family physicians or breast surgeons, who are asked to complete a simple result form.

20.4.9.1.2 Normal Screening Reports. A computer link to the BC Cancer Registry has been set up to allow identification of those women whose most recent screening mammography examinations have been deemed negative but who have been diagnosed subsequently with breast cancer. These "postscreen" cancers are analyzed in detail as described below.

20.4.9.2 Data Analysis

The Program maintains a central computer for data communication among the various centers and for statistical analysis. The case follow-up of procedures (approximately 7000 abnormal results/year) is conducted on an ongoing basis. Data are downloaded and analyzed biannually. Various outcome statistics such as center-specific screening volume, age of screenees, compliance with rescreening, age-specific abnormal call rates, results of diagnostic investigations, biopsy yield ratios, and cancer characteristics

Table 20.1. Cost comparison between 1992, 1993, and 1994 fiscal years

	1992	1993	1994
No. of screens	64964	89390	108490
No. of cancers detected	249	337	372
Total cost	$4173719	$4641412	$5355705
Total cost/screen	$64.25	$51.92	$49.37
Central services	19.85	11.93	10.36
Other operating costs	32.36	29.39	27.02
Professional reading fee	5.58	5.58	5.79
Capital allocation (incl. amortization)	6.46	5.02	4.20
Cost per cancer detected	$16761.92	$13772.74	$14397.05

are analyzed and presented in formal reports. In addition, a detailed cost analysis is performed annually to allow comparison with previous years. A sample cost analysis is presented in Table 20.1.

20.4.9.3 Quality Management

20.4.9.3.1 Radiologist Screener-Specific Procedures. All screening centers hold monthly review sessions in which diagnostic information is available for all cancer and interval cancer cases and a random selection of cases deemed to require additional investigation but proving, ultimately, to be benign. These workshops are valuable, not only as education for the screening radiologist but also as a means of ensuring that the recommended diagnostic workups have been completed and that the appropriate disposition of screenings has been made. Occasionally, for example, the chief screener must contact family physicians to provide specific recommendations for additional studies needed to complete the diagnostic process.

20.4.9.3.2 Postscreen and Interval Cancer Review. All cases which have resulted in a diagnosis of breast cancer, after either a normal screen or an abnormal screen prompting a diagnostic investigation interpreted as benign, are subjected to detailed review. The first level, the blinded review, is conducted by three experienced screeners who review these selected cases intermixed with normal cases in a 1:10 ratio. The blinded review results are tabulated by the Program Evaluator and the same cases are then subjected to a joint review by the same team of interpreters. The joint review is retrospective, however, and is performed with the benefit of diagnostic results. Based upon the results of the two reviews, the cancers are classified as:

1. *Interval*
   a) True – cannot see in retrospect
   b) Missed – can see in retrospect
   c) Technical error
2. *Contradiction*: Cases in which the screening mammography examination was called abnormal but either deemed normal by the diagnostic radiologist, inappropriately investigated by the surgeon, or erroneously deemed benign by the pathologist.
3. *Postscreen noncompliance*: Breast cancers detected more than 1 year after a negative screening mammography examination (BURHENNE et al. 1994).

The results of these analyses are analyzed and presented at the Annual Screening Mammography Scientific Forum.

20.4.10 External Review

A Program External Review radiologist was appointed to report and advise on quality standards of interpretation throughout the Program. A selection of normal and abnormal cases for all screeners is reviewed annually and the results of the review are communicated directly to the radiologist screeners, with subsequent opportunity for discussion with the Executive Director.

20.4.11 Pathology Review

An important feature of quality control is formal pathology review. Specifically, the senior breast pathologist at the BC Cancer Agency reviews specimens for all breast cancers, all borderline lesions, and lobular neoplasms. For new centers, all benign biopsy specimens are reviewed for at least the first 6 months, and longer, if necessary, to establish consistency between the original and review diagnoses. The review involves correlation of screening mammography findings and pathology interpretation. When there is disagreement or discordance between the radiology and pathology reports, a more in-depth review is arranged between the screening team and the review pathologist. This procedure is intended to ensure that primary treatment is appropriate and timely.

20.5 Results

The value of a program of mammography screening will ultimately be measured in terms of mortality reduction. However, during the course of an organized population-based screening program, certain performance indicators can be used to predict mortality reduction. These indicators include population coverage and compliance, referral or abnormal call rate, benign biopsy rate (per 1000 women screened), cancer prevalence (per 1000 women screened), surgical biopsy yield (percentage of biopsies producing cancer diagnosis), and percentage of invasive cancers <10 mm in diameter (WALD et al. 1993). Other performance indicators include incidence of all screen-detected cancers, interval cancers, and cancers in those who do not attend screening, as well as staging characteristics of detected cancers (TABAR et al. 1992).

Alternatively, surrogate end points are recommended as measures to assess the success of screening women aged 40–49, since a study with sufficient statistical power to provide proof for mortality reduction in this age group has not yet been performed. Such surrogate measures include some of those recommended as standard performance indicators for population screening, but also the rate of node-negative cancers, the prevalence/incidence ratio, the interval cancer rate, and characteristics of and death rate from interval cancers (FEIG 1994).

For a broad-based population screening program, central computerization for data collection and analysis is essential. Such a system offers the opportunity for creativity in data analysis and presentation.

20.5.1 Demographics

Demographic information collected on women screened through the Screening Mammography Program of British Columbia includes age, ethnic background, level of education attained, parity and menstrual history, family history of breast cancer, history of previous breast biopsy, and conduct of positive health practices such as annual breast physical examination, breast self-examination, and Pap smear examinations. In addition, women attending the Program for the first time are asked to state whether or not they have had mammography in the 2 years prior to screening.

20.5.2 Mammography Results

The recall or abnormal call rate refers to the rate (number) of women whose screening mammography examinations are regarded as requiring further investigation. Such women are referred for diagnostic mammography, ultrasonography (with or without needle aspiration biopsy), and breast physical examination. Open biopsy will eventually be required for some of these patients, depending on the results of diagnostic examination. The cumulative results of diagnostic investigation within the SMPBC are shown in Table 20.2. A complete analysis of cancer detection results is shown in Table 20.3.

Histologic diagnosis, lesion measurement, and nodal and metastatic status are required for staging, and the TNM staging system of the American Joint Committee on Cancer is used. The characteristics of these cancers as determined by 10-year age groups are shown in Table 20.3. The variation, on a cumulative basis, of abnormal call rate, cancer detection rate, positive predictive value of screening

Table 20.2. Cancer detection by age for screening examinations performed between July 1988 and March 1993

	1989/1990	1990/1991	1991/1992	1992/1993	Cumulative[e]
No. of examinations	9454	31 029	64 964	89 390	201 937
No. of women	9415	30 951	64 717	88 672	128 325
Age <50	3412 (36.2%)	11 548 (37.3%)	22 259 (34.4%)	29 076 (32.8%)	44 933 (35.0%)
Age ⩾50	6003 (63.8%)	19 403 (62.7%)	42 458 (65.6%)	59 596 (67.2%)	83 392 (65.0%)
Abnormal call rate	592 (6.3%)	2 323 (7.5%)	4 169 (6.4%)	6 002 (6.7%)	13 808 (6.8%)
No. of cancers	36	142	258	337	802
Age <50	7 (19.4%)	15 (10.6%)	49 (19.0%)	50 (14.8%)	125 (15.6%)
Age ⩾50	29 (80.6%)	127 (89.4%)	209 (81.0%)	287 (85.2%)	677 (84.4%)
Positive predictive value[a]	6.1%	6.1%	6.2%	5.6%	5.8%
Biopsy yield ratio[b]	32.1%	32.9%	34.7%	35.3%	33.6%
Prevalent cancer rate[c]	5.5/1000 women	5.3/1000 women	5.0/1000 women	4.9/1000 women	8.3/1000 women 5.0/1000 exams.
Incident cancer rate[d]	0.6/1000 women	1.5/1000 women	1.7/1000 women	2.7/1000 women	3.2/1000 women 2.2/1000 exams.
Overall cancer rate	3.8/1000 women	4.6/1000 women	4.0/1000 women	3.8/1000 women	6.2/1000 women 4.0/1000 exams.

[a] Percent of cancers detected in abnormal calls
[b] Percent of cancers detected in open biopsies performed
[c] Participants with no previous screening examination
[d] Participants with previous screening examination
[e] Note that 7000 women screened in 1988 are not considered in the preceding columns; consequently the cumulative figures exceed the totals of the four columns

Table 20.3. Cancer characteristics by age

	Age at last examination				Total
	40–49	50–59	60–69	≥70	
Cancers detected[a]	150	221	323	311	1005
In situ	42 28.0%	58 26.2%	61 18.9%	33 10.6%	194 19.3%
Invasive	108 72.0%	163 73.8%	262 81.1%	278 89.4%	811 80.7%
Invasive tumor size					
≤5 mm	12 11.3%	12 7.5%	22 8.5%	5 1.8%	51 6.4%
6–10 mm	12 11.3%	39 24.2%	70 27.1%	71 26.0%	192 24.1%
11–20 mm	43 40.8%	75 46.6%	129 50.0%	137 50.2%	384 48.1%
>20 mm	39 36.8%	35 21.7%	37 14.4%	60 22.0%	171 21.4%
Unknown	2	2	4	5	13
Median size (mm)	16	15	13	15	15
Axillary lymph node involvement	22 14.7%	32 14.5%	47 14.6%	50 16.1%	151 15.0%
TNM staging[b]					
In situ	41 27.9%	58 26.5%	61 19.1%	33 10.8%	193 19.5%
I	59 40.1%	106 48.4%	189 59.1%	179 58.5%	533 53.7%
II	44 29.9%	55 25.1%	66 20.6%	89 29.1%	254 25.6%
III+	3 2.1%	0 –	4 1.2%	5 1.6%	12 1.2%
Unknown	3	2	3	5	13

[a] Based upon provisional diagnosis if pathology review has not been completed (one in situ and ten invasive cancers)
[b] TNM staging was determined by using mammographic measurement whenever pathologic measurement of the tumor was not available, and by assuming no node involvement (N0) whenever axillary lymph nodes were not assessed, and no distant metastases (M0) unless otherwise informed

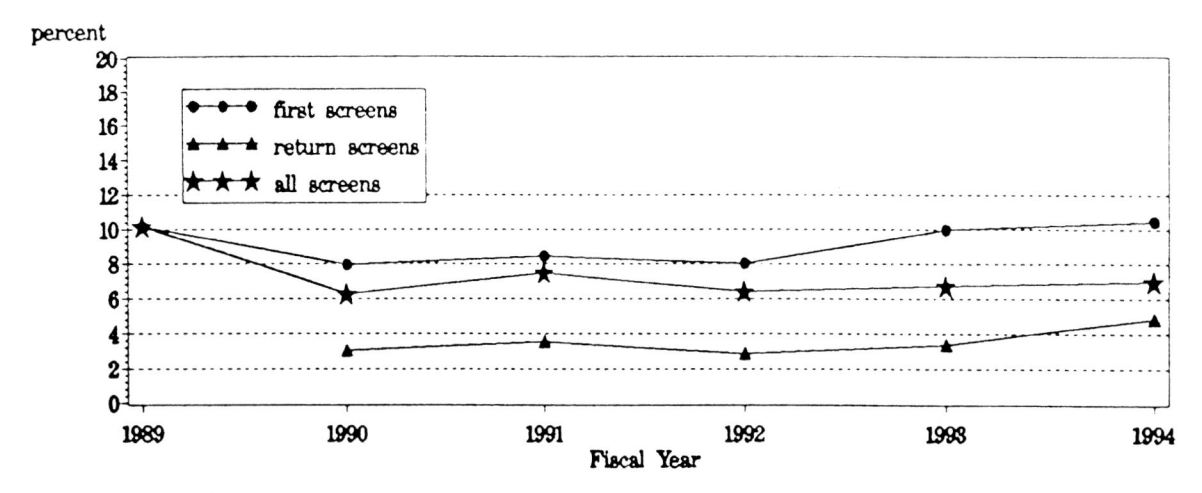

Fig. 20.1. Abnormal call rate

mammography, and biopsy yield ratio is shown in Fig. 20.1–20.4.

20.5.3 Cost Analysis

The Screening Program began as a single 9-month pilot project with a budget of CAN $406 000. The unit cost of a screening examination in this setting, in which rental of the facility and the mammography machine were provided by the institution, was CAN $33.81 (1989).

At present, individual unit costs are calculated based upon total Program costs, including those required to establish new centers and all costs for privately administered screening centers. The current formula for unit cost per screen is illustrated in Table 20.4. The cost per cancer detected, although calcu-

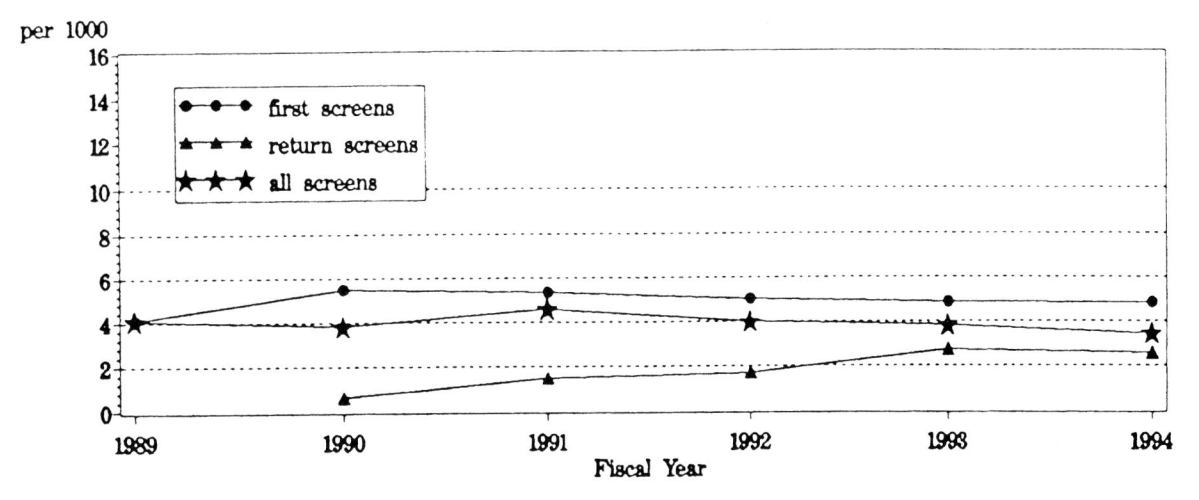

Fig. 20.2. Cancer detection rate

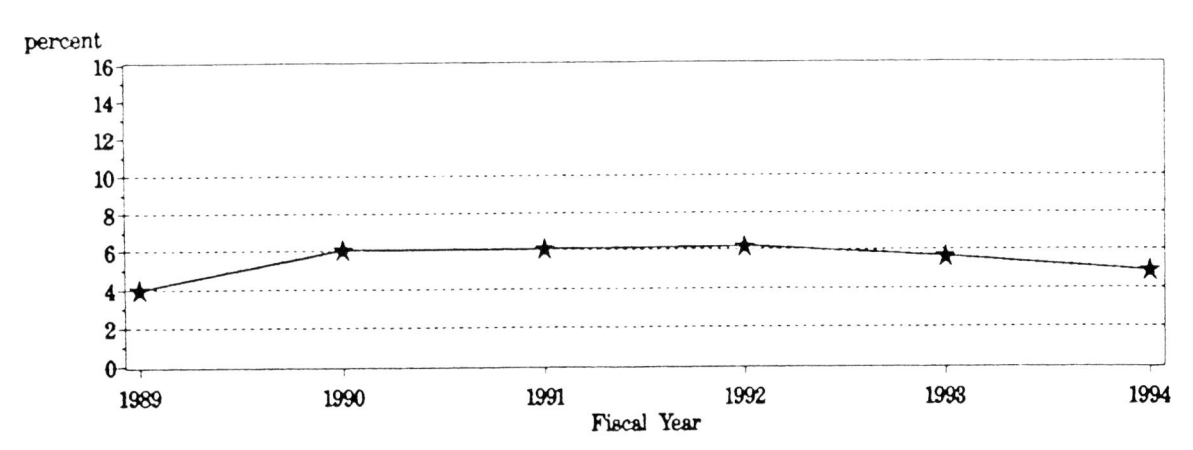

Fig. 20.3. Positive predictive value (PPV) of screening mammography. PPV is the proportion of breast cancers detected in women with an abnormal screening result

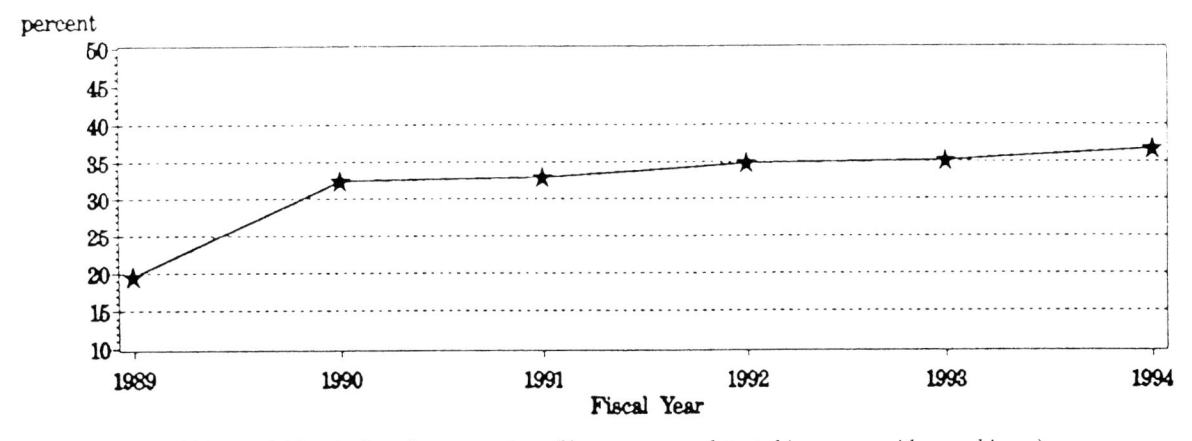

Fig. 20.4. Surgical biopsy yield ratio (i.e., the proportion of breast cancers detected in women with open biopsy)

lated directly from the quotient of the total costs and numbers of cancers detected, will depend upon the decreasing prior probability of cancer in the population as an increasing percentage of women attending the Program undergo incidence (rather than precedence) screening.

20.5.4 Cost-effectiveness

The cost-effectiveness of various medical interventions is becoming increasingly more important with the proliferation of medical technology, in both diagnosis and therapy.

"Cost-effective" is a relative term and implies that the procedure or technology is to be compared with the use of some other technology or with doing nothing. For example, where an intervention improves outcomes and decreases costs, there is a clear answer that the intervention is cost-effective. Conversely, if an intervention results in reduced benefits and increased costs, then the intervention cannot be cost-effective. However, when interventions leads to increased costs, they still may be cost-effective if the added cost is reasonable for the benefit achieved. Under these circumstances, the use of the intervention becomes a societal decision. Such decisions are determined by considerations as to allocation of health care resources and how the cost is to be distributed throughout society (MUSHLIN and FINTOR 1992; HILLMAN 1994).

Cost-effectiveness analysis focuses on the number of lives saved or extended and is expressed as the ratio obtained by dividing the cost by the number of life years saved by the intervention (HILLMAN 1994).

For breast cancer screening, factors such as the cost of the screening examination, screening interval, cost of diagnostic procedures, treatment cost, and prior probability of cancer in the population will all affect cost. However, cost-effectiveness analysis is useful to make judgments as to the value of a given intervention as well as to compare the cost-effectiveness of different interventions.

Recently, cost-effectiveness calculations have been made and compared for Spain, France, the United Kingdom, and the Netherlands. This study used a detailed cost-effectiveness analysis of breast cancer screening in the Netherlands as a starting point. In the Netherlands, screening women aged 50 and older at 2- to 3-year intervals was determined to be the most cost-effective approach (VAN DER MAAS et al. 1989; DE KONING 1991).

The analysis used data on breast cancer incidence, mortality, demography, organization of screening, and price levels in health care to calculate cost-effectiveness based on the assumption that women aged 50–70 are screened at 2-yearly intervals. The calculated costs per year of life gained, assuming an organized national screening system for all countries based on 1990 pound Sterling currency were: United Kingdom 1800, Netherlands 2120, France 5800, and Spain 9700. The figures are highly influenced by the differences in incidence and mortality in the various countries. For example, breast cancer incidence is twice as high in the Netherlands as in Spain and breast cancer mortality is twice as high in the United Kingdom as in Spain. Therefore, the life years gained as a result of screening will be appreciably higher for the Netherlands and the United Kingdom. In addition because screening is conducted differently in France and Spain, as compared with the United Kingdom and Netherlands, when a correction is made for increased costs for a nationwide organization, the relative costs in Spain and France are increased. The great variability in such factors cause the authors to conclude that one uniform screening policy for the European community would not be appropriate.

In 1993, a cost-effectiveness analysis was performed based upon actual experience within the SMPBC. The actual costs of performing screening, the induced costs of various diagnostic procedures, and the medical costs avoided all were compiled directly. Cost-effectiveness calculations were based upon the first 4 years of operation, involving 112 543 screening examination, detection of 455 cancers, and a total cost of CAN $8 148 539. It was elected to make calculations for the entire group screened and also for <50 and ≥50 age groups. Two different assumptions for mortality reduction were used for women younger than age 50: first, a 30% mortality reduction (the same as already observed for women ≥50), and second, a 13% mortality reduction for women <50 derived from a recent meta-analysis (NYSTROM et al. 1993). Specifically, the calculated costs per woman-year of life saved are summarized in Table 20.4.

Most importantly, although it is acknowledged that there is considerable variability in cost-effectiveness calculations throughout the literature, such calculations do allow for comparison of screening mammography with other interventions widely accepted for funding by society. The range of cost-effectiveness for the SMPBC (from approximately CAN $2000 for women ≥50 to the CAN $17 000 estimate for women <50 using the conservative mortal-

Table 20.4. Cost per woman-year of life saved [CAN $ (1993)]

% Mortality reduction assumption	All women	Women ≥50	Women < 50
All: 30	3014	1997	6 280
All: 13			16 935
≥50: 30	3769		
<50: 13			

ity reduction estimate) compares favorably with Canadian costs for left mainstem coronary bypass graft surgery of CAN $5300 (WEINSTEIN and STASON 1982), bone marrow transplant therapy for acute nonlymphocytic leukemia of CAN $13 700 (WELCH and LARSON 1989), treatment of moderate hypertension in a middle-aged man of CAN $9600–$83 000 (WEINSTEIN and STASON 1982), renal transplant surgery of CAN $22 000–$25 000 (STANGE and SUMMER 1978; WELCH and LARSON 1989), and the wide range in liver transplant costs from CAN $56 000 to CAN $312 000 (MUSHLIN and FINTOR 1992). Costs for cervical cancer screening, particularly in the elderly, are in the CAN $3000 range, while similar estimates for cervical cancer screening for younger women (aged 20–39) range from CAN $810 to CAN $6000 (MANDELBLATT and FAHS 1988). Our calculations do not take into consideration the expected social costs of short- and long-term disability (relating to lost years of earning) or the added cost for child care attributable to premature deaths from breast cancer (especially pertinent for women in their 40's) (SCHWARTZ and ROLLINS 1985; MOSKOWITZ 1987). Such additional costs can be expected to reduce further the cost per women-year of life saved. Conversely, our calculations do not take discounting into consideration, which would reduce the future value of benefits and increase the cost estimates (ROSENQUIST and LINDFORS 1994).

Although it has been shown that the most favorable cost-effectiveness is for biannual screening for women aged 50–70 (deKONING et al. 1991), the calculations for women aged 40–49 based upon actual SMPBC data provide an important yardstick for future planning and allocation of health care resources.

20.6 Summary

Mass mammography screening has evolved from the various randomized and nonrandomized controled trials performed over the past several decades, to application of the procedure on a wide scale throughout North America and Europe. The UICC, in 1990, emphasized the importance of strict adherence to high-quality procedures to ensure that the 30% mortality reduction demonstrated in controlled trials can be achieved in wide-scale routine population screening (RUTQVIST et al. 1990).

The ultimate goal of all breast cancer screening is to reduce premature mortality from the disease. It is implicit that if this goal is to be reached, then treatment must be timely and appropriate, and that the option of conservative therapy, where indicated, will be an important side benefit.

In the planning, development, and expansion of the SMPBC, we relied greatly upon the experience and advice of others (TABAR et al. 1985a; BIRD and McLELLAND 1986; SICKLES et al. 1986; SICKLES 1988; BIRD 1989). We view the requirements for success as falling into three main categories:

1. Elements related to planning and organization
2. Elements of service and administration
3. Elements of internal quality control and continuous quality improvement

20.6.1 Planning and Organization

It is our experience that it is critical to involve everyone in the planning process, including physicians, other professional-service providers, and the public. This fosters cooperation between the providers and consumers of the service as well as the cooperation of funding agencies. Similarly, the physicians in the communities where screening will be initiated need to be prepared with up-to-date information on the recommendations for screening as well as the planned program procedures for screening and diagnostic workup. In addition, the provision of screening, particularly to a dispersed population, requires creativity in the design of the screening center models; ideally, the choice of model should suit the community it will serve. Finally, all procedures should be designed to provide the highest quality service at all levels.

20.6.2 Service and Administration

The concept of comprehensive care is essential, with careful integration of screening and diagnostic procedures and emphasis on prompt reporting and communication of results. This requires a high level of cooperation among physicians and a refined team approach. The personnel should individually and collectively seek to maximize true-positive results while minimizing false-positive results.

Monitoring of clinical outcomes and collection of data must not only respect the limited ability of primary care physicians to respond to requests for information but also be meticulous in the recording and coding of results. Similarly, it is essential to maintain internal controls, such as regular reviews of positive and negative cases by radiologists, external reviews, and pathology reviews.

Finally, notwithstanding the emphasis on quality, there should be careful attention to the inverse relationship between volume and unit cost, since funding agencies will scrutinize the economics of screening programs to the same degree that medical professionals will analyze the clinical results of screening.

20.6.3 Quality Control and Continuous Quality Improvement

Quality control and continuous quality improvement imply not only following standard procedures but also adjusting the procedures to suit changing circumstances. Quality control audits should extend from regular cost analyses through careful appraisal of new techniques. In addition, attention should be given to input from consumers at all levels – particularly community physicians and the women who are screened – since high compliance is the key not only to mortality reduction but also to the economic success of screening programs. Some compliance barriers are common to both physicians and women, such as cost and radiation risk; others, such as concern over "excessive" false-positives and false-negatives, relatively low yield, and the perception that mammography is unnecessary in the absence of symptoms, are more physician related. The most significant patient-related barriers are lack of a strong physician recommendation and lack of access (Fox et al. 1985; Hayward et al. 1988; Rimer et al. 1989; American Cancer Society 1990; The NCI Breast Concer Screening Consortium 1990; Vogel et al. 1990; Fox et al. 1991; Gambhir and Bassett 1991; Schofield et al. 1994; Turner et al. 1994). Most of the compliance barriers can be categorized as problems of either awareness or accessibility. Such a classification is helpful in designing efforts to overcome the barriers.

Continuous quality improvement should involve the ongoing assessment of new techniques and other scientific informaton that might affect screening protocols. There should be a built-in review process to ensure that all Program protocols are up to date.

Thus, an organized program of mass mammography screening will depend, for success, on careful planning and organization, insistence upon the highest quality in the administration and service provided, and finally, the devotion of all members of the mammography screening program team to quality maintenance and improvement.

Appendix. SMPBC Quality of Image Audit

DATE: _____   CENTER: _____

Indicate if improvement is required

SMPBC ID Number:										
1. Film Markers Clearly Visible										
• screenee name										
• screenee ID number										
• left and right markers										
2. Positioning										
• craniocaudal										
• mediolateral oblique										
• compression										
• other										
3. Image Quality										
• contrast and density										
• sharpness										
• film-screen contact										
• artifacts										
• image distortion										
• other										

*REVIEWER: Please provide constructive comments using specific ID numbers on the attached sheet and indicate if problems identified are sufficiently significant to warrant:

☐ positioning in-service

☐ interim audit

References

American Cancer Society (1990) 1989 survey of physicians' attitudes and practices in early cancer detection. CA Cancer J Clin 40:77

Austoker J (1991) Organisation of a national screening programme. Br Med Bull 47:416-426

Baker LH (1982) Breast Cancer Detection Demonstration Project: five year summary report. CA Cancer J Clin 32:194-226

Beahrs LH, Shapiro S, Smart C (1979) Report of the working group to review the National Cancer Institute – American Cancer Society Breast Cancer Detection Demonstration Projects. J Natl Cancer Inst 62:640-709

Bird RE (1989) Low cost screening mammography: report on finances and review of 21 716 consecutive cases. Radiology 171:87-90

Bird RE, McLelland R (1986) How to initiate and operate a low cost screening mammography center. Radiology 161:43-47

Bjurstam N, Bjorneld L (1994) Mammography screening in women aged 40-49 years at entry: results of the randomized controlled trial in Gothenburg, Sweden. Syllabus, 26th National Conference on Breast Cancer. American College of Radiology, Reston, VA, p 101

Burhenne HJ (1993) Screening mammography in British Columbia. Roentgenpraxis (Germany) 46:367-370

Burhenne HJ, Warren Burhenne L, Goldberg F et al. (1994) Interval breast cancers in the screening mammography program of British Columbia: analysis and classification. AJR 162:1067-1071

Canadian Cancer Statistics, Statistics Canada (1993) Health & Welfare Canada, pp 55-65

Chamberlain J, Moss SM, Kirkpatrick AE (1993) National health service breast screening programme results for 1991-2. BMJ 307:353-356

Collette HJA, Day NE, Rombach JJ et al. (1984) Evaluation of screening for breast cancer in a non-randomized study (the DOM Project) by means of a case-control study. Lancet 1:1224-1226

DeBruhl ND, Bassett LW, Jessop NW et al. (1994) Mobile mammography: results of national survey. Radiological Society of North America, Chicago, Ill., p 217

de Koning HJ, van Ineveld BM, van Oortmarssen GJ et al. (1991) Breast cancer screening and cost-effectiveness; policy alternatives, quality of life considerations and the possible impact of uncertain factors. Int J Cancer 49:531-537

Eckhardt S, Badellino F, Murphy GP (1995) UICC meeting on breast cancer screening in premenopausal women in developed countries. UICC News IV, 4 December 1995

Elwood JM, Cox B, Richardson AK (1993) Effectiveness of breast cancer screening by mammography in younger women. J Curr Clin Trials 3L:32

Feig SA (1994) Determiniation of mammographic screening intervals with surrogate measures for women aged 40-49 years. Radiology 193:311-314

Feig SA, Hendrick RE (1994) Risk, benefit, and controversies in mammographic screening. RSNA Categorical Course in Physics, pp 121-137

Fletcher SW, Black W, Harris R et al. (1993) Report of the international workshop on screening for breast cancer. J Natl Cancer Inst 85:1644-1656

Fox S, Baum JK, Klos DS et al. (1985) Breast cancer screening: the underuse of mammography. Radiology 156:607-611

Fox SA, Murata PJ, Stein JA (1991) The impact of physician compliance on screening mammography for older women. Arch Intern Med 151:50-56

Frisell J, Eklund G, Hellstrom L et al. (1987) Analysis of interval breast carcinomas in a randomized screening trial in Stockholm. Breast Cancer Res Treat 9:219-225

Gambhir S, Bassett LW (1991) The underutilization of screening mammography: overcoming the barriers. J Prim Care Cancer, October 1991, pp 27-33

Garfinkel LE (1994) Evaluating cancer statistics. CA Cancer J Clin 44:5-6

Hakama M, Elovainio L, Kajantie R et al. (1991) Breast cancer screening as public health policy in Finland. 64:962-964

Hayward RA, Shapiro MF, Freeman HE et al. (1988) Who gets screened for cervical breast cancer? Arch Intern Med 148:1177-1181

Hillman BJ (1994) Outcomes research and cost-effectiveness analysis for diagnostic imaging. Radiology 193:307-310

Klemi PJ, Joensuu H, Toikkanen S et al. (1992) Aggressiveness of breast cancers found with and without screening. BMJ 304:467-469

Kopans DB (1994) Conventional wisdom: observation, experience, anecdote, and science in breast imaging. AJR 162:299-303

Kopans DB, Halpern E, Hulka CA (1994) Statistical power in breast cancer screening trials and mortality reduction among women 40-49 years of age with particular emphasis on the National Breast Screening Study of Canada. Cancer 74:1196-1203

Kron ES, Moskowitz H, McConner D et al. (1989) Mobile mammography: the first six-months experience at Mount Sinai Hospital. Conn Med 53:71-72

Letton AH, Mason EM (1989) Routine breast screening for cancer. Semin Surg Oncol 5:163-167

Mandelblatt JS, Fahs MC (1988) The cost-effectiveness of cervical cancer screening for low-income elderly women. JAMA 259:2409-2413

Mettlin C, Smart CR (1994) Breast cancer detection guidelines for women aged 40 to 49 years: rationale for the American Cancer Society reaffirmation of recommendations. CA Cancer J Clin 44:248-255

Moskowitz M (1987) Costs of screening for breast cancer. Radiol Clin North Am 25:1031-1037

Mushlin AI, Fintor L (1992) Is screening for breast cancer cost-effective? Cancer 69:1956-1962

National Board of Health and Welfare (1990) Official recommendations from the National Board of Health and Welfare. Mammographic screening for early detection of breast cancer. Socialstyrelsen, Stockholm, Sweden

Nystrom L, Rutqvist LE, Wall S et al. (1993) Breast cancer screening with mammography: overview of Swedish randomised trials. Lancet 341:973-978

Palli D, Del Turco MR, Buiatti E et al. (1986) A case-control study of the efficiency of a non-randomized breast cancer screening program in Florence, Italy. Int J Cancer 38:501-504

Pamilo M, Anttinen I, Soiva M et al. (1990) Mammography screening – reasons for recall and the influence of experience on recall in the Finnish system. Clin Radiol 41:384-387

Peeters PHM, Verbeek ALM, Hendriks JHCL et al. (1989) Screening for breast cancer in Nihmegen. Report of 6 screening rounds, 1975-1986. Int J Cancer 43:226-230

Richert-Boe KE, Humphrey LL (1992) Screening for cancers of the cervix and breast. Arch Intern Med 152:2405-2411

Richards MT (1994) Australian experience of mammographic screening. In: Tan L, Siew E (eds) Handbook for the 18th

International Congress of Radiology, Singapore. Continental Press, p 787
Rimer BK, Kasper Keintz M, Kessler HB et al. (1989) Why women resist screening mammography: patient-related barriers. Radiology 172:243–246
Roberts MM, Alexander FE, Anderson TJ et al. (1990) Edinburgh Trial of Screening for Breast Cancer: mortality at seven years. Lancet I:241–246
Rosenquist CJ, Lindfors KK (1994) Screening mammography in women aged 40-49 years: analysis of cost-effectiveness. Radiology 191:647–650
Rubin E, Frank M, Stanley R et al. (1990) Patient initiated mobile mammography: analysis of the patients and the problems. South Med J 83:178–184
Rutqvist LE, Miller AB, Andersson I et al. (1990) Reduced breast cancer mortality with mammography screening – an assessment of currently available data. Int J Cancer 5:76–84
Schwartz RM, Rollins PL (1985) Measuring the cost benefit of wellness strategies. Business Health, October, 24–26
Schofield PE, Cockburn J, Hill DJ et al. (1994) Encouraging attendance at a screening mammography programme: determinants of response to different recruitment strategies. J Med Screen 1:144–149
Seidman H, Gelb SK, Silverberg E (1987) Survival experience in the Breast Cancer Detection Demonstration Project. CA Cancer J Clin 37:258–290
Shapiro S (1977) Evidence of screening for breast cancer from a randomized trial. Cancer 39:2722–2782
Shapiro S, Venet W, Strax P et al. (1982) Ten-to-fourteen-year effect of screening on breast cancer mortality. J Natl Cancer Inst 69:349–355
Shapiro S, Venet W, Strax P et al. (1988) Periodic screening for breast cancer: the Health Insurance Plan Project and its sequelae. Johns Hopkins University Press, Baltimore, pp 1963–1986
Sickles EA (1988) Impact of low cost mammography screening on nearby mammography practices. Radiology 168:59–61
Sickles EA, Kopans DB (1993) Deficiencies in the analysis of breast cancer screening data. J Natl Cancer Inst 85:1621–1624
Sickles EA, Weber W, Galvin HB et al. (1986) Mammographic screening: how to operate successfully at low cost. Radiology 160:95–97
Sickles EA, Ominsky SH, Sollitto RA et al. (1990) Medical audit of a rapid throughput mammography screening practice: methodology and results of 27 114 examinations. Radiology 175:323–327
Smart CR, Hendrick RE, Rutledge JH III, Smith RA (1995) Benefit of mammography screening in women ages 40 to 49 years: current evidence from randomized controlled trials. Cancer 75:1619–1626
Stange PV, Sumner AT (1978) Predicting treatment costs and life expectancy for end-stage renal disease. N Engl J Med 298:372–378
Strax P, Venet L, Shapiro S (1973) Value of mammography in reduction of mortality from breast cancer in mass screening. AJR 117:686–689
Tabar L, Dean PB (1989) The present state of screening for breast cancer. Semin Surg Oncol 5:94–101
Tabar L, Fagerberg G, Eklund G (1985a) Reduction in breast cancer mortality by mass screening with mammography: first results of randomized trial in two Swedish counties. Lancet 1:829–832
Tabar L, Gad A, Holmberg L et al. (1985b) Significant reduction in advanced breast cancer: results of the first seven years of mammography screening in Kopparberg, Sweden. Diagn Imaging Clin Med 54:158–164
Tabar L, Fagerberg G, Duffy SW et al. (1992) Update of the Swedish two-county program of mammographic screening for breast cancer. Radiol Clin North Am 30:187–210
The Essendon Breast X-ray Program Collaborative Group (1992) A mammographic screening pilot project in Victoria 1988–1990. Med J Aust 157:670–675
The NCI Breast Cancer Screening Consortium (1990) Screening mammography: a missed clinical opportunity? JAMA 264:54–58
Thurfjell EL, Lindgren AA (1994) Population-based mammography screening in Swedish clinical practice: prevalence and incidence screening in Uppsala County. Radiology 193:351–357
Turner KM, Wilson BJ, Gilbert FJ (1994) Improving breast screening uptake: persuading initial non-attenders to attend. J Med Screen 1:199–202
UK Trial of Early Detection of Breast Cancer Group (1988) First resuls on mortality reduction in the UK trial of early detection of breast cancer. Lancet II:411–416
UK Trial of Early Detection of Breast Cancer Group (1992) Specificity of screening in United Kingdom trial of early detection of breast cancer. BMJ 304:346–349
UK Trial of Early Detection of Breast Cancer Group (1993) Breast cancer mortality after 10 years in the UK trial of early detection of breast cancer. The Breast 2:13–20
van der Maas, de Koning HJ, van Ineveld BM et al. (1989) The cost-effectiveness of breast cancer screening. Int J Cancer 43:1055–1060
van Dijck JAAM, Verbeek ALM, Hendriks JHCL et al. (1993) The current detectability of breast cancer in a mammographic screening program. Cancer 72:1993–1938
van Ineveld BM, van Oortmarssen GJ, de Koning HJ et al. (1993) How cost-effective is breast cancer screening in different EC countries? Eur J Cancer 29A:1663–1668
Verbeek ALM, Hwnseika JHCL, Holland R et al. (1984) Reduction of breast cancer mortality through mass screening with modern mammography: first results of the Nijmegen Project. Lancet 1:1222–1224
Vogel VG, Graves DS, Coody DK et al. (1990) Breast screening compliance following a statewide low-cost mammography project. Cancer Detect Prev 14:573–576
Wald N, Chamberlain J, Hackshaw A (1993) Report of the European society of mastology breast cancer screening evaluation committee. Tumori 79:371–379
Warren Burhenne LJ (1994)
Warren Burhenne LJ, Hislop TG, Burhenne HJ (1992a) The British Columbia mammography screening program: evaluation of the first 15 months. AJR 158:45–49
Warren Burhenne LJ, Burhenne HJ, Hislop TG (1992b) Result-oriented mass mammography screening. RSNA, Chicago, p 60
Weinstein MC, Stason WB (1982) Cost-effectiveness of coronary artery bypass surgery. Circulation 66:56–66
Welch HG, Larson EB (1989) Cost effectiveness of bone marrow transplantation in acute nonlymphocytic leukemia. N Engl J Med 321:807–812

21 Medicolegal Aspects of Breast Imaging

R.J. Brenner

CONTENTS

21.1	Introduction	367
21.2	Basic Legal Principles	368
21.3	Battery: An Intentional Tort	368
21.4	Law of Negligence	369
21.5	Standard of Care: Basic Duties	370
21.6	Screening Versus Diagnostic Mammography	370
21.7	Reporting	371
21.8	Self-referred Patients	373
21.8.1	Ordering Screening Mammograms	373
21.8.2	Agency	374
21.8.3	Abandonment	374
21.8.4	Negligent Referral	374
21.9	Lawsuits and Conflict Resolution	374
21.10	Conclusions	376
	References	376

21.1 Introduction

The emergence of publicly funded breast cancer screening programs in many countries around the world reflects a scientific basis showing that sufficiently early detection and proper treatment of breast malignancies can favorably impact case fatality rates as well as political, social, and economic forces prioritizing this effort among competing national agendas. Clinical trials from Europe and North America have helped define both the potentials and the limitations of screening programs, as indicated elsewhere in this text. With information available in both scientific and lay publications, women's awareness of the possibility of early detection of breast cancer is perhaps greater than with respect to any other disease.

While such developments have helped to encourage participation in screening mammography programs, they have also created high expectations for cure. A woman whose breast cancer is found at a stage where it has already metastasized is thus more likely to believe that the medical system and those associated with her care have failed, or done something wrong.

The practice of medicine is subject to a number of methods of accountability. Facility accreditation and physician credentialing, case management conferences, and even peer pressure offer forums for the free intellectual exchange of information and ideas in assessing desired performance standards. Most countries afford an aggrieved patient an opportunity for a different forum of accountability; namely, legal redress. Some countries, such as Sweden, have a system of "no fault liability" where compensation following a showing of negligence is made through a patient insurance program (Brahams 1988). Other countries, such as Switzerland, provide a patient the opportunity to submit her case for review by independent university experts who offer impartial opinions with respect to the merits or failures of those taking care of her in a program conducted by the Swiss Medical Association (FMH). Patients who disagree with such determinations are still free to pursue their case in courts of law within a legal system that offers several disincentives for such further action when the review process indicates no negligence. It has been suggested that this kind of system is the basis for relatively few medical malpractice lawsuits being tried in courts in Switzerland (Kuhn 1993).

In the United States, where more than 1 million lawsuits are filed each year, medical malpractice cases afford virtually any aggrieved patient access to the legal system. While some safeguards have been developed in several states, such as mandatory review by a medical panel (Alaska) or limitations on pain and suffering awards (California), the number of lawsuits against physicians in the field of breast cancer evaluation continues to rise. A study in 1995 by a consortium of insurance carriers around the country, the Physicians Insurers Association of America (PIAA), indicated that delay in diagnosis of breast cancer is the most common reason that physi-

---

R.J. Brenner, MD, JD, Director, Breast Imaging, Eisenberg Keefer Breast Center, John Wayne Cancer Institute, St. Johns Hospital and Health Center, 1328 22nd Street, Santa Monica, CA 90404, USA and Associate Clinical Professor, UCLA, Los Angeles, CA 90095-6952 USA

cians are sued and the second leading cause of indemnity payments (PIAA 1995).

It is instructive to review principles of American jurisprudence with respect to cases for malpractice and the diagnosis of breast cancer in order to understand the legal relationships that exist among patients and their medical providers. Such an analysis will provide a basis for understanding similar relationships in other countries, where conflict resolution may be facilitated by different means. Indeed, much of American jurisprudence is based in eighteenth century English law. A study of American legal relationships should prompt both a sensitivity for avoidable problems and a rationale for providing risk management strategies that have universal significance.

21.2 Basic Legal Principles

Like medicine, American law is divided into several fields or specialties. Rules of evidence and procedure vary with different fields of law, which include, for example, contract law, maritime law, and administrative law. The interests of society in general are protected under rules of criminal law. Criminal conviction is predicated on very high standards of proof where the offended party is the "state" and where fines or even incarceration are penalties imposed on guilty defendants. Physicians are occasionally subject to criminal law allegations such as misrepresentation to government reimbursement agencies ("Medicare fraud") but even prosecutions for medical malpractice have (rarely) been pursued under criminal auspices.

Most medical malpractice cases are tried as issues of civil law or, more specifically, tort law. This law defines relationships between any two (or more) parties and generally offers remedies for offenses in the form of restitution, usually resulting in the payment of money. Under tort law, cases may be filed as "intentional torts" such as battery, but the overwhelming majority are pursued as cases in "negligence." The law of negligence defines departures from recognized standards of care perpetrated by one party upon another. Most civil law is derived from two sources: statutory law and common law.

Statutory law is that body of law that is drafted and approved by lawmakers or legislatures at various levels of government, including municipal, state, and national (Congress) bodies. These laws are usually interpreted by regulatory agencies, a dispute with which ultimately may be appealed to a court of law. Laws are codified and can be found in most law libraries. Licensure laws or statutory prescriptions for certain kinds of informed consent are examples of statutory law. The Mammography Quality Standards Act (MQSA), which was passed by Congress in 1992 and will be both interpreted and administered by the Food and Drug Administration (FDA), is an example of statutory law that will set expressed standards for the performance of mammographic examinations in the United States (MQSA 1992).

Most law pertaining to medical malpractice is not covered by statutes and is referred to as common law. American common law, which began in the eighteenth century, was adapted from English common law whereby decisions of judges helped establish proper rules or conduct for society. Certain professions were held to a "public calling" to provide for the safety and welfare of the citizens. Common law is based on the legal principle of *stare decisis* whereby a decision by an appellate court establishes a legal precedent to be followed in that jurisdiction or locale when similar facts or situations arise again. Most appellate decisions are published for purposes of reference and, while they apply specifically to the jurisdiction in which they are rendered, may have relevance to other jurisdictions.

There are relatively few appellate decisions regarding mammographic examinations and interpretations. A review of appellate decisions during the past 25 years in the United States by this author revealed approximately 80 cases dealing with delay in diagnosis of breast cancer, with very few decisions commenting upon the conduct of the breast imaging facility. The approach to evaluating the medical legal aspects of breast imaging, therefore, must be predicated primarily upon fundamental jurisprudential notions, buttressed where possible by appellate court reasoning or statutorily prescribed guidelines.

21.3 Battery: An Intentional Tort

An intentional tort is one in which the offending party intends to commit an act and in fact commits it. Legal redress for such an act requires no proof of harm or motivation. Intentional torts afford the aggrieved party the possibility of "punitive damages" or awards based on punishment and deterrence rather than compensation for harm done. In the United States, punitive damages can be most severe because they generally are not covered by medical malpractice insurance, thereby subjecting the physician to personal financial exposure. The most common intentional tort which is raised in court by aggrieved patients is that of battery. Battery is defined as an unlawful touching of another individual. Normal incidental touchings or those touchings that are an inherent component of the physical examination are not considered battery. Rather considerations of battery arise when an interventional procedure is performed. The defense to the charge of battery is the obtaining of informed consent.

Battery may also exist when the performance of a procedure exceeds that procedure covered by the scope of the consent. For example, informed consent for a cyst aspiration may not provide a defense to battery if, failing to obtain fluid, a large bore core needle biopsy is subsequently performed. In a survey of radiologists performing interventional procedures such as preoperative localization of nonpalpable lesions, a majority of the respondents indicated that they do not obtain informed consent (Reynolds et al. 1993).

Informed consent must be obtained by the person performing the procedure and cannot be delegated to other individuals. Informed consent involves the physician disclosing to the patient material risks of a procedures. Material risks are those which a reasonably prudent person would want to know to make an informed decision and usually include those risks of high frequency and low severity or low frequency and high severity (Cantebury v Spence 1972). In some states, alternatives and the risk of not performing a procedure must also be disclosed. Radiologists are advised to consult their local laws for further requirements of informed consent as well as specific exceptions to obtaining consent.

Most lawsuits emerging from claims for battery or inadequate informed consent are tried under the law of negligence; namely, "the negligent obtaining of informed consent."

21.4 Law of Negligence

The law of negligence governs most medical malpractice cases and is concerned with the conduct of physicians rather than the outcome of their actions. Nonetheless, it is the outcome and especially negative outcome which brings the issue of conduct to a court's attention. Medical negligence, rather than the derogatory connotation that physicians often associate with the word, is a term of art established by four elements. The first element is duty. "One who undertakes gratuitously or for consideration to render services to another which he should recognize as necessary for the protection of the other person or things, is subject to liability to the other for physical harm resulting from his failure to exercise reasonable care or perform his undertaking if such failure to exercise such care increased the risk of such harm . . ." [Restatement (second) of Torts]. This legal definition of duty, which incorporates conduct by a physician either informally or formally, has been interpreted by most courts in similar fashion. The standard of care defined by duty is established by determining what a reasonable physician would do under similar circumstances (Skeffington v Bradley 1962).

Judge Learned Hand, one of the more noted commentators in American jurisprudence, attempted to reduce the abstract principle of "standard of care" to a mathematical relationship. He suggested that the standard of care be determined by the relationship and the likelihood of an untoward event and its severity. The standard of care in interpretation of mammograms is judged therefore by the predictable incidence of malignancy in a given age group and the untoward consequences of undiagnosed breast cancer. Note how this formula applies to encouraging screening mammography in age groups where breast cancer is more prevalent. The formula may also be used to assess potential negligent parameters in the obtaining of informed consent and in fact is generalized in its application to most fields of medicine.

The second element of negligence is breach of duty or breach of the standard of care. The third element is causation. When a defendant's act bears a sufficiently causative relationship to an injury such as delay in diagnosis then negligence has been established. The terms of art often applied in this context include "cause in fact" and "proximate cause." Many courts have adopted the parameter of "substantial factor" in assessing whether or not a defendant's conduct indeed led to a patient's injury.

Negligence is established by the above three elements. Unlike intentional torts, where no harm need be suffered, a negligence lawsuit requires a showing of damages to be "actionable." Usually these damages are assessed in terms of money including the out of pocket expenses consequent to the delay in diagnosis (compensatory damages) as well as pain and suffering and usually loss of consortium (special damages). An emerging measure of damages includes the "loss of chance," a determination indicating a worsened prognosis resulting from a delay in diagnosis caused by the "tort-feasor" or defendant (KING 1981).

Unlike battery, cases in negligence often require experts to help in establishing the standard of care parameters and in the assessment of damages. An emerging national standard of care permits experts from one part of the country to testify in another, although frequently the "locale rule" or local community standard relationships are still relevant (FRANCISCO V PARCHMENT MEDICAL CLINIC 1978). Experts are designated by both the plaintiff and the defendant as consultants to the court but their role as advocates in judicial proceedings has received critical attention (BRENNER 1993).

21.5 Standard of Care: Basic Duties

The duty of the breast imager is a variable one depending on the defined goals of the examination. The fundamental duty of the radiologist and the facility is to obtain satisfactory images and effectively render a reasonable interpretation.

Radiographs are objective evidence in a court of law and inadequately obtained mammograms may subject the radiologist to legal exposure. In 1987, The American College of Radiology instituted a mammography accreditation program which provided voluntary peer review mechanisms to ensure that an imaging facility was capable of producing satisfactory images. This directive was eventually incorporated in the MQSA Act of 1992, the provisions of which not only invited but insisted that all mammography facilities demonstrate evidence of excellent image quality production employing safe, dose-controlled equipment. Such provisions are purported to encourage and assist radiologists in this endeavor, although severe sanctions are available for noncompliance. For many years most states have required radiation safety compliance. These programs, if successful, may serve as a model for other countries. While accreditation is evidence of a facility's ability to perform satisfactory imaging, it is no defense where the particular case in question fails to meet acceptable standards.

Reasonable interpretation is a more difficult parameter to assess. Because even the most expert interpretation will be compromised by inadequate images, the first component of reasonable interpretation relates to the production of satisfactory images discussed previously. Lesions partially obscured by positioning or motion blurriness may be difficult to detect and characterize.

Errors in interpretation include both detection errors and diagnostic errors. The former relate to optimal image production as well as reader error. The latter relate to diagnostic assessment criteria. Reviews of rates and causes of errors have been published suggesting that interval cancers arise from abnormalities that are not detected, improperly diagnosed, or not mammographically demonstrable (BIRD et al. 1992; THURFJELL et al. 1994; RENFREW et al. 1992). Perhaps the most troubling of these circumstances are those abnormalities which are detected but are insufficiently characteristic of a malignant process, in which area a cancer is eventually found. So-called subthreshold features may be the subject of litigation and, in a legal context, emphasize the legal concept of forseeability. The issue of forseeability is an important measure in determining standard of care for radiographic interpretation. The court must determine whether a lesion was sufficiently suspicious as to warrant an interpretation inviting biopsy or whether the lesion's characteristics were sufficiently benign that alternative interpretations and management would be reasonable. Recall that a patient may insist on the removal of a lesion regardless of interpretation. A discussion of the mammographic signs of benign and malignant features appears elsewhere in this text. Types of mammographic abnormalities that have been studied by long-term surveillance provide a basis for alternatives to biopsy for low-suspicion abnormalities (SICKLES 1991).

21.6 Screening Versus Diagnostic Mammography

Screening mammography is essentially a public health effort, an attempt to identify a relatively small population of asymptomatic patients with mammographic abnormalities from the overwhelming number with essentially normal studies. Consequently, low-cost, high-volume-oriented techniques with proven efficacy have been applied to this effort (SICKLES et al. 1986; BIRD and MCLELLAND 1986). Different medical societies in the United States as well as public programs in other countries have attempted to reconcile such methodologies with national strategies and limited funding. Public programs and managed care plans need to incorporate such strategies into benefit packages. In addition to meeting the medical challenge of impacting case fatality rates and presumably realizing the economic as well as social benefits to be derived from such programs, potential legal exposure may emerge when programs do not provide for screening examinations.

At present, no appellate court in the United States has ruled that screening mammography is a standard of care requirement although several trial courts have considered the issue. Only one appellate decision in the past 25 years has taken judicial notice of screening mammography goals (LEVINE V ROSEN 1990).

Legal exposure in screening mammography programs extends, of course, beyond provider benefit packages. The radiologist is charged with the reasonable detection of significant mammographic abnormalities, the failure of which – if it results in delay of diagnosis of cancer – may constitute negligence. Detection error is a source of liability in many fields of radiology, most notably mammography and chest radiography. The radiologic "miss" may arise from the lack of observation of a focal abnormality or from its observation but dismissal as an insignificant finding. Errors are subject to expert review. Because screening mammography is in effect limited to two universally prescribed radiographic views, incomplete assessment should prompt the radiologist to suggest further evaluation of a potentially significant abnormality, in the same way in which courts have instructed clinicians to further evaluate specific clinical findings.

Occasionally specific diagnoses can be rendered from a screening mammogram. A spiculated mass with no accompanying history of trauma or infection is likely to prompt surgical evaluation without additional workup. Given the known history of associated multifocal and multicentric disease, subthreshold abnormalities surrounding a diagnosable lesion on a screening m ammogram may prompt further evaluation under certain circumstances. Likewise the observation of a well-circumscribed 8-mm mass with a central fatty hilus in the upper outer quadrant of the breast may usually be dismissed as an intramammary lymph node (HOMER 1987). Diagnostic or problem-solving mammography affords the breast imager the opportunity to tailor an examination to solve a particular problem identified on either a screening mammogram or a clinical examination. By employing ancillary procedures such as ultrasonography, special views, microfocal spot cones, compression images, computed tomography, and magnetic resonance imaging, the diagnostic examination is an attempt to provide a reasonable interpretation regarding the likelihood of malignancy for a mammographically or clinically detected abnormality.

The screening mammographer is charged primarily with the detection of abnormalities. The diagnostic mammographer is charged with both the detection of abnormalities and the reasonable interpretation of such abnormalities.

Legal consequences necessarily follow from these two aspects of mammography, both of which are essential to a successful screening program. The legal exposure of a radiologist evaluating a palpable abnormality may be somewhat mitigated by the paramount importance of the clinical examination. A palpable mass may require biopsy in spite of a negative or benign mammographic interpretation. On the other hand, ill-defined abnormalities which may not be characterized as dominant masses may be improperly followed if the radiologist erroneously assigns a clearly benign diagnosis such as a simple cyst to the focus of clinical concern. This example emphasizes the importance of specific circumstances by which the courts will evaluate reasonable conduct on the part of all healthcare providers.

Mammographers are encouraged to, and, under MQSA, may be required to assess their skills by means of some form of audit. When a women detelops breast cancer following a series of mammographic and clinical examinations, it may be contended that the radiologist did not apply appropriate skill and reasonable care to the mammographic interpretation. Audits which demonstrate proficiency commensurate with other successful breast imaging institutions, especially when buttressed with cases preceding the one in contention that form a basis for a challenged interpretation, may provide evidence for the reasonableness of a given interpretation.

21.7 Reporting

The reporting of results is related to the type of examination performed. Screening mammography reports often use a standardized form, especially because the goals of public health low-cost high-volume screening combined with the anticipated high percentage of normals favors such a system. Facilities wishing to individually tailor interpretations to each screening mammogram exceed basic legal requirements and incur higher costs.

Diagnostic examinations require a more definitive interpretation and recommendation. While "indeterminate" may be an appropriate conclusion for screening mammograms (inviting further imaging assessment), it is usually an unreasonable interpretation for a diagnostic examination. A group of very malignant appearing calcifications, for example, which are not interpreted as suspicious but rather equivocal or indeterminate may foreseeably invite delay in diagnosis if subsequent management is then left to the discretion of the clinician. Practices are advised to review their diagnostic interpretations in this context, and may use the ACR lexicon diagnostic categories as a standard by which to measure their reporting system. The law permits alternative approaches to medical care in all circumstances so long as they are reasonable and recognized as such. Reporting systems may employ their own terminology and recommendations subject to the test of reasonableness.

Occasionally mammographic reports include general disclaimers and caveats which may or may not be pertinent to the particular examination under study. Comments such as "malignancy cannot be excluded" are considered precatory in a legal sense, offering no defense to a mammographic interpretation incorrectly rendered as benign. Indeed, malignancy can never be excluded without histologic confirmation. Where findings are insufficiently suspicious in an area of palpable concern, radiologists have been encouraged to employ an approach used in other imaging examinations, the "pertinent negative," to alert the clinician that the particular mammographic examination cannot adequately characterize a given area of concern (BRENNER 1993). Pertinent negatives are unlikely to be relevant where clinical findings are absent (MOSKOWITZ 1983).

The fear of lawsuits has prompted some inexperienced mammographers to consider malignancy for an unusually large number of mammographically detected abnormalities. This trend has been abetted by the use of stereotactically guided tissue sampling techniques, often for abnormalities incompletely evaluated. There are no prescriptive guidelines to account for all cases. Appropriate recommendations for tissue sampling, however, require at a minimum a demonstrable lesion. Lawsuits have arisen for improper use of surgery, a phenomenon which may extend to radiologists who, seeking to escape legal exposure, recommend biopsies in a manner inconsistent with reasonable interpretation. The ability to reconcile the importance of early detection of cancer with the multitude of abnormalities detected which are most likely benign is a dilemma pertinent to all aspects of radiology and particularly relevant to mammography because of the large numbers of women subject to this examination during public health oriented screening programs. Second opinions, the use of limited tissue sampling, and mammographic surveillance are examples of mechanisms that may be employed in difficult cases.

When a screening-detected abnormality is found that is significantly suspicious for malignancy, the duty of the radiologist probably extends beyond the simple issuing of a report. As an Ohio court stated, "The communication of a diagnosis so that it may be beneficially utilized may be altogether as important as the diagnosis itself" (BRENNER 1991; ROBERTSON and KOPANS 1989). Consider the asymptomatic patient with a spiculated mass seen on screening mammography where the radiologist is the only individual who knows that a likely cancer exists within the women's breast. Because it is foreseeable that reports may be misfiled or not reach their intended party, radiologists are advised to personally communicate the results of suspicious findings and document such communications in a regular business record (e.g., the report, the patient's medical record). This added "duty" again follows from the formula discussed earlier of Judge Learned Hand.

Mammographic abnormalities which are probably benign and need further assessment should also be communicated to the referring physician, a task which may be accomplished in a different manner derivative of Learned Hand's prescription. Patients whose screening mammograms are not evaluated on site need to be afforded mechanisms to return for further evaluation. This kind of communication is often particularized to the imaging facility and its relationship to the patient and referring physician. Reminder letters inviting further assessment, short-term follow-up, or even annual mammograms have been a favored mechanism for encouraging compliance with recommendations. These may be accomplished by the primary care provider, the referring imaging facility, or both. Because patients may choose not to return to the original screening facility for further study, insuring compliance is often the primary responsibility of the clinical physician. Radiology facilities may encourage physician referrals and patient satisfaction under many circumstances by assisting in such recall efforts.

When further assessment yields a suspicious diagnosis, then direct communication with the referring physician is again essential. The interrelationship among different specialties invites communication problems, often to the detriment of the patient's well-being. Some facilities have chosen to report results directly to the patient, usually employing lay terminology. While this practice was required under the Medicare program for screening mammography (Omnibus Reconciliation Act of 1990), it is not required under MQSA for physician-referred patients. Nonetheless, the benefits of reporting results to patients directly need to be assessed by individual facilities with respect to their relationship to referring physicians and particular patient populations and especially with respect to predicted compliance rates with recommendations (ROBERTSON and KOPANS 1989; DeNEEF and GANDARA 1991).

21.8 Self-referred Patients

Breast imaging occupies a somewhat unique role in radiology. In the United States, radiologic consultation is predicated upon referred patients from primary care physicians, a disease-oriented approach upon which the legal system of evaluating medical malpractice is based. In the United States as well as other countries, women may seek breast care evaluation independent of other forms of medical care. Because fiscally sound screening mammography programs are often dependent upon high-volume strategies, many facilities in the United States have invited self-referred women to attend regular breast screening (MONSEES et al. 1988). The basic medical and legal requirements discussed previously apply to such self-referred practices. However, additional duties attend these practices, which may enjoy a multitude of benefits emphasizing outreach programs.

A number of medical studies, the most prominent of which in the United States has been the Breast Cancer Detection Demonstration Project (BCDDP), have indicated that a significant percentage of breast cancers may be palpable where mammographic features are either undeclared or insufficiently specific to render a diagnosis of malignancy (Breast Cancer Detection Demonstration Project 1987). Breast cancer screening is not synonymous with mammography screening and such facilities are encouraged to provide a mechanism (either onsite or by referral) for physical examination, an important component of any screening program.

The distinction between screening and diagnostic mammography mentioned earlier includes in the latter category patients who have signs or symptoms of breast cancer and thus may benefit from specially tailored examinations. Self-referral facilities may wish to functionally if not structurally designate those components of practice which are dedicated to screening and diagnostic studies, the former often not requiring on-site physician availability.

An important component of such designation for both physician-referred and self-referred facilities is an intake sheet documenting the nature of the examination, patient profile, and patient history. This is an essential component of risk management for patients who suffer breast cancer and claim that earlier examinations were not properly performed for specific complaints. The documentation of the presence or absence of complaints is important for selecting the appropriate type of mammographic examination to be scheduled as well as substantiating, if challenged, the reasons for choosing such a type.

The self-referral facility assumes the position of a primary care physician not only in directing the patient for physical and mammographic examination but also in communicating results. Because there is no intermediary primary care physician, these facilities need to communicate the results of examinations directly to the patient. In this role a number of considerations emerge that are particularly though not exclusively applicable to the self-referral facility.

21.8.1 Ordering Screening Mammograms

As discussed earlier, no appellate court has imposed a duty on the part of a clinician or a radiologist to order a screening mammography. Primary care physicians or radiologists accepting self-referred patients may wish to do so for several reasons including:

1. A number of trial court experts' opinions have indicated the issue as bearing on standard of care.
2. The inference that specialty societies and government-sponsored programs encourage the use of screening mammography as a standard of medical practice.
3. The ordering of a screening mammogram defeats a plaintiff's potential contention that a clinical cancer would have been discovered earlier had the physician ordered a screening mammogram (BRENNER, In Press).

In a manner similar to the recall of patients for additional studies and short-term follow-up mammography, self-referral facilities may wish to employ mechanisms (tickler files) for advising patients of the importance of regular screening mammograms.

21.8.2 Agency

The law of agency governs those errors or omissions committed by personnel under the supervision of and acting for the benefit of a physician or imaging facility. Legal doctrines such as *respondent superior and vicarious liability* attribute the errors of such personnel or "agents" to the person or persons in charge of the facility. Such relationships apply universally but come into focus for self-referral facilities who accept patients who may have no other medical record to refer to if identifying information is misregistered. Consider the situation where films are either batch processed or read at the end of a screening day and where a significant abnormality is detected. Because the patient may have no other treating physician, the inability to contact the patient for purposes of recall and communication of mammographic results because of misinformation obtained by an agent prior to an examination (e.g., clerk) may result in an untoward delay in diagnosis of breast cancer for the patient and legal exposure for the physician and/or facility. Safeguards may be employed such as the documented recertification of demographic information by the patient prior to leaving the facility or instituting further mechanisms for patient communication with the facility following the study. Alternatively self-referral facilities may wish to afford access to immediate diagnostic evaluation for mammographically detected abnormalities.

21.8.3 Abandonment

When a self-referral facility determines that patient care requires medical care beyond the capabilities of the facility, the facility is required to make appropriate referrals and recommendations to the patient. Depending on the acuity of the clinical circumstances, the facility may be required either to more or less insure compliance with such recommendations or to document refusal. Thus when a highly suspicious lesion is seen on mammogram or a malignancy is diagnosed by tissue sampling and a referral is made to a breast surgeon, the facility is responsible for helping insure compliance with this recommendation, again a derivative of Learned Hand's formula. Compliance is often documented in a report issued from the surgeon to the referring physician (or the imaging facility) regarding assessment and future plans. If such reports are not received, other documentation regarding compliance or documented refusal by the patient to comply is necessary to avoid the tort of abandonment.

The relationship of a patient and a physician is not one of parity. The patient may decline to seek physician services at any time whereas the physician, depending on the circumstances, must provide some basis for continuing care to the patient when the relationship is terminated. Depending on the exigencies of the situation, the physician will need to go to greater or lesser lengths in documenting the transference of care. Thus if a facility declines to see a patient for regular screening mammography, simple documentation regarding the patient's and physician's consensual agreement on such termination may be appropriate. On the other hand, where a relationship breaks down under more precarious circumstances – such as that described above where cancer is discovered and needs to be treated accordingly – documented evidence of the successful transference of care may need to meet stricter standards. While these concepts are contrary to the usual notions whereby a primary care physician refers the patient to the radiologist for a consultation, they are neither unduly harsh nor difficult to understand and follow from appropriate principles of patient care management.

21.8.4 Negligent Referral

Another tort exists regarding the referral of patients. When a patient is referred to another consultant (e.g., surgeon) or facility which the referring physician knows or should know may be unable to render suitable care, then the referring physician or facility itself has acted unreasonably and may be subject to the tort of "negligent referral." Loss of staff privileges at hospitals or criminal investigation of a party to which the patient is being referred may prompt the referring physician to further evaluate the basis for a referral. Other less serious considerations such as economic relationships may also invite stricter scrutiny of referral practices.

21.9 Lawsuits and Conflict Resolution

Most states have enacted "Statutes of Limitations" which define a period of time whereby an aggrieved patient may file a lawsuit. The triggering event is usually defined by when the patient has discovered or should have discovered possible negligence in her care. Statutes may begin when the patient discovers that she has breast cancer or, under other circumstances, when adverse events occur regarding breast implant, surgery, or other actionable events.

When a lawsuit is filed the defendant or defendants will receive a "summons and complaint" stating multiple "causes of action." The text of such a complaint is often based on suggested procedural forms available to attorneys. A radiologist receiving such a complaint is advised to seek immediate legal assistance. Radiologists reviewing the text of a formal complaint who are not versed in legal procedure may find the documents intimidating, threatening, and "unfair." The parameters involved in filing such a complaint, however, must meet minimum legal standards to avoid personal legal exposure by the attorney.

When a complaint is received, the insurance carrier and/or risk manager for the practice should be notified immediately. Soon therepafter an attorney will be assigned to the case. The relationship between that attorney and defendant should be one of mutual respect, confidence, and constructive enterprise. A failure of such a relationship should prompt the defendant physician to consider alternative legal representation which may be facilitated by the insurance carrier.

Any conversations occurring outside of the physician–attorney "privileged" relationship are subject to legal discovery. For example, a defendant physician who shows a contested x-ray to a colleague who does not agree with the original interpretation invites evidentiary disclosure of such adverse comments (in an otherwise innocuous discussion) by the process of discovery. All actions related to a case in litigation should be coordinated with the defendant attorney and, in general, any further conversations with the plaintiff patient or plaintiff attorney should be performed with legal representation. While such directives appear harsh, the adversarial nature of the American judicial system prompts such a recommendation. One unfortunate consequence of this directive is that the patien–physician relationship will often be suspended. This, however, does not relieve the physician of providing a transference of care, discussed earlier, to avoid a further charge of abandonment. The defendant physician is advised to "freeze the past episode in time and place." Medical records and any previous films related to the patient should be carefully sequestered. Alteration of medical records, detectable by handwriting experts, or loss of radiographs following the filing of a lawsuit is more likely to compromise the defense of the physician's conduct than any other aspect of the case because the physician's credibility becomes suspect.

The anxiety consequent to the discovery of cancer is shared by the patient as well as her providers. Information material relevant to the case should not be misrepresented or withheld from the patient. As difficult as confronting a possible delay in diagnosis may be, such misrepresentation or concealment may not only adversely affect the credibility of the defendant physician, but may be a basis for extending or "tolling" the Statute of Limitations indefinitely.

Most malpractice cases are settled by mutual consent prior to trial. On the basis of such settlements, insurance companies such as the PIAA have pooled data to help assess the parameters regarding malpractice lawsuits (PIAA 1995). Interestingly, much of this information has been corroborated by review of appellate decisions where, for technical reasons, the facts of the case have been recapitulated (BRENNER 1991; KERN 1992). Table 21.1 reviews the average indemnity awards by various sub-specialties based on the PIAA data. Tables 21.2 and 21.3 indicate the reasons for patient delay and physician delay in the diagnosis of breast cancer. As can be seen, radiologists, who have in the past been infrequently involved in such lawsuits, are now the most commonly named defendants in cases involving delay in breast

Table 21.1. Claim counts and indemnity by specialty (based on PIAA 1995)

Specialty	No. of claims	Total indemnity	Av. indemnity
Radiology	165	$30 079 579	$182 300
Obstetrics/gynecology	154	$42 736 849	$277 512
Family practice	113	$19 744 677	$174 732
Surgical specialty	97	$24 922 537	$256 933
Internal medicine	61	$10 760 227	$176 397
Pathology	11	$3 799 502	$345 409
Other physician	31	$5 084 276	$164 009
Corporation	30	$8 155 226	$271 841
Hospital	13	$1 528 167	$117 551
Total	675	$146 811 040	$217 498

Table 21.2. Suspected reasons for delays in diagnosis due to patients (based on PIAA 1995)

Reason	% of 487 cases
No delay by patient	63.4
Failure to keep follow-up appointment	11.3
Procrastination	7.2
Other health problems involved	5.7
Behavioral/emotional problems	3.3
Socioeconomic issues	3.1
Fearful of examination	1.6
Refused mammogram	1.2
Other/not specified	7.4
Not known	9.2

Table 21.3. Reasons for delays in diagnosis due to physicians (based on PIAA 1995)

Reason	No. of cases
Poor examination by physician	50
Inadequate communication	51
Failure to order mammogram	54
Repeat examinations did not arouse suspicion	55
Distracted by other health problems	55
Failure to react to mammogram	60
Delay in or failure to consult	75
Failure to perform proper biopsy	110
Mammogram misread	110
Negative mammogram report	125
Failure to follow up with patient	150
Physical findings failed to impress	169

cancer diagnosis, and the increasing use of screening mammography is likely to generate an even higher number of lawsuits against radiologists in the future.

21.10 Conclusions

The high public profile enjoyed by mammography and other forms of breast imaging is an important component of promoting compliance with screening recommendations and making successful a recently defined public health effort. A consequence of such efforts has been a rising level of malpractice lawsuits directed against physicians for delay in diagnosis. The combined goals of mass screening and diagnostic imaging invite system problems that may be solved by defining the purpose of a given examination, recognizing potential adverse consequences of variance from reasonable conduct, and developing risk management strategies in clinical practice which address both medical and legal concerns. The lessons derived from the American experience may serve as a model for other countries where legal consequences may be less severe but where medical and public health goals are similar. Appropriate allocation of resources and a well-reasoned, accountable medical approach should position facilities in such a manner as to either reduce or defeat unnecessary legal grievances.

References

Bird RE, McLelland R (1986) How to initiate and operate a low-cost screening mammography center. Radiology 161:43–47

Bird RE, Wallace TW, Yankaskas BC (1992) Analysis of cancers missed at screening mammography. Radiology 184: 613–617

Brahams D (1988) The Swedish medical insurance schemes: the way ahead for the United Kingdom. Lancet 1:43–47

Brahams D (1987) Breast Cancer Detection Demonstration Project: end results. CA Cancer J Clin 37:5–29

Brenner RJ (1991) Medicolegal aspects of breast imaging: variable standards of care relating to differing types of practice. AJR 156:719–723

Brenner RJ (1993) Mammography and malpractice litigation: current status, lessons, and admonitions. AJR 161:931–935

Brenner RJ (1995) Reporting the "missed" radiologic diagnosis: medicolegal and ethical considerations. Breast Disease: A Yearbook Quarterly 6:121–122

Cantebury v Spence (1972) 464 F. 2d 772 (D.C. Circ., 1972) cert denied, 409 U.S. 1064, 935 S. Ct. 560

DeNeef P, Gandara J (1991) Experience with indeterminate mammograms. West J Med 154:36–39

Francisco v Parchment Medical Clinic (1978) P.C., Mich. App. 272 N.W. 2d 736

Homer MJ (1987) Imaging features and management of characteristically benign and probably benign breast lesions. Radiol Clin North Am 25:932–940

Kern KA (1992) Causes of breast cancer malpractice litigation. Arch Surg 127:542–547

King H (1981) Causation, valuation and chance in personal injury torts involving pre-existing conditions and future consequences. Yale Law Journal 90:1353–1397

Kuhn FH (1993) Aussergerichtliche Gutachterstelle der FMH. Schweizerische Ärztezeitung 74:712–713

Levine v Rosen (1990) 19 Phila 529

Monsees B, Destouet JM, Evens RG (1988) The self-referred mammography patient: a new responsibility for radiologists. Radiology 166:69–71

Moskowitz M (1983) The predictive value of certain mammographic signs in screening for breast cancer. Cancer 51:1007–1011

MQSA (1992) Mammography Quality Standards Act, PL 102–539 (Oct 27, 1992)

PIAA (1995) The breast cancer study, Physician Insurers Association of America. Washington DC, June 1995

Renfrew DL, Franken EA, Bernbaum KS (1992) Error in radiology: classification and lessons in 182 cases presented at a problem case conference. Radiology 183:145–150

Restatement (second) of Torts, Section 323(a)

Reynolds HE, Jackson VP, Musick BS (1993) A survey of interventional mammography practices. Radiology 187: 71–73

Robertson CL, Kopans DB (1989) Communication problems after mammographic screening, Radiology 172:443–444

Sickles EA (1991) Periodic mammographic follow-up of probably benign lesions: results in 3184 consecutive cases. Radiology 179:463–468

Sickles EA, Weber HN, Glapin HD, et al. (1986) Mammography screening: how to operate successfully at low cost. Radiology 175:323–326

Skeffington v Bradley (1962) 366 Mich 552, 115 NW 2d 303

Thurfjell EL, Lernevall KA, Taube AAS (1994) Benefit of independent double reading in a population-based mammography screening program. Radiology 191:241–244

Subject Index

Abandonment 374
Abscess(es) 138, 201, 312
Accrediting body requirements 62
Acini 13
Acoustic impedance 185
Acoustic scattering centers 185
Acoustical lens 184
Adaptive histogram equalization 68
Adenofibrolipomas 149
Adenoma 200
Adenosis
 microcystic 91
 microcystic (blunt duct) 26, 92
 sclerosing 17
Age 170
 at first birth 7
 at menarche 7
 at menopause 7
Age group selection 348
American College of Radiology's Mammography Accreditation Program (ACR MAP) 57, 59
Angiogenetic factors 222
Apocrine carcinoma 124
Architectural distortion 160, 185, 186, 303
 spiculated soft tissue 303
Areas of increased density 22
Areola 190
Artefacts/Artifacts 182, 184, 233 (see also Calcium-like artifacts)
 absorption 184, 186
 motion 233
 refraction 183
 scattering 184
 shadowing 182
 slice thickness 182
 summation 245
 susceptibility 272
 time-of-flight 183, 199
Aspiration cytology 304
Attenuation 185
Augmentation mammoplasty 203, 320
 subglandular 320
 subpectoral 320
Augmented breast 86
Automatic exposure control 86

Background pattern(s) 186
 low-echo 186
Base plus fog 44–46
Battery 368

BCDDP (Breast Cancer Detection Demonstration Project) 339
Beam profile 182
Benefit 333
Benign breast conditions 173
Bias 333
Biopsy 30, 167, 182, 241, 272, 299, 304, 335
 aspiration cytology 167, 304
 core (see Core biopsy)
 fine needle 241
 fine-needle aspiration (see Fine-needle aspiration)
 high-speed core 30
 MR-guided 271, 272
 open surgical 167
 percutaneous core 299
 preoperative 272
 rate 335, 341
 ultrasound-guided fine-needle array 182
BIRADS (Breast Imaging Reporting and Data System) 171
Blood pool markers 230
Blood supply 13
Blunt duct disease 26
Blur 35, 36, 38, 46, 48
 subject contrast 35
Blurring
 focal spot size 35
 molybdenum 35
 rhodium target 35
 tungsten 35
BRCA1 7
Breast 186, 299, 319
 augmentation 319
 augmented 86
 conservation 299, 301
 conservation therapy 266, 299, 314
 hormonally stimulated 186
 juvenile 186
 lump 334
 postmenopausal involutional 186
 surgical biopsies 299
Breast cancer 6, 15, 255
 etiology 4
 familial 6
 hereditary 6
 incidence 76, 173, 177
 mortality 178
 multifocality/multicentricity 257
 physical sign 15
 screening 347
 staging 255

Breast cancer radiation induced, mammography radiation dose 173–177
Breast carcinoma 15, 224
 inflammatory 15
Breast conditions
 benign 173
Breast examination
 clinical 349
Breast health awareness 3
Breast implant ruptures 326
Breast implants 319 (see also Silicone, breast implants)
Breast lesions
 nonpalpable 283
Breast masses 137, 149
 nonpalpable 137
 circumscribed 149
Breast parenchyma 189
 graphic types 191
Breast screening programs 10
Breast self-examination 349
Bucky grid (see Grids, moving)

Calcification(s) 25, 105, 125, 126, 149, 153, 163, 168, 299, 306, 308
 amorphous 153
 arterial 126
 arterial, and hyperparathyroidism 126
 in axillary lymph nodes 127
  after BCG innoculation 127
  in tuberculosis 127
 benign 306
 of blood vessels 125
 in cat-scratch disease 127
 coarse 25
 in comedocarcinoma 104
 dystrophic 299, 308
 in metastases 127
 popcorn 149
 in scar tissue 126
 secretory 104, 119
 small arteries of 126
 in small papillary cribriform carcinoma 105
 intraductal 105
  cluster shape 105
   propeller or star form 105
   round/oval shape 105
   triangles or trapezoid form 105
 sutural 308

Calcified foreign bodies 129
   filariasis 129
   gold deposits 129
   paraffin injection 129
   sebaceous glands 130
   silicone bullet fragments 129
   suture material 129
   trichinella 129
Calcium deposit 23
Calcium-like artifacts
   contrast medium 132
   fingerprints 132
   metal chippings 132
   particles of dust 132
   powers 132
   tatoo marks 132
   zinc 132
Cancer 170, 316, 333
   axillary node involvement 335
   circumscribed 170
   detection 90
      cluster shape 91
      early 333
      the form of the clusters 90
      the shapes of individual
         microcalcifications 90
   in situ 335
   incident 338
   inflammatory 316
   interval 335, 348
   invasive 335
   minimal 343
Cancer risk 235
Carcinogenesis 4
   two-stage model 5
Carcinoma in situ 5, 18
Carcinoma in situ (Ductal carcinoma
     in situ (DCIS)) 19
   comedo 19
   cribriform 19
   ductal 19
Carcinoma in situ (Lobular carcinoma
     in situ (LCIS)) 20
   lobular 18, 20
   micropapillary 19
   solid 19, 108
Carcinoma(s) 16, 138, 161, 184, 185,
     233, 254, 299
   adenoid 254
   aprocrine 16, 18
   circumscribed 204, 210
   clinging 97, 106, 110
   colloid 161, 211
   comedo 24
   comedo-type 254
   completely hyperreflective 214
   cribriform 108, 109, 204
   detection rate 266
   diffuse lobular 213
   diffusely infiltrating 204, 211
   ductal 16, 161, 254
   ductal invasive 185, 209
   echogenic 210
      invasive lobular 213
      scirrhous 185, 212
   fine-papillary 204
   fluid-fluid level 211

   hyperechoic 184, 187
   hypervascular 254
   hypoechoic invasive ductal 213
   infiltrating 185, 233, 254
   infiltration zone 209
   inflammatory 204, 212, 254
   intracystic papillary 198, 211
   intraductal 204
      component 214
   invasive 16
      ductal 16, 138, 204, 207, 209, 214
      lobular 18, 30, 138, 209, 210
   lipid-rich 16, 18
   lobular 161, 254
   mainly hyperechoic 214
   mammographically occult 210
   medullary 16, 17, 161, 186, 211, 254
   metaplastic 16, 18
   micropapillary 97, 108, 110, 254
   mucinous 17, 161, 254
   mucinous (colloid) 161, 211
   mucoid 186
   multicentric 213
   non-tumor forming 186
   noninfiltrating, in situ 254, 261
   noninvasive 18
      comedo 206
   not other specified, (NOS) 16
   papillary 16, 17, 24, 254
   recurrent 299
   scirrhous 16, 245
      type 209
   secretory 18
   small papillary 97
   solid 110
   sonographically 210
   spiculated 209
   stellate 204
   tubular 16, 209, 210, 254
   tumor-forming types 186
   recurrent 299
Charcoal marking 272 (see Marking)
Charge coupled devices (CCDs) 70
Chemical shift imaging (CSI) 327
Chemicals 44
Chemosuppression 10
Classification 21
   pathological 21
Clemmesen's hook 4
Collimation
   beam 35
Colour Doppler 223, 225, 226, 227
   angle correction 223
   computer-assisted image analysis 225
   vascular density 223
Comedo carcinoma 110 (see
     Carcinoma)
Comedo mastitis 104, 119
Comedocarcinoma ductal carcinoma
     in situ (DCIS) 91
Committee 350
   academic 351
   administrative 351
   quality management 351
   Screener's Advisory 351

   SMPBC Steering 350
Complex sclerosing lesions 194
   (see Lesions)
Compliance 334, 353
Compressibility 215
Compression 35, 80
   breast 33, 35, 36, 46
   paddle 78
Computed tomography (CT) 254, 331
   contrast-enhanced 254
Computer-assisted detection 68
Computer-assisted image evaluation 233
Contaminations 338
   of study groups 338
Continuous-wave Doppler 221, 222, 226
   pulsatility index 222
   resistance index 222
Contour 188
Contrast 36
   agents 230
   resolution 66
   subject 33–35
Contrast enhancement 232, 235
   delayed 255
   diffuse 235
   dynamic criteria 254
   dysplastic breasts 237
   film 35, 42, 44–46
   focal 235
   medium wash-out 233
   morphological criteria 254
   multifocal, multinodular 235
   rim enhancement 255
Cooper's ligament 183, 190
Core biopsies 296
Core biopsy 161, 241, 272, 294, 295, 296, 297, 304
   computed tomography 293
   fine-needle 304
   indications 294
   large-needle 304
   macrocalcifications 295, 297
   magnetic resonance imaging 293
      guidance 293
   mammographic-stereotaxic
      guidance 291
   needle material 272
   negative predictive value 296
   number of tissue cylinders 297
   positive predictive value 296
   sensitivity 296
   specificity 296
   specimen radiography 295
   stereo pictures 292
   stereotaxic 296
      equipment 291
      localization 292
   tissue sampling 296
      inadequate 296
   ultrasonographically guided 296
Corona halo 209
   hyperreflective 209
Cost 167, 345
Cotton-wool 200

Subject Index

Cribriform carcinoma (see Carcinoma cribriform)
Cyst(s) 154, 170, 196, 197
  atypical 154
    echogenic 197
    fluid-fluid level 197
    lipid 159
    liponecrotic microcysts
      calcified 115
      disappearance and reappearance 122
  oil 125, 149, 203, 308
  simple 154
Cystosarcoma 160

Density 168, 237, 303
  areas of increased 22
  asymmetric 237
  focal asymmetric 168
  radiographic 65
  spiculated 272
Depth-to-width ratio 207
Determinants of breast cancer
  nongenetic 5
Diabetes mellitus 196
  insulin-dependent 196
Diabetic fibrous disease 196
Diagnostic criteria 184, 187
  sonographic 187
Digitization 66
Dissection
  axillary 301
Distortion 168
  architectural 168
Dixon technique 327
DOM project 338
Doppler ultrasonography 221, 222, 225, 254
  amplitude imaging 227
  angle correction 223
  differential diagnosis 225, 226
  duplex 222
  flow velocities 224
  harmonic imaging 227
  monitoring 225
  power 7
  prognostic assessment 225, 226
  pulsatility index 222
  pulsatility/resistance indices 224
  pulsed 222
  resistance index 222
  sums of flow velocities 225
  technical innovations 227
  therapy monitoring 226
  tumor detection 225, 226
  ultrasound contrast agents 227
  vascular density 223
Dose requirements 58, 61
Dual-energy subtraction 68
Duct 97, 168, 194
  dilated 168
  ectasia 104, 194
Duret's crest 183, 188
Dynamic breast imaging 181
Dynamic contrast-enhanced MR 229
Dynamic focusing 184

Early detection 4
Echo pattern(s) 183, 185, 186
  inhomogeneous 186
Echo texture 189
Echo time (TE) 231
Echodense noise 325
Echogenic border 186, 188, 214
  sign 184, 207, 209
Echogenicity 185, 188
Echographic contrast 187
Edema 304
Edge enhancement 67
Elasticity disruption of architecture 184
Elasticity
  movability 186
Equipment requirements 58, 61
Evaluative criteria 188
Examination
  clinical 30
  physical 334
Excitation angles 231
Extended processing 177
Extensive intraductal component (EIC) 301
Extracellular space 254

Family history 6
Fast-spin-echo (FSE) 327
Fat lobules 186
Fat necrosis 125, 138, 159, 160, 162, 203, 243, 308, 315
  spiculated 245
Fat suppression techniques 231
Fibroadenolipomas 149
Fibroadenoma 6, 23, 25, 92, 100, 149, 162, 186, 199, 238
  adenomatous 241
  calcified 199, 200
  calcifications 100
  corkscrew-like 100
  degenerating 23
  forms 100
  hyaline degeneration 199
  intracanalicular 100
  macrocalcifications 199
  myxoid 238
  pericanalicular 100
  progressive calcification 100
  proliferating 238
  sclerosing 199, 200
  sclerotic 199
Fibroadenomatosis 199
Fibrocystic disease 6
Fibrohyalinosis 208
Fibrosing (sclerosing) adenosis 92, 100
Fibrosis 138, 266
  postradiation 266
Fibrotic filaments 209
Fibrous encapsulation 88
Film speed 44–46, 51
Fine-needle aspiration 291, 294, 297, 299
  cytology 291
  indications 294
  magnetic resonance imaging 293

  guidance 293
Fluid collection(s) 303
  postoperative 303
Focal spot-to-(or breast surface-) object distance 33, 35, 36
Focal spot-to-object 36
Focal spots 33, 52
  size 35, 36, 48
Focal zones 184
Follow-up 134, 167
  posttreatment 301
  studies 301

Gadopentetate dimeglumine (Gd-DTPA) 230
Galactocele 154
Galactography 13, 24
Gel bleed 329, 331
Genetic linkage studies 6
GRASS (Gradient-recalled acquisition in the steady state) 327
Gray-scale reversal 67
Grids 36, 46, 53
  dedicated mammographic x-ray units 36
  focused stationary grids 36
  moving-type 36
Growth pattern 185
  macroscopic 185, 186
  multifocal 185
  non-tumor forming types 186
  scirrhous 209
  spiculated 209

Halo 214
  artifacts 68
  hyperreflective 207
  sign 185
Hamartomas 149, 162, 200
Hard copy 66
Health Insurance Plan (HIP) 335
Hematoma(s) 138, 160
Heterogeneity 4
Hormonal replacement therapy 13
Hyalinosis 185, 209
Hyperparathyroidism 124
  bone metastases 124
  renal insufficiency 124
Hyperplasia 6
  atypical 6
    ductal 91, 234, 248
  epithelial 6
Hyperprolactinaemia 25
Hypothyroidism 26

Image quality 183, 333, 335
  echographic 183
Image(s)
  latent 53
  postprocessing 67
  proton-density-weighted 231
  T1-weighted 231
  T2-weighted 231
Imaging sequence(s) 231
  2D gradient,-gradient-echo 231
  3D acquisition 229

Imaging sequence(s) (*Cont.*)
  FFE (Fast-Field-Echo) 231
  FISP 231
  FLASH 2D, 3D 231
  GRASS 231
  MR signal 231
  RARE 231
  spin-echo 230
Impact of MQSA 62 (*see also* MQSA)
  cost of mammography 63
  inspection fee 63
Implant(s) 320, 329
  double-lumen 320
  expander 329
  foam 329
  multicompartmental 329
  rupture(s) 323
    ultrasonography 323
  saline 329
  single-lumen 320
  silicone 329
  stacked 329
Incidence patterns
  age-specific 2
Incidence rate 1
Indian file tumor infiltrates 211
Inflammatory breast disease 174
Intracystic vegetations 235
Intraductal carcinoma (DCIS) 104, 105 (*see* Carcinoma in situ)
  calcifications 104, 105
  clinging 105
  comedocarcinoma 104
  cribriform 104
  micropapillary 104
  roman bridge 104
  small papillary 105
Intraductal noncomedocarcinoma 91
Intraductal proliferation 235
Invasive lobular carcinoma 138 (*see* Carcinoma, Invasive lobular)
Inversion recovery 327
Irradiation 300

Lactiferous sinus 194
Larmor frequency(ies) 229, 327
Legislation 57
Length/width ratio 188
Lesion(s) 149, 167, 243
  pathognomonically benign 149
  probably benign 167
  sclerosing
    complex 194
  spiculated 245
  stellate 243
Lifetime risk 2, 3
  increase in 3
Linguine sign 325, 329
Lipofibroadenomas 149
Lipomas 149, 201
Liponecrotic cysts 126 (*see* Cysts)
Liponecrotic microcysts calcified 125 (*see* Cysts)
  disappearance and reappearance of the same 126 (*see* Cysts)
Lymphatic drainage 15
Lymph node(s) 18, 21, 162, 300
  axillary 300
  local and distant 18
  regional 21
Lobular cancerization 124
Lobular carcinoma in situ (LCIS) 91 (*see* Carcinoma in situ (LCIS))
Lobules 13
Localization 283
  geometric 283
  grid 283
  methods of 283
  prebiopsy 283
  stereotactic 284
  ultrasound 285
Lumpectomy 249, 299, 300

Macrocalcifications 185
Macrocystic disease 235
Magnetic dipole 230
Magnetic resonance imaging (MRI) 229, 326
  dynamic contrast-enhanced 229
  indications 273, 276 ff
Magnevist 230
Magnification 33, 36, 37, 48, 49
Magnification radiography 301, 310
Malignancy grades 18
  cytonuclear 18
  histological 18
Mammography 22, 65, 168
  digital 65
  quality of mammography 57
    medicare 57, 59
    personal requirements 59
    quality control (QC) 58
    requirements 59
  spot-compression magnification 168
  ultrasonography, predictive value
    negative 276 ff
    positive 276 ff
Marking (*see* Charcoal marking)
  charcoal 286
  guide wire 286
  methods
    skin, needle and dye 286
Mass(es) 23, 168
  BIRADS 137
  density 137
  irregular borders 23
  location 137
  margins 137
  shape 137
  spiculated 23
Mastectomy 21, 255, 299, 314
  salvage 299
Mastitis 202
  chronic or interstitial 201
  plasma cell 160
  postpartum 173–175
Mastopathy 185, 191
  macrocystic 92, 94, 192
Matched filters 68
Medical records 62
Medico-legal 376
Menopause 7, 13
  artificial 7

Menstrual cycle 13
Metastases 21, 161, 182, 218, 278
  axillary lymph node 278
  lymph node 182, 268, 335
Microcalcification(s) 20, 22–24, 89, 185, 235, 268, 301, 309
  acinar 92
  of acinar and ductal 124
  after radiotherapy 109
  benign-type 24
  branched 24
  of breast carcinomas 89
  clustered 22, 24
  clustered pleomorphic 206
  ductal 104
  detectability 66
  disappearance of 109
  increase in the number 109
  irregularly linear 24
  lucent-centered 24
  in male breast cancer 119
  malignant-type 24
  outside of the acini and milk ducts 125
  papilloma 119
  papillomatosis 119
  pleomorphic 24, 26, 206, 301
  round facetted 24
  simultaneous occurrence of acinar and ductal 124
  tea-cup shaped 24
  varying density 24
  visualized by ultrasonography 206
Milk ducts 195
  dilated 195
Milk of calcium 150
  cysts 91, 105
Modulation transfer function (MTF) 37, 48, 49
Mole 154
Morbidity 167
Morphological criteria 233
Mortality 3, 333, 348
Mortality rates 1
  reduction 348
Motion unsharpness 78
Mottle 35
  quantum 35, 42, 50
Mammography Quality Standards Act, (MQSA) requirements 59
  accreditation 59
  annual inspection 59
  interim rules 59, 60
    interpreting physicians 60
    medical physicists 61
    personnel requirements 60
    radiologic technologists 61
  legislation 59
  quality standards 59
MR signal 229
Multicentricity 20, 301
Multifocality 20
Myocutaneous flap reconstruction 316

National Breast Screening Study (NBSS) 337

Subject Index

Negligence 369, 374
Negligent referral (see Referral)
Neovascularization 254, 263
Nipple 190
   discharge 25, 26, 195, 258
   shadowing 186, 188
Nodes 149, 170
   intramammary 149, 170
Noise 35
   power spectrum 52
   radiographic 35, 42, 50, 51
Non-Hodgkin's lymphoma 161
Nuclear magnetic spins 229

Object-image receptor distance 35
Oil cysts (see Cysts)
Oil (foreign body) granuloma 253, 254

Papilloma(s) 27, 104, 160, 162, 195, 241
   intracystic 196, 243
   intraductal 195
   proliferating 243
Papillomatosis 27, 243
   clinging 104
   micropapillary 104
   small papillary 104
Paraffin 319
Paramagnetic 230
Parity 7
Partial volume effects 233
Pectoral fascia 189
Phylloid tumor 160
Pleura 190
Positioning
   mammographic 75
Postoperative changes 299
Postoperative status 266
Predictive value 276 ff
   positive 335
Predisposition, genetic 6
Prevalence ratio 335
Prevalence/incidence (P/I) ratio 338
Probabilities
   individualized 10
Probes 182
   hand-held 182
   high-frequency 182
   high-resolution 192
   linear-array 182, 184
   sector scanning 183
   short-focused mechanical 183
   small area 183
   small area high-resolution 185
Prostheses 319
Psammoma bodies 94, 105, 108, 110, 119
Pseudo lesion 85
Pulse length 182
Pulse repetition time (TR) 231

Quality assurance (QA) 57, 59, 61
   medical physicist's QC report 59
   radiologic technologist's QC results 59
Quality control (QC) 46, 53, 335

Quality of life 333
Quality of mammography 57
   (see Mammography)
   medicare 57, 59
Quantum mottle 35 (see Mottle)

Radial folds 329
Radial scar(s) 138, 142, 194 (see Scars)
Radiation 7, 36
   postsurgical changes 299
Radiation therapy 173, 175, 176, 231, 299, 300, 301
Radio-frequency (rf) waves 229
Radiotherapy 251
   postoperative 251
Rapid acquisition techniques 232
Rates (see Mortality rates)
   mortality 1
Reciprocity law failure 39, 52
   cycle 41
   characteristic curve 43
   extended-cycle processing 41
   standard processing 41
Recurrence(s) 266, 303
   extramammary 268
   intramammary 266, 268
   thoracic wall 268
Referral rate 340
   negligent 374
Reflectivity 185
Region of interest (ROI) 187, 233
   reimbursement 57
Relaxation time constant 229
   spin-spin relaxation (T2) 229
   transverse or spin-lattice (T1) 229
Relaxation times 327
   silicone, fat, and water 327
Replacement therapy
   estrogen 8
Replenishment 44
   chemical 44, 45
      flooded replenishment 46
   extended-cycle processing 46
Reporting 371
Resolution 37, 49, 50, 182
   axial 182
   contrast 182
   geometric resolution 38
   in plane 182
   lateral 182
   limiting resolution 50
   spatial resolution 37
Resonance frequency 326
Retraction
   starlike 250
Risk 333
   absolute 333
   factors 5
   relative 5
Risks and benefits 177
Roman bridge structure 106, 110
Rupture 329 (see Silicone implant 329)

Scan 183
   compound 183

linear sector 183
Scanners 181
   automated dedicated breast 183
   bi-plane 183
   compound 181, 183
   electronic 184
   hand-held 183
   high-resolution 181, 184
   immersion 181, 183
   mechanical sector 182, 183
   real-time 181, 184
   water path 183
Scanning technique(s) 183
   compression 214
   dynamic 214
   radial 205
   real-time 184
Scanning planes 181
Scar(s) 16, 203, 243, 301, 303
   intramammary 243, 250
   postoperative 138, 140, 243
   radial 16, 138, 142, 194
Scatter radiation 35–37
Sclerosing adenosis 160 (see Fibrosing (sclerosing) adenosis)
Screen
   incidence 337
   prevalence 337
Screen-film contact 50
Screening 68, 348, 354, 370
   abnormal call rate 356
   benign biopsy rate 356
   cancer prevalence 356
   compliance 356
   cost analysis 358
   cost-effectiveness 360
   costs 348
   data analysis 355
   data collection 355
      analysis 362
   data control 355
   equipment 354
   external review 356
   guidelines 11
   interval(s) 348, 356
   interval cancers 356
   lead time 334
   mammography 80, 349, 370
      diagnostic 370
   mortality reduction 360
   pathology review 356
   performance indicators 356
   planning and organization 361
   postscreen and interval cancer review 356
   postscreen noncompliance 356
   projects 333
   quality control 362
   quality improvement 362
   quality management 356
   Radiologist Screener-specific procedures 356
   radiologists 354
   rate 357
   recall 357
   results 356

Screening (Cont.)
  service and administration 362
  surgical biopsy yield 356
  test 335
Screening benefit vs. risk 177–179
Screening Center 353
Screening Center Models 351
  fixed center 351
  mobile centers 351
Segmentectomy 300
Self-referral 373
Self-selection 333, 334
Sensitivity 238, 333
  of MRI 271, 272, 273 ff
Sequence 327
Side lobes 182
Signal intensities 327
  silicone, fat, water 327 (see also Silicone)
Signal intensity 232, 254
Silicone 203
  breastimplants 205
  contracture 320
  free 203
  granuloma 203, 204
  injections 319
  leakage 203, 320
  rupture 320
  selective sequence 327
Silicone implant 268, 321, 328
  double-lumen 329
  encapsulation 321
  gel bleed 321
  prosthesis 319
  rupture 321
    extracapsular 321, 325
    intracapsular 321, 325
  single-lumen 328
Size
  lesion 170
Skin 189
  lesion 154
  retraction 15
  thickening 304
Snow-storm
  appearance 325
  pattern 203
Sojourn time 344
Sonopalpation 184, 207, 214
Sound
  absorption 183
  transmission 183
Spatial frequency 49
  limiting resolution 50
Spatial resolution 65, 66
Specificity 238, 333
  of MRI 271, 272, 273 ff
Specimen radiography 24, 299, 300, 301
Speckle 185
Spicules 138
  computer-aided diagnosis 138
  desmoplastic response 138
Spin-echo sequence 231
Stability 146
Stand-off devices 182

Standard of care 370
Statistical power 342
Stepladder sign 324, 325
Stereotaxic localization 717
STIR 327
Storage phosphors 69
  imaging plates 70
Study
  active population 343
  case control 333
  clinical 333
  florence 338
  German Mammography 341
  observational 343
  passive population 343
  randomized clinical 333, 335
  Two-County 335
Subtraction technique 233
Summation shadows 170
Superconducting magnet 229
Suppression techniques
  fat, water 327
Surface coil (double breast coil) 229
Surrogate end-points 343
Surrogate measures 343
Surveillance 167
Suture material 308
Symptom 4

Tail of Spence 77
Tea-cup appearance 153
Tea-cup phenomenon 94
Tear-drop sign 329
Terminal-ductal lobular units (TDLU) 13
Thermography 254
Time
  lead 339
  sojourn 344
  volume doubling 344
Time-gain control (TCG)
Time-signal-intensity profile 233, 255
Tissue
  components 185
  compression 186
  elasticity 186
  fibrous adenoid 185
  glandular 186
TNM classification 18
Transducer(s) 182, 184
  annular-array 182
  high frequency 184
  single element 183
Transmission frequency 183
Trial
  Canadian 337
  Edinburgh 337
  Swedisch 335
  TEDBC 340
Tube target 33
  molybdenum 34, 35
  rhodium 35
  subject contrast 34
  tungsten 34, 35
Tumor 254

  benign 254
  biology 344
  hypovascular 254
Tumor size 210
  histopathologic diameter 210
  pathological measurements 210
  sonographic diameter 210
Tumor angiogenesis factor 254
Tumor recurrence 299
Tumor spread 18
Tumor vasculature 222
  immunohistochemical endothelium stain 226

Ultrasonography 168, 181, 303, 311
  basic technical principles 182
  diagnostic value of breast cancer diagnosis 212
  high-resolution real-time 182, 215
Ultrasound
  angiography 227
  velocity 185
Unsharp masking 67

Video display monitors 66
View 80, 90, 150, 303, 310, 315, 321
  anterior compression 83, 85
  caudocranial 86
  change of angle 83, 85
  cleavage 83, 86
  craniocaudal 80
  displaced 321
  exaggerated craniocaudal 82, 83, 84
  implant 321
  lateral 85
  magnification 83, 84
  mediolateral oblique 81
  modified compression 83, 86
  spot compression 83, 84
  spot compression magnification 150
  tailored 83
  tangential 303, 310
  tangential spot 84
  uncompressed axillary 315

Water path 184
Wide tumor excision 299
Wires 301
Women's Health Initiative 9
World population 1
  age-standardized 1

X-ray films 33, 39, 51
  breast compression 33
  characteristic curves 43, 48
  direct exposure 33
  film processing 33, 39, 44, 52
    cycle, film processing 41
    extended-cycle 41, 42, 46
    standard processing 41, 42
  industrial type 33
X-ray units 33, 52
  dedicated 33, 36
Xeromammography 338

List of Contributors

DORIT D. ADLER, MD
Associate Professor of Radiology
and Associate Director, Division of Breast Imaging
Department of Radiology
University of Michigan Hospitals, TC-2910P
1500 E. Medical Center Drive
Ann Arbor, MI 48109-0326
USA

LAWRENCE W. BASSETT, MD
Iris Cantor Center for Breast Imaging
165-43 Department of Radiological Sciences
200 UCLA Medical Plaza
Los Angeles, CA 90095-6952
USA

MICHAEL BAUER, MD
Professor
Münsterplatz 6
79098 Freiburg i. Br.
Germany

R. JAMES BRENNER, MD, JD
Director, Breast Imaging
Eisenberg Keefer Breast Center
John Wayne Cancer Institute
St. Johns Hospital and Health Center
1328 22nd Street
Santa Monica, CA 90404
and Associate Clinical Professor
UCLA
Los Angeles, CA 90095-6952
USA

MIREILLE J.M. BROEDERS, MSc
Department of Medical Informatics,
Epidemiology and Statistics
Katholieke Universiteit Nijmegen
P.O. Box 9101
6500 HB Nijmegen
The Netherlands

NANETTE D. DEBRUHL, MD
Iris Cantor Center for Breast Imaging
165-43 Department of Radiological Sciences
200 UCLA Medical Plaza
Los Angeles, CA 90095-6952
USA

STEFAN DELORME, MD
Department of Radiological Diagnostics
and Therapy
Deutsches Krebsforschungszentrum
Im Neuenheimer Feld 280
69120 Heidelberg
Germany

G.W. EKLUND, MD
15251 SE 58th Street
Bellevue
WA 98006
USA

STEPHEN A. FEIG, MD
Professor of Radiology, Jefferson Medical College
Director, Breast Imaging
Department of Radiology
Thomas Jefferson University Hospital
1100 Walnut Street
Philadelphia, PA 19107
USA

D. VON FOURNIER, MD
Professor
Universitäts-Kliniken
Abteilung Gynäkologische Radiologie
Voßstraße 9
69115 Heidelberg
Germany

MICHAEL FRIEDRICH, MD
Professor
Abteilung für Radiologie und Nuklearmedizin
Kraukenhaus Am Urban
Dieffenbachstraße 1
10967 Berlin
Germany

HANS-JOACHIM FRISCHBIER, MD
Professor
Universitäts-Frauenklinik
Strahlenabteilung
Martinistraße 52
20246 Hamburg
Germany

DAVID P. GORCZYCA, MD
Iris Cantor Center for Breast Imaging
165-43 Department of Radiological Sciences
200 UCLA Medical Plaza
Los Angeles, CA 90095-6952
USA

ARTHUR G. HAUS
195 Crossroads Lane
Rochester, NY 14612
USA

R. EDWARD HENDRICK, PhD
Associate Professor and Chief
Division of Radiological Sciences
Department of Radiology, C278
University of Colorado
Health Sciences Center
4200 E. 9th Avenue
Denver, CO 80262
USA

HANS JUNKERMANN, MD
Universitäts-Kliniken
Abteilung Gynäkologische Radiologie
Voßstraße 9
69115 Heidelberg
Germany

M. LANYI, MD
Martinweg 8
94072 Bad Füssing
Germany

ELLEN B. MENDELSON, MD
Director, Mammography and Women's Imaging
Department of Radiology
The Western Pennsylvania Hospital
4800 Friendship Avenue
Pittsburgh, PA 15224
USA

JÖRG-WILHELM OESTMANN, MD
Professor
Klinikum der Georg-August-Universität
Röntgendiagnostik I
Robert-Koch-Straße 40
37075 Göttingen
Germany

ETTA D. PISANO, MD
Associate Professor of Radiology
and Chief of Breast Imaging
Department of Radiology
CB# 7510, Room 503, Old Infirmary Building
University of North Carolina at Chapel Hill
Chapel Hill, NC 27599-7510
USA

INGRID SCHREER, MD
Universitäts-Frauenklinik
Strahlenabteilung
Martinistraße 52
20246 Hamburg
Germany

R. SCHULZ-WENDTLAND, MD
Universitätskliniken
Abteilung Gynäkologische Radiologie
Universitätsstraße 21
91054 Erlangen
Germany

EDWARD A. SICKLES, MD
Professor, Department of Radiology, Box 1667
University of California Medical Center
San Francisco, CA 94143-1667
USA

PD Dr. Dipl.-Phys. JOACHIM TEUBNER
Klinkum Mannheim
Institut für Klinische Radiologie
Theodor-Kutzer-Ufer
68167 Mannheim
Germany

CORINNE E. TOBIN, MD
Nassau Radiologic Group, P.C.
120 Mineola Blvd.
Mineola, NY 11501
USA

List of Contributors

Peter Tontsch
Munsterplatz 6
79098 Freiburg i. Br.
Germany

Tulusan A.H, MD
Professor
Direktor der Frauenklinik
Klinikum Bayreuth
Preuschwitzstraße 101
95445 Bayreuth
Germany

A.L.M. Verbeek, MD, PhD
Professor
Department of Medical Informatics
Epidemiology and Statistics
Katholieke Universiteit Nijmegen
P.O. Box 9101
6500 HB Nijmegen
The Netherlands

Linda J. Warren Burhenne, MD
Executive Director
Screening Mammography Program of British Columbia
Suite # 414, 750 West Broadway
Vancouver, BC V5Z 1H3
Canada

MEDICAL RADIOLOGY – Diagnostic Imaging and Radiation Oncology

Titles in the series already published

Diagnostic Imaging

Innovations in Diagnostic Imaging   Edited by J.H. Anderson

Radiology of the Upper Urinary Tract   Edited by E.K. Lang

The Thymus – Diagnostic Imaging, Functions, and Pathologic Anatomy   Edited by E. Walter, E. Willich and W.R. Webb

Interventional Neuroradiology   Edited by A. Valavanis

Radiology of the Pancreas   Edited by A.L. Baert, co-edited by G. Delorme

Radiology of the Lower Urinary Tract   Edited by E.K. Lang

Magnetic Resonance Angiography   Edited by I.P. Arlart, G.M. Bongartz and G. Marchal

Contrast-Enhanced MRI of the Breast   S.H. Heywang-Köbrunner and R. Beck

Radiological Diagnosis of Breast Diseases   Edited by M. Friedrich and E.A. Sickles

Radiology of the Trauma   Edited by M. Heller and A. Fink

Spiral CT of the Chest   Edited by M. Rémy-Jardin and J. Rémy

Biliary Tract Radiology   Edited by P. Rossi Co-edited by M. Bezzi

Radiation Oncology

Lung Cancer   Edited by C.W. Scarantino

Innovations in Radiation Oncology   Edited by H.R. Withers and L.J. Peters

Radiation Therapy of Head and Neck Cancer   Edited by G.E. Laramore

Gastrointestinal Cancer – Radiation Therapy   Edited by R.R. Dobelbower, Jr.

Radiation Exposure and Occupational Risks   Edited by E. Scherer, C. Streffer and K.-R. Trott

Radiation Therapy of Benign Diseases – A Clinical Guide   S.E. Order and S.S. Donaldson

Interventional Radiation Therapy Techniques – Brachytherapy   Edited by R. Sauer

Radiopathology of Organs and Tissues   Edited by E. Scherer, C. Streffer and K.-R. Trott

Concomitant Continuous Infusion Chemotherapy and Radiation   Edited by M. Rotman and C.J. Rosenthal

Intraoperative Radiotherapy – Clinical Experiences and Results   Edited by F.A. Calvo, M. Santos and L.W. Brady

Radiotherapy of Intraocular and Orbital Tumors   Edited by W.E. Alberti and R.H. Sagerman

Interstitial and Intracavitary Thermoradiotherapy   Edited by M.H. Seegenschmiedt and R. Sauer

Non-Disseminated Breast Cancer Controversial Issues in Management   Edited by
G.H. FLETCHER and S.H. LEVITT

Current Topics in Clinical Radiobiology of Tumors   Edited by H.-P. BECK-BORNHOLDT

Practical Approaches to Cancer Invasion and Metastases
A Compendium of Radiation Oncologists Responses to 40 Histories   Edited by
A.R. KAGAN with the Assistance of R.J. STECKEL

Radiation Therapy in Pediatric Oncology   Edited by J.R. CASSADY

Radiation Therapy Physics   Edited by A.R. SMITH

Late Sequelae in Oncology   Edited by J. DUNST and R. SAUER

Mediastinal Tumors. Update 1995   Edited by D.E. WOOD and C.R. THOMAS, Jr.

Thermoradiotherapy and Thermochemotherapy
Volume 1: Biology, Physiology, and Physics
Volume 2: Clinical Applications
Edited by M.H. SEEGENSCHMIEDT, P. FESSENDEN and C.C. VERNON

Carcinoma of the Prostate. Innovations in Management   Edited by Z. PETROVICH,
L. BAERT, and L.W. BRADY

Printing and Binding: Universitätsdruckerei H. Stürtz AG, Würzburg